NEURODEGENERATIVE DISEASES – PROCESSES, PREVENTION, PROTECTION AND MONITORING

Edited by **Raymond Chuen-Chung Chang**

Neurodegenerative Diseases – Processes, Prevention, Protection and Monitoring
Edited by Raymond Chuen-Chung Chang

Published by InTech

Janeza Trdine 9, 51000 Rijeka, Croatia

Publishing Process Manager Ivana Zec

Technical Editor Teodora Smiljanic

Cover Designer InTech Design Team

Additional hard copies can be obtained from orders@intechopen.com

Neurodegenerative Diseases – Processes, Prevention, Protection and Monitoring,
Edited by Raymond Chuen-Chung Chang
p. cm.
ISBN 978-953-307-485-6

For EU product safety concerns:
IN TECH d.o.o., Prolaz Marije Krucifikse Kozulić 3, 51000 Rijeka, Croatia,
info@intechopen.com or visit our website at intechopen.com.

Meet the editor

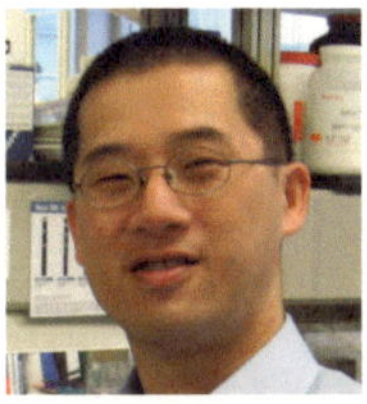

Dr Chang did his BSc training in Biochemistry in Hong Kong. Then he furthered his MPhil training in neurochemistry and neuroanatomy at the same university. He received a research scholarship by German Academic Exchange Service (DAAD) to pursue his doctoral training in neurophysiology and clinical neuroscience at the University of Munich, Germany. Afterwards, he continued his postdoctoral training in neuropharmacology and molecular neuroscience at NIH, USA. He has published over 80 peer-reviewed papers and book chapters in neurodegeneration, neuroimmunology and drug discovery in these areas. Dr Chang is now the Scientific Advisory Board member in International AD/PD Symposium, Scientific Review Committee for Alzheimer Association in USA, editorial board member in many different journals including Journal of Alzheimer's Disease. Dr. Chang's research interest is to investigate molecular mechanisms of neurodegeneration in Alzheimer's disease, Parkinson's disease, ALS, glaucoma and aging-related macular degeneration (AMD) so that pharmacological targets can be found.

Contents

Preface

We have different forms of neurodegenerative diseases. Most of them are aging-associated such as Alzheimer's disease (AD), Parkinson's disease (PD), glaucoma, aging-related macular degeneration (AMD) and aging-related hearing loss. Some are related to genetic such as Huntington's disease (HD), amyotrophic lateral sclerosis (ALS) and Frontotemporal dementia. Some are related to autoimmune responses such as multiple sclerosis (MS). Although the primary reasons for different neurodegenerative diseases are very different and occur in different regions of the central nervous system (CNS), the degenerative processes share high similarity. Therefore, prevention and protective measures are very similar. This is the reason why we can collect different chapters together in this book.

The first section of this book discusses toxic proteins in neurodegenerative diseases. Mis-folded/unfolded proteins escaped from regulatory control of chaperons usually create lots of problems to neurons. At early state, those aggregated proteins may block axonal transport by impairing the dynamic of cytoskeletal proteins. One should note that axonal transport along the track, microtubules, are extremely important for neurons. At late state, aggregated proteins choke ubiquitin-proteasomes system (UPS) and may also impair autophagic-lysosomal pathway to degrade them.

Having set the general landscape of neurodegenerative processes, the key factor to promote the processes is oxidative stress. Therefore, a whole section is dedicated to oxidative stress. We have chapters to discuss how and why oxidative stress contributes to neurodegeneration. We have also chapters to discuss how docosahexaenoic acid (DHA) elicits neuroprotection and current therapeutic methods to reduce oxidative stress. It is hope that reduction of oxidative stress can delay and prevent progression of neurodegeneration.

Then, how different stresses activate different signaling pathways to inform neurons to undergo the death pathways is discussed. It is apparently a vast variety of different signaling pathways leading to neurodegeneration. We collect chapters to discuss phospholipase A2 and apoptosis-signaling kinase-1 (ASK1) in this section. These two signaling pathways are partly activated by oxidative stress. We have a chapter to discuss how connexin hemichannels contribute to degenerative processes.

The processes of neurodegeneration are greatly affected by neighboring glial cells. Activation of astrocytes into gliosis or morphological changes of microglia can serve as pathological markers to inform cerebral inflammation. How microglia affected by calcium will be discussed. More importantly, how activation of microglia is regulated by CD200 is also discussed in this chapter.

Neurodegeneration is a result of multi-factorial factors contributing the fate of neurons. Among these factors, increasing lines of study pay attention to hormonal control and metabolism of brain cells or even the whole body metabolism. Vascular endothelia growth factor-B (VEGF-B) has recently been found to be a potential neuroprotective agent. We have a chapter to discuss its recent development.

The last section of this chapter integrates prevention, protection and monitoring of neurodegenerative diseases. We have chapter to discuss a natural product for prevention. Two chapters discuss how brain volume and acid-sensing channels help us to monitor degenerative processes. We have a chapter to discuss immunization. More importantly, we have a chapter to introduce how medical device helps monitoring disease progression.

Collectively, this book can give us a comprehensive overview of neurodegeneration from the processes, prevention, protection and monitoring. It is hope that we can collect a wide scope of neurodegeneration in a book to illustrate the principle of neurodegeneration. I am very pleased to be the editor of this book.

Raymond Chuen-Chung Chang, PhD
Assistant Professor and Laboratory Head
Laboratory of Neurodegenerative Diseases
Department of Anatomy
The University of Hong Kong Alzheimer's Disease Research Network
Research Centre of Heart, Brain, Hormone and Healthy Aging
LKS Faculty of Medicine
The University of Hong Kong
Pokfulam, Hong Kong SAR,
China

Part 1

Toxic Proteins and Disturbance of Neuronal Functions in Neurodegeneration

1

What is the Link Between Protein Aggregation and Interneuronal Lesion Propagation in Neurodegenerative Disease?

Garth F. Hall
Department of Biological Sciences, University of Massachusetts Lowell, USA

1. Introduction

During the past 10-15 years it has become clear that most major neurodegenerative diseases (Alzheimer's disease, Parkinson's disease, ALS, tauopathies, prion diseases and trinucleotide repeat diseases - henceforth to be referred to collectively as AANDs) share cellular and systemic features that suggest a common underlying mechanism of pathogenesis. At the cellular level, our understanding of the common aspects of AAND pathogenesis can be most simply summarized in terms of the downstream consequences of uncontrollable protein oligomerization and aggregation in postmitotic cells. The aggregated proteins block or disrupt normal proteosomal turnover and autophagy and become abnormally modified over time, generating toxicity via multiple pathways (mitochondrial damage, increased intracellular Ca++, caspase activation etc.) eventually leading to neurodegeneration and neuron death. This hypothesis is consistent with a key genetic similarity between these diseases - e.g. that familial forms are typically caused by autosomal dominant mutations that favor aggregation (in the case of asyn, tau, PrP and SOD1) or formation (in the case of APP and CAG repeat sequences) of disease-specific, aggregation-prone proteins. These similarities have suggested to many that a single central defect (i.e. the failure of normal protein folding) lies at the heart of most or all of the diseases listed above, and has led to them being categorized be some as "protein misfolding diseases".

While the importance of aggregate formation (and its attendant cellular dysfunctions) in each of these diseases is well established and has been intensively studied, our understanding of the intercellular and systemic aspects of these diseases is less detailed. That said, enough has been learned about their roles in neuronal biology and pathobiology and in the neuropathogenesis of AANDs to generate a general consensus that AAND development is 1) not cell autonomous and 2) that AANDs have another common hallmark- the progressive involvement of synaptically connected regions of the CNS over time in disease-specific patterns. Furthermore, it has become clear that important synergistic interactions between specific aggregation-prone proteins (tau and asyn (83), PrP and APP/Abeta (134), PrP and tau (216), PrP and asyn (95) may occur at both at the cellular and interneuronal level that affect the pathogenesis of specific AANDs. However, while neurofibrillary lesions develop according to characteristic, disease-specific sequences between highly interconnected regions of the brain in some AANDs (e.g. AD, tauopathies and LBD), the mechanisms by which the tendency toward aggregate formation is propagated between neurons as the disease progresses remains unclear, as does the degree to which such mechanisms contribute to disease pathogenesis as a whole. Similarly, there is still a gap between what we now know about the normal (mostly as monomer) and toxic (mostly as oligomers and aggregates) functions of each of these proteins at the cellular level. We know a good deal about the factors that favor AAND oligomerization, but very little about how oligomerization actually occurs in human disease. In particular, we have no real idea how these factors might 1) interact synergistically to drive cytotoxicity and degeneration and 2) are related to the mechanisms by which interneuronal toxicity is propagated between neurons in different parts of the brain. This review will attempt to integrate relatively recent findings about the interactions between the 3 most widely studied of these proteins (i.e. tau, alpha synuclein and the prion protein) both with each other and with cellular mechanisms associated with unconventional protein secretion into a framework that will account for common pathogenic features of these diseases and suggest future avenues of inquiry. For the sake of clarity, the discussion will be focused on asyn, tau and PrP and their interactions with APP/Abeta, and will omit a detailed consideration of other diseases that may have similar pathogenetic features (e.g ALS, Huntington's disease) and associated aggregation-prone proteins (SOD1, polyglutamine expansions, TDP-43, FUS), except when these become relevant to the discussion of general mechanisms. It will be guided by the example of PrP misprocessing and prion diseases, where the key link between intracellular protein aggregation, interneuronal transfer and the spread of neurofibrillary lesions through the brain has already been definitively established and which provides hints as to where to look for similar links in other AANDs.

Overview of common neuropathological and genetic aspects of AAND pathogenesis at the cellular and systemic levels

The predominant focus of basic research over the past 2 decades into the pathogenesis of all of the major AANDs has been on 1) the mechanisms responsible for protein aggregate formation and 2) the nature of cytotoxic changes that accompany and result from the aggregation of each of the proteins being discussed. As a consequence, aggregation-associated events and downstream consequences of aggregation such as the failure of protein turnover mechanisms in long-lived postmitotic cells such as neurons are among the best-characterized cytopathological features of neurodegenerative diseases. This work has generated a broad consensus that aggregation causes the failure of normal protein turnover mechanisms and the consequent development of abnormal toxic routes of protein disposal are central pathogenic events of the degenerative diseases that afflict the human central nervous system as it ages. Common toxic elements downstream of protein aggregation in AANDs include: 1) aggregation associated damage to protein turnover mechanisms, 2) mitochondrial dysfunction and or maldistribution leading to apoptosis-associated changes due to low ATP, generation of oxidative stress and abnormal Ca++ fluxes and 3) aggregate-mediated sequestration of normal proteins resulting in a loss of the normal function associated with sequestered proteins.

The classic example of a neuropathogenesis pattern suggestive of lesion spread in AANDs (outside of prion diseases) is provided by Alzheimer's Disease (AD). Ever since the seminal studies of Heiko and Eva Braak (27), it has been apparent that the neurofibrillary degenerative changes of AD develop in a characteristic sequence that closely follows the clinical progression of symptoms (11, 203). The earliest changes occur in specific limbic regions concerned with olfaction, spatial localization and episodic memory formation and consolidation (transentorhinal, entorhinal, pyriform cortices), functions that are typically compromised in the earliest clinical (and even preclinical) phases of AD. This is followed by the progressive involvement of limbic and paralimbic centers including the hippocampus, adjacent allocortical regions of the medial temporal lobe (e.g. subiculum), the insula and anterior cingulate cortex. Again, these neuropathological changes match the development of AD symptoms quite closely, with changes in emotional processing and short term memory becoming evident by the time AD can be recognized as such in the clinic, together with the onset of cognitive changes. The most prominently affected limbic centers are strongly interconnected with one another synaptically as well as functionally (203), as would be necessary for lesion propagaion via transsynaptic toxicity transfer. The areas affected in this "limbic stage" of mild AD make up only a small proportion of the brain by volume (24), but make and receive major inputs to and from large neocortical regions that become involved in later (isocortical) stages of AD, which could account for the sudden expansion of AD neurofibrillary lesions at the onset of Braak Stage 5 (24, 202). Although some regions of the brain (e.g. the primary sensory and motor cortices) are almost never involved significantly in AD despite being strongly interconnected with highly vulnerable limbic centers, it seems likely that this is due to cell specific or even connectivity-specific factors (8) that may delineate individual AANDs from one another (63, 59, 109, 116).

The progressive involvement of synaptically interconnected brain regions seen in AD is mirrored in non-AD tauopathies such as frontotemporal dementia (FTD), Pick's Disease (PiD) progressive supranuclear palsy (PSP) and corticobasal degeneration (CBD) and involve some of the same parts of the brain (prefrontal/frontal cortex temporal cortex, insula) although the areas of initial involvement are different from AD and from each other (9, 10, 11, 63). Similarly, Parkinson's Disease (PD) and PD-associated dementing syndromes such as Lewy Body Disease (LBD) share a common set of vulnerable loci (dopaminergic neurons in the substantia nigra, brainstem autonomic nuclei, olfactory bulb and neocortical loci) but vary significantly in the initial nidus of vulnerability and the degree of involvement of other parts of the brain (48, recently reviewed in 3, 50, 59). Also, the progression of Lewy Body containing lesions in LBD and PD differs significantly from that seen in AD in that it is not tightly linked to overall clinical or neuropathological severity (28). Overall, significant overlap between the areas vulnerable to synucleinopathies with those involved in early stages of AD (nucleus of Meynert, olfactory bulb, various isocortical loci) and in non-AD tauopathies (basal ganglia, isocortex). Familial prion diseases (fatal familial insomnia, Creutzfeld Jacob disease (CJD), Gerstmann-Schenker-Straussler syndrome) show a similar pattern (lesion evolution via a subset of synaptically connected areas from characteristic initiation loci) with a common set of vulnerable loci (thalamus, neocortex, ANS, cerebellum) that partly overlaps those of the other ANDDs (illustrated in Figure 1).

Another distinctive feature of AANDs as a group is the manifestation of each syndrome in both sporadic and familial forms, with exonic or intronic mutations in a specific aggregation-prone protein being sufficient to generate a (usually) dominant allele capable of replicating all aspects of the (usually more common) sporadic disease with high penetrance (197). Perhaps the most interesting aspects of this pattern are a) the degree of similarity between sporadic and familial disease forms, and b) the greater tendency of sporadic, but not familial, disease forms to show asymmetrical development, especially in non AD tauopathies (59, 143). These emphasize the importance of both selective vulnerability and synaptic connectivity as common factors in these diseases, and is consistent with the intriguing relationship between acquired, sporadic and familial forms of prion diseases such as Creutzfeld-Jacob disease (CJD), where the point of origin is clearly different in each case, but common aspects of vulnerability and synaptic connectivity are sufficient to generate a common clinical presentation (CJD), despite the presence of characteristic differences in lesion form (175). A similar relationship may hold between certain non-AD tauopathies and clinically identical diseases (both called FTDP or FTDP-17) involving loss of function changes in RNA-binding proteins (TDP-43, progranin) involved in the localization and translation of cytoskeletal proteins (hnnRPs), including tau and neurofilament proteins (147). Here, TDP-43 and or progranin may be activating downstream elements of a common

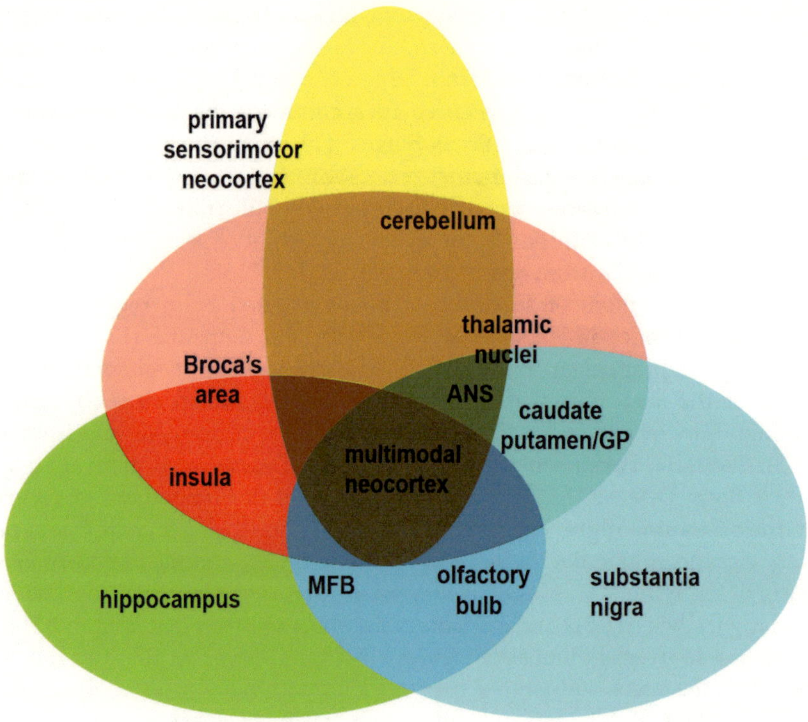

Fig. 1. Schematic illustrating the relationship between the characteristically vulnerable regions in AD, (green) nonAD tauopathies (pink), familial prion diseases (yellow) and synucleinopathies (blue). Regions typically involved in multiple AAND disease classes are shown in overlapping areas. Individual syndromes from all of these diseases eventually involve polymodal (associative) isocortical areas and thus cause dementia, even though severe cognitive changes may be absent or develop very late in other members of each group (e.g. Parkinson's Disease, fatal familial insomnia). Vulnerable areas in familial and sporadic forms of each AAND are identical, with familial syndromes beginning earlier and progressing faster than sporadic ones. Characteristic areas of vulnerability for frontotemporal syndromes (FTDP-U) that involve TDP-43 and FUS rather than tau aggregates and acquired forms of prion disease (vCJD, kuru) are virtually identical to non AD tauopathies (pink) and familial prion diseases (yellow), respectively, possibly owing to the presence of "prion like" motifs in these proteins (53). ANS: autonomic nervous sytem, MFB: medial forebrain bundle/nucleus of Meynert, GP: globus pallidus

misprocessing pathway that can also lead to the spread of tau-based lesions in the same overall pattern, rather than recruiting tau directly. Such a pathway might involve the mislocalization of proteins important in the maintenance of neuronal polarity from the axon to the soma and dendrites via a failure of hnnRP-mediated mRNA localization. This possibility is particularly intriguing since a) hnnRP interactions with the 3′ UTR of the mRNA encoding tau have been shown to be responsible for both tau localization to the axon (12, 146) and the generation of neuronal polarity (147) and b) the neuropathology of AD and non-AD tauopathies suggests that polarity loss plays a role in tauopathy pathogenesis (107, 1741). Overall, the common neuropathological and genetic features of AANDs involving tau, asyn and PrP are largely consistent with the existence of a common lesion propagation mechanism (or several closely related mechanisms) that involves direct interneuronal transfer of a toxic factor between adjacent and transsynaptic neurons.

Linking aggregation to lesion spreading – The case of the prion protein

The prototypic (and most extreme) example of an aggregation-prone protein that propagates its misfolded state at the protein, cellular and even organismal level is of course the prion protein (PrP), the misfolding of which mediates a class of mostly rare neurological degenerative diseases (transmissable spongiform encephalopathies) of humans and other mammals, the best known of which are CJD, scrapie, and kuru. Due to the pioneering work of Tikva Alper, Carlton Gadjusek and (particularly and most recently) Stanley Prusiner and co-workers over the past 50 years, and after rigorous verification by often highly skeptical investigators, there is now a general consensus that the so called "Prion hypothesis" proposed by Prusiner 30 years ago has correctly predicted key peculiarities of prion disease transmission such as the effect of PrP knockouts (31) and thus correctly describes the pathogenesis of these diseases (reviewed in 3, 49, 175). The Prion Hypothesis states that individual molecules of a single, widely expressed protein (the prion protein, or PrP) becomes misfolded and misprocessed in a manner that makes it adopt a neurotoxic conformation (PrP^{Sc}), but more importantly, permits it to transmit this conformation on to other prion proteins in the normal (PrP^{C}) conformation. The peculiar and controversial history of prion biology thus provides us with a highly verified example of how the misprocessing of an aggregation-prone protein into a toxic form can result in the interneuronal propagation of a protein with self regenerating, neurotoxic characteristics, and thus effect the spreading of neurofibrillary lesions to adjacent, presynaptic or postsynaptic neurons. The likely relevance of PrP misprocessing mechanisms to the pathogenesis of tauopathies, synucleinopathies, and other AANDs is further underscored by recent demonstrations that immensely subtle differences in PrP misprocessing and PrP^{Sc} structure appear to mediate the distinctive clinical and neuropathological manifestations of the various prion diseases (18, 40, 49, 168). In addition, recent studies of the normal cellular functions of PrP^{C} suggest that it is involved in the function of the actin-rich subcortical cytoskeleton and its interactions with microtubules, cellular membrane trafficking, cell adhesion and signal transduction in a variety of cell types (reviewed in 3, 53). In neurons, PrP^{C} appears to play a critical (if subtle) role in synaptic plasticity and most interestingly, in the propagation of HIV infection in the CNS (149, 180). The similarities in the cellular function, localization and misprocessing of PrP, APP/Abeta, asyn and tau identify likely points of interaction between these proteins, and synergy in their misprocessing, which are discussed futher below.

		APP/Abeta (AD, DS)	tau (PiD, PSP, CBD)	Asyn (PD, LBD)	PrP^{Sc} (CJD, GSS, FFI, kuru, vCJD)
Etiology	Sporadic	Most (80%)	Varies	Most (95%)	Probably most (CJD)
	Dominant	APP (1%) PS1, PS2	tau (exonic, isoform splicing)	Asyn LRRK2	PrP
	Recessive	–	–	DJ1, Pink1, Parkin	–
Risk Factors	Genetic	APP expression (DS) APoE4 isoform	tau expression (H1 haplotype)	diverse loci in mitochondria	PrP129
	Environmental	TBI, axotomy	TBI, axotomy	ROS-generating toxins	PrP^{Sc} in diet, iatrogenic risk
Neuropathology					
	Neuronal vulnerability factors	plasticity large size glutamatergic	3R/4R isoforms tau expression NF expression	dopaminergic High ROS	varies with mutation (FFI/CJD/GSS) Cerebellum (kuru, vCJD)
	Neuritic Sprouting	dystrophic neurites neuropil threads	neuropil threads	dystrophic neurites	dystrophic neurites
	Connectivity-based pathogenesis	yes	yes	yes	yes
Propagation	Clinical	no	no	yes	yes
Interneuronal transfer (human protein)	secretion	in situ culture	in situ culture	culture	culture
	secretion mechanism	exosome	exosome*	exosome	exosome
	uptake	culture	in situ culture	culture	in situ
	transmission	in situ (IP injection)	in situ	in situ	in situ
	transmitted toxicity	in situ (tangles) culture	in situ culture	culture	in situ culture
Synergy	Clinical	PD, LBD	PD, LBD	AD, tauopathy	Unclear
	Neuropathology	PD, LBD (tau)	Asyn Abeta	tau, Abeta	tau, Abeta
	Protein interaction	Asyn PrP tau (binding)	Asyn (coaggregation) PrP (binding) APP (binding)	tau (coaggregation) Abeta PrP	Asyn Abeta tau

Table 1. Comparison of the pathobiological characteristics of 4 aggregation-prone proteins responsible for most aggregation-associated neurodegenerative diseases (AANDs) in humans The table summarizes aspects of disease-associated misprocessing of 4 aggregation-prone proteins (amyloid precursor protein/beta amyloid (APP/Abeta) tau, alpha synuclein (asyn) and prion (PrP)) discussed in the text that are relevant to both aggregate formation and lesion propagation in major human neurodegenerative diseases (Alzheimer's Disease (AD) Down's Syndrome (DS), Pick's Disease (PiD), progressive supernuclear palsy (PSP), corticobasal degeneration (CBD), Parkinson's disease (PD), Lewy Body disease (LBD), Creutzfeld-Jakob disease (CJD), Gerstmann Straussler Schenker disease (GSS), fatal familial insomnia (FFI), kuru and variant CJD (vCJD). *publication in review (185)

2. Common structural/functional features of AAND proteins favoring aggregation and intercellular transfer

General molecular and cellular considerations

The abnormal and irreversible oligomerization and/or aggregation of specific proteins (e.g. tau, asyn, PrP) is the central common feature in AAND cytopathogenesis and by itself accounts for many of the other common cellular features of these diseases (a good review of the subject can be found in 196). Familial AANDs are typically induced by intronic, autosomal dominant mutations that either directly favor aggregation (tau, asyn, PrP), favor events that lead to generation of the aggregation-prone form of the protein (e.g. cleavage, abnormal association with other proteins, abnormal glycosylation or phosphorylation), or both (tau, PrP) (3, 50, 202). Exceptions to the autosomal dominant pattern include recessive mutations responsible for loss of function effects in protein turnover pathways (e,g, parkin 126). These genetics suggest that AAND pathology is due to a gain of function leading to aggregate formation and downstream toxicity involving the poisoning or overloading of proteasomal or autophagy-based protein turnover. A common structural feature among these proteins relevant to their tendency to aggregate is the co-existence in each one of a "core" domain which can form beta sheet interactions plus at least one other domain that inhibits this tendency, resulting in a balance between a normal conformation (rich in alpha helix or "random coil") conformation and an abnormal beta sheet-rich conformation that favors aggregation (50, 5, 156). Key common features in the cellular functions of tau, asyn and PrP include interaction with both chaperone proteins and with signal transduction elements, which might be expected of proteins capable of both aggregation and transcellular movement, respectively. Moreover, all three proteins are frequently associated with cellular membranes under normal conditions, especially in synapses (29, 71, 76, 148, 212, 213, 233) where they interact with APP (an integral membrane protein) and/or Abeta (93, 171), and are substrates for lipid raft-associated Srk family tyrosine kinases (e.g. fyn - 95, 137, 188, syk - 136 and abl - 37). In particular, the luminal localization of each protein in endosomes and/or trafficking vesicles associated with unconventional secretion (35, 78, 140, 142), reviewed in 215), and the interactions (in some cases copolymerization) that can occur between them (83, 134, 171, 216, 217) make endosomal pathways a highly plausible candidate site that might mediate the synergistic misprocessing of these proteins. An endosome-mediated common misprocessing pathway is also consistent with the availability of templating polyanionic ligands such as membrane-associated proteoglycans favoring further aggregation and toxicity (51, 52, 91, 106, 111), and the ready diversion of endocytosed proteins to unconventional secretion pathways (68, 70, 733, 102, 116, 124, 140, 175, 215).

Tau, asyn and PrP are all "switch" proteins that alternate between 2 states based on regulated charge/charge modifications. Under normal circumstances, asyn, tau and PrP function as soluble monomers that interact extensively with other proteins in the both in the cytosol and in association with cellular membranes. Soluble PrP^{C} and asyn contain alpha helical and random coil domains, and take up a predominantly random coil conformation in aqueous solution (186, 219, 231). In cells, tau normally extends along microtubules, where it stabilizes them by preventing classic dynamic instability via binding to them at multiple sites in its aggregation prone-microtubule binding domain (MTBR) (33). Tau:MT binding is itself dynamic (186), and tau interacts with fyn kinase, actin and protein chaperones via loci that overlap the MTBR when not bound to MTs (95, 107, 189). Monomeric asyn exists in both membrane-associated and cytosolic loci, and like tau, can bind to both actin and tubulin (4). As with tau, disease-causing mutations in asyn cause it to preferentially bind to membrane-associated proteins (69). Both membrane and MT-associated asyn have been found to aggregate (4, 139), in some cases forming clusters of microvesicles (195). PrP possesses an aggregation-prone domain (octopeptide repeat) that appears to be oligomerized reversibly during endocytosis. Unlike tau, it also possesses a separate N terminal MT-binding domain (231). All three proteins possess-aggregation-prone domains via which they aggregate resulting in a significant increase in beta sheet structure (156, 187, 231). Deletion analyses of all three proteins show that the removal or inactivation of non-aggregating domains (the N terminus of PrP, the tau N and C termini, the asyn C terminus) may tip this balance toward aggregate formation (1, 38, 112, 226). Post-translational regulation of each protein via phosphorylation may also do this (5, 41, 42, 80), either because it blocks the binding of the aggregation-prone domain to its normal cellular ligand, thereby permitting self assembly (156), or by favoring conversion of soluble oligomer to insoluble higher-order aggregates (187). Familial disease mutations may mimic these changes (13, 66, 80) as well. Overall, while tau, asyn and PrP are capable of aggregate formation and normally interact with both MTs and membrane associated components, the details of how oligomer formation and membrane association is related to normal function vary considerably. A key common feature relevant to the appearance of gain-of-function properties leading to interneuronal propagation in AANDs is the existence of self-binding/assembly capable and assembly-inhibiting domains in each protein that are normally balanced in favor of monomeric functions. This can thus act as a "switch" between normal and abnormal processing pathways which may be mutated to favor oligomer formation in familial AANDs, or alternatively, be "flipped" by derangement of regulatory elements (e.g. kinase/phosphatase and protease activities) that induce these posttranslational processing events in sporadic AAND pathogenesis.

Protein misprocessing in AANDs becomes irreversible and opens processing pathways associated with cellular membranes. A key feature of almost all AANDs involving tau, asyn and PrP is that they can occur as both familial and sporadic syndromes, which suggests that a common AAND pathogenesis mechanism must involve self-regenerating alteration in cellular function that is largely irreversible. Initial stages of oligomerization (e.g. dimerization) are most likely insufficient to do this, since all 3 proteins are normally found in a variety of reversible folding states, including low level oligomers, and are ligands for membrane-associated signal transduction kinases that reversibly oligomerize downstream elements (205). However, the binding of these proteins to templating ligands is likely to create higher-order oligomers that could become subject to irreversible structural changes such as proteolytic cleavage (90, 226, 234) and covalent crosslinking (62, 118, 161, 192). The nature of ligands shown to be capable of doing this currently includes 1) the proteins themselves, in the case of PrP^{Sc} (175) and mutant asyn (227), 2) polyanions such as heparan sulfate proteoglycans (HSPGs) (106, 225) or RNA (57, 119) and 3) other aggregation-prone proteins (83, 93, 95, 216). Other effectively irreversible changes in the cellular environment may be produced by downstream toxic effects of the initial aggregates, such as protease activation (7, 169), possibly aided by ionophore formation (39, 84, 133), or the recruitment of monomers into existing toxic aggregates via sequestration (6, 120). Endocytosed proteins that bind to the membrane via charge-charge interactions will undergo an acidification of their environment that may favor templating interactions and oligomer formation (67) Hyperphosphorylation, cleavage and aggregation of wild type tau isoforms can be induced simply by increasing the concentration of protein that is not MT-associated and thus vulnerable to misfolding (reviewed by 13, 203), causing the release of tau to the cytosol. This kind of release likely accompanies Abeta or axotomy-induced MT loss (32, 101), and thus could account for some of the dependence of tau misprocessing on Abeta generation and traumatic head injury in AD (151, 178).

While aggregate formation is a central event in the misprocessing of aggregation-prone proteins that drive AAND pathogenesis, it remains unclear how it is connected to the diversion of these proteins into the unconventional secretion pathways that might account for the interneuronal transmission of neurofibrillary lesions that appears to occur in these diseases. One possibly relevant property common to tau, asyn and PrP is their tendency to associate with membranes (29, 40, 53, 67, 173, 230, 233) and bind to membrane associated molecules such as HSPGs and fatty acids (44, 222, 225, 232). HSPG binding favors oligomer and fibril formation (52, 91, 120, 225) and may facilitate interactions with APP, which also interacts with HSPGs in cholesterol rich microdomains (lipid rafts 64, 193). Such interactions seem to be favored in AAND pathogenesis, since APP, tau and asyn colocalize with HSPGs in AAND neuropathological lesions (51, 59, 109 197). HSPGs may facilitate interactions between asyn and tau (both localized to elements on the inside of the membrane) and PrP^{C}, which is typically found on the exterior surface attached via a GPI anchor (163, 232) and may themselves mediate transcellular protein movement, as has been suggested by studies of morphogen movement during *Drosophila* development (166), possibly by trapping interacting proteins in the extracellular space (232). Raft-associated interactions appear to be important in disease-associated misprocessing of tau, asyn and PrP mediated via fyn (131, 138, 188, 221), in aggregation (195, 230) and in disruption of signal transduction pathways in CNS dendrites (108, 117). Lipid association also drives oligomer and filament formation of Abeta, tau and PrP (44, 208, 221). In a very recent study by Binder and colleagues (170), a mAb specific for tau oligomer identified the presence of arachidonic acid as one of the requirements for early oligomer formation in cell culture. Similarly, the presence of membrane anchors and raft localization motifs plays an essential role in the development of characteristic lesion morphology of PrP-mediated disease (40); the removal of the GPI anchor has been shown to produce novel syndromes in transgenic models (43), while the removal of all of the multiple raft localization motifs on PrP blocks lesion formation and propagation entirely (16, reviewed in 209).

The relationship between asyn misprocessing and membrane localization in AANDs may be more complex than that of PrP and tau, since some, but not all disease-inducing mutations block raft-asyn association (75). Like PrP and tau, asyn is localized to lipid raft microdomains in presynaptic terminals, where it accumulates in dystrophic neurites associated with Parkinson's Disease and Lewy body dementia (81). Similarly, asyn fibrillization is favored by interactions with unsaturated fatty acids (173) but unlike tau, this is inhibited by saturated fatty acids (233). A particularly intriguing recent finding by Fang et. al. demonstrated a direct link between oligomerization and unconventional secretion in a study showing that higher-order oligomerization can drive exosome-mediated secretion of a wide variety of oligomerized proteins (70). This is particularly interesting given that tau, asyn and PrP are all substrates for fyn and related raft-associated srk tyrosine kinases (136, 138, 188), and that such interactions are associated with AAND pathogenesis (19, 110) and have potentially self-regenerative features (i.e. by activating both the tyrosine kinase and its substrate 179). Such activation can result in fyn-mediated endocytosis via the caveolar pathway (204) or direct release of microvesicles to the extracellular space mediated via the SH4 domain of fyn (or other srk kinases) (34, 210). Regulation of endocytosis and exocytosis in neuronal growth cones by srk family kinases regulates endothelial apical endocytosis (77) and has been described in the marine snail Aplysia (223) suggesting that this is an evolutionarily conserved role for fyn-like Srk family kinases in diverse tissues. Developmental programs requiring high levels of localized membrane addition (e.g. neurite outgrowth) are dependent on the local presence of both srk family kinases and aggregation-prone proteins such as tau (20, 21) asyn (17) or Abeta (172) and are often abnormally reactivated in AANDs (26, 108, 174).

3. Cytopathological features linking aggregation and secretion in ANDDs

We have discussed the generation of abnormal tau, asyn and PrP oligomers as the most likely proximate cause of neurodegeneration in AANDs and proposed a common set of membrane-associated ligands for these proteins (e.g. HSPGs, signal transduction pathway kinases, fatty acids) which might mediate common aspects of their misprocessing, including their oligomerization, cellular colocalization and diversion into unconventional secretion pathways. Several features peculiar to neuronal AAND pathobiology that seem particularly likely to be important are discussed below.

Misprocessing of APP to Abeta 1-42 in early endosomes

So far, this discussion has focused the discussion on tau, asyn and PrP as aggregation-prone proteins immediately responsible for downstream neurotoxicity, and has ignored the contribution of aberrant APP misprocessing to Abeta in AAND pathogenesis, despite its well established importance in the pathogenesis of AD in particular (32, 94). However, it has now generally regarded as established that APP misprocessing to Abeta is the initiating event in the pathological cascade leading to AD, even if much of the proximate cytotoxicity driving neurodegeneration is mediated by tau (87, 125, 177, 180). The high cholesterol environment of rafts appears to be necessary for AAND associated misprocessing both in cell culture and in *in situ* AD models (64, 120, 198, 208). Furthermore, Abeta production and toxicity appears to play an important role in AANDs involving asyn and PrP as well as tau (48, 58, 134, 164, 198). Most important for the present analysis is the major site of Abeta production from APP - the early endosome. Endosomal production of Abeta 1-42 RNAi experiments have shown that APP endocytosis requires the raft marker flotillin2 in neurons, and furthermore, that misprocessing of wild type APP to Abeta 1-42 is blocked by inhibition of endocytosis (191), as is the secretion of Abeta to the extracellular space (46). APP is recruited to rafts by the raft-associated tyrosine kinase fyn (155), where its interactions with tau, asyn and PrP may play a role in both oligomerization and raft patching (163) leading to secretion of these proteins via either endocytosis and eventually exosome-mediated release (68, 70, 73, 176, 185), or microvesicle shedding (145, 163). This similarity should result in extensive opportunities for co-oligomerization between tau, asyn and possibly PrP in endosomal processing, resulting in diversion of oligomerized proteins to the exosome pathway - schematized in Figure 3.

AAND-associated proteins interact with APP in lipid rafts and may affect A beta production. There is some reason to believe that tau may influence APP misprocessing to

Abeta in association with endosomes, since tau binds to and may modulate the activity of presenilin 1, an intrinsic membrane protein which serves as the gamma secretase responsible for completing the cleavage of APP to Abeta (207), and is the site of most mutations responsible for autosomal dominant familial AD. Similarly, PrP^{C} is normally endocytosed via a raft specific, flotillin2/clathrin dependent pathway (204), and it has been suggested that the conversion of PrP^{C} to PrP^{Sc}, like APP cleavage to Abeta, occurs during endosome formation. There is indeed some evidence that PrP conversion to misfolded PrP^{Sc} forms can increase the misprocessing of APP by increasing the activity of the so-called beta secretase, which cleaves APP to a extracellularly released fragment and a "C99" transmembrane domain (14). Asyn interactions with APP have also been shown to greatly increase the level of Abeta secretion from PC12 cells (121). Conversely, the observation that Abeta activates the srk family kinase Abl resulting in tau phosphorylation at sites crucial to disease-associated tau aggregation (34), is also consistent with the possibility that Abeta-induced tau misprocessing may occur in the context of endosome formation.

AAND-associated protein misprocessing may favor exosomal secretion by damaging autophagy-mediated protein turnover mechanisms. It has long been suspected that alterations in protein turnover mechanisms play a significant role in the cytopathogenesis of AANDs. Under normal conditions, much of the proteolytic turnover of small cytosolic proteins such as tau, asyn and very likely PrP as well is accomplished via the ubiquitin/proteosome pathway (88, 181, 218). The aggregation of these proteins blocks this pathway, apparently due to the steric limitations of the proteosome, resulting in the ubiquitination of tau and Asyn aggregates typically seen in AANDs (158, 220). This provokes the upregulation of the macroautophagy (or simply autophagy) pathway, producing endosomal and lysosomal hypertrophy (35, 36, 165, 167) presumably due to the diversion of proteosome-mediated turnover of AAND associated proteins to the autophagy pathway. It is now becoming clear that aberrant autophagy pathway function is a general phenomenon in AANDs, and increasingly appears that autophagy pathway insufficiency rather than overactivity is the key cytopathological factor (105, 220), reviewed in (153). Since autophagy can function to remove cytosolic debris from cells via lysosomes as well as recycle cytosolic components, this may provide a secretion route for aggregated or misprocessed proteins in AANDs, especially if lysosome-mediated proteolysis is compromised (see Figure 2). Specific inhibition of autophagy combined with tau overexpression results in tau aggregate formation even in cultured neuronal cells, with tau aggregates (104) and toxic cleavage fragments (129) accumulating in lysosomal compartments. Blockade of normal retrograde axonal transport of lysosomes in AD (23) or by specific mutation (178) appears to inhibit autolysosome function indirectly by preventing amphisome-lysosome fusion in the soma, which may favor secretion by diverting incompletely degraded cytoskeletal material into exosomal secretion pathways (Figure 2). Such secretion has been described as "exophagy" in yeast (2). It is quite possible that this kind of diversion into exosomal secretion pathways may apply generally in AANDs, as autophagy disruption also occurs to a significant extent in association with asyn, Abeta, and PrP^{Sc}-positive lesions in AANDs (154, 164). Moreover, the tendency of AAND associated proteins to disrupt retrograde transport of autophagosomes (229) could very well promote exosomal secretion of these proteins from ectopic locations in the distal axons, providing a mechanism for the long distance lesion propagation seen in AD (203) and other AANDs (9-11) - see further discussion below).

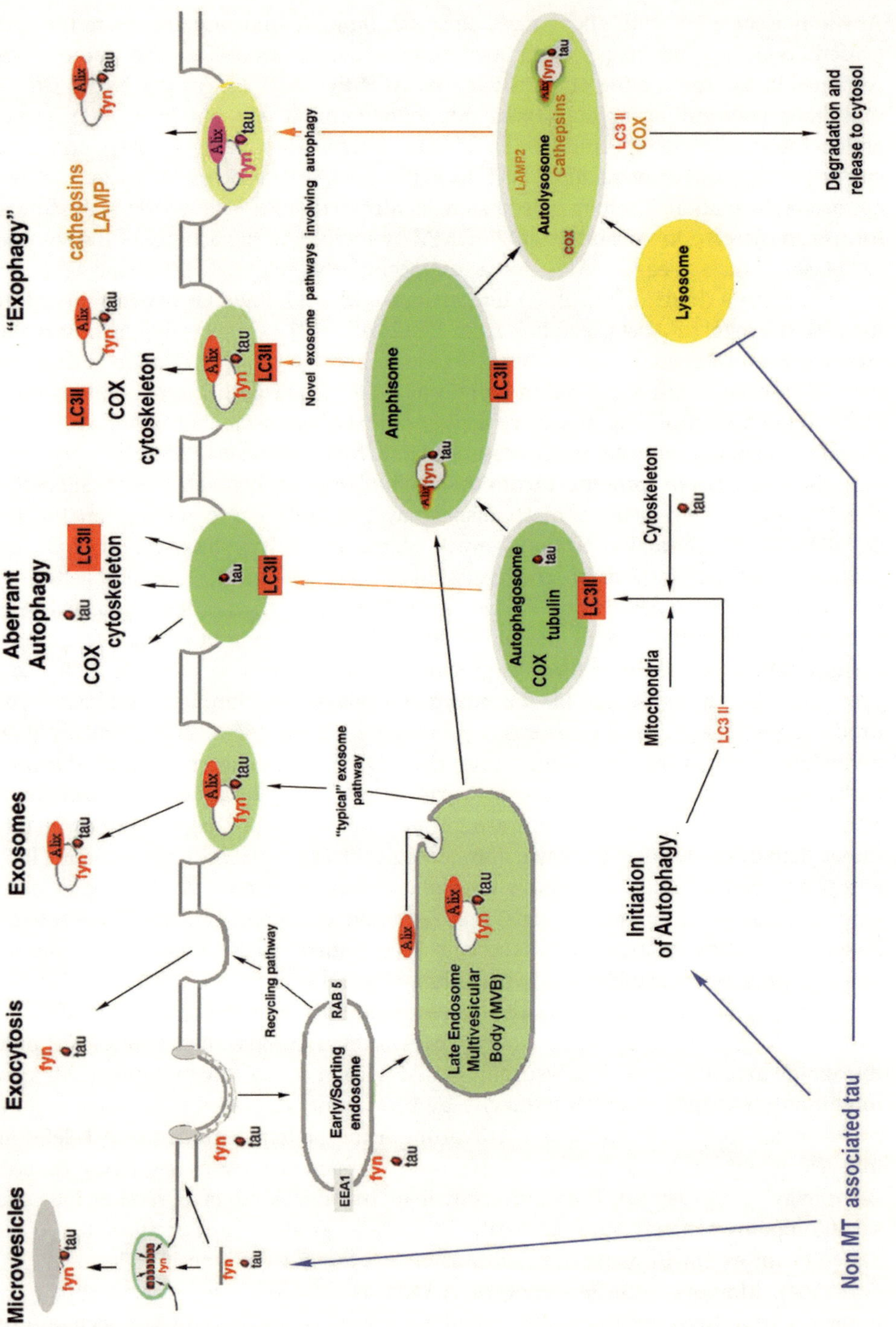

Fig. 2. Overview of possible secretion routes for AAND-associated proteins based on current literature Unconventional secretion has now been demonstrated for tau, asyn, PrP and Abeta in various model systems

This schematic illustrates how an aggregation-prone cytosolic protein with alternative membrane-associated ligands (in this case tau and fyn, respectively) might become aberrantly included in one of several possible vesicle trafficking pathways leading to unconventional release if it is released from its normal cytosolic ligand (microtubules) due to disease-associated conditions, which include hyperphosphorylation and microtubule loss, and which can be mimicked by overexpression (142). While tau is shown in this figure, the exosomal secretion pathways for Asyn, A beta, and PrP appear to be similar, especially since misprocessing of each of these proteins favors membrane-associated misprocessing (1) in association with the activation of autophagy (2) combined with disruption of downstream autophagic mechanisms that are necessary for the complete degradation of proteins in the autophagosome (3). While the secretion mechanism that has been identified for any of these proteins is nominally the "classic" exosomal pathway, marked by the presence of exosome-enriched proteins (e.g. Alix), it is likely that exosome secretion occurs via a number of closely related pathways that are associated to a greater or lesser degree with macroautophagy and lysosome-mediated protein turnover. Some of these pathways are indistinguishable from (or even included in) the "classical" exosome pathway (which does not involve lysosomal processing) and can be identified only via the identification of autophagosomal marker proteins (e.g cleaved LC3 (LC3II), cytoskeletal/mitochondrial proteins (COX, tubulins) and/or lysosomal markers (LAMP2, cathepsins) copurifed with exosomal/MVB markers and the AAND-associated protein in question. Involvement of autophagy-associated mechanisms to form a hybrid "exophagy" pathway (2) is particularly likely if misprocessing is associated with aggregate-induced impairment of autophagy, as occurs in AANDs. Secretion pathways are elaborated from Abrahamsen et. al. (2) and Nickel (163). (1) microvesicle shedding- this pathway is driven by srk kinase activity and oligomer-mediated "patching", but does not involve endocytosis, (2) endosome recycling pathway, (3) classic exosome pathway, (4) non-exosomal autophagosome dumping (commonly seen with tau overexpression models), (5-6) "exophagy" pathways either without autophagolysosomal formation.

Unconventional secretion may be linked to axonal transport and neuronal polarity defects caused by AAND-associated protein misprocessing. Another attractive area to look for common links between AAND associated aggregation and secretion of tau, PrP, asyn and APP is that of axonal transport and axonal identity. Each of these proteins is normally axonally localized (22, 127, 150), and the misprocessing of each protein has been shown to disrupt axoplasmic transport in AANDs and AAND models, (157, 162, 199, 200, reviewed in 183), while disruption of dynein/dynactin mediated transport produces a phenocopy of AAND-like syndromes (132). General abnormalities in axonal transport are likely relevant to common neuropathological characteristics of AANDs, such as the anterograde and retrograde propagation of lesions between distant areas of the brain and the disproportionate involvement of large neurons, presumably due to their inherently increased vulnerability to mitochondrial misdistribution and growth factor deprivation (160, 190, 206).

The reported nature of the disruptions of axonal transport has most often involved the obstruction of axonal transport and accompanied by neurodegeneration via what may be effectively an axotomy syndrome related to synapse loss and growth factor deprivation (157, 195) However, the more interesting possibility, at least with respect to lesion propagation, is that misprocessed tau, asyn or PrP could be itself aberrantly transported along the axon in ways that could account for disease-specific features of AANDs. There is a great deal of circumstantial and correlative evidence in favor of a major role for axonal transport of vesicle-associated pathogens within the CNS, which closely resembles the movement of infectious prions within the brain (3, 53, 215). Interneuronal movement of HIV has recently been shown to involve PrP^{C} mediation (181) and the binding of a raft-localizing domain that also mediates Abeta and PrP^{Sc} localization to rafts (149), lending direct support to the operation of this mechanism in AANDs. The transfer of PrP^{Sc} from the gut to the CNS in diseases such as kuru and vCJD involves passage through lymphatic tissues where intercellular movement of both proteins and viral particles occurs via exosomes (215) the unconventional secretion pathway common to asyn, Abeta, PrP and tau (68, 73, 176, 185). Each of these proteins is associated with axonally transported vesicles (71, 76, 123, 127, 140, 141, 150, 230), sometimes in colocalization with (71) or functionally linked with one another (134) in synapses. Moreover, exosome release of PrP has recently been tied to synaptic function with specific neurotransmitters (135), illustrating one mechanism by which specific anterograde and or retrograde pathways might be targeted. The possible operation of common a "prion like" propagation of vesicle-associated misprocessed protein in AAND pathogenesis is further strengthened by the demonstrations that Abeta toxicity can be propagated from the peritoneal cavity to the CNS in a manner similar to ingested prions (65), and that vesicle-associated tau can be dendritically transported and secreted in an *in situ* tauopathy model (123, 141). Finally, numerous studies of LBD, AD and CJD pathology in human patients and/or disease models have now documented the selective colocalization of axonally transported tau and asyn in dystrophic neurites associated with neurofibrillary lesions (neuritic plaques) produced by APP and/or PrP based amyloids (81, 82, 109) suggesting that synergistic interactions associated with vesicle formation (presumably during endocytosis or endosomal processing) may play a role in the lesion overlap and risk synergy so often seen in AAND neuropathology and epidemiology.

Is polarity loss connected to the misprocessing and secretion of tau and other AAND-associated proteins?

Another aspect of axonal function that is of particular relevance to tauopathies and AD, but may well be involved in any or all of the AANDs under discussion, is the selective effect of tau misprocessing on axonal identity, process outgrowth and synaptic connectivity in AD and non-AD tauopathies. Tau is normally axonally localized in neurons (22) and plays a well-established role in axonal outgrowth (20, 34, 60, 235, reviewed in 91) and in the generation of axonal identity in at least some CNS neuron types (21, 34). Much of this developmental activity of tau involves interactions with the plasma membrane and signal transduction elements rather than MTs (20, 115, 235), and appears to be partly recapitulated in AD and tauopathy pathogenesis with the outgrowth of axonlike processes (neuropil threads). Another aspect of AD pathogenesis that reflects developmental tau function is the loss of neuronal polarity seen in the neuropathology of AD and non-AD tauopathies, which is manifested in a) the progressive movement of tau from the axons to the somatodendritic compartment with the development of neurofibrillary pathology (15, 89) and b) the origination of many tau-positive neuropil threads from the dendrites of neurons in AD (107, 174).

The link between AAND neuropathology and polarity loss accounts for important neuropathological and etiological peculiarities of AD, including: a) the mislocalization and trapping of signal transduction elements essential to the establishment of axonal identity and neuronal polarity, such as CRMP-2 (159, 228) and PAR1/MARK kinase (21), and b) the greatly increased risk (up to 19 fold) that traumatic brain injury (TBI) and chronic injury caused by multiple concussions (CTE) poses for the development of neurodegenerative disease, AD in particular (152). Torsion and stretching injury to the brain resulting in occult axotomy of long tracts in the CNS is a major pathological feature in CTE (212), and can occur very close to the soma of the axotomized neuron without killing it (194). Such injury results in the accumulation of axonally transported asyn, APP, PrP and in some cases tau at the proximal axon stump of injured neurons that are reminiscent of axonal swellings containing these proteins in AANDs (15, 162, 212).

Studies in lower vertebrate (98, 99, 101) and mammalian (45, 144, 182) systems have consistently suggested that polarity loss induced by proximal axotomy could be a mechanism capable of linking axonal injury and the development of AAND-like neuropathology. Proximal axotomy induces ectopic axonlike sprouting (98, 182), the aberrant phosphorylation and missorting of cytoskeletal proteins (99, 100) and thus reproduces key aspects of AD neuritic pathology (26, 107, 174). Missorting of axonal elements such as tau can produce AD-like loss of function degenerative changes in the axon such as synapse loss (54) as well as somatodendritic hyperphosphorylated tau accumulation, which it does even at low levels of overexpression in murine transgenics (30, 86). Interestingly, tau induced neuropathology in tauopathy models produces a number of toxic changes in the dendrites that might shed light on the link between tau misprocessing and interneuronal tau transfer. Tau expression in models causes progressive dendritic degeneration (101) and has specific effects on dendritic MT number (103) and function (61) that resemble both AD pathology (27, 151) and the effects of proximal axotomy (72, 182 , 200, 101). A recent result of particular interest in this context is the recent demonstration by Ittner and co-workers (117) that ectopically localized dendritic tau mediates Abeta toxicity in a transgenic mouse tauopathy model. This finding highlights the possibility that Abeta-mediated tau misprocessing might be initiated by the aberrant juxtaposition of (normally axonal) tau with membrane-associated signal transduction partners that are present in dendrites, causing abnormalities in tau processing that lead to aggregation and eventually secretion, possibly via interactions with synaptic Abeta (71, 135). The dependence of neuronal polarization and axonal outgrowth on normal interactions between tau and localized membrane-associated tyrosine kinases (20, 21, 55) and the sensitivity of dendritic integrity to disruption of dendritic signal transduction pathways by mislocalized PrP (115) suggests that the relocalization of key proteins in AANDs might be a generally applicable mechanism in the misprocessing of AAND proteins by which normal cellular functions and interactions are replaced by abnormal ones by missorting events associated with damage to axonal transport and identity mechanisms.

4. Summary and conclusions

The aggregation of the AAND-associated proteins tau, asyn, PrP and APP/Abeta appears to be triggered by one or more post-translational events (cleavage/phosphorylation/ glycosylation) that redistribute charges so as to change the predominant secondary structure from an unfolded/alpha helical pattern to a beta pleated sheet pattern. This change is associated with and driven by familial disease mutations, and may also be favored by the interaction with hydrophobic elements in cellular membranes and/or the binding of perimembranous polyanions (e.g. HSPGs), raising the interesting (and heretofore largely ignored) possibility that aggregate formation in AANDs may depend at least in part on interactions with cellular membranes. The relationship between membrane associated misprocessing and the cytopathogenesis of AANDs is summarized in Figure 3.

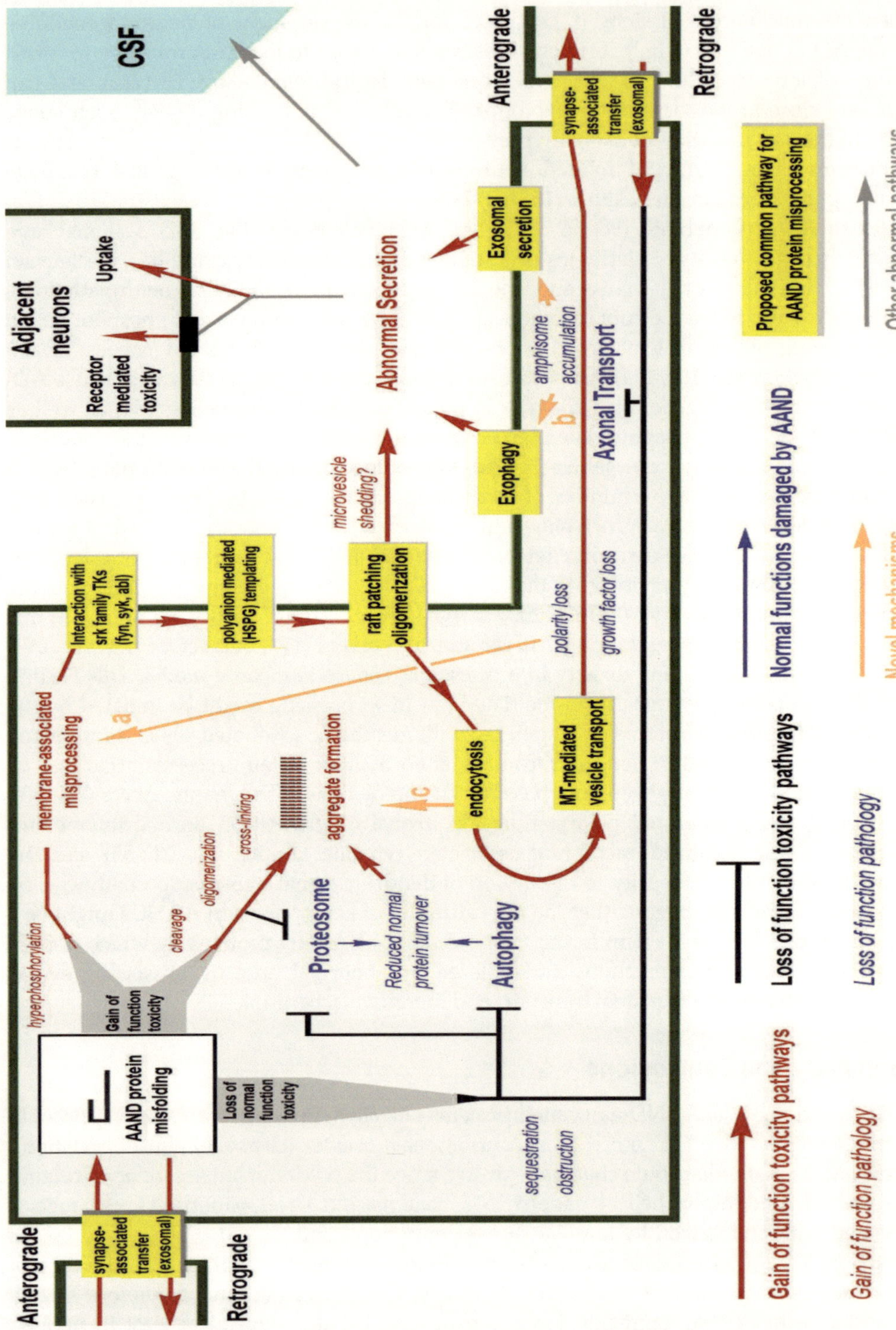

Fig. 3. Summary of common cellular misprocessing pathways linking aggregation and interneuronal transfer of AAND-associated proteins

Hypothetical scheme by which the initial misfolding of AAND-associated proteins (tau asyn, PrP and Abeta) produces intracellular aggregates and other typical AAND cytopathological features in combination with the propagation of this pathology to adjacent, presynaptic and postsynaptic neurons. AAND cytopoathology is produced via a combination of pathological gain of function and loss of function toxicity pathways as indicated. Recent evidence for a common membrane associated misprocessing route that causes the diversion of endocytosed proteins into abnormal vesicle trafficking pathways is highlighted, as it links oligomeri formation with interneuronal transfer and offers multiple opportunities for the colocalization and synergistic interaction (e.g. co-oligomerization) between AANDs at the cellular level necessary to explain the clinical and neuropathological evidence for synergy between AANDs. The classical cytosolic route for aggregate formation is also shown. Novel relationships suggested by recent studies (peach - see text for discussion) that account for key common and/or specific AAND features and could be fruitful foci of future research include links between a) axonal damage, protein mislocation due to polarity loss, and aberrant toxic interactions with dendritic signalling pathways and b) membrane-associated oligomerization and aggregate formation are shown as well, as c) the possible link between damage to axonal transport (failure of normal autophagosome/lysosome colocalization) and unconventional secretion.

Current evidence indicates that initial protein misprocessing in AANDs becomes irreversible due to cleavage and/or crosslinking events that are favored by and occur during the oligomerization/aggregation process and that novel emergent pathological interactions due to polymerization eventually become dominant in the affected neuron, leading both to the dysfunction and death of the aggregate-containing neuron and the spreading of the aggregation tendency to other neurons, where the degenerative cycle is repeated. The retrograde and/or anterograde transfer of membrane associated, oligomerized, toxic protein to other neurons involves axonal propagation of endosome-derived vesicles via transport mechanisms that may have been altered by aggregate-mediated toxicity. Lesion spreading occurs either 1) via a toxic consequence of aberrant neuronal function, such as the loss of transneuronal trophic factor transmission or the increased generation of toxic byproducts of degeneration, or 2) via the actual transfer of misprocessed proteins from one neuron to another. Evidence supporting the latter possibility (that lesion spread occurs via actual protein transfer in AANDs) has accumulated recently, as specific secretion, uptake, transfer and interneuronal toxicity transfer has now been observed for each of these proteins (47, 57, 73, 74, 75, 85, 123, 124, 128, 135, 140 - summarized in Table 1) and a common unconventional secretion pathway (i.e. exosome-mediated secretion) has been identified for PrP and Abeta (73, 176) and (quite recently) asyn and tau (68, 185). A hypothetical common misprocessing pathway for these proteins in AANDs is schematized in Figure 3.

The focus of this discussion has been on the shared characteristics of tau, asyn, PrP and Abeta that could allow each to a) associate with signal transduction elements in membrane raft domains and b) interact and oligomerize in association with elements capable of driving endocytosis (HSPGs, each other, possibly RNA, possibly via acidification driven charge-charge interactions) under circumstances which allow entry to exosomal secretion pathways, possibly via modifications induced in protein turnover mechanisms (autophagy) by aggregate toxicity. In particular, I have focused on whether this hypothesis is consistent with the now voluminous evidence that AANDs involving tau, asyn, PrP and APP misprocessing overlap one another in their etiology and pathogenesis, and whether and how well this hypothesized common link between aggregation and lesion propagation accounts for the peculiarities of a specific protein–disease pair (tau and AD). While the necessarily general nature of this analysis precludes the accurate identification of emergent common mechanisms of AAND pathogenesis in any detail, it is hoped that it can provide a framework that may help guide further investigation in this rapidly changing field.

5. References

[1] Abraha, A., Ghoshal, N., Gamblin, T. C., Cryns, V., Berry, R. W.,Kuret, J., and Binder, L C-terminal inhibition of tau assembly in vitro and in Alzheimer's disease. *J. Cell Sci.* 2000; 113: 3737–3745.

[2] Abrahamsen H and H Stenmark (2011) Protein Secretion: Unconventional Exit by Exophagy *Current Biology,* 20: R4-8

[3] Aguzzi A, Sigurdson C, Heikenwaelder M. Molecular mechanisms of prion pathogenesis. *Ann Rev Pathol* 2008; 3: 11–40.

[4] Alim M.A., Q.L. Ma, K. Takeda, T. Aizawa, M. Matsubara, M. Nakamura, A. Asada, T. Saito, H. Kaji, M. Yoshii, S. Hisanaga and K. Ueda, Demonstration of a role for alpha-synuclein as a functional microtubule-associated protein, *J. Alzheimer's Dis.* 2004; 6:435–442.

[5] Alonso AC, Zaidi T, Novak, M, Grundke-Iqbal I, Iqbal K. Hyperphosphorylation induces self-assembly of tau into tangles of paired helical filaments and straight filaments *Proc Natl Acad Sci USA* 2001; 98: 6923–6928.

[6] Alonso, AD, Grundke-Iqbal I, Barra HS, Iqbal K. Abnormal phosphorylation of tau and the mechanism of Alzheimer neurofibrillary degeneration: sequestration of microtubule associated proteins 1 and 2 and the disassembly of microtubules. *Proc Nat Acad Sci USA* 1997; 94: 298-303.

[7] Amadoro G, Serafino AL, Barbato C, Ciotti MT, Sacco A, Calissano P, Canu N. Role of N-terminal tau domain integrity on the survival of cerebellar granule neurons. *Cell Death Differ* 2004; 11: 217–230.

[8] Arendt T. Disturbance of neuronal plasticity is a critical pathogenetic event in Alzheimer's disease Reversible paired helical filament-like phosphorylation of tau is an adaptive process associated with neuronal plasticity in hibernating animals. *Int. J. Devl Neuroscience* 2001; 19: 231–245

[9] Armstrong RA, Cairns NJ, Lantos PL. Clustering of Pick bodies in Pick's disease. *Neurosci Lett* 1998;242:81–4.

[10] Armstrong RA, Cairns NJ, Lantos PL. Dementia with Lewy bodies: clustering of Lewy bodies in human patients. *Neurosci Lett* 1997;224:41–4.

[11] Armstrong RA, Cairns NJ, Lantos PL. . What does the study of spatial patterns tell us about the pathogenesis of neurodegenerative disorders? *Neuropathology* 2001; 21: 1–12.

[12] Aronov S, Aranda G, Behar L, Ginzberg I. 2001. Axonal *tau* mRNA localization coincides with tau protein in living neuronal cells and depends on axonal targetting signal. *J. Neurosci.* 21: 6577-6587.

[13] Avila J. Tau phosphorylation and aggregation in Alzheimer's disease pathology. *FEBS Lett* 2006; 580:2922-2927.

[14] Baier M, Apelt J, Riemer C, Gültner S, Schwarz A, Bamme T, Burwinkel M, Schliebs R. 2008 Prion infection of mice transgenic for human APPSwe: increased accumulation of cortical formic acid extractable Ab(1-42) and rapid scrapie disease development. *Int J Dev Neurosci.* 26(7):821-4.

[15] Bancher C., Brunner C., Lassman H, Budka H. Jellinger K, Wiche G, Seitelberger F, Grundke-Iqbal I, Iqbal K, Wisniewski HM. Accumulation of abnormally phosphorylated tau precedes the formation of neurofibrillary tangles in Alzheimer's disease. *Brain Res* 2109; 477: 90–99.

[16] Baron GS, Caughey B. Effect of glycosylphosphatidylinositol anchordependent and -independent prion protein association with model raft membranes on conversion to the protease-resistant isoform. *J Biol Chem* 2003;278:15983–92.

[17] Beggs HE, Soriano P, Maness PF (1994) NCAM-dependent neurite outgrowth is inhibited in neurons from Fyn-minus mice. *J Cell Biol* 127, 825-833.

[18] Bessen RA, Kocisko DA, Raymond GJ, Nandan S, Lansbury PT, Caughey B (1995) Non-genetic propagation of strain-specific properties of scrapie prion protein. *Nature* 375:698–700.

[19] Bhaskar K, Hobbs GA, Yen SH, Lee G: Tyrosine phosphorylation of tau accompanies disease progression in transgenic mouse models of tauopathy. *Neuropathol Appl Neurobiol;* 2010; 36(6):462-77

[20] Biernat J, Mandelkow EM. The development of cell processes induced by tau protein requires phosphorylation of Serine 262 and 356 in the repeat domain and is inhibited by phosphorylation in the proline-rich domains. *Mol Biol Cell* 1999; 10:727-740.

[21] Biernat J. et al. Protein kinase MARK/PAR-1 is required for neurite outgrowth and establishment of neuronal polarity. *Mol Biol Cell* 2002; 13: 4013–4028.

[22] Binder LI, Frankfurter A, Rebhun LI. The distribution of tau polypeptides in the mammalian central nervous system. *J Cell Biol* 1985; 101:1371–1378.

[23] Boland BA, Kumar A, Lee F-M, Platt J, Wegiel J, Yu WH, Nixon, RA. Autophagy induction and autophagosome clearance in neurons: relationship to autophagic pathology in Alzheimer's disease. *J Neurosci* 2008; 28: 6926–6937.

[24] Braak H, Alafuzoff I, Arzberger T, Kretzschmar H, Del Tredici K, Staging of Alzheimer disease neurofibrillary pathology using paraffin sections and immunocytochemistry, *Acta Neuropathol* 112, 2006, pp.389-404

[25] Braak E, Braak H, Mandelkow EM. A sequence of cytoskeleton changes related to the formation of neurofibrillary tangles and neuropil threads. *Acta Neuropathol* 1994; 87: 554-567.

[26] Braak H, Braak E. Neuropil threads occur in dendrites of tangle- bearing nerve cells. *Neuropathol Appl Neurobiol* 1988; 14:39-44.

[27] Braak H, Braak E. Neuropathological staging of Alzheimer-related changes. *Acta Neuropath* 1991; 82: 239-259.

[28] Braak, H., Ghebremedhin, E., Rueb, U., Bratzke, H. and K. del Tradici Stages in the development of Parkinson's disease-related pathology *Cell Tissue Res.* 2005; 318: 121–134.

[29] Brandt, R., Léger, J., and Lee, G. Interaction of tau with the neural plasma membrane mediated by tau's amino-terminal projection domain. *J. Cell Biol.* 1995; 131:1327-1340.

[30] Brion JP, Tremp G, Octave JN. Transgenic expression of the shortest human tau affects its compartmentalization and its phosphorylation as in the pretangle stage of Alzheimer's disease. *Am J Pathol.* 1999; 54: 255-270.

[31] Büeler HR, Aguzzi A, Sailer A, Greiner RA, Autenried P, Aguet M, Weissmann C. Mice devoid of PrP are resistant to scrapie. *Cell* 73: 1339–1347, 1993.

[32] Busciglio J, Lorenzo A, Yeh J, Yankner BA. Amyloid fibrils induce tau phosphorylation and loss of microtubule binding. *Neuron* 1995; 14: 879–888.

[33] Butner KA, Kirschner, MW. Tau protein binds to microtubules through a flexible array of distributed weak sites. *J Cell Biol* 1991; 122:717–730.

[34] Caceres A, Kosik KS. Inhibition of neurite polarity by tau antisense oligonucleotides in primary cerebellar neurons. *Nature* 1990; 343: 461–463.

[35] Cataldo AM, Barnett JL, Berman SA, Li J, Quarless S, Bursztajn S, Lippa C, Nixon RA. Gene expression and cellular content of cathepsin D in Alzheimer's disease brain: evidence for early up-regulation of the endosomal-lysosomal system. *Neuron* 1995; 14: 671-680.

[36] Cataldo AM, Petanceska S, Terio NB, Peterhoff CM, Durham R, Mercken M, Mehta PD, Buxbaum J, Haroutunian V, Nixon RA. Abeta localization in abnormal endosomes: association with earliest Abeta elevations in AD and Down syndrome. *Neurobiol Aging* 2004;25:1353–1272.

[37] Cancino, G.I., et al., c-Abl tyrosine kinase modulates tau pathology and Cdk5 phosphorylation in AD transgenic mice. *Neurobiol.Aging* 2009; 32: 1249-1351.

[38] Caughey B, Raymond GJ, Ernst D, Race RE (1991) N-terminal truncation of the scrapie-associated form of PrP by lysosomal protease(s): implications regarding the site of conversion of PrP to the protease-resistant state. *J Virol* 65: 6597–6603.

[39] Caughey, B. and P. Lansbury Protofibrils, Pores, Fibrils, and Neurodegeneration: Separating the Responsible Protein Aggregates from The Innocent Bystanders. *Annu. Rev. Neurosci.* 2003. 26:267–98

[40] Caughey B, Baron GS. 2006. Prions and their partners in crime. *Nature* 443:803–10

[41] Chang E, Kim S, Schafer KN, Kuret J: Pseudophosphorylation of tau protein directly modulates its aggregation kinetics. *Biochim Biophys Acta*; 2011;1814(2): 388-95.

[42] Chen L. and M.B. Feany, Alpha- synuclein phosphorylation controls neurotoxicity and inclusion formation in a *Drosophila* model of Parkinson disease, *Nat. Neurosci.* 8 (2005), pp. 657–663.

[43] Chesebro B, Race B, Meade-White K, LaCasse R, Race R, et al. (2010) Fatal Transmissible Amyloid Encephalopathy: A New Type of Prion Disease Associated with Lack of Prion Protein Membrane Anchoring. *PLoS Pathog* 6(3): e1000800.

[44] Chirita CN, Necula M, Kuret J. Anionic micelles and vesicles induce tau fibrillization in vitro. *J Biol Chem* 2003; 278:25644-50.

[45] Cho EY, So KF. Characterization of the sprouting response of axon-like processes from retinal ganglion cells after axotomy in adult hamsters: a model using intravitreal implantation of a peripheral nerve. *J Neurocytol* 1992; 21: 589–603.

[46] Cirrito, J. R., Kang, J. E., Lee, J., Stewart, et. al. Endocytosis is required for synaptic activity-dependent release of amyloid-beta in vivo. *Neuron* 2008; 58, 42-51.

[47] Clavaguera F, Bolmont T, Crowther RA, Abramowski D, Frank S, Probst A, Fraser G, Stalder AK, Beibel M, Staufenbiel M, Jucker M, Goedert M, Tolnay M. Transmission and spreading of tauopathy in transgenic mouse brain. *Nat Cell Biol* 2009; 11: 909-913.

[48] Clinton LK, Blurton-Jones M, Myczek K, Trojanowski JQ, LaFerla FM. Synergistic Interactions between Abeta, tau, and alpha-synuclein: acceleration of neuropathology and cognitive decline. *J Neurosci.* 2010; 30(21): 7281-9.

[49] Collinge, J and AR Clarke A General Model of Prion Strains and Their Pathogenicity *Science* 2007; 318, 930-936.

[50] Cookson, M Alpha-Synuclein and neuronal cell death *Molecular Neurodegeneration* 2009: 4:9 1-13

[51] Cotman, S.L., Halfter, W., and Cole, G.J. Agrin binds to β-amyloid (Aβ), accelerates Aβ fibril formation, and is localized to Aβ deposits in Alzheimer's disease brain. *Mol. Cell Neurosci.* 2000; 15: 183–210.

[52] Cohlberg, J.A., Li, J., Uversky, V.N., and Fink, A.L. Heparin and other glycosaminoglycans stimulate the formation of amyloid fibrils from α-synuclein in vitro. *Biochemistry,*2002 41: 1612–1621.

[53] Cushman M, Johnson B, King O, Gitler A, and J Shorter Prion-like disorders: blurring the divide between transmissibility and infectivity *Journal of Cell Science* 2010 123: 1191-1201 2Cohlberg

[54] Dawson HN, Cantillana V, Jansen M, Wang H, Vitek MP, Wilcock DM, Lynch JR, Laskowitz DT.Loss of tau elicits axonal degeneration in a mouse model of Alzheimer's disease. *Neuroscience.* 2010;169(1):516-31.

[55] Dawson HN, Ferreira A, Eyster MV, Ghoshal N, Binder LI, Vitek MP Inhibition of neuronal maturation in primary hippocampal neurons from tau deficient mice. *J Cell Sci* 2001 121:1249-1257.

[56] Deleault NR, Lucassen RW, Supattapone S RNA molecules stimulate prion protein conversion. *Nature* 2003 425:717–720.

[57] Desplats P, et al. Inclusion formation and neuronal cell death through neuron-to-neuron transmission of α-synuclein. *Proc Natl Acad Sci USA* 2009 106:13004–13005.

[58] Dickson, D.W.Tau and synuclein and their role in neuropathology.Brain Pathol.1999. 9, 657–661.

[59] Dickson DW, Neuropathology of non Alzheimer degenerative disorders, Int J Clin Exp Pathol, 3, 2010, pp. 1-22.

[60] DiTella M, Feiguin F, Morfini G, Caceres A. Microfilament associated growth cone component depends upon tau for its intracellular localization. *Cell Motil Cytoskel* 1994; 29:124–130.

[61] Dixit R, Ross JL, Goldman YE, Holzbaur EL. Differential regulation of dynein and kinesin motor proteins by tau. Science 2008; 319:1086-9.

[62] Dudek SM, Johnson GV. Transglutaminase catalyzes the formation of sodium dodecyl sulfate-insoluble, Alz-50-reactive polymers of tau. *J Neurochem* 1993; 61:1229-62.

[63] Dugger BN, Tu M, Murray ME, Dickson DW: Disease specificity and pathologic progression of tau pathology in brainstem nuclei of Alzheimer's disease and progressive supranuclear palsy. *Neurosci Lett*; 2011; 491(2):122-6.

[64] Ehehalt R, Keller P, Haass C, Thiele C, Simons KAmyloidogenic processing of the Alzheimer beta-amyloid precursor protein depends on lipid rafts. *J Cell Biol* 2003 160:120–123.

[65] Eisele,Y.S., U. Obermuller, G. Heilbronner, F. Baumann, S.A. Kaeser and H. Wolburg *et al.*, Peripherally applied Abeta-containing inoculates induce cerebral beta-amyloidosis, *Science* 2010; 330: 980–982.

[66] El-Agnaf, O. , Jakes R, Curran, MD. and Wallace, A. Effects of the mutations Ala30 to Pro and Ala53 to Thr on the physical and morphological properties of alpha synuclein protein implicated in Parkinson's disease. *FEBS Lett.* 1998; 440: 67-70.

[67] Elbaum-Garfinkle S, Ramlall T, Rhoades E. The role of the lipid bilayer in tau aggregation. *Biophys J.* 2010 98:2722-30.

[68] Emmanouilidou E, Melachroinou K, Roumeliotis T, Garbis SD, Ntzouni M, Margaritis LH, Stefanis L, Vekrellis K. Cell-produced alpha-synuclein is secreted in a calcium-

dependent manner by exosomes and impacts neuronal survival. *J Neurosci.* 2010; 30:6838-51.

[69] Esposito A, Dohm CP, Kermer P, Bähr M, Wouters FS. 2007 Alpha-Synuclein and its disease-related mutants interact differentially with the microtubule protein tau and associate with the actin cytoskeleton. *Neurobiol Dis.* 26(3):521-31.

[70] Fang, Y., Wu, N., Gan, X., Yan, W., Morrell, J. C., and Gould, S. J. (2007). Higher-order oligomerization targets plasma membrane proteins and HIV gag to exosomes. *PLoS Biol* 5, e158.

[71] Fein JA, Sokolow S, Miller CA, Vinters HV, Yang F, Cole GM, Gylys KH. Co-localization of amyloid beta and tau pathology in Alzheimer's disease synaptosomes. *Am. J. Pathol* 2008; 172: 1683-1692.

[72] Fenrich KK, Skelton N, MacDermid VE, Meehan CF, Armstrong S et al. Axonal regeneration and development of de novo axons from distal dendrites of adult feline commissural interneurons after a proximal axotomy. *J Comp Neurol* 2007; 502:1079–1097.

[73] Fevrier B, Vilette D, Archer F, Loew D, Faigle W, Vidal M, Laude H, Raposo G. Cells release prions in association with exosomes. *Proc Natl Acad Sci USA* 2004; 101: 9683-9688.

[74] Fevrier, B., and Raposo, G. Exosomes: endosomal-derived vesicles shipping extracellular messages. *Curr Opin Cell Biol* 2004; 16: 415-421.

[75] Fortin DL, Troyer MD, Nakamura K, Kubo S, Anthony MD, Edwards RH: Lipid rafts mediate the synaptic localization of alphasynuclein. *J Neurosci* 2004, 24:6715-6723.

[76] Fournier J-G, Escaign-Haye F, Villemeur TBD and Robain O Ultrastructural localisation of cellular prion protein in synaptic boutons of normal hamster hippocampus. *CR Acad Sci (Paris)*, 1995; 318, 339–344.

[77] Freedman, S. D., Katz, M. H., Parker, E. M., and Gelrud, A. Endocytosis at the apical plasma membrane of pancreatic acinar cells is regulated by tyrosine kinases. *Am J Physiol* 1999; 276, C306-311.

[78] Friedrich RP, Tepper K, Rönicke R, Soom M, Westermann M, Reymann K, Kaether C, Fändrich M. Mechanism of amyloid plaque formation suggests an intracellular basis of Abeta pathogenicity. *Proc Natl Acad Sci U S A.* 2010 107(5):1942-7.

[79] Frost B, Jacks RL, Diamond MI. Propagation of tau misfolding from the outside to the inside of a cell. *J Biol Chem* 2009; 284: 12845-12852.

[80] Fujiwara, H., Hasegawa, M., Dohmae, N., Kawashima, A., Masliah, E., Goldberg, M.S., Shen, J., Takio, K., Iwatsubo, T. alpha-synuclein is phosphorylated in synucleinopathy lesions. *Nat. Cell Biol.* 2002; 4, 160–164.

[81] Galvin JE, Uryu K, Lee VM, Trojanowski JQ Axon pathology in Parkinson's disease and Lewy body dementia hippocampus contains alpha-, beta-, and gamma-synuclein. *Proc Natl Acad Sci USA* 1999; 96:13450–13455.

[82] Giaccone, G, Mangieri M., Capobianco R, Limido L, Hauw JJ, Haïk S, Fociani P, Bugiani O, Tagliavini, F. Tauopathy in human and experimental variant Creutzfeldt-Jakob disease. *Neurobiol. Aging,* 2008 , 29:1864-1873.

[83] Giasson BI, Forman M, Higuchi M, Golbe L, Graves C, Kotzbauer P, Trojanowski JQ, Lee V.M-Y. Initiation and synergistic fibrillization of tau and alpha synuclein. *Science* 2003; 300: 636-640.

[84] Glabe, C.G., Kayed, R., Sokolov, Y., Hall, J., 2004. Common structure and mechanism of soluble amyloid oligomer pathogenesis in degenerative diseases. Neurobiol. Aging 25, 75.

[85] Gomez-Ramos A, Diaz-Hernandez M, Cuadros R, Hernandez F, Avila, J. Extracellular tau is toxic to neuronal cells. *FEBS Lett.* 2006; 580: 4842–4850.

[86] Gotz J, Probst A, Spillantini MG, Schafer T, Jakes R, Burki K, Goedert M Somatodendritic localization and hyperphosphorylation of tau protein in transgenic mice expressing the longest human brain tau isoform, *Embo J.* 1995; 14: 1304-1313 .

[87] Gotz J, Chen F, van Dorpe J, Nitsch RM: Formation of neurofibrillary tangles in P301l tau transgenic mice induced by Abeta 1-42 fibrils. *Science* 2001; 293: 1601-1605.

[88] Grune T, Botzen D, Engels M, Voss P, Kaiser B, Jung T, Grimm S, Ermak G, Davies KJ. (2010) Tau protein degradation is catalyzed by the ATP/ubiquitin-independent 20S proteasome under normal cell conditions. *Arch Biochem Biophys.* 500(2):181-8.

[89] Grundke-Iqbal I, Iqbal K, Tung YC, Quinlan M, Wisniewski HM, Binder LI. Abnormal phosphorylation of the microtubule-associated protein tau in Alzheimer cytoskeletal pathology. *Proc Natl Acad Sci USA* 2106; 83: 4913– 4917.

[90] Guillozet-Bongaarts AL, Garcia-Sierra F, Reynolds MR, Horowitz PM, Fu Y, Wang T, Cahill ME, Bigio EH, Berry RW, Binder LI. Tau truncation during neurofibrillary tangle evolution in Alzheimer's disease. *Neurobiol Aging* 2005; 26:1015-22.

[91] Goedert M, Jakes R, Spillantini MG, Hasegawa M, Smith MJ, Crowther RA. Assembly of microtubule-associated protein tau into Alzheimer-like filaments induced by sulphated glycosaminoglycans. *Nature* 1996; 383: 550-553.

[92] Gonzalez-Billault C, Engelke M, Jimenez-Mateos EM, Wandosell F, Caceres A, Avila J. Participation of structural microtubule-associated proteins (MAPs) in the development of neuronal polarity. *J Neurosci Res* 2002; 67: 713–719.

[93] Guo JT, Arai J, Miklossy J, McGeer P. Tau and A beta forms soluble complexes that may promote self aggregation of both into the insoluble forms observed in Alzheimer's disease *Proc Natl Acad Sci USA* 2006; 103: 1953-1958.

[94] Haass C, Lemere CA, Capell A, Citron M, Seubert P, Schenk D, Lannfelt L, Selkoe DJ. 1995. The Swedish mutation causes early-onset Alzheimer's disease by β-secretase cleavage within the secretory pathway. *Nat Med* 1: 1291–1296.

[95] Haïk S, Privat N, Adjou KT, Sazdovitch V, Dormont D, Duyckaerts C, Hauw JJ. Alpha-synuclein-immunoreactive deposits in human and animal prion diseases. *Acta Neuropathol.* 2002 103(5):516-20.

[96] Hall GF. Cellular responses of identified lamprey central neurons to axonal and dendritic injury. *Ann NY Acad Sci* 1993; 679: 43-64.

[97] Hall GF. Neuronal Morphology: Development and maintenance of neuronal polarity. *Encyclopedia of Neuroscience, ed Adelman & Smith* 1999; 1409-1413.

[98] Hall GF, Poulos A, Cohen MJ. Sprouts emerging from the dendrites of axotomized lamprey central neurons have axonlike ultrastructure. *J Neurosci* 1989; 9: 588-599.

[99] Hall, G. F. and K. S. Kosik Axotomy-induced neurofilament phosphorylation is inhibited *in situ* by microinjection of PKA and PKC inhibitors into identified lamprey neurons. *Neuron* 1993; 10: 613-625.

[100] Hall GF, Yao J. and Lee G. Tau overexpressed in identified lamprey neurons in situ is spatially segregated by phosphorylation state, forms hyperphosphorylated, dense

aggregations and induces neurodegeneration. *Proc Nat Acad Sci USA* 1997; 94: 4733-4738.

[101] Hall GF, Yao J, Selzer M, Kosik KS. Cytoskeletal correlates to cell polarity loss following axotomy of lamprey central neurons *J Neurocytol* 1997; 26: 733-753.

[102] Hall GF, Lee S, Yao, J. Neurofibrillary degeneration can be arrested in an in vivo cellular model of human tauopathy by application of a compound which inhibits tau filament formation in vitro. *J. Mol. Neurosci* 2002; 19: 253-260.

[103] Hall GF, Chu B, Lee G, Yao J. Human tau filaments induce microtubule and synapse loss in vertebrate central neurons. *J Cell Sci* 2000; 120: 1373-1387.

[104] Hamano T, Gendron TF, Causevic E, Yen SH, Lin WL, Isidoro C, Deture M, Ko LW. Autophagic-lysosomal perturbation enhances tau aggregation in transfectants with induced wild-type tau expression. *Eur J Neurosci* 2008; 27: 1119-30.

[105] Hara T, Nakamura K, Matsui M, Yamamoto A, Nakahara Y, Suzuki-Migishima R, Yokoyama M, Mishima K, Saito I, Okano H et al.: Suppression of basal autophagy in neural cells causes neurodegenerative disease in mice. *Nature* 2006, 441:885-889.

[106] Hasegawa M, Smith MJ. Goedert M. Tau proteins with FTDP-17 mutations have a reduced ability to promote microtubule assembly. *FEBS Lett* 1998; 437: 207-210.

[107] He HJ, Wang XS, Pan R, Wang DL, Liu MN, He RQ. The proline rich domain of tau plays a role in interactions with actin. *BMC Cell Biol* 2009; 10: 81-93.

[108] Helmke S, Pfenninger KH (1995) Growth cone enrichment and cytoskeletal association of non-receptor tyrosine kinases. *Cell Motil Cytoskeleton* 30, 194-207.

[109] Higashi S, Iseki E, Yamamoto R, Minegishi M, Hino H, Fujisawa K, Togo T, Katsuse O, Uchikado H, Furukawa Y, Kosaka K, Arai H. Concurrence of TDP-43, tau and alpha-synuclein pathology in brains of Alzheimer's disease and dementia with Lewy bodies. *Brain Res* 2007; 1254: 284-294.

[110] Ho GJ, Hashimoto M, Adame A, Izu M, Alford MF, Thal LJ, Hansen LA, Masliah E. Altered p59Fyn kinase expression accompanies disease progression in Alzheimer's disease: implications for its functional role. *Neurobiol Aging* 2005; 26:625-35.

[111] Hooper NM. Glypican-1 facilitates prion conversion in lipid rafts. 2011 *J Neurochem*.16(5):721-5.

[112] Horowitz PM, LaPointe N, Guillozet-Bongaarts AL, Berry RW, Binder LI. N-terminal fragments of tau inhibit full-length tau polymerization in vitro. *Biochemistry* 2006; 45: 12859–12866.

[113] Hundt C *et al.* (2001) Identification of interaction domains of the prion protein with its 37-kDa/67-kDa laminin receptor. *EMBO J*, 20, 5876–5886.

[114] Ihara, Y. Massive somatodendritic sprouting of cortical neurons in Alzheimer's Disease. *Brain Res* 2108; 459: 138-144.

[115] Ishikura N, Clever J, Bouzamondo-Bernstein E, Samayoa E, Prusiner SB, Huang E, DeArmond SJ. Notch-1 activation and dendritic atrophy in prion diseases. *PNAS.* 2005;102:886–891.

[116] Iqbal KC, Alonso A, Chen S, Chohan MO, El-Akkad E, Gong CX, Khatoon S, Li B, Liu F, Rahman A, Tanimukai H, Grundke-Iqbal I. Tau pathology in Alzheimer disease and other tauopathies. *Biochim. Biophys. Acta,* 2005; 1739: 210-210.

[117] Ittner LM, Ke YD, Delerue F, Bi M, Gladbach A, van Eersel J, Wölfing H, Chieng BC, Christie MJ, Napier IA, Eckert A, Staufenbiel M et al. Dendritic function of tau mediates amyloid-beta toxicity in Alzheimer's disease mouse models. *Cell* 2010; 142: 387-97.

[118] Johnson GV, Cox TM, Lockhart JP, Zinnerman MD, Miller ML, Powers R. Transglutaminase activity is increased in Alzheimer's disease brain. *Brain Res* 1997; 751: 323-329.

[119] Kampers T, Friedhoff P, Biernat J, Mandelkow EM. RNA stimulates aggregation of microtubule-associated protein-tau into Alzheimer-like paired helical filaments, *FEBS Lett* 1997; 399: 344- 349.

[120] Kawarabayashi T,Shoji M, Younkin L, Wen-Lang L, Dickson D, Murakami T, Matsubara E, Abe K, Ashe K. Younkin S. Dimeric amyloid beta protein rapidly accumulates in lipid rafts followed by apolipoprotein E and phosphorylated tau accumulation in the Tg2576 mouse model of Alzheimer's disease. *J. Neurosci.* 2004; 24: 3801–3809.

[121] Kazmierczak A, Strosznajder JB, Adamczyk A. 2008 A-Synuclein enhances secretion and toxicity of amyloid beta peptides in PC12 cells. *Neurochem Int.* 53(6-8):263-9.

[122] Kempf M, Clement A, Faissner A, Lee G, Brandt R. Tau binds to the distal axon early in development of polarity in a microtubule- and microfilament-dependent manner. *J Neurosci* 1996; 16:5583-5592.

[123] Kim W, Lee S, Jung C, Ahmed A, Lee G, Hall GF. Interneuronal transfer of human tau between Lamprey central neurons in situ. *J Alz Dis* 2010; 19:647-64.

[124] Kim W, Lee S, Hall GF. Secretion of human tau fragments resembling CSF-tau inAlzheimer's disease is modulated by the presence of the exon 2 insert. *FEBS Lett* 2010; 584:3085-8.

[125] King ME, Kan H, Baas PW, Erisir A, Glabe C, Bloom GS. Tau-dependent microtubule disassembly initiated by prefibrillar beta-amyloid. *J Cell Biol* 2006; 175: 541–546.

[126] Kitada T, Asakawa S, Hattori N, Matsumine H, Yamamura Y, Minoshima S, Yokochi M, Mizuno Y, Shimizu N. Mutations in the parkin gene cause autosomal recessive juvenile parkinsonism. *Nature.* 1998 392(6676):605-8

[127] Koo EH, Sisodia SS, Archer DR, Martin LJ,Weidemann A, Beyreuther K, et al. Precursor of amyloid protein in Alzheimer disease undergoes fast anterograde axonal transport. *Proc Natl Acad Sci USA* 1990; 87:1561–5.

[128] Kordower, J., Y Chu, R Hauser, T Freeman and CW Olanow (2008) Lewy body-like pathology in long-term embryonic nigral transplants in Parkinson's disease *Nature Medicine* 14, 504–506.

[129] Khurana V, Elson-Schwab I, Fulga TA, Sharp KA, Loewen CA, Mulkearns E, Tyynelä J, Scherzer CR, Feany MB: Lysosomal dysfunction promotes cleavage and neurotoxicity of tau in vivo. *PLoS Genet*; 2010; 6(7):e1001026

[130] Lachenal, Gaelle (2011) Release of exosomes from differentiated neurons and its regulation by synaptic glutamatergic activity. *Molecular and Cellular Neuroscience* 46(2)

[131] Lambert MP, Barlow AK, Chromy BA, Edwards C, Freed R, Liosatos M, Morgan TE, Rozovsky I, Trommer B, Viola KL, Wals P, Zhang C, Finch CE, Krafft GA, Klein WL. Diffusible, nonfibrillar ligands derived from Abeta1-42 are potent central nervous system neurotoxins. *Proc Natl Acad Sci USA* 1998; 95: 6448–6453.

[132] LaMonte BH, Wallace KE, Holloway BA, Shelly SS, Ascano J, Tokito M, Van Winkle T, Howland DS, Holzbaur EL: Disruption of dynein/dynactin inhibits axonal transport in motor neurons causing late-onset progressive degeneration. *Neuron* 2002, 34:715-727.

[133] Lashuel, H.A., Petre, B.M., Wall, J., Simon, M., Nowak, R.J., Walz, T., Lansbury Jr., P.T., 2002. Alph-synuclein, especially the Parkinson's disease-associated mutants, forms pore-like annular and tubular protofibrils. J. Mol. Biol. 322, 1089- 1102.

[134] Lauren, J, Gimbel, DA, Nygaard HB, Gilbert JW and Strittmatter SM. Cellular prion protein mediates impairment of synaptic plasticity by amyloid-beta oligomers. *Nature* 2009; 457:1128-32.

[135] Lazarov O, Lee M, Peterson DA, and Sisodia, SS. Evidence that synaptically released beta-amyloid accumulates as extracellular deposits in the hippocampus of transgenic mice. *J. Neurosci.* 2002; 22: 9785-9793.

[136] Lebouvier T, Scales TM, Hanger DP, Geahlen RL, Lardeux B, Reynolds CH, Anderton BH, Derkinderen P. The microtubule-associated protein tau is phosphorylated by Syk. *Biochim Biophys Acta* 2008; 1783: 188–92

[137] Lee G, Newman ST, Gard DL, Band H, Panchamoorthy G. Tau interacts with src-family non-receptor tyrosine kinases. *J. Cell Sci* 1998; 111: 3167-3177.

[138] Lee G, Thangavel R, Sharma VM, Litersky JM, Bhaskar K, Fang SM. Do LH, Andreadis A, Van Hoesen G, and Ksiezak-Reding H. Phosphorylation of tau by fyn: implications for Alzheimer's disease. *J. Neurosci* 2004; 24: 2304–2312.

[139] Lee HJ, Choi C, Lee SJ. Membrane-bound alpha-synuclein has a high aggregation propensity and the ability to seed the aggregation of the cytosolic form. *J. Biol. Chem.* 2002; 277 (1): 671–8.

[140] Lee HJ, Patel S, and Lee, SJ Intravesicular localization and exocytosis of α-synuclein and its aggregates. *J. Neurosci.*, 2005; 25, 6016–6024.

[141] Lee S, Jung C, Lee G, and Hall GF Exonic point mutations of human tau enhance its toxicity and cause characteristic changes in neuronal morphology, tau distribution and tau phosphorylation in the lamprey cellular model of tauopathy. *J. Alz. Dis.*, 2009; 16, 99-111.

[142] Lee S, Kim W, Li Z and Hall GF Accumulation of vesicle-associated human tau in distal dendrites drives degeneration and tau secretion in an in situ cellular tauopathy model *Int J. Alz Dis* 2011 accepted.

[143] Lee VM, Goedert M, Trojanowski JQ. Neurodegenerative tauopathies. *Annu Rev Neurosci* 2001; 24:1121-59.

[144] Linda H, Risling M, Cullheim S. 'Dendraxons' in regenerating motoneurons in the cat: do dendrites generate new axons after central axotomy? *Brain Res* 2112; 358:329–333.

[145] Lindwasser W and M Resh Multimerization of Human Immunodeficiency Virus Type 1 Gag Promotes Its Localization to Barges, Raft-Like Membrane Microdomains *J.Virol,* 2001; *75: 7913-7924*

[146] Litman P, Barg J, Rindzoonski L, Ginzburg I. Subcellular localization of tau mRNA in differentiating neuronal cell culture: Implications for neuronal polarity. *Neuron* 1993; 10: 627-638.

[147] Liu, Y. and Szaro, B. hnRNP K Post-transcriptionally Co-regulates Multiple Cytoskeletal Genes Needed for Axonogenesis *Development* (in press)

[148] Maas, T., Eidenmuller, J., and Brandt, R. (2000) Tau's interaction with the neural membrane cortex is regulated by phosphorylation at sites that are modified in paired helical filaments. *J. Biol. Chem.* 275, 15733–15740.

[149] Mahfoud R, Garmy N, Maresca M, Yahi N, Puigserver A and J. Fantini, Identification of a common sphingolipid-binding domain in Alzheimer, prion, and HIV-1 proteins, *J. Biol. Chem.* 2002; 277: 11292–11296.

[150] Maroteaux L, Campanelli JT, Scheller RH: Synuclein: a neuronspecific protein localized to the nucleus and presynaptic nerve terminal. *J Neurosci* 2108, 8:2804-2815.

[151] McKee AC, Kowall NW, Kosik KS. Microtubular reorganization and dendritic growth response in Alzheimer's disease *Ann Neurol*. 1989; 26: 652-659.

[152] McKee AC, Cantu R, Nowinski C, et al. Chronic traumatic encephalopathy in athletes: progressive tauopathy after repetitive head injury. *J Neuropathol Exp Neurol* 2009; 68:709–35.

[153] Menzies F. Moreau, K. and D. Rubinsztein Protein misfolding disorders and macroautophagy *Current Opinion in Cell Biology* 2011; 23:190–197

[154] Michiorri S, Gelmetti V, Giarda E, Lombardi F, Romano F, Marongiu R, Nerini-Molteni S, Sale P, Vago R, Arena G et al.: The Parkinson-associated protein PINK1 interacts with Beclin1 and promotes autophagy. *Cell Death Differ* 2010; 17: 962-974.

[155] Minami S, Hoe H, Burns M, Matsuoka Y and G Rebeck Fyn kinase regulates phosphorylation and localization of APP and Dab1 to lipid rafts *J. Neurochem.* 2011; 125: 879–890

[156] Mocanu MM, Nissen A, Eckermann K, Khlistunova I, Biernat J, Drexler D, Petrova O, et al. The potential for beta-structure in the repeat domain of tau protein determines aggregation, synaptic decay, neuronal loss, and coassembly with endogenous Tau in inducible mouse models of tauopathy. *J Neurosci* 2008; 28: 737-748.

[157] Morfini GA, Burns M, Binder LI, Kanaan NM, LaPointe N, Bosco DA, et al. Axonal transport defects in neurodegenerative diseases. *J Neurosci* 2009; 29: 12776-86.

[158] Mori H., Kondo J., and Ihara Y. (2107). Ubiquitin is a component of paired helical filaments in Alzheimer's disease, *Science*235, 1641–1644.

[159] Morita T, Sobue K. Specification of Neuronal Polarity Regulated by Local Translation of CRMP2 and Tau via the mTOR-p70S6K Pathway *J. Biol Chem* 2009; 284: 27734–27745.

[160] Mufson EJ, Kroin JS, Sendera TJ, Sobreviela T. Distribution and retrograde transport of trophic factors in the central nervous system: functional implications for the treatment of neurodegenerative diseases. *Prog Neurobiol* 1999; 57: 451- 484.

[161] Nemes Z, Devreese B, Steinert PM, Van Beeumen J. Fesus L. Cross-linking of ubiquitin, HSP27, parkin, and alpha-synuclein by gamma-glutamyl-epsilon-lysine bonds in Alzheimer's neurofibrillary tangles. *FASEB J*. 2004; 18:1205–7.

[162] Newell, KL, Boyer P, Gomez-Tortosa, E, Hobbs W, Hedley-Whyte, ET, Vonsattel, JP, Hyman, BT. alpha-Synuclein immunoreactivity is present in axonal swellings in neuroaxonal dystrophy and acute traumatic brain injury. *J. Neuropathol. Exp. Neurol.* 1999; 58, 1353–1358.

[163] Nickel W. Unconventional secretory routes: direct protein export across the plasma membrane of mammalian cells. *Traffic* 2005; 6: 607–614.

[164] Nixon, R. A. (2005). Endosome function and dysfunction in Alzheimer's disease and other neurodegenerative diseases. *Neurobiol Aging* 26, 373–382.

[165] Nixon RA, Wegiel J, Kumar A, Yu WH, Peterhoff C, Cataldo A, Cuervo AM. Extensive involvement of autophagy in Alzheimer disease: an immuno-electron microscopy study. *J Neuropathol Exp Neurol* 2005; 64: 120–122.

[166] Nybakken K, Perrimon N.Heparan sulfate proteoglycan modulation of developmental signaling in Drosophila *Biochimica et Biophysica Acta* 2002; 1573: 280–291

[167] Pan, T., S. Kondo, W. Le, J. Jankovic, The role of autophagy–lysosome pathway in neurodegeneration associated with Parkinson's disease, *Brain* 131 (2008) 1969–1978.

[168] Parchi P, Castellani R, Capellari S, Ghetti B, Young K, et al. Molecular basis of phenotypic variability in sporadic Creutzfeldt-Jakob disease. *Annal Neurol.* 1996;39:767–778.

[169] Park SY, Ferreira A. The generation of a 17 kDa neurotoxic fragment: an alternative mechanism by which tau mediates beta-amyloid-induced neurodegeneration. *J Neurosci* 2005; 25: 5365-5375.

[170] Patterson, K. C Remmer, Y Fu, S Brooker, N Kanaan, L Vana, S Ward, J Reyes, K Philibert, M Glucksman, and LI Binder Characterization of Prefibrillar Tau Oligomers in Vitro and in Alzheimer Disease *J. Biol. Chem.* 2011 286: 23063-23076.

[171] Pérez, MR, Cuadros M, Benítez J, Jiménez J. Interaction of Alzheimer's disease amyloid ß peptide fragment 25-35 with tau protein, and with a tau peptide containing the microtubule binding domain *J Alz Dis* 2004; 6: 461-467.

[172] Perez MR, Zheng H, Lex H, Van der Ploeg T and Koo E. The b-Amyloid Precursor Protein of Alzheimer's Disease Enhances Neuron Viability and Modulates Neuronal Polarity *J. Neurosci.* 1997; 17(24):9407–9414

[173] Perrin RJ, Woods WS, Clayton DF, George JM (2001) Exposure to long chain polyunsaturated fatty acids triggers rapid multimerization of synucleins. *J Biol Chem* 276: 41958–41962.

[174] Perry G, Kawai M, Tabaton M, Onorato M, Mulvihill P, Richey P, Morandi A, Connolly JA, Gambetti P. Neuropil threads of Alzheimer's disease show a marked alteration of the normal cytoskeleton. *J Neurosci* 1991; 11:1748-1755.

[175] Prusiner SB, Scott MR, DeArmond SJ and Cohen FE (1998) Prion protein biology. *Cell,* 93, 337–348.

[176] Rajendran L, Honsho M, Zahn TR, Keller P, Geiger KD, Verkade P, Simons K. Alzheimer's disease beta-amyloid peptides are released in association with exosomes. *Proc Natl Acad Sci USA* 2006; 103: 11242-11247.

[177] Rapoport M, Dawson HN, Binder LI, Vitek MP, Ferreira A. Tau is essential to beta-amyloid-induced neurotoxicity. Proc Natl Acad Sci USA 2002; 99: 6364–6369.

[178] Ravikumar B, Acevedo-Arozena A, Imarisio S, Berger Z, Vacher C, O'Kane CJ, Brown SD, Rubinsztein DC: Dynein mutations impair autophagic clearance of aggregate-prone proteins. *Nat Genet* 2005, 37:771-776.

[179] Reynolds CH, Garwood CJ, Wray S, Price C, Kellie S, Perera T, Zvelebil M, Yang A, Sheppard PW, Varndell IM, *et al.*: Phosphorylation regulates tau interactions with Src homology 3 domains of phosphatidylinositol 3-kinase, phospholipase Cgamma1, Grb2, and Src family kinases. *J Biol Chem* 2008, 283:18177-18186.

[180] Roberson ED, Scearce-Levie K, Palop J.J, Yan F, Cheng IH, Wu T, Gerstein H, Yu GQ, Mucke L. Reducing endogenous tau ameliorates amyloid beta-induced deficits in an Alzheimer's disease mouse model. *Science* 2007; 316: 750-754.

[181] Roberts TK, Eugenin EA, Morgello S, Clements JE, Zink MC, Berman JW. PrPC, the cellular isoform of the human prion protein, is a novel biomarker of HIV-associated neurocognitive impairment and mediates neuroinflammation. *Am J Pathol.* 2010; 177(4):1848-60.

[182] Rock KL, Gramm C, Rothstein L, Clark K, Stein R, Dick L, Hwang D, Goldberg AL. (1994) Inhibitors of the proteasome block the degradation of most cell proteins and the generation of peptides presented on MHC class I molecules. *Cell* 78(5): 761-71.

[183] Rose PK, MacDermid V, Joshi M, Neuber-Hess M. Emergence of axons from distal dendrites of adult mammalian neurons following a permanent axotomy. *Eur J Neurosci* 2001; 13:1236–1246.

[184] Roy, S., Zhang, B, Lee, V. M.-Y. & Trojanowski, J. Q. Axonal transport defects: a common theme in neurodegenerative diseases. *Acta Neuropathol.* 109, 5–13 (2005).

[185] Saman S. and Hall GF (2011) Analysis of tau associated proteins in secreted exosomes - clues to tau-mediated neurodegeneration? *Alzheimer's and Dementia*, in press.

[186] Samsonov A, Yu JZ, Rasenick M, Popov SV. Tau interaction with microtubules in vivo. *J Cell Sci* 2004; 124: 6129-41

[187] Sandal M, Valle F, Tessari I, Mammi S, Bergantino E, Musiani F, Brucale M, Bubacco L, Samorì B (2008). Conformational equilibria in monomeric α-synuclein at the single-molecule level. *PLoS Biol.* 6 (1): e6.

[188] Santuccione A, Sytnyk V, Leshchyns'ka I, Schachner M. Prion protein recruits its neuronal receptor NCAM to lipid rafts to activate p59fyn and to enhance neurte outgrowth. *J Cell Biol* 2005; 169: 341–354.

[189] Sarkar M, Kuret J, Lee G. Two motifs within the tau microtubule binding domain mediate its association with the hsc70 molecular chaperone. *J Neurosci Res* 2008; 86: 2763-73.

[190] Schindowski K, Belarbi K, Buee L. Neurotrophic factors in Alzheimer's disease: role of axonal transport *Genes, Brain and Behavior* 2008; 7(Suppl. 1): 43–56.

[191] Schneider, A. et al. (2008) Flotillin-dependent clustering of the amyloid precursor protein regulates its endocytosis and amyloidogenic processing in neurons. *J. Neurosci.* 28, 2874–2882

[192] Shmerling, D. *et al.* Expression of amino-terminallytruncated PrP in the mouse leading to ataxia and specific cerebellar lesions. *Cell* 93, 203–214 (1998).

[193] Simons M, Keller P, De Strooper B, Beyreuther K, Dotti CG, Simons K.Cholesterol depletion inhibits the generation of beta-amyloid in hippocampal neurons. *Proc Natl Acad Sci* USA 1998; 95:6460–4.

[194] Singleton, RH., Zhu J, Stone JR., Povlishock JT. Traumatically induced axotomy adjacent to the soma does not result in acute neuronal death. *J Neurosci* 2002; 22: 791–802.

[195] Soper, J. H., Roy, S., Stieber, A., Lee, E., Wilson, R. B., Trojanowski, J. Q., Burd, C. G. and Lee, V. M.(2008). Alpha-synuclein-induced aggregation of cytoplasmic vesicles in Saccharomyces cerevisiae. *Mol. Biol. Cell* 19, 1093-1103.

[196] Soto C, Estrada L. Protein Misfolding and Neurodegeneration *Arch Neurol.* 2008 65(2):184-189

[197] Spillantini, M.G., Bird, T.D., Ghetti, B. Frontotemporal dementia and parkinsonism linked to chromosome 17: a new group of tauopathies. *Brain Pathol.* 1998; 8 (2): 387–402.

[198] Spillantini, M. G., Tolnay, M., Love, S. & Goedert, M. Microtubule-associated protein tau, heparan sulphate and alpha synuclein in several neurodegenerative diseases with dementia. *Acta Neuropathol.*1999; 97: 585-594.

[199] Stamer K, Vogel R, Thies E, Mandelkow E, Mandelkow EM. Tau blocks traffic of organelles, neurofilaments, and APP vesicles in neurons and enhances oxidative stress. *J. Cell Biol* 2002; 156: 1121-1063.

[200] Stokin GB, Lillo C, Falzone TL, Brusch RG, Rockenstein E, Mount SL, Raman R, Davies P, Masliah E. Williams DS, Goldstein LS. Axonopathy and transport deficits early in the pathogenesis of Alzheimer's disease. *Science* 2005; 307: 1282–1288.

[201] Stone MC, Nguyen MM, Tao J, Allender D.L, Rolls MM. Global Up-Regulation of Microtubule Dynamics and Polarity Reversal during Regeneration of an Axon from a Dendrite. *Mol Biol Cell* 2010; 21: 767–777.

[202] Stoothoff W, Johnson GV. Tau phosphorylation: physiological and pathological consequences *Biochimica et Biophysica Acta* 2005 1739 280-297.

[203] Su JH, Deng G, Cotman CW. Transneuronal degeneration in the spread of Alzheimer's disease pathology: immunohistochemical evidence for the transmission of tau hyperphosphorylation. *Neurobiol Dis* 1997; 4: 365–375.

[204] Sunyach C, Jen A, Deng J, Fitzgerald KT, Frobert Y, Grassi J, McCaffrey MW, Morris R The mechanism of internalization of glycosylphosphatidylinositol-anchored prion protein. *EMBO J* 2003; 22: 3591–3601.

[205] Sverdlov, M., Shajahan, A. N., and Minshall, R. D. Tyrosine phosphorylationdependence of caveolae-mediated endocytosis. *J Cell Mol Med* 2007; 11: 1239-1340.

[206] Swerdlow RH, Khan SM. A "mitochondrial cascade hypothesis" for sporadic Alzheimer's disease. *Med Hypotheses.* 2004; 63:8–20.

[207] Takashima A., Murayama M., Murayama O., Kohno T., Honda T., Yasutake K., et al. Presenilin 1 associates with glycogen synthase kinase-3 beta and its substrate tau. *Proc. Natl. Acad. Sci. USA* 1998; 95: 9637–9641.

[208] Taraboulos A, Scott M, Semenov A, Avrahami D, Laszlo L, Prusiner SB, Avraham D (1995) Cholesterol depletion and modification of COOH- terminal targeting sequence of the prion protein inhibit formation of the scrapie isoform. *J Cell Biol* 129:121–132.

[209] Taylor, D and N Hooper Role of lipid rafts in the processing of the pathogenic prion and Alzheimer's amyloid-beta proteins. *Seminars in Cell & Developmental Biology* 18 (2007) 638–648.

[210] Tournaviti, S., Hannemann, S., Terjung, S., Kitzing, T. M., Stegmayer, C., Ritzerfeld, J., Walther, P., Grosse, R., Nickel, W., and Fackler, O. T. (2007). SH4-domain-induced plasma membrane dynamization promotes bleb-associated cell motility. *J Cell Sci* 120, 3820-3829.

[211] Uchida Y, Ohshima T, Sasaki Y, Suzuki H, Yanai S, Yamashita N, Nakamura F, Takei K, Ihara Y, Mikoshiba K, et al. . Semaphorin3A signalling is mediated via sequential Cdk5 and GSK3beta phosphorylation of CRMP2: implication of common phosphorylating mechanism underlying axon guidance and Alzheimer's disease. *Genes Cells* 2005; 10:165–179.

[212] Uryu K, Chen XH, Martinez D, et al. Multiple proteins implicated in neurodegenerative diseases accumulate in axons after brain trauma in humans. *Exp Neurol* 2007; 208:185–92.

[213] Uversky VN. Neuropathology, biochemistry, and biophysics of alpha-synuclein aggregation. *J. Neurochem.* 2007; 103 (1): 17–37.

[214] Uversky VN, Fink AL Amino acid determinants of alpha-synuclein aggregation: putting together pieces of the puzzle *FEBS Lett.* 2002; 522(1-3):9-13.

[215] Vella L, R Sharples, R Nisbet, R Cappai and A Hill The role of exosomes in the processing of proteins associated with neurodegenerative diseases, *Eur. Biophys. J.* 2007; 37: 323–332.

[216] Wang XF, Dong CF, Zhang J, Wan YZ, Li F, Huang YX, Han L, Shan B., Gao C, Han J, Dong XP. Human tau protein forms complex with PrP and some GSS- and fCJD-related PrP mutants possess stronger binding activities with tau in vitro. *Mol. Cell Biochem.* 2010; 310: 49-55.

[217] Waxman EA, Giasson BI: Induction of intracellular tau aggregation is promoted by α-synuclein seeds and provides novel insights into the hyperphosphorylation of tau. *J Neurosci*; 2011 31(21):7604-18

[218] Webb JL, Ravikumar B, Atkins J, Skepper JN, Rubinsztein DC:Alpha-Synuclein is degraded by both autophagy and the proteasome. *J Biol Chem* 2003, 278:25009-25013.

[219] Weinreb, PH, Zhen, W, Poon, AW, Conway, KA. & Lansbury, PT. 1996 NACP, a protein implicated in Alzheimer's disease and learning, is natively unfolded. *Biochemistry* 1996; 35, 13710-13715.

[220] Williams AL, Jahreiss S. Sarkar S. Saiki FM, Menzies B. Ravikumar B, Rubinsztein DC. Aggregate-prone proteins are cleared from the cytosol by autophagy: therapeutic implications. *Curr Top Dev Biol* 2006; 76: 89–101.

[221] Williamson R, Scales T, Clark BR, Gibb G, Reynolds CH, Kellie S, Bird IN, Varndell IM, Sheppard PW, Everall I, Anderton BH: Rapid tyrosine phosphorylation of neuronal proteins including tau and focal adhesion kinase in response to amyloid-beta peptide exposure: involvement of Src family protein kinases. *J Neurosci* 2002, 22:10-20.

[222] Wilson, D. M. & Binder, L. I. Free fatty acids stimulate the polymerization of tau and amyloid beta peptides. *Am. J. Pathol.* 1997; 161,: 2321-2335.

[223] Woodring PJ, Litwack ED, O'Leary DD, Lucero GR, Wang JY, Hunter T (2002) Modulation of the F-actin cytoskeleton by c-Abl tyrosine kinase in cell spreading and neurite extension. *J Cell Biol* 156, 879-892.

[224] Wu, B, B Decourt, M Zabidi, L Wuethrich, W Kim, Z Zhou, K MacIsaac, and D Suter Microtubule-mediated Src Tyrosine Kinase Trafficking in Neuronal Growth Cones. *Molec. Biol Cell* 2008; 19, 4611-4627,

[225] Yin S. et al. Human prion proteins with pathogenic m10utations have common conformational changes resulting in enhanced binding to glycosaminoglycans. *Proc. Natl. Acad. Sci. U. S. A.* 2007; 104: 7546–7551.

[226] Yin H, Kuret J. C-terminal truncation modulates both nucleation and extension phases of tau fibrillization. *FEBS Lett* 2006; 580: 211-215.

[227] Yonetani M, Nonaka T, Masuda M, Inukai Y, Oikawa T, Hisanaga S, Hasegawa M. 2009 Conversion of wild-type alpha-synuclein into mutant-type fibrils and its propagation in the presence of A30P mutant. *J. Biol. Chem* 284(12):7940-50.

[228] Yoshida, H., A. Watanabe, and Y. Ihara. Collapsin response mediator protein-2 is associated with neurofibrillary tangles in Alzheimer's disease. *J Biol Chem* 1998; 273: 9761–9768.

[229] Yue Z, Wang QJ, Komatsu M. Neuronal autophagy: going the distance to the axon. *Autophagy.* 2008; 4(1):94-6.

[230] Zabrocki P, Bastiaens I, Delay C, Bammens T, Ghillebert R, Pellens K, De Virgilio C, Van Leuven F, Winderickx J: Phosphorylation, lipid raft interaction and traffic of alpha-synuclein in a yeast model for Parkinsonism. *Biochim Biophys Acta* 2008, 1783:1767-1780.

[231] Zahn R. The octapeptide repeats in mammalian prion protein constitute a pH-dependent folding and aggregation site. *J Mol Biol.* 2003; 334(3): 477-88.

[232] Zehe C., Engling A., Wegehingel S., Schäfer T., and Nickel W. Cell-surface heparan sulfate proteoglycans are essential components of the unconventional export machinery of FGF-2. *Proc. Natl. Acad. Sci. U S A* 2006; 103: 15479-15484.

[233] Zhu M, Li J, Fink AL (2003). The association of alpha-synuclein with membranes affects bilayer structure, stability, and fibril formation. *J. Biol. Chem.* 278 (41): 40186–97.

[234] Zilka N, Filipcik P, Koson P, Fialova L, Skrabana R, Zilkova M, Rolkova G, Kontsekova E, Novak M. Truncated tau from sporadic Alzheimer's disease suffices to drive neurofibrillary degeneration in vivo. *FEBS Lett* 2006; 580:3582-8.

[235] Zmuda J, Rivas R. Actin disruption alters the localization of tau in the growth cones of cerebellar granule neurons *J Cell Sci* 2000; 120: 2797-2809.

2

Roles of Microtubules in Maintenance of Nerve Cell Networks

Kentaro Yomogida, Shumi Yoshida-Yamamoto and Hiroshi Doi
Department of Food Science and Nutrition,
School of Human Environmental Sciences,
Mukogawa Women's University
Nishinomia
Japan

1. Introduction

Recent topics of neural networking studies

Various higher brain functions such as reflex, memory, emotion, imagination and so on, are supported by complicated neuronal networks. To keep the precise connections of the wires is very important for the central nerve functions. The discovery of neural stem cell provided us many clues to understand the mechanism of neural networking. Now, we know that the networking neurons and the supportive neuroglia cells are yielded from the neural stem cells by regulation of several specific bHLH transcription factors (Sakamoto. M., et al., 2003, Liu, Y. et al., 2004, Parras, C.M. et al., 2002). In these processes, the networking cells project axons to connect the dendrite of counterpart cells precisely. Since the connections between differentiated nerve cells must be kept for the functions, the morphological disruptions lead to some neural disorders. Recent brilliant studies about the microtubule dynamics enhance our understandings of the mechanism of neural network maintenance and the disorders.

1.1 Neural networking and neural stem cell during neural development

During early neural development, neural stem cells transform from neuroepithelial cells into radial glial cells (Hatakeyama, J. et al., 2004). The radial glial cell in ventricular zone, projected a long radial glial process to cerebral membrane, self-renews and produces an immature neuron (Miyata T., et al., 2004). The immature neuron transforms into multipolar cell with many process containing actin fibers. Cyclin-dependent kinase 5 (Cdk5) regulates the formation of these process and the transform of multipolar cell into bipolar locomotion cell having a leading process (Kawauchi, T., et al., 2006). The bipolar locomotion cells move to the precise layer along the radial glial fiber, and differentiate into mature networking neurons. To construct an ordered six layer structure of mammalian cerebral cortex, the locomotion of these neural stem cell linage cells is strictly regulated by Reelin signal pathway affecting microtubule dynamics (Liu, J.S., 2011). So, some disorders of the microtubule regulation can cause structural errors of neural network development.

1.2 Maintenance of neural network in adult hippocampus

In adult hippocampus, it was shown that neurogenesis also occurs constantly (Eriksson, PS. et al. 1998). Like early neural development, these new neurons are produced from radial glia cells (Fukuda, S., et al., 2003). Since the neurogenesis and activity-dependent synaptic plasticity are accelerated by long term learned behavior (Bruel-Jungernab, E., et al., 2006), it can participate in functional remodeling of neural networks during the formation of memories. A recent interesting study indicates microtubule transport systems in the dendrites play important roles in maintenance of the synaptic plasticity (Okada, D., et al., 2009). It suggests that the healthy microtubule kinetics is needed to maintenance the neural networking during the formation of memories. What microtubule is all about?

2. The kinetics of microtubules and cell functions

2.1 Function of microtubules

The cytoskeleton is the essential infrastructure of all cells; it consists of microtubules, actin microfilament, and intermediate filaments. Microtubules are a major component of the cytoskeleton and form a highly organized network of intermingled filaments in eukaryotic cells. Microtubules are important components of several subcellular structures, including the mitotic apparatus, cilia, flagella, and neurons. Microtubules are fundamentally composed of a protein called tubulin. Tubulin is made of α- and β-tubulin. The molecular weight of each is about 50 kDa. There are many microtubule-associated proteins (MAPs) (Wade, R.H., 2009) in addition to the tau protein, which contributes to the formation of microtubules. The tau protein is enriched in axons. Two types of high-molecular-weight MAPs (200-300 kDa) and the lower-molecular-weight ones (~55 kDa) have been isolated from the brain. For example, MAP2 is found in the cell body and dendrites. In addition, microtubules interact with many proteins, including motor proteins, such as kinesin and dynein.

Microtubules play many roles in cellular processes, such as cell division, cell motility, and morphogenesis, and they are required for brain function. Purich and Kristofferson (1984) have reviewed microtubule assembly. Wade has described the function of the cell division of microtubules in detail (Wade, R.H., 2009). The motor proteins kinesin and dynein use microtubules as pathways for transport and are also involved in cell division. Microtubules organize the spatial distribution of organelles. Actin and microtubule cytoskeletons determine cell shape and polarity during morphogenesis and promote stable cell-cell and cell-matrix adhesions through their interactions with cadherins and integrins, respectively (Hall, A., 2009).

2.2 Polymerization of tubulin: Microtubule assembly

Tubulin is widely distributed in eukaryotic cells, and the specific self-assembly of tubulin results in microtubule formation. Microtubules are hollow tubes approximately 25nm in diameter. Tubulin is composed of two subunits of α- and β-tubulins that bind one mole of guanosine triphosphate (GTP) each. GTP binding to α-tubulin is present at the non-exchangeable site in α-tubulin, and that binding to β-tubulin is at an exchangeable site in β-tubulin. Some reports have focused on microtubule assembly kinetics (Detrich, et al., 1985; Barton, J.S., et al., 1987; Caplow, M., and Shanks, J., 1990). The polymerization mechanism of tubulin is fundamentally due to the polymer self-assembly theory of Oosawa and Kasai (1962). Magnesium is required for tubulin polymerization (Weisenberg, R.C., 1972; Olmsted

J.B., and Borisy, G.G., 1975), and calcium inhibits microtubule assembly. The assembly kinetics of the microtubule protein is altered by the ionic strength, temperature, and magnesium ion but not by the pH (Barton, J.S., et al., 1987). Timasheff and Grisham have reviewed in detail an *in vitro* assembly process from tubulin and the mechanism of microtubule assembly (Timasheff, S.N., and Grisham, L.M., 1980).
On the growth of microtubules, Mitchison and Kirshner (1984) proposed a behavior called dynamic instability. Horio and Hotani (1986) confirmed alternate phases of growth and shrinkage of microtubule assembly using a light optical technique.
Post-translational modifications of tubulin building generate functional diversity of microtubules. Hammond et al. (2008) have reported that tubulin modifications influence microtubule-associated proteins, such as severing proteins, plus-end tracking proteins, and molecular motors. In this way, tubulin modifications play an important role in regulating microtubule properties, such as stability and structure, as well as microtubule-based functions, such as ciliary beating, cell division, and intracellular tracking (Hammond, J.H., et al., 2008).

2.3 Relationship between microtubule assembly and GTP hydrolysis

Tubulin used in our experiments was prepared from bovine brain by the modified procedure of Lee et al. (Weisenberg, R.C., and Timasheff, S.N., 1970; Lee, J.C., et al., 1973; Na, G.C. and Timasheff, S.N., 1981). Microtubule assembly was monitored by turbidity at 350 nm using a spectrophotometer with a recorder. GTP hydrolysis accompanies microtubule formation. GTP bound at an exchangeable site is hydrolyzed. GTPase activity was evaluated by the measurement of GDP produced using HPLC with an ODS column (Seckler, R., et al., 1990). We examined the effects of the magnesium ion on microtubule assembly and the GTPase activity of tubulin. GTPase activity was clearly observed at a 2 mM magnesium ion concentration, while the formation of microtubules under the same conditions was not observed (Doi, H., et al., 1991). Microtubule assembly and GTPase activity were examined in the presence of 0.1 mM calcium ion as well. GTPase activity was apparently observed at 2min after heating at 37 °C, while there was no turbidity. The results described above indicate that the GTPase activity of tubulin occurs before microtubule assembly. The facts support the results of O'Brien et al. (O'Brien, E.T., et al., 1987) rather than those of Carlier (Carlier, M.-F., 1982).

3. Some evidence of nerve cell dysfunction caused by the microtubules disorder

Here, we present some evidence of nerve cell dysfunction caused by the microtubules disorder. Our series of experiments using a neural cell line PC12 demonstrated that the oxidative damage of microtubules causes the morphological abnormality cell (Yamanaka, Y., et al., 2008).

3.1 Function of microtubules in neuronal cells

In neurons, microtubules play a variety of roles in brain function. As in many other cells, microtubules form organized structures within a cell that can act as structural scaffolds. With respect to specific for neuron, microtubules have three functions. First, the stabilization of microtubules is sufficient to induce axon formation during neuronal development, and they act as signal molecules for initial neuronal polarization (Witte H et al., 2008). Second, the development of dendritic spines that are major sites of excitatory synaptic input is regulated by microtubules (Gu, J., et al., 2008). Third, microtubules participate in the trafficking of synaptic cargo molecules that are essential for synapse formation, function, and plasticity. Cargos are transported between axons and dendrites mediated by motor proteins moving along microtubules to their plus or minus ends (Hirokawa N and Takemura, R., 2005). The motor proteins are the minus-end directed dynein and plus-end directed kinesins (Schliwa, M., 2003, Vale, R.D., 2003). On the other hand, several studies have shown the importance of the actin-based transport mechanism at excitatory synapses. Actin, which is abundant in highly dynamic structures, such as growth cones and dendritic spines, receives the cargo following passage of the microtubules. Neuronal transmission is achieved partly by collaboration of both microtubules and actins.

As reported above, it is clear that microtubules play an essential role in neuronal development, function, and transmission. Disruption of neuronal microtubules means functional failure of brain. Indeed, microtubule dysfunction and impairment of neurotransmission were observed in neurodegenerative diseases, such as Alzheimer's disease (refer to Chapter 4) and Parkinson's disease. The Alzheimer brain is characterized by the presence of aberrant amyloid plaques, neurofibrillary tangles, and alpha-synuclein. Neurofibrillary tangles are composed of paired helical filaments made from abnormally formed tau protein. In the normal brain, tau binds to microtubules and, thereby, stabilizes neuron structure and promotes tubulin assembly into microtubules. However, hyperphosphorylation of tau is assumed to be the cause of the formation of paired helical filaments; namely, it could result in the self-assembly of tangles of paired helical filaments and straight filaments. α-Synuclein is a microtubule-associated protein (MAP) that is colocalized with tubulin in Lewy's bodies. The deposition of α-synuclein as fibrillary aggregates in neurons or glial cells is observed in a Lewy variant of Alzheimer's disease (Spillantini, M.G., et al., 1997) and Parkinson's disease (Lücking, C.B. and Brice, A., 2000). It has been reported that α-synuclein could promote tubulin polymerization in microtubules (Alim MA et al., 2004), whereas other studies have indicated that α-synuclein inhibits tubulin polymerization (Chen L et al., 2007, Zhou RM et al., 2010).

Cumulative evidence suggests that neurodegenerative diseases are associated with neuronal cytoskeletal alterations. These findings suggest that elucidating the biology of the cytoskeleton could be a target for drug therapy.

3.2 The PC12 cells as a model for neurite outgrowth

To study the behavior of the neuronal microtubules, PC12 would be an appropriate cultured cell line. It can enable us to conduct a visual assessment of neurite behavior from formation to disruption.

The adrenal pheochromocytoma (PC12) cell line has been well studied as a model for neurite outgrowth. It was originally isolated from a tumor in the adrenal medulla of a rat in 1976 (Greene, L. A., and Tischler, A. S., 1976). One of the main characteristics of PC12 cells is to differentiate into sympathetic neuron-like phenotypes in response to nerve growth factor (NGF) (Figure 1A, 1B). The mechanism of NGF-induced neuronal differentiation has not been fully elucidated; however, it has been reported that the regulator of G-protein signaling (RGS) proteins associates TrkA with activated signaling proteins of the Ras/pErk1/2 pathway (Willard, M.D., et al., 2007, Nusser, N., et al., 2002).

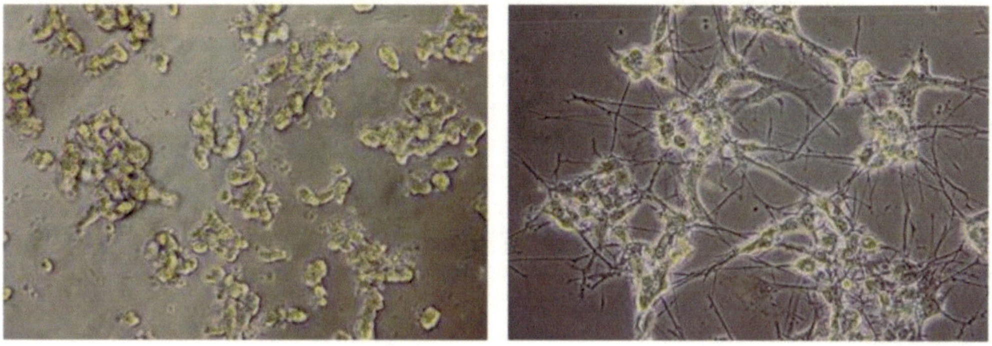

(A) (B)

Fig. 1. Phase contrast microscopic observation of PC12 cells (A)before differentiation (B) after differentiation. For differentiation, the undiffereantiated cells were treated with 100 ng/mL NGF. NGF induced the apparent morphological transformation of PC12 cells into neuronal-like cells within 3days

3.3 The oxidative damage to PC12 cells

Many studies have demonstrated that lipid peroxidants are present in the AD brain (Keller. J. N., and Mattson, M. D., 1998; Markesbery, W. R., and Carney, J. M., 1999;). We tried to verify whether lipid peroxidation was induced in PC12 cells by exogenously added phosphatidylcholine hydroperoxides (PCOOH) which is a primary product of lipid peroxidation. Lipid peroxidation was measured according to the method of Hedley and Chow (1992), which utilizes time-resolved flow cytometry. Table 1 shows the fluorescence of undifferentiated and differentiated cells before and after exposure to PCOOH for 24 or 48 h. Compared with that of undifferentiated cells, the fluorescence of differentiated cells was significantly decreased in the presence of 100 μM PCOOH for 48 h ($P < 0.05$). The fluorescence of undifferentiated cells exposed to the same concentration of PCOOH was slightly but not significantly affected. These results suggest that PCOOH induces membrane lipid peroxidation in PC12 cells before and after differentiation. The levels of peroxidation were higher in the membranes of differentiated cells than in those of undifferentiated cells. It is likely that differentiated cells are more sensitive to oxidative stress. Considering that lipid peroxidation was certainly induced in differentiated PC12 cells, this experimental system may be useful as a model for AD brain cells.

Conc. of PCOOH (μM)	Before Differentiation (%)		After Differentiation (%)	
	24h	48h	24h	48h
0	100	100	100	100
100	88.8	79.2	84.9	63.8*

Table 1. Relative fluorescent intensity of *cis*-parinaric acid bound by the cell membrane

Neurites consist mainly of microtubules, whose function is significantly based on the ability of tubulin to polymerize and depolymerize. To examine the effect of PCOOH on microtubule formation from tubulin, we measured the GTPase activity of PC12 cells. GTPase activity is an indicator of microtubule formation and, therefore, provides the degree of microtubule assembly (O'Brien, E.T. et al., 1987; Seckler, R., et al., 1990; Doi, H., et al.,

1991). The specific activity of GTPase derived from differentiated cells was significantly decreased in the presence of 50 μM PCOOH ($P < 0.01$) (Figure 2). In the case of exposure to 100 μM PCOOH, the value was decreased by one-tenth compared to that in the absence of PCOOH. In undifferentiated cells, the specific activity of GTPase decreased by half in the presence of 50 μM PCOOH (Figure 3). The difference in sensitivity might be due to the presence or absence of neurites. Although GTP hydrolysis accompanies the polymerization reaction (Doi, H., et al., 1991), GTP resynthesis does not occur in the reverse reaction of depolymerization (David-Pfeuty, T., et al., 1977). Thus, PCOOH disrupts existing microtubules and inhibits new microtubule formation from tubulin.

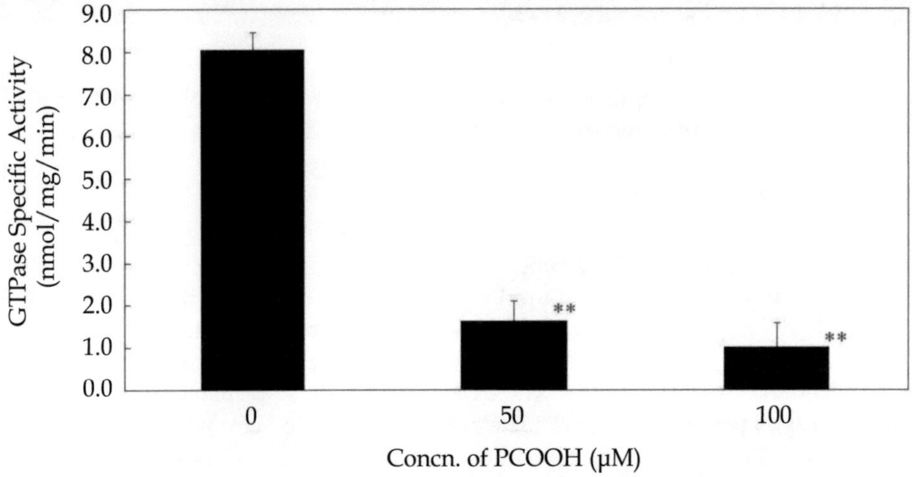

Fig. 2. GTPase-specific activity of the differentiated cells incubated with PCOOH at various concentrations for 24 h. The data represent means ± SD, **$P < 0.01$ compared with the control value

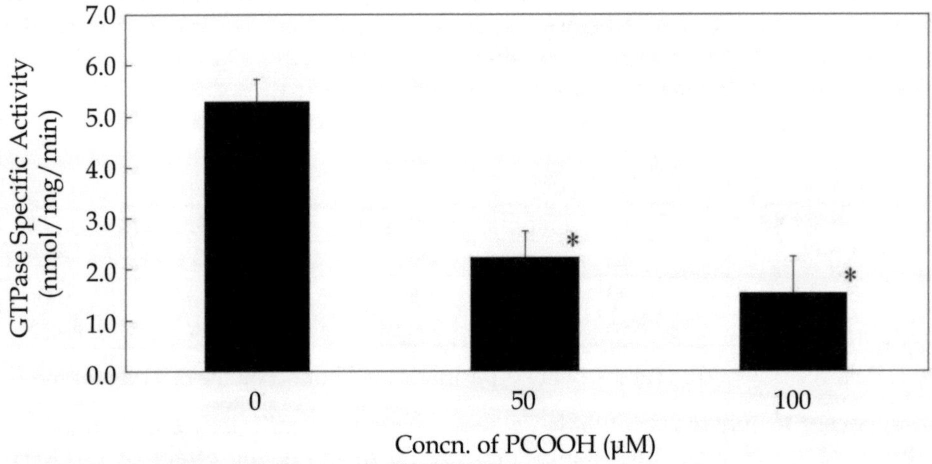

Fig. 3. GTPase-specific activity of the undifferentiated cells in the same condition as that described in Figure 2. The data represent means ± SD, *$P < 0.05$ compared with the control value

To visualize PCOOH-induced damage to the tubulin, we performed immunofluorescence microscopy using an antibody to monoclonal mouse anti-α-tubulin clone B-5-1-2. Undifferentiated or differentiated cells were individually cultured with 250 μM of PCOOH for 6 h. After that, the cells were stained by the antibody to monoclonal mouse anti-α-tubulin clone B-5-1-2 and the antibody to Cy3-conjugated sheep anti-mouse IgG. As shown in the photographs in Figure 4A, the undifferentiated cells looked like grape clusters, and the cell shape was clear. However, after exposure to PCOOH, the cell shape was drastically changed (Figure 4B), becoming too vague to identify. The fluorescence emitted from cells was weakened. PCOOH may have induced cell shape alteration by the degradation of tubulin, which was more marked in differentiated cells than in undifferentiated cells. Although the extended neurites were observed clearly in the absence of PCOOH (Figure 4C), they disappeared when exposed in PCOOH for 6h (Figure 4D). The shape of the small cell was vague, as it was in undifferentiated cells, and the fluorescence emitted from cells became extremely weak. The fact that neurites composed of microtubules are easy to be injured may account for the higher vulnerability of differentiated cells.

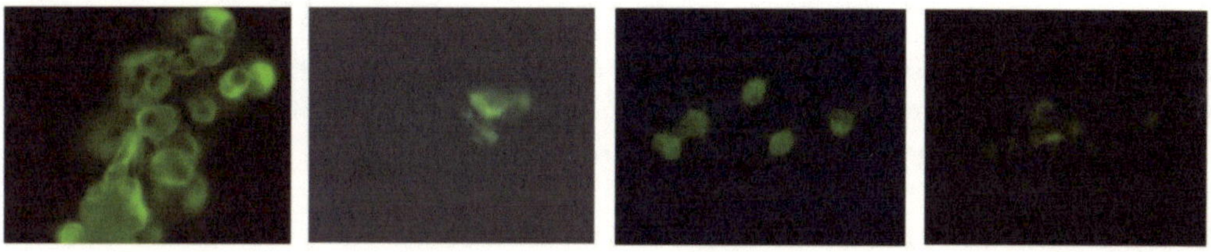

(A) (B) (C) (D)

Fig. 4. Fluorescence microscopic observation of cells after tubulin antibody staining. Representative fields are shown: undifferentiated cells before (A) and after exposure to PCOOH for 6h (B), and differentiated cells before (C) and after exposure to PCOOH for 6h (D)

Furthermore, we tried to verify that the tubulin depolymerization induced by PCOOH could be attenuated by antioxidant. Differentiated cells were cultivated with 5 μM retinol or ascorbic acid beforehand and then exposed to PCOOH. The GTPase activity of cell extracts derived from cells treated with retinol was three-fold higher than that of untreated control cells (Figure 5). Incorporation of antioxidants in cells before exposure to PCOOH protected tubulin depolymerization. This experimental data might lead to the development of an effective strategy to prevent some neurodegenerative diseases.

4. Ageing of central nerve system and the microtubules disorder caused by neural malnutrition

As people get older, the brain functions decline in varying degree. Although the causes are still unknown, the neurogenesis in hippocampus is decreased dramatically with ageing (Cameron, HA., et al., 1999). The other hand, we can detect neurofibrillary tangles in aged entorhinal cortex or brain cortex of neurodegenerative disorder. These tangle formation are concerned with aggregation of tau, which is a microtubule binding protein. In this section, we will discuss the factors determining the ageing-related neural functional decline in Alzheimer's disease from the aspect of the axonal microtubules disorder caused by neural malnutrition.

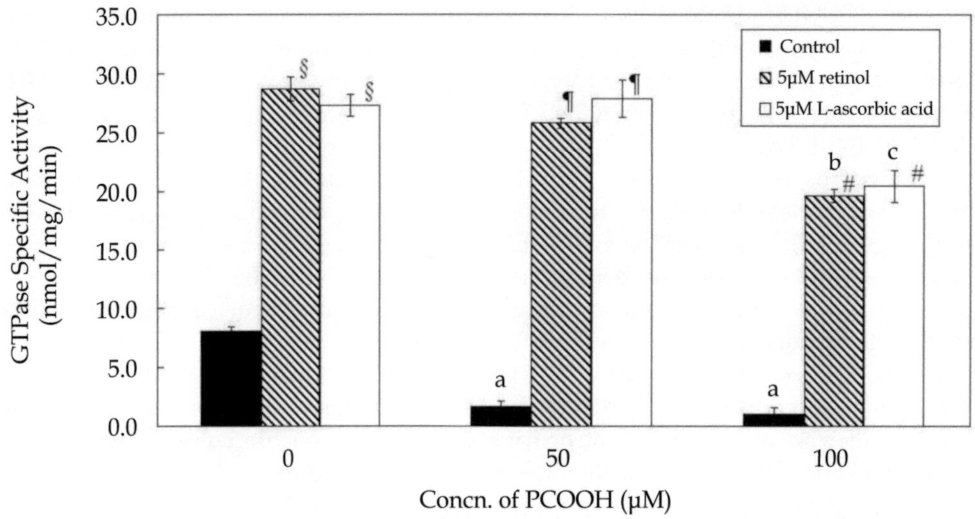

Fig. 5. GTPase-specific activity of the differentiated cells incorporated 5 μM retinol or 5μM ascorbic acid before exposure to PCOOH. The data represent means ± SD, §, ¶, #P<0.01 compared with the corresponding control value, a<0.01 compared with the data without PCOOH, b,c<0.05 compared with the data without PCOOH

4.1 Microtubule degeneration and Alzheimer's disease

Alzheimer's disease (AD) is characterized by neuronal cell death and two kinds of deposits, neurofibrillary tangles (NFT) and senile plaques. Abnormal microtubule-binding tau proteins were isolated from AD by Liu et al. (1991). As is well known, in an AD brain, aberrant accumulation of amyloid-β-protein (Aβ) occurs ahead of the accumulation of paired helical filament in NFT. Imahori and Uchida (1997) observed extensive phosphorylation of tau and programmed cell death in a primary culture of embryonic rat hippocampus with Aβ (Imahori, K., and Uchida, T., 1997). There are several important reports on the phosphorylation of tau protein in AD by the group of Iqbal (Alonso, A.D.C., et al., 1994; Gong, C-X., et al., 1994; Iqbal, K., et al., 1994; Gong, C-X., et al., 1995). Glycogen synthase kinase -3β(GSK-3β) is responsible for most of the abnormal hyperphosphorylation of tau observed in paired helical filaments, which are diagnostic for AD (Imahori, K. and Uchida, T., 1997). The tau protein is a microtubule-associated protein that contributes to the formation of microtubules. It is considered that hyperphosphorylated tau is free from microtubules and induces the destruction of the cytoskeleton.

It is possible that microtubules are related to many neurodegenerative diseases in addition to AD. In the brain with Alzheimer's disease, glycation end products are observed. Microtubule-associated protein T is glycated at the tubulin binding site (Ledesma, et al., 1995). The facts observed in microtubule-associated proteins of tau and T appear to indicate that they play a role in microtubule assembly. Furthermore, microtubule assembly is not likely to take place when tubulin has been modified.

4.2 Lipid hydroperoxides in neurodegenative disease

A part of the oxygen introduced in cell produces reactive oxygen species as a by-product in an electron transport system because of NADPH-dependent oxidase. Materials in cell are

exposed by oxidative stress, and then oxidative modifications of lipid in the cell membrane and DNA are introduced. The role of oxidative stress in Alzheimer's disease has been reported in several studies, some of which showed elevated markers of oxidative stress, including lipid oxidation products (Sultana, R., et al., 2006). Oxidized lipid hydroperoxides are a characteristic of neurodegenerative disease, and oxidized lipid by-products were enriched in the brain with Alzheimer's disease (Yoo, M-H., et al., 2010).
Hydroperoxides of phospholipid were detected in brain samples from patients with Alzheimer's disease using oxidative lipidomics (Tyurin, V.A., et al., 2008).

4.3 Inhibition of microtubule assembly by lipid hydroperoxides

We have investigated the effect of lipid hydroperoxides on microtubule assembly (Kawakami, M., et al., 1993; Kawakami, M., et al., 1998). Lipid hydroperoxides were prepared from soybean phosphatidylcholine by photosensitized oxidation in methanol, with methylene blue being added to the phosphatidylcholine-methanol solution as a sensitizer (Kawakami, M., et al., 1998). Microtubule formation was inhibited dose-dependently by lipid peroxides. This result suggests the possibility that the interaction between tubulin and lipid peroxides may be the cause of some brain diseases. Matsuyama and Jarvik speculated that microtubule integration was a key to Alzheimer's disease (Matsuyama, S.S. and Jarvik, L.F., 1989).
Bizzozero et al. (2007) also indicated by *in vitro* experiments that lipid hydroperoxides were most likely responsible for protein oxidation. Lipid peroxidation scavengers, such as butylated hydroxytoluene, prevent the carbonylation of cytoskeletal brain protein-induced glutathione depletion (Bizzozero, O.A., et al., 2007).

4.4 The mechanism of tubulin modification by phosphatidylcholine hydroperoxides

We examined the concentration-dependent effects of phosphatidylcholine hydroperoxides on the ability of tubulin to polymerize into microtubules (Kawakami, M., et al., 2000). The results demonstrated that even very low concentrations of peroxides were sufficient to interfere with tubulin and, therefore, microtubule function. In the fluorescence spectra of tubulin before and after interaction with phosphatidylcholine hydroperoxides, a red shift in the emission maximum was observed. This fact indicates a conformational change upon the reaction, namely, that fluorescent aromatic amino acids become easier to dissolve on reaction with phosphatidylcholine hydroperoxides. The interaction mechanism may be a hydrophobic one because no effect on electric conductivity was observed, indicating that modulation of ionic binding was not involved.

4.5 Possibility of recovery of tubulin function deteriorated by lipid hydroperoxides

The effects of lipid hydroperoxides on microtubule assembly were studied in an *in vitro* assay system, as were the protective effects of vitamin A derivatives (β-carotene, retinal, and retinol). All vitamin A derivatives had the ability to protect against the inhibitory effects of lipid hydroperoxides, presumably owing to their antioxidant activities. This suggests a mechanism for the ability of vitamin A to inhibit cell ageing.
Glutathione and cysteine were used as water soluble reductants (Kawakami, M., et al., 1999). Tubulin GTPase activity deteriorated by lipid hydroperoxides was restored by the addition of water soluble reductants as well. These chemicals also have a protective effect on cellular ageing by the reduction of materials oxidized *in vivo*.

The detection of microtubule assembly-promoting material was tried using tubulin GTPase activity as the assay of microtubule assembly. Kawaguchi, M., et al. (2007) found a peptide with a molecular weight of 1340.8 from Japanese classified barley flour.

4.6 Polymerization and calcium binding to tubulin-colchicine complex

Calcium plays important roles as a messenger in a signal transaction by changing its concentration. The calcium concentration is continually changing, while the concentration is fundamentally very low in a cell. This means that the change affects the functions of many cell constituents.

Calpain is a neutral cysteine proteinase activated by calcium in cytozol, and it converts p35 to p25 (Lee, M-S., et al., 2000). In the brain of AD patients, p25 is stimulated. P25 induces the activation of cyclin-dependent kinase 5 (CDK5). CDK5 is also a factor for the hyperphosphorylation of tau. Indirubins, which are inhibitors of CDK5/p25, repress cell death (Leclerc, S., et al., 2001).

We are interested in the effect of calcium on tubulin polymerization because calcium is an inhibitor of microtubule assembly. Another reason may be the contribution of calpain, which is regulated by calcium, to AD. Instead of tubulin, the tubulin-colchicine complex was used (Doi, H., et al., 2003a). The high affinity sites of calcium took part in the polymerization of the complex in the GTP state, while the low ones participated in the depolymerization. The complex had 2 high-affinity sites with a dissociation constant of 11.5×10^{-6} M and 16 low-affinity sites with a dissociation constant of 2.27×10^{-4} M in the GTP state. In the case of the GDP state, the dissociation constant of the high-affinity site was 7.2 x 10-6 M, and that of the-low affinity site was not observed. The ultracentrifugal experiment indicated a slightly more compact structure in the GTP state compared with the GDP state. The partial specific volumes of the tubulin-colchicine complex in the state of GTP were 0.739 and 0.744 ml/g in imidazole and BES buffers, respectively (Doi, H., et al., 2000b). The sedimentation coefficient $S^0_{20.w}$ increased from 5.38 S with no calcium to 5.75 and 6.08 S with calcium concentrations of 0.1 and 0.5 mM, respectively, in the absence of the magnesium ion. In an imidazole buffer, the sedimentation coefficients $S^0_{20.w}$ were 5.82 and 6.06 S in the presence of 0 and 2 mM $MgCl_2$, respectively. These results indicate that the tubulin-colchicine complex causes the calcium affinity to become low after polymerization with its conformational change. This means that the assembly induces the stability of microtubules from calcium.

5. The microtubules disruption and some neurodegenerative diseases

Finally, we will discuss the association between the microtubules disorders and other some neurodegenerative diseases. Each neurodegenerative disease has specific aberrant intracellular structures like neurofibrillary tangles of AD (Chiti, F. and Dobson, C.M., 2006). Recently, TRA DNA-binding protein of 43kD (TDP-43) has been spotlighted as a common factor associated with the formation of these aberrant structure (Neumann, M. et al., 2006, Arai, T. et al., 2006, 2009, Fujishiro, H. et al. 2009, Schwab, C. et al., 2008). Although several diseases show only TDP-43 intracellular accumulation, TDP-43 is combined with other protein such as tau in many neurodegenerative diseases. It suggests that TDP-43 is a causal factor of microtubules disruption in these diseases. Although the intrinsic or extrinsic causes of many neurodegenerative diseases have been investigated aggressively, the breakdown of microtubules maintenance system by lack of brain blood flow has not been understand well.

Since neurons require sufficient energy supply for maintaining their high-performance, the lack of energy might damage the microtubule dynamics. As mentioned above, the microtubules disruption can be a trigger of neural degeneration. Further investigation for causes of microtubule disruption in neurons might be contribute for our understanding neurodegenerative disease.

6. Acknowledgements

This work was supported in part by a Grant-in-Aid for Scientific Research (C) from the Japan Society for the Promotion of Science (to HD) (No. 20500731 and No. 23500985). In addition, this work was partially supported by the Research Center for Elderly Nutrition and Development, Mukogawa Women's University (recipients: HD and YK).

7. References

Alim, M.A., Takeda, K., Aizawa, T., Matsubara, M., Asada, A., Saito, T., Kaji, H., Yoshii, M., Hisanaga, S., and Ueda, K., (2004) Demonstration of a role for alpha-synuclein as a functional microtubule-associated protein. J. Alzheimers Dis. 6, 435-442; discussion 443-439.

Alonso, A.D.C., Zaidi, T., G-Iqbal, I., and Iqbal, K, (1994) Role of abnormally phosphorylated tau in the breakdown of microtubules in Alzheimer disease. Proc. Natl. Acad. Sci. USA, 91, 5562-5566.

Arai, T., Hasegawa, M., Akiyama, H., Ikeda, K., Nonaka, T., Mori, H., Mann., D., Tsuchiya, K., Yoshida, M., Hashizume, Y., Oda, T., (2006) TDP-43 is a component of ubiquitin-positive tau-negative inclusions in frontotemporal lobar degeneration and amyotrophic lateral sclerosis. Biochem. Biophys. Res. Commun., 351, 602-611

Arai, T., Mackenzie, I.R., Hasegawa, M., Nonoka, T., Niizato, K., Tsuchiya, K., Iritani, S., Onaya, M., Akiyama, H., (2009) Phosphorylated TDP-43 in Alzheimer's disease and dementia with Lewy bodies. Acta Neuropathol., 117, 125-136

Barton, J.S., Vandivort, D.L., Heacock, D.H., Coffman, J.A., and Trygg, K.A., (1987) Microtubule assembly kinetics. Changes with solution conditions. Biochem. J., 247, 505-511.

Bizzozero, O.A., Reyes, S., Ziegler, J., and Smerjac, S., (2007) Lipid peroxidation scavengers prevent the carbonylation of cytoskeletal brain proteins induced by glutathione depletion. Neurochem. Res., 32, 2114-2122.

Bruel-Jungernab, E., Davis, S., Rampon C, Laroche, S., (2006) Long-term potentiation enhances neurogenesis in the adult dentate gyrus. J. Neurosci., 26, 5888-5893

Caplow, M., and Shanks, J., (1990) Mechanism for oscillatory assembly of microtubules. J. Biol. Chem., 265, 1414-1418.

Carlier, M.-F, (1982) Guanosine-5'-triphosphate hydrolysis and tubulin polymerization. Mol. Cell Biochem., 47, 97-113.

Chen, L., Jin, J., Davis, J., Zhou, Y., Wang, Y., Liu, J., Lockhart, P.J., and Zhang, J., (2007) Oligomeric alpha-synuclein inhibits tubulin polymerization. Biochem. Biophys. Res. Commun. 356, 548-553.

Chiti, F., Dobson, C.M., (2006) Protein misfolding, functional amyloid, and human disease. Annu. Rev. Biochem., 75, 333-336

Correia SS, Bassani S, Brown TC, Lisé MF, Backos DS, El-Husseini A, Passafaro M, Esteban JA., (2008) Motor protein-dependent transport of AMPA receptors into spines during long-term potentiation. Nat Neurosci., 11, 457-466

David-Pfeuty, T., Erickson, H.P., and Pantaloni, D. (1977). Guanosinetriphosphatase activity of tubulin associated with microtubuleassembly. Proc. Natl. Acad. Sci. USA. 74, 5372-5376.

Delcroix, J.D., Valletta, J., Wu, C., Howe, C.L., Lai, C.F., Cooper, J.D., Belichenko, R.V., Salehi, A., and Mobley, W.C., (2004) Trafficking the NGF signal: implications for normal and degenerating neurons. Prog. Brain Res. 146, 3-23.

Detrich H.W., Jordan, M.A., Wilson, L., and Williams Jr., R.C., (1985) Mechanism of microtubule assembly. Changes in polymer structure and organization during assembly of sea urchin egg tubulin. J. Biol. Chem., 260, 9479-9490.

Doi, H., Imanishi, T., Iwami, K., and Ibuki, F., (1991) Is microtubule assembly not associated with GTP hydrolysis ? Agric. Biol. Chem., 55, 245-246.

Doi, H., Kawaguchi, M., and Timasheff, S. N. (2003a) Polymerization and calcium binding of the tubulin-colchicine complex in the GDP state. Biosci. Biotechnol. Biochem., 67, 1643-1652.

Doi, H., Kawaguchi, M., and Timasheff, S. N. (2003b) Ultracentrifugal behaviors of the tubulin-colchicine complex in the state of GTP in different buffers. J. Biol. Macromol., 3, 117-125.

Eriksson, P.S., Perfilieva, E., Björk-Eriksson, T., Alborn, A.M., Nordborg, C., Peterson, D.A., Gage, F.H., (1998) Neurogenesis in the adult human hippocampus. Nature Med., 4, 1313-1317

Fujishiro, H., Uchikado, H., Arai, T., Hasegawa, M., Akiyama, H., Yokota, O., Tsuchiya, K., Togo, T., Iseki, E., Hirayasu, Y., (2009) Accumulation of phosphorylated TDP-43 in brains of patients with argyrophilic grain disease. Acta Neuropathol., 117, 151-158

Fukuda, S,, Kato, F., Tozuka, Y., Yamaguchi, M., Miyamoto, Y., Hisatsune, T., (2003) Two distinct subpopulations of nestin-positive cells in adult mouse dentate gyrus. J Neurosci., 23,9357-66.

Gong, C-X., Shaikh, S., Wang, J-Z., Zaidi, T., G-Iqbal, I., and Iqbal, K. (1995) Phosphatase activity toward abnormally phosphorylated τ: Decrease in Alzheimer's disease brain. J. Neurochem., 65, 732-738.

Gong, C-X., Singh, T.J., G-Iqbal, I., and Iqbal, K, (1994) Alzheimer's disease abnormally phosphorylated τ is dephosphorylated by protein phosphatase 2B(calcineurin). J. Neurochem., 62, 803-806.

Greene, L.A., and Tischler, A.S. (1976) Establishment of a noradrenergic clonal line of rat adrenal pheochromocytoma cells which respond to nerve growth factor. Proc. Natl. Acad. Sci. U S A. 73, 2424-2428.

Gu, J., Firestein, B.L., and Zheng, J.Q., (2008) Microtubules in dendritic spine development. J. Neurosci. 28, 12120-12124.

Hall, A., (2009) 1The cytoskeleton and cancer. Cancer Metastasis Rev., 28, 5-14.

Hammond, J.H., Cai, D., and Verhey, K.J., (2008) Tubulin modification and their cellular functions. Curr. Opinion Cell Biol., 20, 71-76.

Hatakeyama, J. et al., (2004) Hes genes regulate size, shape and histogenesis of the nervous system by control of the timing of neural stem cell differentiation. Development, 131, 5539-5550

Hedley, D., and Chow, S. (1992) Flow cytometric measurement of lipid peroxidation in vital cells using parinaric acid. Cytometry 13, 686-692.

Hirokawa, N., and Takemura, R. (2005) Molecular motors and mechanisms of directional transport in neurons. Nat. Rev. Neurosci. 6, 201-214

Horio, K., and Hotani, H., (1986) Visualization of the dynamic instability of individual microtubules by dark-field microscopy. Nature, 321, 605-607.

Imahori, K., and Uchida, T. (1997) Physiology oad pathology of tau protein kinases in relation to Alzheimer's disease, J. Biochem., 121, 179-188.

Iqbal K., Singh, T.J., and G-Iqbal, I., (1994) Mechanism of neurofibrillary degeneration in Alzheimer's disease. Mol. Immunol., 9, 119-123.

Kawakami, M., Kanazawa, K., and Doi, H., (1993) Effects of Lecithin peroxides on microtubule assembly. J. Jap.Soc.Nutri. and Food Sci., 46, 89-91.

Kawakami, M., Ward, L., and Doi, H., (1998) Inhibition of tubulin guanosine-5′-triphosphate by lipid peroxides: Protective effects of vitamin A derivatives. J. Am. Oil Chem. Soc., 75, 635-641.

Kawakami, M., Ward, L., and Doi, H., (2000) Mechanisms of tubulin modification by phosphatidylcholine hydroperoxides. Lipids, 35, 205-211.

Kawakami, M., Nakano, M., Kiyohara, T., and Doi, H., (1999) The protective effects of SH reductants (glutathione and cysteine) on tubulin GTPase activity deteriorated by lipid peroxides. Bull. Mukogawa Women's Univ., Nt. Sci., 47, 29-34.

Kawaguchi, M., Sekiguchi, A., Yamanaka, Y., and Doi., H., (2007) Purification of microtubule assembly promoting material from Japanese classified barley flour. Food Clin. Nutr., 2, 27-34. (Article in Japanese)

Kawauchi, T., Chihama, K., Nabeshima, Y., Hoshino, M., (2006) Cdk5 phosphorylates and stabilizes p27kip1 contributing to actin organization and cortical neuronal migration. Nat. Cell Biol., 8, 17-26.

Keller, J.N., and Mattson, M.P. (1998) Roles of lipid peroxidation in modulation of cellular signaling pathways, cell dysfunction, and death in the nervous system. Rev. Neurosci. 9, 105-116.

Leclerc, S., Garnier, M., Hossel, R., Marko, D., Bibb, J. A., Snyder, G. L., Greengard, P., Biernat, J., Wu, Y-Z., Mandelkow, E-M., Eisenbrand, G., and Meijer, L., (2001) Indirubins inhibit glycogen synthase kinase-3β and CDK5/P25, two protein kinases involved in abnormal tau phosphorylation in Alzheimer's disease. J. Biol. Chem., 276, 251-260.

Ledesma, M.D., Bonay, P., and Avila, J., (1995) T protein from Alzheimer's disease patients id glycated at its tubulin-binding domain. J. Neurochem., 65, 1658-1664.

Lee, J.C., Frigon, R.P. and Timasheff, S.N. (1973) The chemical characterization of calf brain microtubule protein subunits. J. Biol. Chem., 248, 7253-7262.

Lee, M-S., Kwon, Y. T., Li, M., Peng, J., Friedlander, R. M., and Tsai, L-H., (2000) Neurotoxicity induces cleavage of p35 to p25 by calpain. Nature, 405, 360-364.

Liu, JS., (2011) Molecular genetics of neuronal migration disorders. Curr Neurol Neurosci Rep., 11, 171-8

Liu, W-K., K-Reding, H., and Yen, S-H., (1991) Abnormal tau proteins from Alzheimer's disease brain. J. Biol. Chem., 266, 21723-21727.

Liu, Y., Encinas, M., Comella, J.X., Aldea, M., Gallego, C., (2004) Basic helix-loop-helix proteins bind to TrkB and p21(Cip1) promoters linking differentiation and cell cycle arrest in neuroblastoma cells. Mol. Cell. Biol., 24, 2662-2672

Lücking, C.B., and Brice, A. (2000) Alpha-synuclein and Parkinson's disease. Cell Mol. Life Sci. 57, 1894-1908

Markesbery, W.R., and Carney, J.M. (1999) Oxidative alterations in Alzheimer's disease. Brain Pathol. 9, 133-146.

Matsuyama, S. S., and Jarvik, L. F. , (1989) Hypothesis: Microtubules, a key to Alzheimer disease. Pro. Natl. Acad. Sci., USA, 86, 8152-8156.

Mitchison, T., and Kirshner, M., (1984) Dynamic instability of microtubule growth. Nature, 312, 237-242.

Miyata, T., et al., (2004) Asymmetric production of surface-dividing and non-surface-dividing cortical progenitor cells. Development, 131, 3133-3145

Na, G.C. and Timasheff, S.N. (1981) Interaction of calf brain tubulin with glycerol. J. Mol. Biol., 151, 165-178.

Neumann, M., Sampathu, D.M., Kwong, L.K., Truax, A.C., Micsenyi, M.C., Chou, T.T., Bruce, J., Schuck, T., Grossman, M., Clark, C.M., McCluskey, L.F., Miller, B.L., Masliah, E., Mackenzie, I.R., Feldman, H., Feiden, W., Kretzschmar, H.A., Trojanowski, J.Q., Lee ,V.M., (2006) Ubiquitinated TDP-43 in frontotemporal lobar degeneration and amyotrophic lateral sclerosis. Scinece, 314, 130-133

Nusser, N., Gosmanova, E., Zheng, Y., and Tigyi, G., (2002) Nerve growth factor signals through TrkA, phosphatidylinositol 3-kinase, and Rac1 to inactivate RhoA during the initiation of neuronal differentiation of PC12 cells. J. Biol. Chem. 277, 35840-35846

O'Brien, E.T. , Voter, W.A., and Erickson, H.P., (1987) GTP hydrolysis during microtubule assembly, Biochemistry, 26, 4148-4156.

Okada, D., Ozawa, F., Inokuchi, K., (2009) Input-specific spine entry of soma-derived Vesl-1S protein conforms to synaptic tagging. Science, 324, 904-909

Olmsted, J.B., and Borisy, G.G., (1975) Ionic and nucleotide requirements for microtubule polymerization in vitro. Biochemistry, 114, 2996-3005.

Oosawa, F., and Kasai, M., (1962)A theory of linear and helical aggregations of macromolecules. J. Mol. Biol., 4, 10-21.

Parras, C.M., Schuurmans, C., Scardigli, R., Kim, J., Anderson, D.J., Guillemot, F., (2002) Divergent functions of the proneural genes Mash1 and Ngn2 in the specification of neuronal subtype identity. Genes Dev., 16, 324-38.

Purich, D.L., and Kristofferson, D., (1984) Microtubule assembly: A review of progress, principles, and perspectives. Advances in Protein Chemistry, 36, 133-212.

Sakamoto., M., Hirata, H., Ohtsuka, T., Bessho, Y., Kageyama, R., (2003) The basic helix-loop-helix genes Hesr1/Hey1 and Hesr2/Hey2 regulate maintenance of neural precursor cells in the brain. J.Biol. Chem., 278, 44808-44815

Schlager M.A., Hoogenraad C.C., (2009) Basic mechanisms for recognition and transport of synaptic cargos. Mol. Brain, 2, 25-36.

Schliwa, M., and Woehlke, G. (2003) Molecular motors. Nature 422, 759-765

Schwab, C., Arai, T., Hasegawa, M., Yu, S., McGeer, P.L., (2008) Colocalization of transactivation-responsive DNA-binding protein 43 and huntingtin in inclusions of Huntington disease. J. Neuropathol. Exp. Neurol., 67, 1159-1165

Seckler, R., G.-M.Wu, and Timasheff, S.N. (1990), Interactions of tubulin with guanylyl-(β-γ-methylene)diphosphate. Formation and assembly of a stoichiometric complex, J. Biol. Chem., 265,7655-7661.

Spillantini, M. G., Schmidt, M.L., Lee, V.M., Trojanowski, J.Q., Jakes, R., and Goedert, M., (1997) Alpha-synuclein in Lewy bodies. Nature 388, 839-840

Sultana, R., Perluigi, M., and Butterfield, D.A., (2006) Protein oxidation and lipid peroxidation in brain of subjects with Alzheimer's disease: insights into mechanism.

Vale, R.D. (2003) The molecular motor toolbox for intracellular transport. Cell 112, 467-480

Timasheff, S.N., and Grisham, L.M., (1980) In vitro assembly cytoplasmic microtubules. Ann. Rev. Biochem., 49, 565-591.

Tyurin, V.A., Tyurina, Y.Y., Kochanek, P.M., Hamilton, R., DeKosky, S.T., Greenberger, J.S., Bayir, H., and Kagan, V.E., (2008) Oxidative lipidomics of programmed cell death. Methods Enzymol., 442,375-393.

Vale, R.D. (2003) The molecular motor toolbox for intracellular transport. Cell 112, 467-480

Wade, R.H., (2009) On and around microtubules: An over view. Mol. Biotechnol., 43, 177-191.

Wang Z, Edwards JG, Riley N, Provance DW Jr, Karcher R, Li XD, Davison IG, Ikebe M, Mercer JA, Kauer JA, Ehlers MD., (2008) Myosin Vb mobilizes recycling endosomes and AMPA receptors for postsynaptic plasticity. Cell, 135, 535-548.

Weisenberg, R.C., (1972) Microtubule formation in vitro in solutions containing low calcium concentrations. Science, 177, 1104-1105.

Weisenberg, R.C., and Timasheff, S.N. (1970) Aggregation of microtubule subunit protein. Effects of divalent cations, colchicines and vinblastine. Biochemistry, 9, 4110-4116.

Willard, M.D., Willard, F.S., Li, X., Cappell, S.D., Snider, W.D., and Siderovski, D.P., (2007) Selective role for RGS12 as a Ras/Raf/MEK scaffold in nerve growth factor-mediated differentiation. EMBO J. 26, 2029-2040

Detrich, H.W., Jordan, M.A., Wilson, L., and Williams, Jr., R.C., (1985) Mechanism of microtubule assembly. Changes in polymer structure and organization during assembly of sea urchin egg tubulin. J. Biol. Chem., 260, 9479-9490.

Witte, H., et al. (2008) Microtubule stabilization specifies initial neuronal polarization. J. Cell Biol. 180, 619-632

Yamanaka Y., Yoshida S., Doi H., (2008) NGF-Induced neurite outgrowth of PC12 cells in the presence of phosphatidylcholine hydroperoxides; Implication for ageing. Mech. Ageing Dev., 129, 215-222

Yoo, M-H., Gu, X., Xu, X-M., Kim, J-Y., Carison, B. A., Patterson, D., Cai, H., Gladyshev, V.N., and Hatfield, D.L., (2010) Delineating the role of glutathione peroxidase 4 in protecting cells against lipid hydroperoxide damage and in Alzheimer's disease. Antioxid. Redox Signal, 12, 819-827.

Yoshimura A, Fujii R, Watanabe Y, Okabe S, Fukui K, Takumi T. , (2006) Myosin-Va facilitates the accumulation of mRNA/protein complex in dendritic spines. Curr. Biol., 16, 2345-2351.

Yamanaka Y., Yoshida S., Doi H., (2008) NGF-Induced neurite outgrowth of PC12 cells in the presence of phosphatidylcholine hydroperoxides; Implication for ageing. Mech. Ageing Dev., 129, 215-222

Zhou, R.M., Huang, Y.X., Li, X.L., Chen, C., Shi, Q., Wang, G.R., Tian, C., Wang, Z.Y., Gao, C., and Dong, X.P., (2010) Molecular interaction of alpha-synuclein with tubulin influences on the polymerization of microtubule in vitro and structure of microtubule in cells. Mol. Biol. Rep. 37, 3183-3192

Part 2

Oxidative Stress and Neurodegeneration

3

Oxidative Stress and Neurodegenerative Disease

Selva Rivas-Arancibia, Cesar Gallegos-Ríos, Nancy Gomez-Crisostomo, Ever Ferreira-Garcidueñas, Dulce Flores Briseño, Luz Navarro and Erika Rodríguez-Martínez
Universidad Nacional Autónoma de México, Facultad de Medicina, Departamento de Fisiología
México

1. Introduction

In an oxidation-reduction balance, the antioxidant and oxidant molecules are in equilibrium in the organism. When a free radical increase causes an increase in the activity of the antioxidant systems, this leads to a state of redox homeostasis. The oxidation-reduction balance loss in the organism, caused by an excess of oxidants or a deficit in the antioxidant system, is defined as an oxidative-stress state, which is characterized by high levels of reactive species.

The oxidative-stress state has an important role in the development of many degenerative diseases, such as autoimmune disease, cancer, cardiac disease, and diabetes, but it also has a crucial role in the neurodegenerative diseases, such as Alzheimer's (Pan et al., 2011), Parkinson's (Sevcsik et al., 2011), Huntington's (Lee et al., 2011), lateral amyotrophic sclerosis (Zhao et al., 2011), multiple Sclerosis (Witherrick et al., 2010), and other processes related to pathological aging (Flovd et al., 2011).

Brain plasticity allows certain mental functions to work normally, e.g the learning and memory process. The synapses that form between the neurons are highly organized and are specific structures that permit fast and highly selective interactions between the cells in response to the constant environmental changes that produce neuroplasticity (Bruel-Jungerman et al., 2011). This allows the cells of the nervous system to be both functional and continuously structurally modified to establish new dendrites and synaptic connections. The brain plasticity process can be altered by oxidative stress, which produces oxidative damage, loss of process, synapse deaths, and alteration in the formation of new cells (Rivas-Arancibia et al., 2010).

The synaptic transmission involves the liberation of neurotransmitters from the presynaptic neurons and their detection by a specific receptor on the surface of the membrane of the postsynaptic neuron. Under conditions of homeostasis, the synaptic plasticity is regulated by changes in the amount of receptors in the postsynaptic membrane, changes in the form and size of the dendrite spines, and kinetic modulation of the protein synthesis and degradation.

The reactive species produce oxidation of lipids, proteins, and DNA in the cell, unfolding the proteins. The oxidation of the molecules that form the cell membrane alters its selective permeability, which leads to a loss of osmotic balance.

Smythies (1999) proposed the redox hypothesis of learning and neurocomputing. This hypothesis suggests that redox signals may control a mechanism involved in brain plasticity, in which the growth and elimination of synapses and dendrite spines depend on the redox state. The fate of a synapse depending in part on the redox balance means that if the oxidant-environmental cell produces an oxidative-stressed state, and the reactive oxygen species (ROS) cause elimination of spines. This has been demonstrated in alcoholism and neurodegenerative diseases (Götz et al, 2001). If the cell's environmental are antioxidant, synapses are preserved (Smythies, 1999) and increase the number of synapses, facilitating plastic brain phenomena. The central nervous system (CNS) is especially sensitive to the oxidants because of its high lipid content, high consumption of oxygen, and low levels of antioxidant enzymes. The hippocampus, substantia nigra, and the striatum are particularly vulnerable to oxidative stress (Rivas-Arancibia et al., 2010; Santiago-López et al., 2010). The vulnerability of these structures is probably caused by the neurochemical and metabolic characteristics of neural network. The hippocampus contains neurotransmitters such as acetylcholine and glutamate, and also has the ability to produce new neurons in the dentate gyrus, which make it susceptible to redox changes. This response is in part modulated by oxidative changes and an excess of reactive species block neurogenesis (Rivas-Arancibia et al., 2010). In the substantia nigra and the striatum, the normal metabolism of dopamine involves many oxidative reactions. In a state of redox balance, the dopamine oxidation does not disrupt normal metabolism of dopamine, because oxidized dopamine is converted by a complex series of reactions to neuromelanin. The loss of the redox balance causes oxidation of cytoplasmic dopamine in the presence of transition metals, with the formation of superoxide, hydrogen peroxide, and the hydroxyl radical. The dopaminergic neurons in the substantia nigra are involved in different functions such as learning and memory processes and motor control. With a loss of redox equilibrium, these neurons easily suffer oxidative damage and begin to produce a chain of events, in which the synthesis and metabolic path of dopamine contribute to the increase of the oxidative stress state because of quinone formation, making the nigroestriatal pathway much more vulnerable to damage in comparison to other brain structures (Santiago López et al., 2010).

2. Free radicals, reactive species formation, and cell signaling

A free radical is a species containing one or more unpaired electrons with the ability to exist independently (Halliwell, 2006, 2007). Free radicals are highly reactive, but despite their chemical reactivity, this reactivity changes over a wide spectrum. The first organic free radical was identified by Gomberg in 1900, the methyl triphenyl radical. More than 50 years ago, free radicals were described in living systems in a classic work by Commoner & Townsed published in Nature (1954). Subsequently, it was proposed that free radicals of oxygen (or reactive species of oxygen), could be formed as products of the enzymatic reactions of cell metabolism. At that time the theory was that the reactive oxygen species (ROS) could be the direct cause of many diseases, including cancer and almost any neurodegenerative process (Harman, 1956). In the 1960s and 1970s, free radicals began to be considered as important elements in biological systems. Among other findings, the enzyme superoxide dismutase (SOD) was discovered that converts the free radical superoxide ($\bullet O_2^-$) into hydrogen peroxide (H_2O_2) (McCord & Fridovich, 1969). This finding convincingly proved the importance of the free radical in biological systems. The simplest of the free radicals is the hydrogen atom, with a single proton and a single unpaired electron. The elimination of a hydrogen atom from a biological molecule produces an unpaired electron on the atom or molecule to which the hydrogen atom was originally bonded.

The diatomic molecule of oxygen (O_2) is regarded as a radical because it has two unpaired electrons, each located in a different orbital, but the two have the same spin. This is why O_2 has a relatively low reactivity in contrast with other highly reactive radicals. The radicals can be formed by the loss of a single electron or by the gain of a single electron, each action from some stable molecule. A radical could donate its unpaired electron to another molecule or could also trap an electron from another molecule turning the latter into a free radical. The unpaired electrons increase the chemical reactivity of the molecule. It is the manifestation of the free radical to get to the most energetically stable state through pairing with another electron. Thus, many radical-radical and radical-molecule reactions take place as soon as two molecules of the reaction are found. In addition the molecules would be changed by this type of reaction. The high reactivity of free radicals causes their half-life to be brief, on the order of milliseconds, varying according to the type of free radical.

3. How are the reactive species formed?

In biological systems, free radicals and the intermediate products of the biological metabolism are formed. Both free radicals and metabolites are called reactive species. Those most often found are reactive oxygen species (ROS) and reactive nitrogen species (RNS). There are also reactive iron species (RIS) and reactive copper species (RCS) (Valko et al., 2007).

3.1 Reactive oxygen species (ROS)

About 60 years ago, it was not thought that the ROS were part of the biological system reactions because of their high reactivity and low selectivity. More than 90% of the oxygen that enters into the cells is used for the production of energy. The mitochondria produce more than 80% of the adenosine triphosphate (ATP) necessary in animal cells. During this process, four electrons are added to each molecule of O_2 resulting in the formation of two molecules of H_2O. During the phosphorylation oxidative process, 1% to 5% of the O_2 used by the mitochondria via complex I and III (Buetler et al., 2004) escape the respiratory chain to form the superoxide anion. Some of these molecules contain an unpaired electron, thus a free radical. The intermediate products have several levels of reactivity with non free radical species. Different ROS often coexist, and it is difficult to identify the specific species as responsible for a given biological effect. For example, different reactive oxygen species formed from the elimination of the superoxide can participate in different types of reactions during which cellular metabolism can suffer a oxidation or reduction process.

3.1.1 Superoxide anion

This is a relatively unreactive species but potentially toxic. It can start reactions that give rise to other reactive ROS. This new anion can be formed as a product of many reactions catalyzed enzymatically, as in flavoprotein reactions (Xanthine oxidase, aldehyde oxidase, purine oxidase) (Behar et al., 1979; Korycka-Dahi & Richardson, 1981), oxidases and hydroxylases (diamino oxidase, galactose oxidase, cytochrome p450), and also those that can be formed in nonenzymatic reactions of oxygen with cysteine (Sáez et al., 1982) or riboflavin, as happens in the mitochondrial respiratory chain (Boveris, 1972).

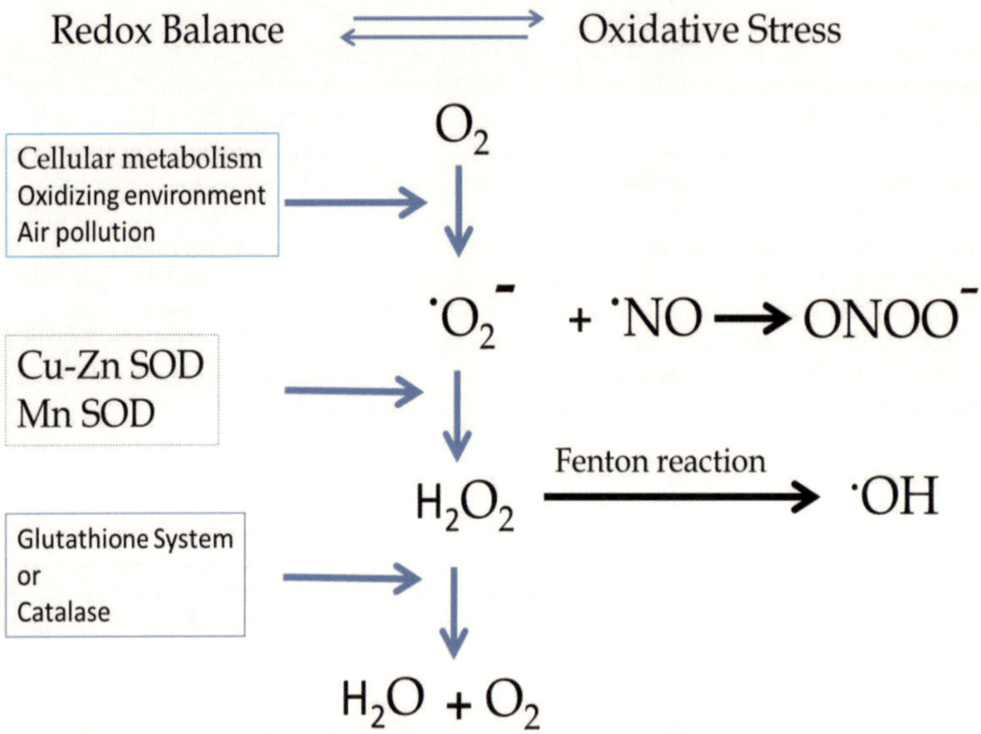

Fig. 1. Schematic oxidation-reduction reactions. Note the reduction reactions in a redox balance (left), and oxidation reactions in an oxidative stress condition (right)

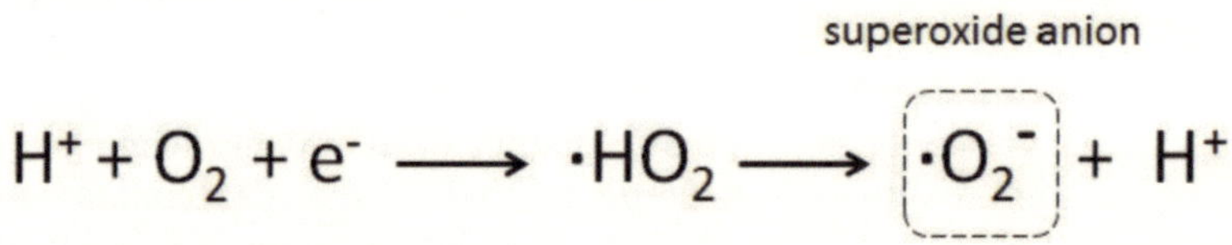

Reaction 1. Formation of Superoxide anion

3.1.2 Hydrogen peroxide (H_2O_2)

Hydrogen peroxide is not a free radical, but it is a reactive oxygen species that can easily diffuse through the membranes. In biological media it is formed by two pathways; 1) After the direct reduction of the oxygen by two electrons (reaction 2) and 2) By the catalyzation of the superoxide anion with SOD (reaction 3).

Many enzymes produce hydrogen peroxide from oxygen, such as xanthine oxide reductase, superoxide dismutase, glucose oxidase, D-amino acid oxidase, uricase (Battaner et al., 1990; Fridovich, 1986; Janolino & Swaisgood, 1975; Romero-Alvira et al., 1987) and may also result from chemical reactions such as the autoxidation of ascorbic acid catalyzed by copper (Korycka-Dahi & Richardson, 1991).

$$O_2 + 2e^- + 2H^+ \longrightarrow \underset{\text{hydrogen peroxide}}{H_2O_2}$$

Reaction 2. Reduction of oxygen

$$\underset{\text{superoxide anion}}{\cdot O_2^-} + 2H^+ \xrightarrow{\text{SOD}} \underset{\text{hydrogen peroxide}}{H_2O_2} + O_2$$

Reaction 3. Dismutation of superoxide anion

3.1.3 Hydroxyl (•OH)

This is the most reactive species, with an average life estimated of about 10^{-9} seconds (Liochev & Fridovich, 1994). Because of Its high reactivity its chemical action is confined to the vicinity of the site of production. It can be formed in vivo as a result of high-energy radiation (x-ray, gamma ray), which can cause homolytic breakage of water. UV light does not have enough energy to split a water molecule but it can split oxygenated water into two molecules of the hydroxyl radical. At the biological level, the most important hydroxyl radical formation is the Fenton reaction (Halliwel & Guteridge, 1992) (reaction 4).

$$\underset{\text{hydrogen peroxide}}{H_2O_2} + \underset{\text{ferrous ion}}{Fe^{2+}} \longrightarrow \underset{\text{ferric ion}}{Fe^{3+}} + \underset{\text{hydroxyl}}{OH^-} + \underset{\text{hydroxyl radical}}{\cdot OH}$$

Reaction 4. Hydroxyl radical formation. Fenton reaction

Hydrogen peroxide and the superoxide radical can form the hydroxyl radical by the Haber-Weiss reaction (Wardman, 1996) (Reaction 5):

$$\underset{\text{hydrogen peroxide}}{H_2O_2} + \underset{\text{superoxide}}{\cdot O_2^-} \longrightarrow O_2 + \underset{\text{hydroxyl}}{OH^-} + \underset{\text{hydroxyl radical}}{\cdot OH}$$

Reaction 5. Hydroxyl radical formation, the Haber-Weiss reaction. This reaction is catalyzed by metals such as iron or copper

3.1.4 Peroxyl radical (ROO•)

The peroxyl radicals are probably the most abundant in biological systems, and they are not as reactive as the ROS. They originate from the addition of oxygen to any hydrocarbon radical (reaction 6). This radical has a relatively long half-life (on the order of seconds).

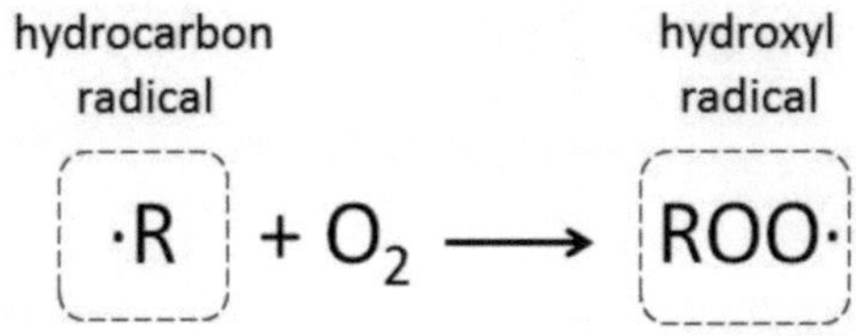

Reaction 6. Production of the peroxyl radical

3.1.5 Oxygen singlet ($^1O_2$)

This is an excited form of molecular oxygen. It is not a free radical and it is formed in vivo by the action of light on oxygen molecules in the presence of photoactivators, such as riboflavin (Aurand et al., 1977). Its half-life is about 10^{-6} seconds, depending on the nature of the surrounding matrix. It can interact with other molecules by transferring to them its excitation energy or by chemically combining with them. It can form in the oxidation of NADPH in the microsomes by the activity of several enzymes such as xanthine oxidase, lactoperoxidase, lipoxygenase, and prostaglandin synthetase.

3.1.6 Nitric oxide (•NO)

It is a lyophilic and water-soluble gas, with an average half-life of 3 to 5 seconds. Enzymatically formed from arginine, its reaction is catalyzed by nitric oxide synthase (NOS). The NOS has three isoforms. The neuronal nitric oxide synthase (nNOS) or type I, the inducible nitric oxide synthase (iNOS) or type II, and the endothelial nitric oxide synthase (eNOS) or type III. They are constitutively expressed. Their activity is regulated by the intracellular concentration of calcium (Bredt et al., 1991). The inducible nitric oxide synthase (iNOS) or type II is expressed in the macrophages when they are stimulated by cytokines, lipopolysaccharides, or other immune substances. It is also is found in other tissues, such as brain tissue and endothelium (MacMicking et al., 1997). Its expression is regulated at both the transcriptional and posttranscriptional level, which involves the transcription by redox signaling as an increase in reactive species and cytokines, such as nuclear factor kappa B (NF-kB) and the MAP kinases (MacMicking et al., 1997). Nitric oxide plays a fundamental role in the regulation of local blood flow, inhibits platelet aggregation, is a neurotransmitter, and is produced by activated macrophages that contribute to the primary immune defense. Another effect of the •NO radical is its ability to react with the iron of intracellular protein, mainly mitochondrial. Most of the enzymes that possess a heme prosthetic group can be inactivated by nitric oxide. Nitric oxide can react with nucleic acids leading to mutations and DNA breakage and it can also cause necrosis (Tang et al., 2011).

The •NO radical has an important antiinflammatory action, and it has the ability to cause cellular and tissue dysfunction by a proinflammatory effect. To understand this double effect it has been proposed that the regulatory and antiinflammatory effects of nitric oxide occur when it has a direct impact on a biological molecule (Grisham et al., 1999), which occurs under physiological conditions in which the production of •NO is low and a redox balance is present. However, upon the loss of the redox balance when the concentration of •NO increases, the •NO has indirect effects through metabolites associated with RNS, and they may react with oxygen or the superoxide radical, which occurs during oxidative stress and an inflammatory response (Tweedie et al., 2011).

3.1.7 Peroxynitrite (•ONOO-)

Nitric oxide can generate the peroxynitrite anion (•ONOO-) by reaction with the superoxide anion (Gryglewsli et al., 1986; Miles et al., 1996).

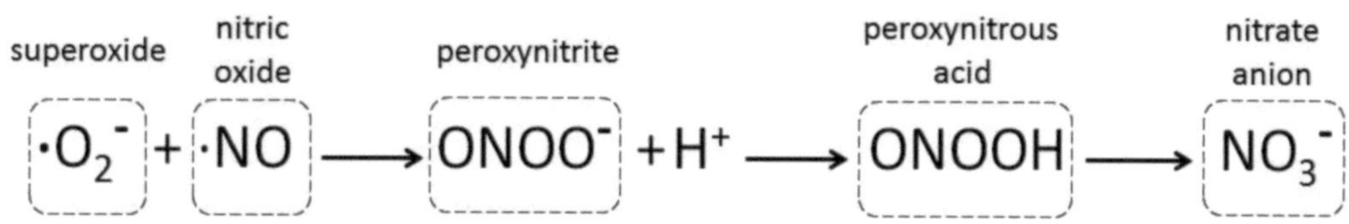

Reaction 7. Formation of peroxynitrite anion

4. Free radical production

There are many ways by which organisms are exposed to the effects of oxygen free radicals. Free radicals can be produced through several chemical processes, both within and outside the organism. The same cell is potentially more than one source of production of a free radical. Depending on the origin of its production, the peroxynitrite can be in equilibrium with its conjugate acid (ONOOH). In neutral solution it is a powerful oxidizing agent able to nitrate tyrosine residues, nitrating and oxidizing guanosine, degrade carbohydrates, initiate lipid peroxidation, and fragment DNA (Beckman & Koppenol, 1994, 1996).

The production of $\bullet O_2$- and •NO in vivo is different. The peroxynitrite production always occurs when there is an excess of one or the other (Grisham et al., 1999). Some authors established that both reactions of oxidation and nitration mediated by the peroxynitrite are influenced largely by the relative flow of production of $\bullet O_2^-$ and •NO (Jourd'Heuil et al., 2001). They also established that the highest rates of oxidation occur with an excess of •NO, producing oxidation through the •OH and from the peroxynitrite $\bullet NO_2$ formed. However, the reaction of peroxynitrite with CO_2 is the most important way that the peroxynitrite decomposes in vivo (Lymar & Hurst, 1995), forming the end product $\bullet N_2O_3$, which is a potent nitrating agent.

In addition to the reactions of oxidation, the peroxynitrite has the ability to nitrate phenolic compounds under physiological conditions, such as the rings of tyrosine (Goldstein et al., 2000). Tyrosine residues are oxidized by the radical derivatives of the peroxynitrite forming the radical tyrosyl, which in turn reacts with •NO to form 3-nitrotyrosine. The nitration mediated by peroxynitrite in vivo might be inhibited by a relative overproduction of $O_2^{-\bullet}$ because of competition between them by the radical tyrosyl, by which the formation of 3-nitrotyrosine would be inhibited when the rate of formation of $\bullet O_2^-$ exceeded that of •NO (Goldstein et al., 2000) in the exogenous and endogenous sources (Freeman & Crapo, 1982).

4.1 Exogenous ROS production

Many antineoplastic agents (Dedon & Goldberg, 1982), such as the adriamycin, bleomycin, daunorubicin, and other antibiotics (Doroshow & Hochstein, 1982) depend on quinoide groups or joining metals for their activity. Some of the effects of these drugs have been attributed to their ability to reduce oxygen to superoxide, the hydroxyl radical, and hydrogen peroxide. The irradiation of organisms by electromagnetic radiation (x-rays and gamma rays) or by particle radiation (electrons, protons, deuterons, and neutrons) also cause free radicals (Bielsky & Gebieki, 1977).

Environmental factors, such as photochemical air pollutants as ozone, hyperoxia, pesticides, tobacco smoke, solvents, anesthetics, and aromatic hydrocarbons are a source of reactive species. These agents have free radicals, such as in tobacco smoke, or become reactive species with cellular metabolism and detoxification processes (Mason, 1982). An important source of reactive species that deserves special importance is environmental pollution (Searing & Rabinovitch, 2011; Bhalla, 1999) because it has been shown that an oxidation environment, in which we live in polluted cities, is associated with chronic-degenerative diseases. An example is ozone pollution (Bhalla & Gupta, 2000). Studies have shown that ozone pollution causes serious damage to human health and is a determining factor in the progression of neurodegenerative diseases (Zawia et al., 2009; Schwela, 2000). This gas acts to produce ROS in the body, causing an increase in oxidants, increasing the state of oxidative stress in the organism and thus contributing to increase the neurodegenerative process in the patient (Cretu et al., 2010).

4.2 Endogenous ROS production

Autoxidation of small molecules. There are a variety of soluble components able to produce phosphorylation in the cell, such as thiols, hydroquinone, catecholamines, flavins, and tetrahydropterins. In all these, the superoxide radical is the radical primarily formed by the dioxygen reduction by these molecules (Baccarini, 1978). Hydrogen peroxide is also produced as a byproduct from the disproportionation of the superoxide radical, either spontaneously or enzymatically catalyzed by superoxide dismutase (SOD).

4.2.1 Soluble enzymes and proteins

Enzymes, such as xanthine oxide reductase, aldehyde oxidase, flavinprotein dehydrogenase, and tryptophan dioxygenase, generate free radicals during their catalytic cycle (Massey et al., 1989). During ischemia, calcium stimulates the activation of proteases leading to changes in the activation of these enzymes (Warner et al., 2004) causing cell damage and death.

4.2.2 Mitochondrial electronic transport chain

In healthy tissue, one of the main sources of free radicals are the mitochondria. This is because these organelles are responsible for more than 90% of cellular oxygen consumption and the radicals in biological systems always, ultimately are generated by the metabolism of oxygen by this route.

Most mitochondrial hydrogen peroxide comes from the disproportionation of the superoxide radical (Boveris & Chance, 1973). The generation of the superoxide radical by mitochondria occurs when the conveyors of the respiratory chain, located in the inner mitochondrial membrane, are highly reduced (Turrens & Boveri, 1980).

Four complexes are responsible for electronic transport in the respiratory chain. The production of radicals has been observed in the mitochondria isolated in complex I (Turrens & Boveri, 1980) and in complex III (Boveris & Chance, 1973). For complex I, the most likely candidates as free radical generators seem to be iron-sulfide centers, whereas complex III has been discussed intensively to determine if they could be a semiquinone (Boveris & Chance, 1973) or cytochrome b (Nohl & Jordan, 1986; Turrens, 2003; Ghouleh et al., 2011).

4.2.3 Electronic transport of the endoplasmic reticulum and nuclear membrane systems

Both systems of intracellular membranes contain cytochromes P450 and b5, which can oxidize unsaturated fatty acids (Capdevila et al., 1981; Ghouleh et al., 2011) and xenobiotics (Chignell, 1979). The cytochromes P450 and b5 are the most powerful oxidizers in vivo, although they can also act as reducing agents. There are several actions that activate molecular oxygen species (Ghouleh et al., 2011) generating oxygen electrophílics in turn by radicals that can be released into the cell (Dolphin, 1988).

4.2.4 Peroxisomes

Peroxisomes are cellular sources of the production of hydrogen peroxide because of their high concentration in oxidases, none of which uses superoxide as a precursor. These enzymes include the D-aminoacid oxidase, urate oxidase, L-a-hydroxyacidic oxidase, and acyl-fatty-Coenzyme A oxidase (Boveris et al., 1973).

Peroxisomal catalase is the enzyme that metabolizes most of the hydrogen peroxide generated by the peroxisomes oxidases (Freeman & Crapo, 1982; Frei, 1994).

4.2.5 Plasma membrane

Free radicals generated extracellularly must cross the plasma membrane before reacting with other cellular components and can then start toxic reactions. Unsaturated fatty acids present in the membrane and transmembrane proteins with oxidizable amino acids are likely to be altered by free radicals. These reactions affect the properties of the membranes by changing their permeability and decreasing the potential of the membranes, making secretory functions stop, and inhibiting metabolic processes in the cells. All this is caused by lipid peroxidation or the oxidation of important structural proteins (Freeman & Crapo, 1982).

5. Antioxidant systems and loss of redox balance

In the presence of the oxygen, organisms have been forced to develop mechanisms for their protection against the ROS. Antioxidants are biological substances that are able to compete for oxidizable substrates and inhibit oxidation (Halliwell & Gutteridge, 1984). Antioxidant systems can be divided into enzymatic and nonenzymatic (Somogyi et al., 2007). The first are the SOD, glutathione peroxidase, catalase, and thioredoxin. Nonenzymatic types include vitamins, proteins, and amino acids, which are less reactive but in greater concentration in contrast to the enzymatic types, which have a high reactivity with the ROS, but are in lower concentrations.

Antioxidant systems counteract the activity of the ROS, thus maintaining the oxidation-reduction balance. These systems can be endogenous and exogenous. The most important endogenous antioxidant systems are the enzymes superoxide dismutase, catalase, and glutathione peroxidase.

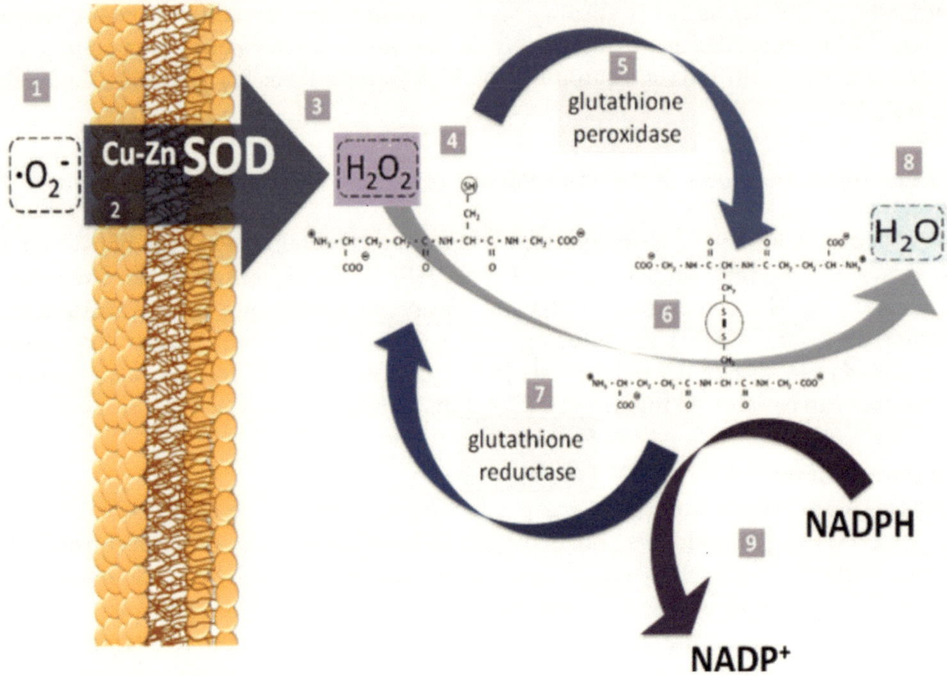

Fig. 2. Shows an oxygen free radical (1), which in the presence of the enzyme Cu-Zn SOD (2) gives rise to peroxides (3) that react with reduced glutathione (4) and are catalyzed by the enzyme glutathione peroxidase (5) resulting in oxidized glutathione (6) and water (7). The peroxides (3) that can be toxic to the cell are removed. The oxidized glutathione (6) in the presence of glutathione reductase (8) and NADPH (9), which hosts an electron, allows the oxidized glutathione to return to its reduced form

5.1 Endogenous systems

5.1.1 Superoxide dismutase (SOD)

The catalytic role of the SOD was discovered by McCord and Fridovich in 1969. The SOD is an enzyme that catalyzes the reduction of the superoxide anion, which is produced in the body as the resulting product of oxidative phosphorylation, either derived from UV radiation or during inflammation, by transforming the superoxide anion into a product such as hydrogen peroxide that is metabolized easily to water by glutathione peroxidase (GPx) and catalase (CAT).The SOD is present in different forms, such as copper-zinc SOD and manganese SOD (Mn-SOD). The Cu-Zn SOD is found in the cytosol and the cell membrane, has a molecular mass of 32 kDa with two identical subunits. The Mn-SOD is located in the mitochondrial matrix (Grisham et al., 1999; Halliwell & Gutteridge, 1989; Ohno et al., 1994) and has a molecular mass of 88 kDa with four identical subunits (Ohno et al., 1994). It acts as a first line of defense in the detoxification of the superoxide anion and seems to be involved in processes of tumor removal or cellular differentiation.

5.1.2 The glutathione antioxidant system

The glutathione antioxidant system is formed by reduced glutathione and the activity of the enzyme glutathione reductase that reduces the oxidized glutathione and glutathione peroxidase, which along with the reduced glutathione contributes to the elimination of peroxides. Glutathione (GSH) is a tripeptide compound of glutamic acid, cysteine, and glycine that has many important functions within cells (Fig. 3). Glutathione serves as a reducer, conjugates to drugs to make them more soluble in water, is involved in the transport of amino acids across cell membranes (γ-glutamyl cycle), is a substrate for the peptide-leukotrienes, serves as a cofactor for some enzyme reactions, and as an aid in the reorganization of protein bridges.

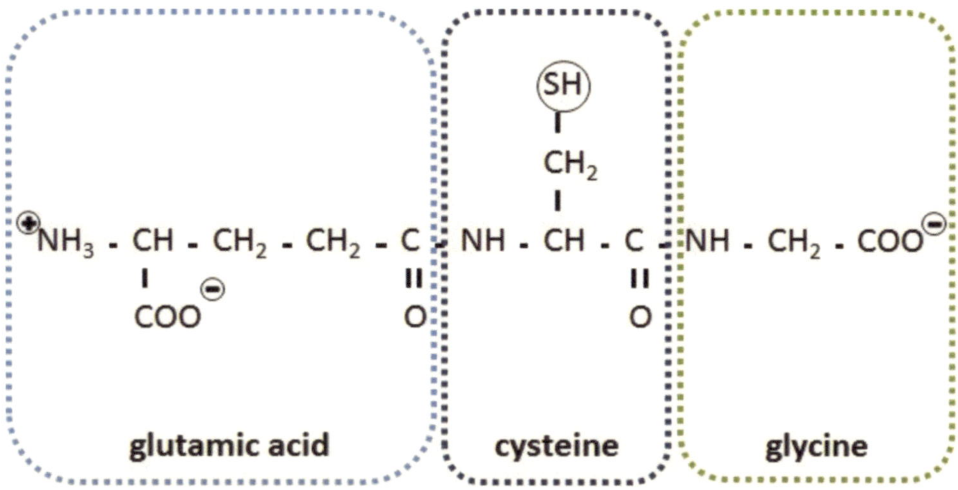

Fig. 3. Structure of glutathione

The role of GSH as a reducing agent is important especially in a highly oxidizing environment. The sulfhydryl of GSH can be used to reduce peroxides. The resulting form of oxidized GSH consists of two molecules of disulfide linked together (GSSG). Glutathione reductase uses NADPH as the cofactor to reduce GSSG to two molecules of GSH. Therefore, the pentose phosphate pathway is important to produce the NADPH required for glutathione reductase. Glutathione peroxidase is a selenium-dependent enzyme that catalyzes the reduction of H_2O_2 or lipoperoxide (L-OOH) using the reduced glutathione (GSH).

Oxidized glutathione is reduced by glutathione reductase that uses NADPH (from the pentose phosphate pathway) as an electron donor, thus maintaining the ratio GSH /GSSG (Fig. 4). There are at least three forms of glutathione peroxidase dependent on selenium; an intracellular form, extracellular (GPx-C), or plasma (GPx-P) that has specific activity for phospho-lipoperoxides (GPx-PH), usually associated with the membrane and although its activity is the same, has structural differences. The GPx-C and GPx-P are tetrameric enzymes composed of four identical subunits with each containing a selenium atom attached covalently to a molecule of cysteine. The sequence of amino acids in the subunits of the GPx-C is different from the sequence of the GPx-P. The separate subunits have no catalytic activity. The GPx-PH is a monomer enzyme that also has an atom of selenium and catalytic activity (Stepanik & Ewing, 1993). The GPx-C has higher affinity for H_2O_2 than for lipoperoxides, and the GPx-P has a similar affinity for the two substrates. The GPx-C and GPx-P are used as substrates for H_2O_2 and the lipoperoxides. They are not able to use the phospholipoperoxides (PHL-OOH) that are the major substrates for the GPx-PH (Maiorino et al., 1991).

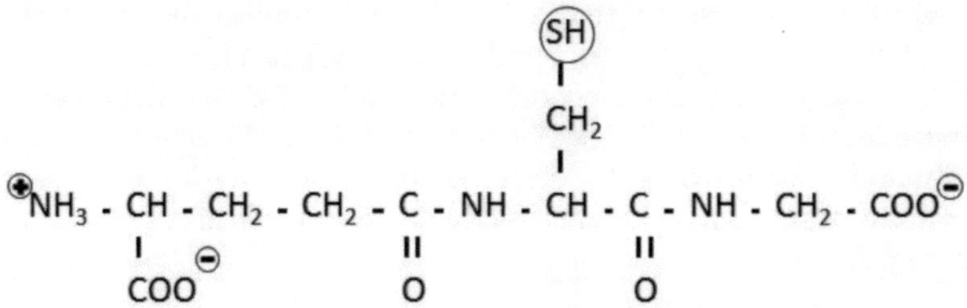

(a)

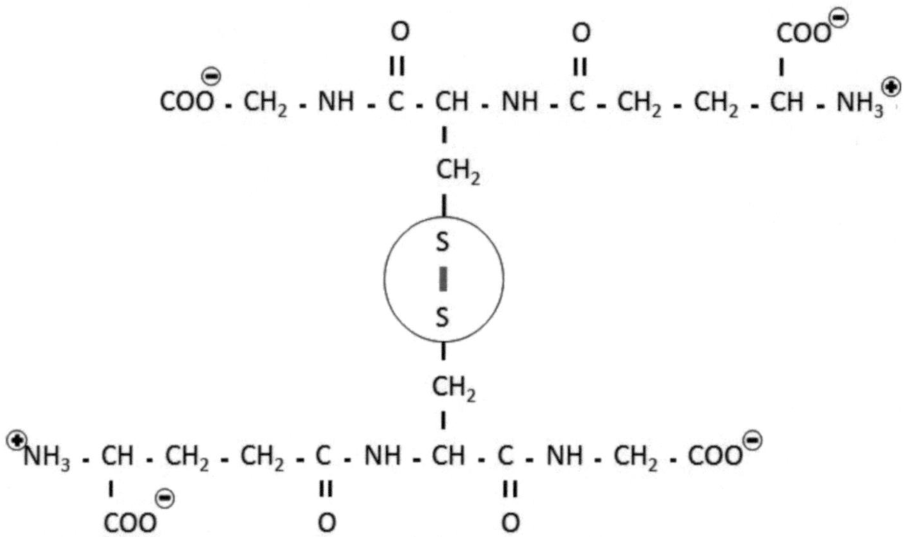

(b)

Fig. 4. (a) Reduced glutathione structure (GSH). (b) Oxidized glutathione structure (GSSG)

5.1.3 Catalase

Catalase (CAT) or hydrogen peroxide oxidoreductase is one of the more abundant enzymes in nature and is widely distributed in the human body. Its activity varies depending on the tissue, highest in the liver and kidneys, lowest in connective tissue and the lining, and practically nonexistent in the nervous tissue. At the cellular level it is located in the mitochondria and peroxisomes, except in erythrocytes, where it is located in the cytosol. This enzyme is a tetrameric metaloprotein of four identical subunits that are held together by noncovalent interactions. Each subunit contains a prosthetic group of protoporphyrin IX. Catalase is involved in the destruction of hydrogen peroxide generated during cellular metabolism. It has two features; the catalytic and the peroxidative. Both can be represented by reaction 9.

The general reaction covers the substrate reduction taking hydrogen atoms from a donor, and the products are the reduced substrate and the oxidized donor. In the catalytic reaction, the donor is another molecule of H_2O_2. This reaction can only be accomplished by the enzyme in its tetrameric form.

$$H_2O_2 + H_2R \xrightarrow{CAT} 2\,H_2O + R$$

Reaction 9. Destruction of hydrogen peroxide by catalase

$$H_2O_2 + H_2O_2 \xrightarrow{CAT} 2\,H_2O + O_2$$

Reaction 10. Catalytic reaction of the enzyme catalase on hydrogen peroxide

In the peroxidative reaction the enzyme can be used as donors of hydrogen to methanol, ethanol, formic acid, and formaldehyde. This reaction can be with monomers, dimers, and tetramers. Glutathione peroxidase (GPx) and glutathione reductase (GRd) are part of an antioxidant system (GPx-GRd), and catalase (SOD-CAT). It has been observed that both systems fail to act simultaneously. The CAT acts in the presence of high concentrations of H_2O_2, and the GPx at low concentrations, which shows an inverse correlation in the activity of two enzymes.

5.2 Exogenous systems

Antioxidant vitamins, along with glutathione, comprise a group of reducing agents able to donate electrons to oxidized species such as free radicals and the lipoperoxides, thus neutralizing their destructive oxidative potential (Chao et al., 2002).The most significant exogenous antioxidant systems are vitamins A, C, and E, and some metals such as copper and selenium. The last is a cofactor for the enzyme glutathione peroxidase.

Vitamin A. It can be derived from retinol of animal origin and comes from different plant carotenes. The main sources of vitamin A are fish liver oils, liver of mammals, and milk. In plants it exists in the form of carotene (provitamin). It has an important role in vision. In the form of retinoic acid, vitamin A is effective in the treatment of acne and other skin conditions.

Vitamin E is a substituted lipid isoprenoid of the tocopherol family. Its biologically active form is D-alpha tocopherol, whose phenolic hydroxyl is responsible for the antioxidant effects. Vitamin B12 is plentiful in the yolk of eggs, whole milk, the offal of mammals, and fish oils. It is essential for humans (Mayes, 1997). The activity of vitamin E is one of the first barriers against the peroxidation of the polyunsaturated fatty acids. Mitochondrial, endoplasmic reticulum, and plasma membrane phospholipids have affinities to alpha-tocopherol, so it is highly concentrated in these sites (Nenzil et al., 2001). Tocopherols act by interrupting free radical chain reactions because of their ability to transfer a phenolic hydrogen to a peroxide free radical. Vitamin E can be in the form of phenoxy or phenoxyl free radical, in unreversible intermediate reactions that presuppose the transformation of the vitamin to its final harmless products. Tocopherols and selenium act synergistically allowing the organism to have its antioxidant activity (Hoenyet et al., 2005). Selenium is required for the normal pancreatic function (Rayman, 2000), which is necessary for the proper digestion of lipids. Though it is known that the levels of vitamin E are correlated with the ability to digest and absorb lipids. Because of its hydrophobic nature a deficiency of tocopherols is found in processes such as hepatic cholestasis and cystic fibrosis or bowel resections. Recent work shows the close relationship of the increase in the requirement of vitamin E and selenium with the intake of unsaturated fatty acids, aging, and the degenerative diseases such as atherosclerosis (Penn et al., 2003), Alzheimer's disease (Butterfield et al., 2002), or prostatic carcinoma (Thomas, 2004).

Vitamin C or L-ascorbic acid is a derivative of glucose. It is essential in the human diet. It is a lactone, in which the hydroxyl associated with the double bond groups function as agents with a high reducing potential, allowing it to participate in the direct reduction of oxygen, thus functioning as a donor substrate in the reactions of the peroxidases (Mayes, 1997). The mechanism of action of this vitamin yields a higher antioxidant level because it includes the inhibition of the formation of the superoxide radical or nitrosamines during digestion. In addition, it is the agent that reduces the phenoxy radical formed during vitamin E activity (Chao et al., 2002). Vitamins C and E are classified as antioxidant switches because they act by stopping the formation of free radical chain reactions (Shite et al., 2001), trapping them and reducing them, unlike the preventive antioxidants (which include peroxidase enzymes) to prevent the initiation of the sequence of reactions. Tocopherols work in an environment of high oxygen partial pressure, whereas beta-carotene works at low O_2 partial pressures.

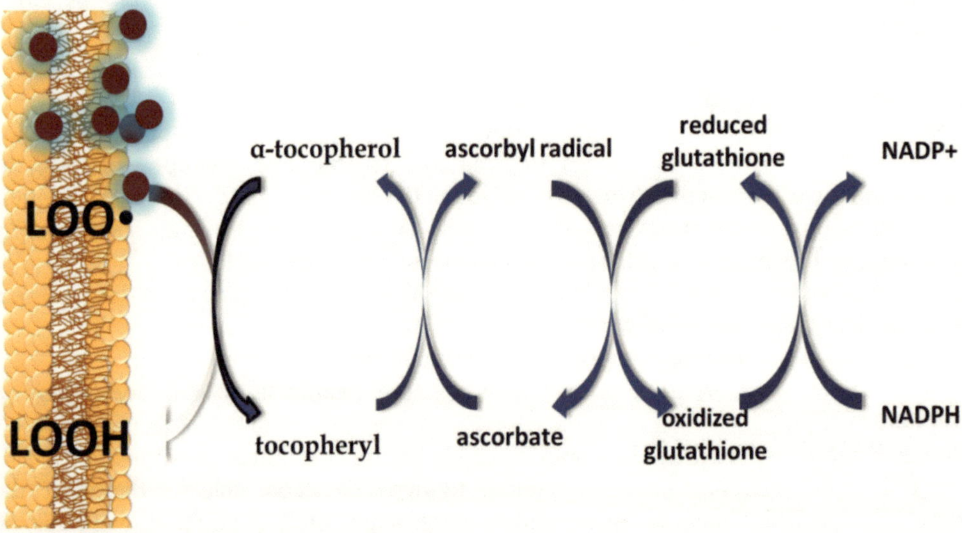

Fig. 5. Action of tocopherol on lipid peroxides and regeneration in the presence of ascorbate and reduced glutathione

6. Role of the reactive species in cellular signaling

The mechanisms of oxidation-reduction and free radicals play an important role in cell physiology (Kovacik & Wells, 2006), from the renewal of membranes, cellular plastic phenomena, cell migration, synthesis and release of some hormones, increase in transcription of cytokines during inflammatory processes, the participation in cell signaling (Stone & Yang, 2006; Biniert et al., 2006), and the mechanisms of second messengers (Smythies, 1999; Chiarugi & Fiaschi, 2007).

The ROS are characterized by their dual nature, which depends on the redox state of the organism. In a balanced oxidation-reduction reaction, the main effects of the ROS in the cell are through their actions in signaling pathways. These oxidant signals can easily be offset through antioxidant systems, To restablish a redox equilibrium, the ROS causes the expression of antioxidant enzymes and related defense mechanisms. At low concentrations the ROS are involved in many physiological functions. It has been suggested that the main effects of the ROS in cells are through interactions they have with different signaling pathways and not by their direct action on macromolecules (Maher, 2000). Both phenomena do coexist. There is evidence that living organisms have not only adapted to coexist with free radicals but they also have generated several mechanisms for using free radicals in different physiological functions (Halliwell & Gutterdge, 2007; Kirkwood, 2005).

Infectious diseases possibly were a mechanism of natural selection in the early stages of human civilization. The ROS participate directly in the defense mechanism against infections. They are part of a respiratory burst and are important modulators of the inflammatory response. Resident glia in the brain in normal situations are produced by ROS and its role in the brain is to counter cell damage. In addition, they participate in other functions, such as the regulation of vascular tone, the monitoring of the oxygen pressure, and the expansion of signal transduction. Signal transduction mediated by reactive species regulates the response to oxidative stress, which keeps the redox balance within homeostatic limits (Droge, 2002). For all this, the homeostatic regulation of the oxidation-reduction balance has a special importance of keeping the delicate balance between the adaptive advantages of the biological use of free radicals and their harmful effects. One of the most important discoveries is that the ROS can regulate gene expression of several bacterial genes, which is generated by H_2O_2 (Christman et al., 1985). For mammals, small amounts of $\bullet O_2^-$ and H_2O_2 increase the production of interleukin 2 (IL-2), which is an important factor of lymphocyte growth, possibly as a response to the activation of the nuclear factor kappa B (NFκB) that occurs in the presence of the ROS (Schreck et al., 1992).

The term "redox signaling" is used to describe a process of regulation, that involves processes of oxidation-reduction. This type of signaling is used by a wide range of microorganisms, including bacteria, and its most common use by the cell is the generation of antioxidant defenses to restore the original state of redox homeostasis after a temporary exposure to the ROS (Droge, 2002). The interaction of various components of antioxidant systems (Mendiratta et al., 1998a, 1998b) is effective for the recycling of components and is sufficient to cope with the stress caused by the ROS for long periods in the life of an organism (Soberman, 2003). Aging and particularly inflammatory, chronic diseases cause an alteration in the maintenance of redox state, which causes mechanisms of progressively aggravated pathology.

As mentioned, the ROS generate cellular events, such as the activation of the pathway of the MAP. These consist of four subfamilies sensitive to the ROS and are identified as kinases regulated by extracellular signaling (ERK1-2), kinase c-Jun NH2 - terminal (JNK), and kinase p38 kinase big MAP type 1 (BMK1 or ERK5). Each family has its trigger mechanism and then modulates specific cellular functions (Suzaki et al., 2002). We will discuss the physiological role of the ROS and the path of the BMK1 or ERK5 kinase in neuronal cells. There is evidence, found in experiments in PC12 cells, of different intracellular signaling steps identified in the path of the MAP kinases, where the ROS are involved (Suzaki et al., 2002).

The activation of the pathway of the BKM1 stimulated by the ROS depends on the presence of c-Src, a protein kinase encoded by the gene Src, and that becomes involved in the internalization of the signals to the nucleus through the phosphorylation of other proteins, including second messengers. When the ROS present in the cells interact with the c-Src, this causes activation of the kinase, which in turn has an immediate effect on the activation of the BMK1 through key intermediates to continue the internalization of the signal initiated by the ROS. Below is shown the cascade of the MEKK3 and MEK5 kinases (Suzaki et al., 2002). The BMK1-ERK5 possesses a amino acid motif TEY of physiological importance because it is on this site where atoms join with the phosphorous kinase MEK5 (Lee et al., 1995; Zhou et al., 1995). This, when phosphorylated, acquires the ability to cause the activation of the MEF2C and MEF2A, both belonging to the family of MEF2 transcription factors, and to cause the translocation at the nucleus, which is involved in the expression of genes of c-Jun and c-Fos, themselves part of the family of the AP1 (Silva, 2001). Components of this family have a common binding site on the DNA that results in the expression of neuropeptides and neurotrophins, synthesis and expression of receptors to various ligands, activation of transcription factors, the synthesis of various enzymes involved in the production of neurotransmitters, such as thyroxine hydroxylase, a limiting enzyme in the production of catecholamines and the formation and polymerization of proteins to the cytoskeleton (Silva, 2001). In endothelial cells, oxidative stress is involved in the formation

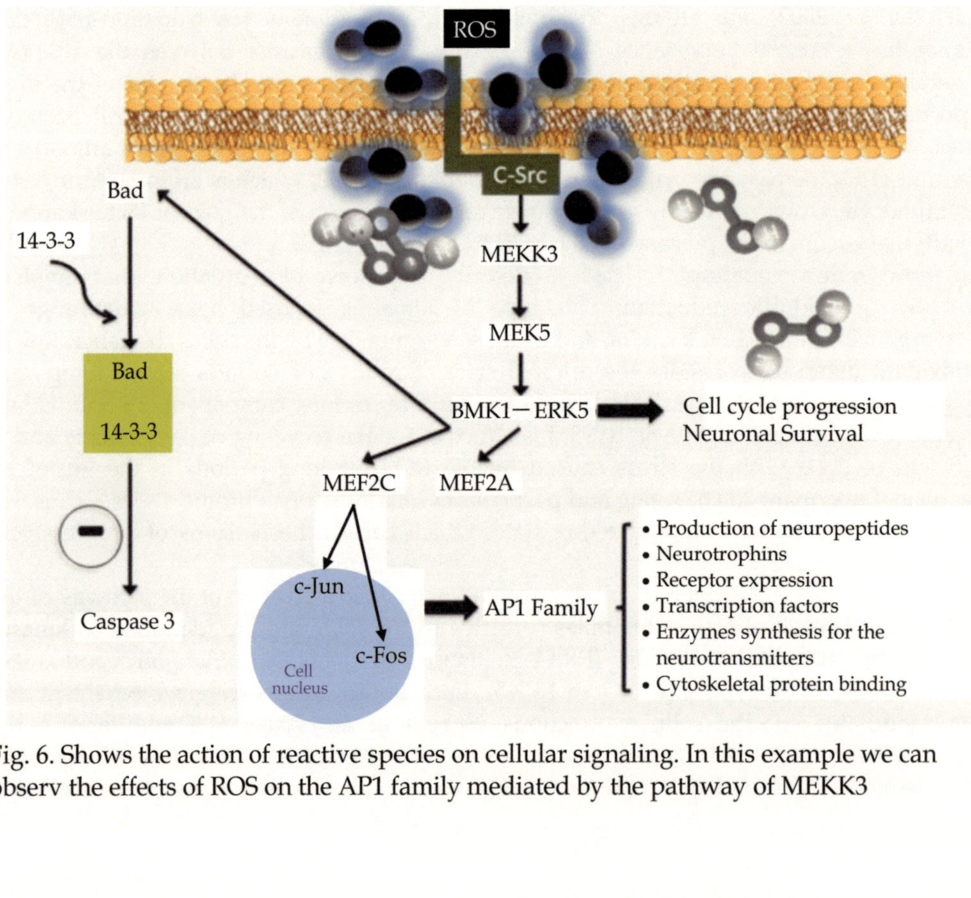

Fig. 6. Shows the action of reactive species on cellular signaling. In this example we can observ the effects of ROS on the AP1 family mediated by the pathway of MEKK3

of BMK1 (Yan, 1999) and this is able to phosphorylate Bad, a protein involved in the signaling of apoptosis. The scaffold 14-3-3 protein binds to Bad when it is phosphorylated and stops it from having proapoptotic activity. The nonphosphorylated Bad is able to travel to the mitochondria, causing the release of cytochrome C, a crucial step for the activation of caspase 3 (Xinchun et al., 2004). This evidence can suggest that the protective role and antiapoptotic action of BMK1-ERK5 is generated by the ROS (Liu et al., 2003).

7. Inflammation response and oxidative stress

The inflammatory response is a natural and important process in the repair of tissues and a fundamental mechanism of defense of the organism against infections and harmful agents. When the inflammatory response is not limited a process of chronic inflammation is established. In the animal model of oxidative stress, caused by exposure to ozone on healthy animals, chronic oxidative stress is able to cause an inflammatory response and dysregulation of the same answer (Rivas-Arancibia et al., 2010). It is widely reported that chronic inflammation produces ROS that lead to a state of oxidative stress. This change in the redox balance, causing activation of the signaling pathways of the cell, causes a perpetually inflammatory state. Maintaining the redox balance is important for cell signaling and adequate transcriptional activity (Chung et al., 2009). The ROS and other reactive species regulate the expression of proinflammatory cytokines, such as TNFα, IL-1β, IL-6, and IL-8, and the cell-adhesion molecules, such as the adhesion intercellular-1 (ICAM-1) and E-selectin molecules. Several biological states cause an increase in the amount of proinflammatory cytokines. Aging causes an increase in the levels of cytokines such as TNF-α, IL-1β, IL-6, gamma interferon (IFNγ), the beta-transforming growth factor (TGFβ), and acute phase proteins (Bruunsgaard et al., 2003). High levels of IL-6 have been associated with neuronal atrophy and chronic inflammatory states such as diabetes type 2 and atherosclerosis (Devaux et al., 1997; Willette et al., 2010). The C-reactive protein (CRP) levels increase with ageing, and high levels of chronic diseases are found associated with ageing, heart disease, and Alzheimer's disease (Ridker et al., 2001).

Activation of transcription factors that are sensitive to redox signals generate the production of inflammatory mediators, such as interleukin-1β (IL-1β), Interleukin-6 (IL-6), necrosis tumor-α factor (TNF-α), cycle-oxygenase-2 (COX-2), lipoxygenase (LOX), and inducible nitric oxide synthase (iNOS), and the cell adhesion molecules(CAMs) (VCAM-1, ICAM-1, and P- and E-selectin) (Salminen & Kaarniranta, 2010). NF-κB is a transcription factor activated by a wide variety of stimuli, such as oxidative stress, infection, and inflammation. This activation plays a key role in regulating the immune response (Salminen & Kaarniranta, 2010). NF-κB is composed of a heterodimericprotein complex containing a DNA-binding domain and a domain of acidic transactivation formed by the heterodimer polypeptides RelA-p65 and p50. Normally NF-κB is linked to a protein of the IκB family in cytoplasm, which inhibits its activation (Baldwin, 1996). When IκB is degraded, the NF-κB is freed and causes its translocation to the nucleus, where the NF-κB can bind to a promoter and start the transcription of specific genes that encode for proinflammatory mediators. Activation of tNF-kB is usually transient, but chronic activation produces changes in the inflammatory response. Protein-generated NF-kB and COX-2, TNF-α,e, and IL-1β and IL-6 are also potent activators of the same pathway, creating a vicious cycle (Handel et al., 1995, Fisher et al., 1996). There is evidence showing that aging increases the degradation of

NF-kB because of phosphorylation of IKB by NIK-IKK and MAPKs (Kim et al., 2000). There are other transcription factors involved in the inflammatory response. The family of the forkhead box O (FOXO) is evolutionarily conserved and integrated by FOXO1, FOXO3a, FOXO4, and FOXO6 in mammals (Van der Heide et al., 2004). The FOXO activation causes the transcription of genes involved in the regulation of the cell-cycle metabolism, cell death, and resistance to oxidative stress (Hedrick, 2009). The activation of these factors of transcription is regulated by growth factors through the phosphorylation of protein kinase B (PKB) (also known as Akt). This formation of phosphoinositide 3-kinase (PI3K) leads to the translocation of FOXO in the cytoplasm to the nucleus (Salih & Brunet, 2008). Both protein-kinase PI3K and Akt are able to mediate many signals of cell survival through inhibition of apoptosis processes (Lawlor and Alessi, 2001). However, little is known about how PI3K-Akt regulates levels of the ROS in cells. FOXO1 reduces the degree of oxidative stress increasing the amount of mRNA coding for Mn-SOD and catalase (Burgering & Medema, 2003). FOXO3a and FOXO4 protect quiescent cells in vitro from oxidative stress. FOXO3a directly activates the transcription of antioxidant enzymes Mn-SOD, catalase, and peroxiredoxin 3 (Prx3) (Marinkovic et al., 2007). This suggests that FOXO also has an important role in the redox balance. Both PI3K and Akt protein kinase are able to mediate many signals of cell survival through inhibition of apoptosis processes (Lawlor & Alessi, 2001).

The hypothesis of molecular inflammation can facilitate a better understanding of the aging process and related diseases such as dementia, cancer, osteoporosis, gingivitis, and vascular diseases.

8. Loss of the redox balance

The free radicals interact with other cell components, such as proteins, DNA, and lipids, to form multiple catabolic products. An example of these is lipid peroxidation resulting in lipid hydroperoxides and aldehydes that interact with the sulfhydryl groups of proteins causing the loss of protein functionality and thus perpetuating cell damage. The increased levels of calcium and nitric oxide stimulates the production of inflammatory interleukins causing gliosis and increasing the state of oxidative stress. This causes damage and cell death (Sugaya et al., 1998; Ryter et al., 2007), thus establishing a cycle through a chain of oxidative reactions that involve both neurons and glia. These are involved in the maintenance of the damage that extends into adjacent tissue cells.

8.1 The role of mitochondria in oxidative stress

Mitochondria play a critical role in maintaining cellular homeostasis. This organelle is an important cellular source of energy in producing ATP. In addition they maintain the intracellular levels of calcium within appropriate ranges to mediate cell signaling and control neuronal excitability and synaptic function. In the brain there is a metabolic coupling between vascular substrates, providing oxygen and glucose and the metabolic needs of the brain tissue, formed by neurons and glia alike (Foster et al., 2006).The sequence of events that occurs after neural stimulation includes an initial decrease of oxygen in areas of high demand for this gas (for example, those first stimulated) and a large further increase of oxygen associated with a wide field of arterial vasodilatation. These events are closely related to mitochondrial activity through the production of H_2O_2 as a signaling molecule (Foster et al., 2006).

Like other cells, nerve cells use ATP as a source of energy for biochemical processes involved in various cell functions, and produce ROS as a result of oxidative phosphorylation. The electrical excitability and structural changes, coupled with the synaptic complexity of neurons yields unusual demands in cellular systems that produce or respond to ATP and ROS. Mitochondria in axons and presynaptic terminals provide for sources of ATP to pump ions that are concentrated in these structures to quickly restore the subsequent ion gradients for depolarization and neurotransmitter release. Mitochondria also play a role in the regulation of synaptic functions because of their ability to regulate calcium levels and the production of ROS (Mattson & Liu, 2002).

Neurons in the brain are highly vulnerable to metabolic changes so that a mitochondrial disorder, which causes a decrease in the production of ATP, represents a clear threat to the viability of the neurons and glial cells, the functionality of neural networks, and consequently the normal functions of the brain can be changed. The alteration in the regulation of calcium levels by the failures of the mitochondrial buffer and the release of mitochondria-bound calcium contributes to a severe injury of brain tissue in response to excitotoxicity by glutamate, oxidative stress, or metabolic damage such as trauma. Similarly, an abnormal increase in the generation of ROS by the mitochondria also puts at risk cell viability because many shock-mechanism absorbers might be overwhelmed (Kann & Kovács, 2007).The result is an oxidative damage to the structural and regulatory proteins of the cell membranes that modulate the redox state, and can lead to abnormal activity in various ionic channels. Another event that puts cell viability at risk is the formation of the mitochondrial permeability-transition pore (mPTP), which occurs in response to a mitochondrial overload of calcium in the presence of high levels of ROS. The mitochondrial permeability-transition pore is characterized by an increase in nonspecific permeability in the inner mitochondrial membrane, loss of membrane potential, a possible rupture of the outer membrane, and a severe mitochondrial swelling. When the opening of the mPTP is transitory, the release of cytochrome C from the intermembranal space can activate the caspase cascade that leads to apoptosis. If the opening of the mPTP is prolonged, the mitochondrial content is reduced by quickly causing necrosis (Kann & Kovács, 2007).

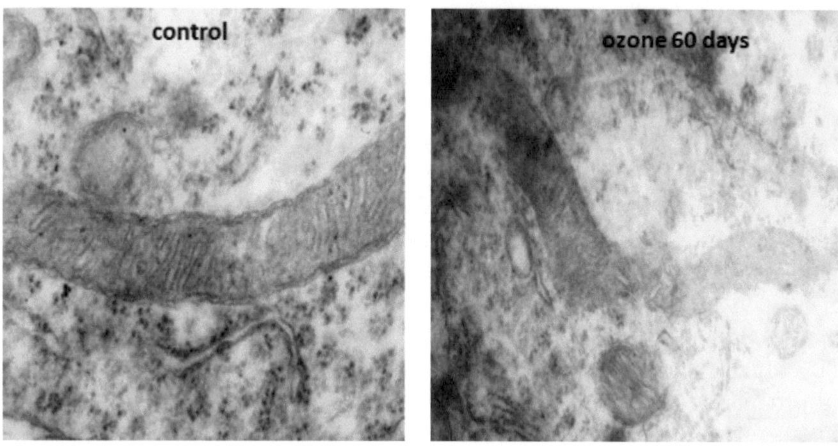

Fig. 7. Electronic microphotography that shows the effects of an oxidative stress state caused by ozone exposure on the neuron mitochondria of the rat hippocampus (30.000x). Observe the loss of the external mitochondrial membrane and damage of the mitochondrial crests after exposure to ozone (right)

9. Oxidative stress state and neurodegenerative process in an animal model

9.1 Ozone as a model for oxidative stress

Various methods have been used to deal with the study of oxidative stress and its biological significance in the organism. This ranges from biochemistry, cell culture, and animal models to clinical studies. Ozone exposure causes the generation of ROS (Chen & Qu, 1997; Kennedy et al., 1992; Pryor, 1994; Pryor & Church, 1991; Romieu et al., 1998, Saintot et al., 1999) and the formation of relatively stable products (Bocci, 2006; Pryor et al.,1995) able to oxidize DNA, proteins (Kanofsky & Sima, 1993), and lipid membranes (Postlethwait et al., 1998), which if they are not offset causes damage and cell death. In the epithelial lining of the lung, the fluid is characterized by high concentrations of antioxidants, mainly ascorbic acid and glutathione (GSH) (Bocci, 2006). To react with these antioxidants a portion of the inhaled ozone is destroyed. The pulmonary antioxidant defenses are able to neutralize the damage, depending on the dose and exposure time, but when they are overwhelmed a chain of chemical reactions begins that leads to the formation of ROS, caused by secondary exposure to ozone. The ROS pass into the blood, and through the bloodstream reach all the organism, producing a state of widespread oxidative stress (Rivas-Arancibia et al., 2000, 2003). The mechanism of toxicity of ozone is explained as a cascade of reactions (Pryor et al., 1995) in which inhaled ozone reacts with molecules in the fluid of the epithelial lining producing ROS and toxic byproducts, which in turn are able to cause other reactions in the blood. This cascade of reactions is responsible for the toxic effects of ozone both in the lung microenvironment and throughout the body (Ballinger et al., 2005; Bocci, 2006; Pryor et al., 1995). Although the majority of the studies on the effects of oxides of carbon, sulphur, nitrogen, and ozone were made in animals, they indicate that damage may be caused in humans when air pollution increases. Oxidative stress caused by acute or prolonged exposure to ozone causes alterations in the brain plasticity that are manifested by the deficit in the learning processes, memory, and motor activity behavior (Rivas-Arancibia et al., 2000; Dorado-Martínez et al., 2001). Exposure to low doses of ozone over a long time causes a process of progressive neurodegeneration (Angoa-Pérez et al., 2006; Pereyra-Muñoz et al., 2006, Rivas-Arancibia 2010).

Brain tissue is most vulnerable to oxidative damage caused by its high consumption of oxygen, a high metabolic rate, and low levels of antioxidant enzymes, such as SOD, glutathione peroxidase, and catalase. A large increase of lipid peroxidate levels is caused by an increase in ROS, because of the brain's high content of polyunsaturated fatty acids that are highly susceptible to oxidation. Different brain structures show differences in their response to oxidative damage (Hermida-Ameijeiras et al., 2004).

There is clear evidence that air pollution causes an oxidizing environment for humans. High levels of contamination in highly populated cities are correlated with the rise of a number of pathologies, such as autoimmune, degenerative, and neurodegenerative diseases. When using a model of oxidative stress, produced by ozone exposure to low doses (0.25 ppm) for 4 hours daily for different times (7, 15, 30, 60, and 90 days), healthy animals developed a process of progressive neurodegeneration that depends on the exposure time (Angoa-Perez et al., 2006; Pereyra-Muñoz et al., 2006; Rivas-Arancibia et al., 2010, Santiago-Lopez et al., 2010).

The increase in the levels of oxidized lipids, proteins, carbohydrates, and nucleic acids are used as indicators of the state of oxidative stress. Levels of antioxidant enzymes and their activity are used as indicators of antioxidant capacity. The determination of oxidized biomolecules and the activity of antioxidant systems clearly determine the redox state in which an individual is found, e.g. we can find high levels of oxidized lipids or proteins, but these can be accompanied by an increase in the activity of the SOD and glutathione peroxidase, or an increase in the levels of reduced glutathione. This indicates that oxidative stress is compensated for because the increase of the prooxidants is accompanied by an increase in the antioxidant systems, which leads to a balanced redox system and tissue changes that are reversible. If the oxidation of the biomolecules increases and there is a decrease in the activity of antioxidant systems, we can then infer that there is a loss of redox balance that produces a state of oxidative stress. This is important to define because many experimental models do not consider these effects and the results are often contradictory. As an example of the models that used ozone, the administration of high doses of this gas in animals may cause a strong antioxidant response and then the increase in the levels of antioxidants has a repair effect on the organism. However, in Wistar rats more than 2-years old, this response causes a severe neuronal and endothelial damage because older animals have a decreased antioxidant activity level in a chronic oxidatively stressed state, and this also occurs in chronic-degenerative diseases.

Another important factor is the dose and exposure time. In healthy young animals exposed to low doses of ozone for 4-h daily for a prolonged time, a chronic oxidative stress state is generated that causes a process of progressive neurodegeneration. This degenerative process becomes irreversible after 30 days of exposure to this gas. Though animals are no longer exposed to ozone the damage continues to make progress. The progressive neurodegeneration process is shown in figures 8,9,10 in which oxidative stress, depending on the time of exposure to ozone, increases the immunoreactivity to p53 and the translocation of p53 to the nucleus, indicating an increase in cell death by apoptosis.

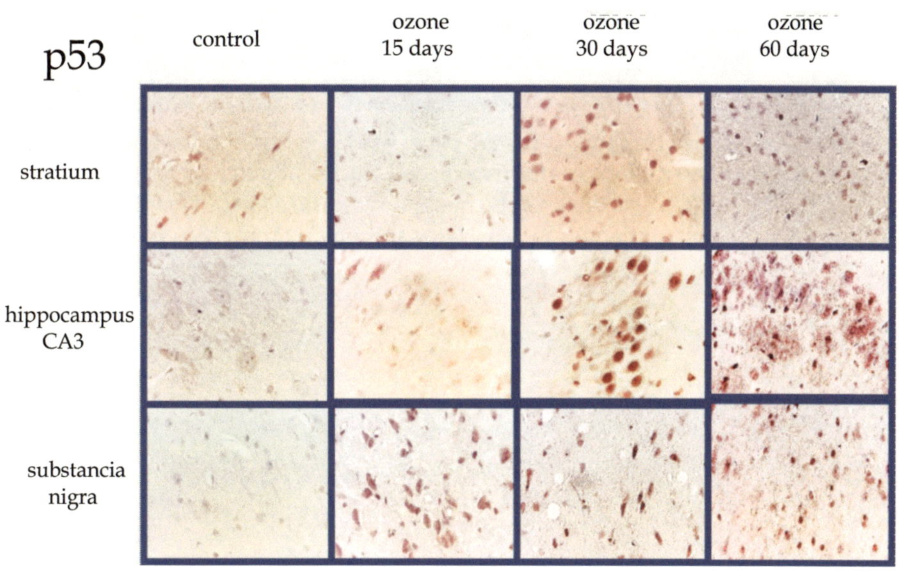

Fig. 8. The effect of oxidative stress on P53 immunoreactivity caused by chronic exposure to low ozone doses for different times (15, 30, and 60 days) in different brain structures (striatum, hippocampus, and substatia nigra). Note immunoreactivity increases in the nucleus as a function of the time of exposure to ozone

This result shows that oxidative stress by itself is able to produce damage and neuronal death, which is accompanied by the loss of regulation of the inflammatory response and by changes in astrocytes and microglia.

We can therefore conclude that oxidative stress caused by ozone produces a state of progressive neurodegeneration, which is characterized by neuronal death, changes in the microglia, loss of regulation of the inflammatory response, and loss of the ability of brain to be repaired.

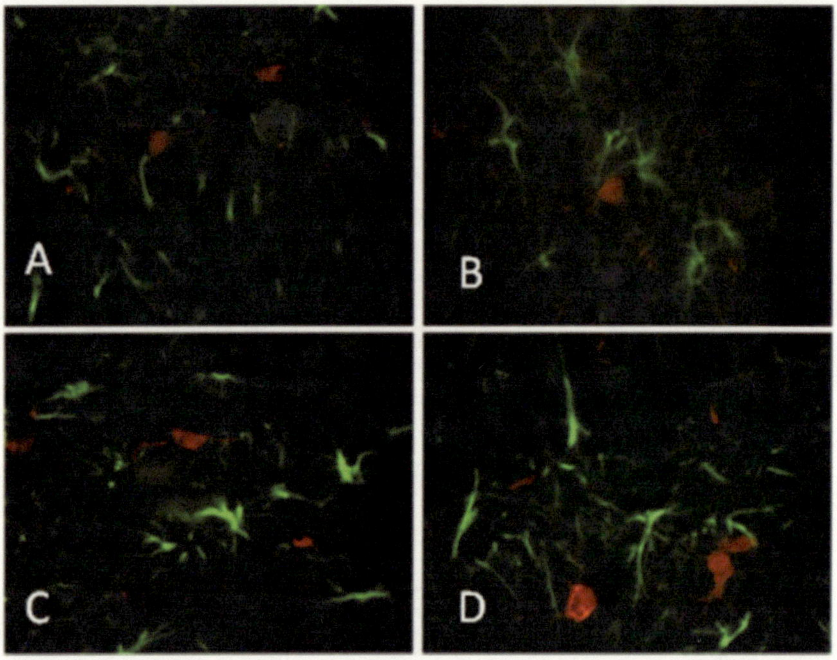

Fig. 9. Double micrograph that shows the effects of oxidative stress on astrocytes (green) and microglia (red) in the rat hippocampus exposed chronically to low ozone doses. Control (A) 30 days (B) 60 days (C), and 90 days (D) of ozone exposure (40x). Note that oxidative stress causes morphological changes in astrocytes and phenotypic changes in microglia

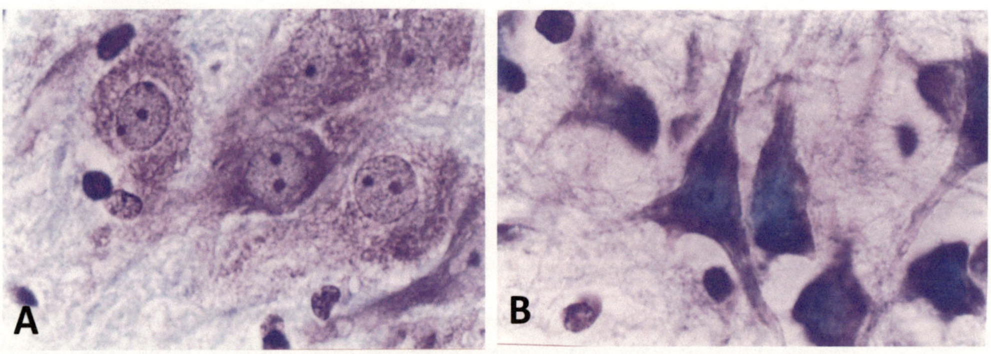

Fig. 10. Micrograph that shows the effects of oxidative stress on the hippocampal neurons of the rat exposed to ozone for 30 days. Control (A) and 30 days of ozone exposure (B) (100x)

10. Neurodegenerative diseases

Neurodegenerative diseases (diseases in which nerve cells degenerate and die) have a variety of symptoms, can affect different parts of the brain, and the causes are multifactorial and still are not entirely clear. All of them have in common the altered mitochondrial function, increased oxidative damage, presence of abnormal aggregates of proteins and proteasomes, alteration in the metabolism of iron, and changes and dysregulation of inflammation and exitotoxicity. All these form a vicious cycle and can initiate cell death and quickly recruit other cells in its destructive purpose. Oxidized proteins are usually removed by the proteasomes. Inhibition of the proteasomes by a redox state alteration leads to an accumulation of abnormal proteins and ROS production. The ROS-producing agents can initiate neurodegeneration because the ROS causes damaged mitochondria, producing an increase in the Ca^{2+}, and inhibiting the function of the proteasomes. The iron in several areas of the brain increases with age and with other metals promotes oxidation, and with this the aggregation of various proteins.

10.1 Oxidative stress and Alzheimer's disease

Alzheimer's disease is characterized by the pathogenic presence of intracellular tangles of tau protein containing hyperphosphorylated and extracellular senile plaques formed primarily by β-amyloid oligomers. Different scenarios have been proposed that explain the causes involved in the development of the disease; one is oxidative stress. There are several studies suggesting that accumulation of free radicals in excess formed during normal metabolism is able to cause oxidation of proteins, DNA and RNA, lipid peroxidation, and modification of sugars, thus generating massive neuronal death in the hippocampus, associated with parts of the neocortex (Praticò, 2008). The formation of senile plaques is caused by the intracellular and extracellular accumulation of insoluble beta amyloid in the brain. The peptide beta amyloid is generated by the splitting of the amyloid precursor protein (APP) that involves the enzymes alpha, beta, and gamma secretases (Rajendran, 2008). There are multiple forms of oligomerization that can be found in the beta amyloid peptide. This peptide can play various physiological and pathological roles depending on

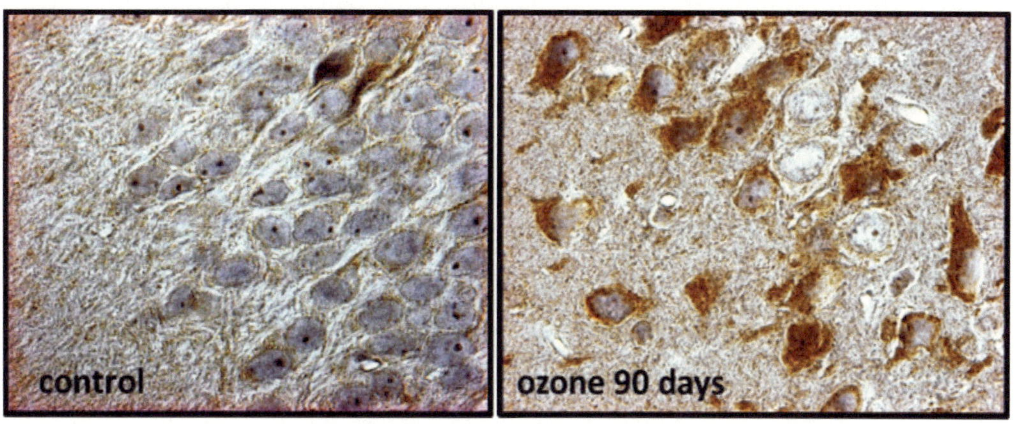

Fig. 12. Microphotography that shows the effects of a chronic, oxidative-stress state on the expression of the insoluble form of β-amyloid 1-42 immunoreactivity in a healthy rat exposed to low ozone doses for 4 h daily for 90 days

the path of its formation. The beta amyloid may deposit in specific regions of brain as amyloid plates that form. Break up of the APP is in two phases; a nonamyloidogenic pathway and an amyloidogenic pathway (Rajendran, 2008). In the nonamyloidogenic pathway, the alpha secretase cleaves in the position of the amino acid 83 from the side carboxyl terminal producing a long ectodominion amino (N) - terminal (sAPPα). The result of this process is the formation of C83, which is retained by the membrane to be cut by the gamma secretase forming short fragments of p3. The breakdown by the alpha secretase occurs in the region of beta amyloid.

The amyloidogenic pathway is an alternate way of rupturing of the APP that leads to the generation of beta amyloid. This path is caused by the beta secretase that cuts in the amino acid 99 allowing the release of sAPPβ in the extracellular space. Subsequently the rupture of this fragment between residue 38 and 43 by γ-secretase releases an intact peptide Aβ. The full length of the β-amyloid peptide is 40 residues ($A\beta_{40}$), with 10% a variant of 42 residues ($A\beta_{42}$). This latter variant is more hydrophobic and easily causes formation of fibrils and is the form of this peptide which predominates in beta amyloid plaques (Rajendran, 2008; Tillement et al., 2010).

Lower levels of the intracellular β-amyloid peptide produce the internalization of the amyloid precursor protein. This internalization is mediated by a low density receptor-related lipoprotein 1B (LRP1B), one of the members of the LDL family, This receptor typically joins the precursor protein of amyloid in the plasma membrane to prevent the internalization of the beta amyloid peptide by reducing its production. The failure of these mechanisms and the association of the tau protein causes the internalization of extracellular protein neurons, which gives rise to the production and outsourcing of the insoluble beta amyloid isoform.

Synthesis of soluble β-amyloid is altered during this phase and increases the synthesis of the insoluble, unfolded β-amyloid as part of the insoluble plates of the β-amyloid. The loss of redox homeostasis, both endogenous or exogenous, produces a state of chronic oxidative stress that increases the production of ROS and RNS, causes a reduced expression or activity of antioxidant systems, accelerates ageing, and plays a key role in the pathogenesis and the course of Alzheimer's disease by the altering of many signaling metabolic pathways in the cell by promoting mutations or altering the postransductional mechanisms. The chronic disruption of the oxidation-reduction balance, causes bad protein folding, products of advanced glycosylation, overload of peroxidation of saturated fatty acids (hydroxynonenal, HNE) (Liu, 2008), oxidation of cholesterol, disturbances in the insulin receptor to cause insulin resistance, and oxidation of LDL receptors involved in the reentry of peptide or the APP (Liu, 2008). We can infer that Alzheimer's is the final manifestation of a series of oxidative alterations of metabolism, which involve different biomolecules, in which the loss of the oxide-reduction balance plays a decisive role in the formation of the phosphorylated tau protein and insoluble beta amyloid .

10.2 Environmental toxics and Parkinson's disease

The initiation and development of the Parkinson disease's (PD) is still uncertain. The pathophysiology is complex and multifactorial and often differs among affected individuals. A large number of studies have provided evidence that loss of redox regulation contributes to all forms of PD, but it has not yet been determined whether the ROS are a primary event or a consequence of the pathogenic factors. An overproduction of ROS is unquestionably an important mediator in cell death in PD (Berg, 2004). It has been suggested that the PD pathogenesis may involve two processes; damage from a specific disease or that combined with damage associated with normal aging. The PD is the result of neurodegeneration in specific areas of the brain (substantia nigra, pars compact, and putamen) resulting in a decrease of dopamine (Cui, 2004). Factors involving dopamine, neuromelanin, increase in the deposits of iron in the substantia nigra, a decrease of ferritin and glutathione (GSH), a deficiency in the role of the complex I mitochondrial respiratory chain, mitochondrial dysfunction and excitotoxicity may be the cause or result of the ROS. Toxins such as paraquat, MPTP, and rotenone have proven to increase the risk of PD in humans. Studies with animal models and cells reveal the oxidative and inflammatory properties of these toxins, and their ability to activate glial cells that subsequently destroy the neighboring dopaminergic neurons. The activity of the complex I mitochondria is deficient in the substance nigra (SN) in PD and can be associated with a genetic abnormality or be the result of oxidative stress. The postulate of a defect in the mitochondrial DNA is still uncertain. It has been shown in the culture of dopaminergic cells that the decrease of glutathione, from the selective loss in the activity of the mitochondrial complex I is an important feature of PD.

10.2.1 Dopaminergic system

Dopamine (DA) is a catecholamine that plays an important role in the human brain as an inhibitory neurotransmitter, particularly involved in the regulation of motor function. It is synthesized in the nerve terminals from tyrosine, the precursor of the amino acid dopaminergic neurons. The synthesis begins with the formation of L-DOPA, through the action of tyrosine hydroxylase and the biopteridines. The former enzyme is the limiting enzyme in the synthesis of dopamine. The activity is strictly controlled. L-DOPA is metabolized to form DA by an aromatic amino acid decarboxylase. In the nerve terminals, the DA is stored in synaptic vesicles with an acid content because it prevents the autoxidation of the DA until it is released. The action ends with the uptake of DA by a membrane transporter and the subsequent reuse or catabolism by the enzyme monoamino-oxidase (MAO) or the catechol-o-methyltransferase (COMT). Within the brain, dopaminergic systems are involved in processes of motivation, learning, memory, and motor control. It is estimated that dopamine is > 80% of the total content of catecholamines in the brain. The greatest risk of the DA is that this catechol group oxidizes easily through a process that involves the transfer of an electron to oxygen. Thus, this oxidation results in the formation of an superoxide anion, hydrogen peroxide, hydroxyl radical, and other ROS that are able to generate a state of oxidative stress and start a process of neurodegeneration.

10.2.2 Dopamine as a source of ROS in the CNS

Mechanisms through which the DA stimulates the production of ROS have been proposed. These depend on the presence or absence of enzyme mediators. It is known that the DA of the SN and the striatum (STR) is deaminated by the enzyme MAO located in the outer membrane of the mitochondrion. This reaction has resulted in the production of a superoxide radical, hydroxyl radical, and hydrogen peroxide (Graham, 1978). Proposed mechanisms through which the DA stimulates the production of ROS depend on the presence or absence of enzyme mediators.

The endogenous dopamine-derived N-methyl(R)salsolinol is one of the most studied derivatives of DA for two reasons. It is present in the human brain and can easily become a neurotoxin able to cause cell death. It has been proposed that this compound can be formed by an enzymatic pathway that involves a synthase or a nonenzymatic pathway by the condensation of the DA with acetaldehyde (Naoi et al., 1996).Another derivative of the DA is the tetrahydropapaveroline (THP), which is obtained from enzymatic catabolism. The THP by itself is able to cause necrosis in neuroblastom cells and is related to the pathogenesis of Parkinson's disease. Derivatives of the metabolism of DA act as proneurotoxins in the development of Parkinson's disease. It is known that certain components of tobacco smoke may react with these proneurotoxins preventing its activation. This may explain the beneficial effect of smoking on the incidence of Parkinson's disease (Hermida-Ameijeiras et al., 2004).

10.2.3 The autoxidation of dopamine

Another mechanism through which DA can contribute to the formation of ROS is its spontaneous autoxidation. The DA is a molecule of the catechol group that can easily oxidize nonenzymatically to form a series of electrochemical type quinoide species. The initial step in the oxidation of the DA involves a reaction with molecular oxygen to form two molecules of the superoxide anion and DA-o-quinone. The formation of the superoxide anions during the autoxidation of the DA leads to the production of hydrogen peroxide by the dismutation of superoxide. The DA-o-quinone then undergoes an intramolecular clyclization to form 5,6-dihydroxiquinoline, which is subsequently oxidized by the DA-o-quinone to form dopaminochrome. This compound undergoes a rearrangement to form 5,6-dihydroxyindole, which in turn is oxidized to an indole quinone. The next

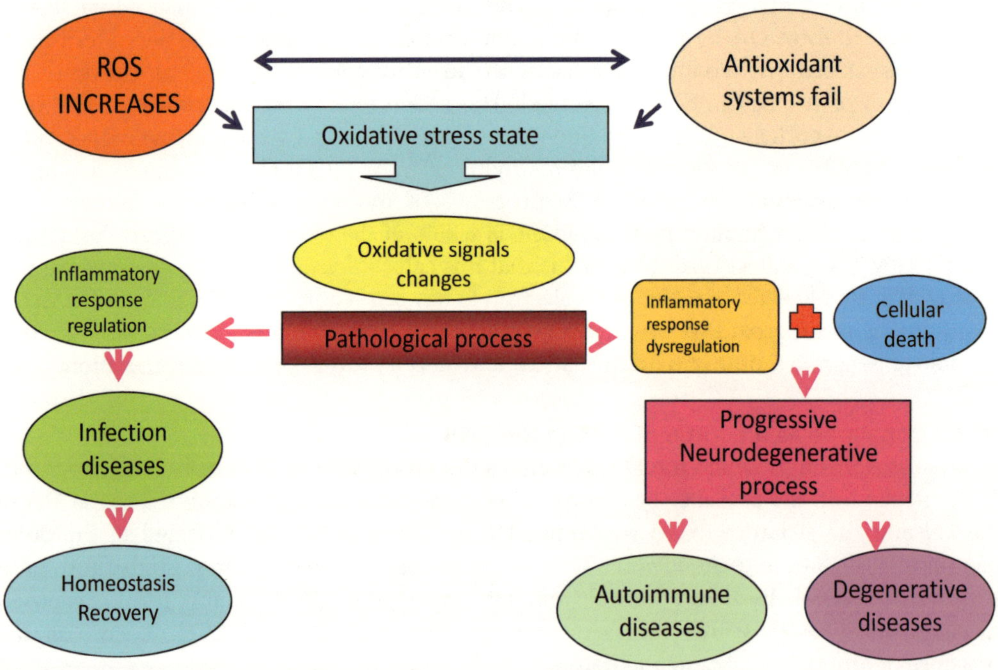

Fig. 13. Showing the effect of oxidative stress on the pathological process and the pathway that is followed depending on the regulation or nonregulation of the inflammatory responses

polymerization process eventually leads to the generation of a dark pigment called neuromelanin. The dark appearance of the SN is caused by the presence of this pigment containing products derived from the oxidation of the cysteinyl-DA. When the autoxidation of the DA takes place in the presence of L-cysteine, the DA-o-Quinone undergoes a nucleophilic attack by the thiol of the amino acid group to form cysteinyl-DA. This differs from normal oxidation of the DA to form neuromelanin (Hermida-Ameijeiras et al., 2004).

11. Conclusions

In a balanced oxidation-reduction system, reactive species have an effect as signaling or a regulator of both the glia and neurons in internal signaling pathways, act as regulators of the immune response, which includes inflammatory response, and as regulators of the cell cycle, neuroplasticity, and metabolism. The short-term loss of the oxidation-reduction balance causes an increase in the activity of antioxidant systems to counteract the oxidative stimulus. The endogenous increase of the antioxidant systems play a restorative role of the organism. An enlightening physiological example of this is the repairing role of exercise in chronic degenerative diseases, which is explained by a rise in free radicals as a consequence of an increase in endogenous antioxidant systems.

The loss of the redox balance (as shown in the model of oxidative stress caused by ozone) implies a loss of regulation of the inflammatory response, which then causes a reparative and self-limiting response. This becomes a perpetual response, a vicious cycle, in which there is mitochondrial failure that leads to a lack of ATP, an increase in the state of oxidative stress, loss of regulation of inflammatory markers, blocking of antioxidant systems, inability to synthesize new proteins, disorders of the proteasome, accumulation of misfolded proteins, and the conformational change in key receptors involved in metabolism and cell signaling. All of them, established slowly over time, can produce chronic degenerative diseases and neurodegenerative diseases as a manifestation of a series of alterations caused by multiple factors, including that of the establishment of a state of chronic-oxidative stress. This plays a key role in the loss of the regulation of cell signaling, of the different responses that lead to neuronal death and loss of brain repair and the altering of the process of neurogenesis. All these are clinically manifested into neurodegenerative diseases long after the vicious cycle has started. The discovery of early oxidative markers specific to each neurodegenerative disease can allow an early diagnosis and break the vicious cycle established by oxidative stress. This can be seen occurring in the near future for the treatment and detection of these diseases.

12. Acknowledgment

Acknowledgment to Dirección General de Apoyo al Personal Académico (IN219511-3 to S R-A). The authors thank Gabino Borgonio-Perez for his invaluable technical support. Thanks to Dr. Ellis Glazier for editing this English-language text.

13. References

Angoa-Pérez, M. Jiang, H. Rodriguez, A. Lemini, C. Levine, RA. Rivas-Arancibia, S. (2006). Estrogen counteracts ozone-induced oxidative stress and nigral neuronal death. *Neuroreport*, 24, 17, 6, pp. 629-33.

Aurand, LW. Boone, NH. Giddings, GG. (1977). Superoxide and singletoxigen in milk peroxidation. *J. Dairy Sci*, 60, 3, pp. 363-369.

Baccarini, DP. (1978). Coupled oxidation of NADPH with thiols at neutral pH. *Arch. Biochem. Biophys*, 191, pp. 315-357.

Baldwin, AS Jr. (1996). The NF-kappa B and I kappa B proteins: new discoveries and insights. *Annu Rev Immunol*, 14, pp. 649-683.

Ballinger, CA. Cueto, R. Squadrito, G. Coffin, JF. Velsor, LW. Pryor, WA. Postlethwait, EM. (2005). Antioxidant-mediated augmentation of ozone-induced membrane oxidation. *Free Radic Biol Med*, 15, 38, 4, pp. 515-26.

Battaner, E. Catalán, J. López, MF. De Luis, JM. Ruiz, CA. Galán, M. (1990). Resolution of amin acid racemates with D amino acid oxidase. Storage stabilityof theenzyme. 5 thMediterranean Congress on Chemical Engineering. Barcelona.

Beckman, JS. Koppenol, WH. (1996). Nitric oxide, superoxide, andperoxyinitrite: the good, the bad and ugly. *Am. J. Physio*, 271, pp. C1424-C1437.

Beckman, JS. Ye, YZ. Anderson, P. Chen, J. Accavetti, MA. Tarpey, MM. White, CR. (1994). Extensive nitration of protein tyrosines in hymanatheroscleosis detected by immunohistochemistry. *Biol.Chem. Hoppe. Seyler*, 375, pp. 81-88.

Beckman, KB. Ames, BN. (1998). The free radical theory of anging matures. *Physiol. Rev.* 78, pp 547-581.

Behar, D. Czapski, G. Rabami, J. Dorfman, IM. Schwarz, HA. (1979). The acid disociation constant and decay kinetics of parthydroxyl radical. *J. Phys. Chem*, 72, pp. 3209-3215.

Berg, D. Youdim, MB. Riederer, P. (2004). Redox imbalance. *Cell Tissue Res*, 318, pp. 201-13.

Bhalla, DK. (1999). Ozone-induced lung inflammation and mucosal barrier disruption: Toxicology, mechanisms and implications. *J. Toxicol. Environ. Health B*, 2, pp 31–86.

Bhalla, DK. Gupta, SK. (2000). Lung injury, inflammation, and inflammatory stimuli in rats exposed to ozone. *J Toxicol Environ Health A*, 25, 59, 4, pp. 211-28.

Bielsky, BH. Gebieki, JM. (1977). Application of radiation chemistry tobiology. *Free radicals in biology. W.A., P., Academic Press*, 3, pp. 1-19.

Biniert, GP. Schjoerring, JK. Jahn, TP. (2006). Membrane transport of hydrogen peroxide. *Biochim Biophys Acta*, 1758, pp. 994-1003.

Bocci V. (2006). Is it true that ozone is always toxic? The end of a dogma. *Toxicol Appl Pharmacol*, 1, 216, 3, pp. 493-504.

Boveris, A. Chance, B. (1973). The mitocondrial generation of hydrogen peroxide. *Biochem J*, 134, pp. 707-716.

Bredt, D. S. Hwang, P. M. Glatt, C. E. Lownstein, C. Reed, R R. Synder, SH. (1991). 450 Reductase. *Nature* , 351, pp. 714-718.

Bruel-Jungerman, E. Lucassen, PJ. Francis, F. (2011). Cholinergic influences on cortical development and adult neurogenesis. *Behav Brain Res*, 10, 221, 2, pp. 379-88.

Bruunsgaard, H. Andersen-Ranberg, K, Hjelmborg, JB. Pedersen, BK. Jeune, B. (2003a). Elevated levels of tumor necrosis factor alpha and mortality in centenarians. *Am J Med*, 115, pp. 278-283.

Buetler, TM. Krauskopf, A. Ruegg UT. (2004). Role of superoxide as a signaling molecule. *News Physiol Sci*, 19, pp. 120–123.

Burgering, BM. Medema, RH. (2003). Decisions on life and death: FOXO Forkhead transcription factors are in command when PKB/Akt is off duty. *J Leukoc Biol*, 73, pp. 689-701.

Butterfield, DA, Castegna, A, Pocernick, CB. (2002). Nutritional approaches to combat oxidative stress in Alzheimer's disease. *J Nut Biochem*, 13, pp. 444-61.

Capdevila, L. Parkhill, L. Chacos, N. Okita, R. Masters, BBS. Estabrook, RW. (1981). The oxidative metabolism of arachidonic acid by purifiedcytocromes P450. *Biochem. Biophys. Res. Commun*, 101, pp. 1357-1362.

Chao, JC. Yuen, MD. Chen, PY. Chien, SW. (2002). Vitamin C and E supplements improve the impaired antioxidant status and decrease plasma lipid peroxides in hem dialysis patients. *J NutBiochem*, 13(11, pp. 653-63.

Chen, LC. Qu, Q. (1997). Formation of intracellular free radicals in guinea pig airway epithelium during in vitro exposure to ozone. *Toxicol Appl Pharmacol*, 143, 1, pp. 96-101.

Chiarugi, P. Fiaschi, T. (2007). Redox signalling in anchorage-dependent cell growth. *Cell Signal*, 19, pp. 672-682.

Chignell, CF. (1979). Spin labelling in pharmacology. *Espin labeling. NewYork, Academic Press*. 2, pp. 223-228.

Christman, MF. Morgan, RW. Jacobson, FS. Ames, BN. (1985). Positive control of a regulon for defences against oxidative stress and some heat-shock proteins in Salmonella typhimurium. *Cell*, 41(3), pp. 753-62.

Chung, HY. Cesari, M. Anton, S. Marzetti, E. Giovannini, S. Seo, AY. (2009). Molecular inflammation: underpinnings of aging and agerelated diseases. *Ageing. Res Rev*, 8, pp. 18-30.

Chung, HY. Cesari, M. Anton, S. Marzetti, E. Giovannini, S. Seo, AY. (2009). Molecular inflammation: underpinnings of aging and agerelated diseases. *Ageing Res Rev*, 8, pp. 18-30.

Commoner, B. Townsend, J. Pake, GE. (1954). Free radicals in biological materials. *Nature*, 9:174(4432), pp. 689-91.

Creţu, DI. Sovrea, A. Ignat, RM. Filip, A. Bidian, C. Creţu, A. (2010). Morpho-pathological and physiological changes of the brain and liver after ozone exposure. *Rom J Morphol Embryol*, 51, 4, pp. 701-6.

Cui, K. Luo, X. Xu, K. Ven Murthy, MR. (2004). Role of oxidative stress in neurodegeneration: recent developments in assay methods for oxidative stress and nutraceutical antioxidants. *Prog Neuro psychopharmacol Biol Psychiatry*, 28, pp. 771-99.

Dedon, P. C. y I.H., Goldberg. (1982). Free radical mechanisms involved in theformation of sequence-dependent bristanded DNA lesions by the antitumorantibiotics bleomycin. *Chem. Res. Toxicol*, 5(3), pp. 311-332.

Devaux, B. Scholz, D. Hirche, A. Klovekorn, WP. Schaper, J. (1997). Upregulation of cell adhesion molecules and the presence of low grade inflammation in human chronic heart failure. *Eur Heart J*, 18, pp. 470-479.

Dolphin, D. (1988). The generation of free radicals during the normal and abnormal functioning of citocromes P450. *Basic Life Sci*, 49, pp. 491-500.

Dorado-Martínez, C. Paredes-Carbajal, C. Mascher, D. Borgonio-Pérez, G. Rivas-Arancibia, S. (2001). Effects of different ozone doses on memory, motor activity and lipid peroxidation levels, in rats. *Int J Neurosci*, 108, 3-4, pp. 149-61.

Doroshow, J. Hochstein, P. (1982). Redox cycling and the mechanism ofaction of antibiotics in neoplasicdiseades. *Pathology of Oxigen. New York,Academic Press*, pp. 245-253.

Droge, W. (2002). Free radicals in the physiological control of cell function. *Physiol Rev*, 82(1), pp. 47-95.

Floyd, RA. Towner, RA. He, T. Hensley, K. Maples, KR. (2011). Translational research involving oxidative stress and diseases of aging. *Free Radic Biol Med*, 51, 5, pp. 931-41.

Foster, KA. Galeffi, F. Gerich, FJ. Turner, DA. Müler, M. (2006). Optical and pharmacological tools to investigate the role of mitochondria during oxidative stress and neurodegeneration. *Prog Neurobiol*. 79:136-171.

Freeman, BA. Crapo, J. (1982). Free radicals and tissue injury. *Lab. Invest*, 47, pp. 412-426.

Frei, B. (1994). Reactive oxygen species an antioxidant vitamins: Mechanismsof action. *Am. J. Med*, 97, 3A, pp. 5S-13S.

Fridovich, I. (1986). Oxygen Radicals, Hydrogen Peroxide and OxygenToxicity. Free Radicals and Biology. Pryor, W. A. *New York, AcademicPress*. 1, pp. 239-246.

Ghouleh, I. Khoo, NK. Knaus, UG. Griendling, KK. Touyz, RM. Thannickal, VJ. Barchowsky, A. Nauseef, WM. Kelley, EE. Bauer, PM. Darley-Usmar,V. Shiva, S. Cifuentes-Pagano, E. Freeman, BA. Gladwin, MT. Pagano, PJ. (2011). Oxidases and peroxidases in cardiovascular and lung disease: New concepts in reactive oxygen species signaling. *Free Radic Biol Med*, 1, 51, 7, pp. 1271-88.

Goldstein, S. Czapski, G. Lind, J. Merényi, G. (2000). Tyrosin nitration bysimultaneous generation of NO• and O2• - under physiological conditions.How the radicals do the job. *J. Biol. Chem*, 275, pp. 3031-3036.

Gomberg, M. (1900). An instance of trivalent carbon: triphenylmethyl. *J. Am. Chem. Soc*, 22, 11, pp. 757–771.

Götz, ME. Janetzky, B. Pohl,i S. Gottschalk, A. Gsell, W. Tatschner, T. Ransmayr, G. Leblhuber, F. Gerlach, M. Reichmann, H. Riederer, P. Böning, J. (2001). Chronic alcohol consumption and cerebral indices of oxidative stress: is there a link?. *Alcohol Clin Exp Res*, 25, 5, pp. 717-25.

Graham., DG. (1978). Oxidative pathways for catecholamines in the genesis of neuromelanin and citotoxic quininas. *Mol. Pharmacol*, 14, pp. 633-643.

Grisham, MB. Jourd´heuil, D. Wink, DA. (1999). Nitric Oxide I. Physiological chemistry of nitric oxide and its metabolites: implications in inflammation. *Am. J. Physiol*, 276, pp. G315-G321.

Gryglewsli, RJ. Palmer, RMJ. Moncada, S. (1986). Superoxide anion isinvolved in the breakdown of endotrhelium-derived vascular relaxing factor. *Nature*, 320, pp. 454-456.

Gutteridge, JM. Halliwel, B. (1989). Iron toxicity and oxygen radicals. *Baillieres Clin Hematol*, 2, 2, pp. 195-256.

Halliwel, B. Gutteridge, J.M. (1984). Lipid peroxidation, oxygen radicals, cell damage and antioxidant therapy. *Lancet*, 23, pp. 1396-98.

Halliwell, B. (2006). Oxidative stress and neurodegeneration: where are we now?. *J Neurochem*, 97, pp. 1634 58.

Halliwell, B. Gutteridge, JM. (1989). *Free radicals in biology and medicine*. Oxford, Clarendon Press.

Halliwell, B. Gutteridge, JM. (1992). Bologically relevant metal ion-dependent OH generation. *FEBS LETT*, 307, pp. 108.

Halliwell, B. Gutteridge, JM. (2007). *Free radicals in biology and medicine*. 4th ed. Oxford University Press, Oxford.

Handel, ML. McMorrow, LB. Gravallese, EM. (1995). Nuclear factor-kappa B in rheumatoid synovium. Localization of p50 and p65. *Arthritis Rheum*, 38, pp. 1762-1770.

Harman, D. (1956). Aging: a theory based on free radical and radiation chemistry. *J Gerontol*, 11, 3, pp. 298-300.

Hedrick, SM. (2009). The cunning little vixen: Foxo and the cycle of life and death. *Nat Immunol* 10:1057-1063.

Hermida-Armeijeiras, A. Méndez-Álvarez, E. Sánchez-Iglesias, S. Sanmartín-Suárez, C. Soto-Otero, R. (2004). Autoxidation and MAO-mediated metabolism of dopamine as potential cause of oxidative stress: role of ferrous and ferric ions. *Neurochem. Int*, 45, pp. 103-116.

Hoenyet, KMJ. Dagneli, PC. Delaere, KPJ. (2005). Effect of a nutritional supplement containing vitamin E, Selenium, vitamin C and Coenzyme Q10 on serum PSA in patients with hormonally untreated carcinoma of the Prostate. *European Urology*, 47, pp. 433-40.

Janolino, VG. Swaisgood, HE. (1975). Isolation and characterization of sulfhydryl oxidase from bovine milk. J. Biol. Chem, 250, pp. 2532-2538.

Jourd´heuil, D. Jourd´heuil, FL. Kutchukian, PS. Musah, RA. Wink, DA. Grisham, MB. (2001). Reaction of Superoxide and Nitric Oxide withPeroxinitrite.*J. Biol. Chem*, 276, pp. 28799-28805.

Kann, O. Kovacs. R. (2007). Mitochondria and neuronal activity. *Am J Physiol Cell Physio*, 292, pp. C641-657.

Kanofsky, JR. Sima, PD. (1993). Singlet-oxygen generation at gas-liquid interfaces: a significant artifact in the measurement of singlet-oxygen yields from ozone-biomolecule reactions. *Photochem Photobiol*, 58(3), pp. 335-40.

Kennedy, CH. Church, DF. Winston, GW. Pryor, WA. (1992). tert-Butyl hydroperoxide-induced radical production in rat liver mitochondria. *Free Radic Biol Med*, 12, 5, pp. 381-7.

Kim, HJ. Kim, KW. Yu, BP. Chung, HY. (2000). The effect of age on cyclooxygenases-2 gene expression: NF-kappaB activation and IkappaBalpha degradation. *Free Radic Biol Med*, 28, pp. 683-692.

Kirkwood, TB. (2005). Understanding the odd science of aging. *Cell*, 120, pp. 437 47.

Korycka-Dahi, M. Richardson, T. (1981). Initiation of oxidative changes infoods. Symposium: oxidative changes in milk. *J. Dairy. Sci*, 63, pp. 1181-1208.

Kovacik, P. Pozos, RS. (2006). Cell signaling (mechanism and repoductive toxicity): redox chains, radicals, electrons, relays, conduit, electrochemistry, and other medical implications. *Birth Defects Res C Embryo*, 78, pp. 333-344.

Lawlor, MA. Alessi, DR. (2001). PKB/Akt: a key mediator of cell proliferation, survival and insulin responses?. *J Cell Sci*, 114, Pt 16, pp. 2903-2910.

Lee, J. Kosaras, B. Del Signore, SJ. Cormier, K. McKee, A. Ratan, RR. Kowall, NW. Ryu, H. (2011) Modulation of lipid peroxidation and mitochondrial function improves neuropathology in Huntington's disease mice. *Acta Neuropathol*, 121, 4, pp. 487-98.

Lee, JD. Ulevitch, RJ. Han, J. (1995). Primary structure of BMK1: a new mammalian map kinase. *Biochem Biophys Res Commun*, 15, 213, 2, pp. 715-24.

Liochev, SI. Fridovich, I. (1994). The role of O2.- in the production of HO. :in vitro and in vivo. *Free Radical Biol. Med*, 16, pp. 29-33.

Liu, L. Cavanaugh, JE. Wang, Y. Sakagami, H. Mao, Z. Xia, Z. (2003). ERK5 activation of MEF2-mediated gene expression plays a critical role in BDNF-promoted survival of developing but not mature cortical neurons. *Proc Natl Acad Sci, U S A*, 100, 14, pp. 8532-7.

Liu, L. Komatsu, H. Murray, IV. Axelsen, PH. (2008). Promotion of amyloid beta protein misfolding and fibrillogenesis by a lipid oxidation product. *J Mol Biol*, 4, 377, 4, pp. 1236-50.

Lymar, SV. Hurst, JK. (1995). Role of compartmentation in promotingtoxicity of leukocyte-generated strong oxidants. *J. Am. Chem. Soc*, 117, pp. 8867-8868.

MacMicking, J. Xie, QW. Nathan, C. (1997). Nitric oxide and macrophagefunction. *Annu. Rev. Immunol*, 15, pp. 323-350.

Maher, P. Schubert, D. (2000). Signaling by reactive oxygen species in the nervous system. *Cell Mol Life Sci*, 57, pp. 1287-305.

Maiorino, M. Chu, F. Ursoni, F. (1991). GPx-PH is the 18 KDaSelenio protein expressed in human tumor cell lines. *Journal of Biological Chemistry*, 266, 12, pp. 7728 - 32.

Marinkovic, D. Zhang, X. Yalcin, S. Luciano, JP. Brugnara, C. Huber, T. (2007). Fox03 is required for the regulation of oxidative stress in erythropoiesis. *J Clin Invest*, 117, pp. 2133-2144.

Mason, RP. (1982). Free radical intermediates in the metabolism oftoxicological significance. *Free radicals biology*. Pryor, W. A. New York,Academic Press, pp. 262-165.

Massey, V. Shopfer, L. M. Nishino, T. Nishino, T. (1989). Differences inprotein structure of xanthine dehydrogenase and xanthine oxidase revealed byreconstitution with flavin active site probes. *J. Biol. Chem*, 264, pp. 10567-10573.

Mattson, MP. Liu, D. (2002). Energetics and oxidative stress in synaptic plasticity and neurodegenerative disorders. *Neuromolecular Med*, 2, pp. 215-231.

Mayes, PA. (1997). Estructura y función de vitaminas liposolubles. *Bioquímica de Harper*. El Manual Moderno, S. A, pp. 728-31.

McCord, JM. (2000). Evolution of free radicals and oxidative stress. *Am. J. Med*, 108, pp. 652-659.

McCord, JM. Fridovich, I. (1969). Superoxide dismutase. An enzymic function for erythrocuprein (hemocuprein). *J Biol Chem*, 244, 22, pp. 6049-55.

McCord, JM. Fridovich, I. (1969). The utility of superoxide dismutase in studying free radicals reaction. I. Radicals generated by the interaction of sulfite, dimethyl sulfoxide, and oxygen. *J Biol Chem*, 244(22), pp. 6056-63.

Mendiratta, S. Qu, ZC. May, JM. (1998b). Enzyme-dependent ascorbate recycling in human erythrocytes: role of thioredoxin reductase. *Free Radic Biol Med*, 25, pp. 221–228.

Mendiratta, S. Qu, ZC. May, JM. (1998a). Erythrocyte ascorbate recycling: antioxidant effects in blood. *Free Radic Biol Med*, 24, pp. 789–797.

Miles, AM. Bohle, DS. Glassbrenner, PA. Hansert, B. Winks, DA. Grisham, MB. (1996). Modulation of superoxide-dependent oxidation andhydroxylation reations by nitric oxide. *J. Biol. Chem*. 271: 40-47.

Naoi, M. Maruyama, W. Dostert, P. Hashizume, Y. Nakahara, D. Takahashi, T. Ota, M. (1996). Dopamine-derived endogenous 1(R),2(N)-dimethyl-6,7-dihydroxy- 1,2,3,4-tetrahydroisoquinoline, N-methyl-(R)-salsolinol, induced parkinsonism in rat: biochemical, pathological and behavioral studies. *Brain Res*, 19, 709, 2, pp. 285-95.

Nenzil, J. Weber, C. Kontush, A. (2001). The role of vitamin E in Atherogenesis. *Atherosclerosis*, 157, 2, pp. 257-83.
Nohl, H. Jordan, W. (1986). The mitochondrial site of superoxide formation. Biochem. Biophys. *Res. Commun*, 138, pp. 533-539.
Ohno, H. Suzuki, K. Ffujii, J. Yamashita, H. Kizaki, T. Oh-ishi, S. Taniguchi, N. (1994). Exercise and Oxygen Toxicity. *Amsterdam, Elsevier Publishers*.
Pan, XD. Zhu, YG. Lin, N. Zhang, J. Ye, QY. Huang, HP. Chen, XC. (2011). Microglial phagocytosis induced by fibrillar β-amyloid is attenuated by oligomeric β-amyloid: implications for Alzheimer's disease. *Mol Neurodegener,*. 30, 6, pp. 45.
Penn, MS. Sapp, SK. Hsu, A. Topol, EJ. (2003). Use of antioxidant vitamins for the prevention of cardiovascular disease. *Lancet*, 361, 9374, pp. 2017-23.
Pereyra-Muñoz, N. Rugerio-Vargas, C. Angoa-Pérez, M. Borgonio-Pérez, G. Rivas-Arancibia, S. (2006). Oxidative damage in substantia nigra and striatum of rats chronically exposed to ozone. *J Chem Neuroanat*. 31, 2, pp. 114-23.
Postlethwait, EM. Cueto, R. Velsor, LW. Pryor, WA. (1998). O3-induced formation of bioactive lipids: estimated surface concentrations and lining layer effects. *Am J Physiol*, 274(6 Pt 1), pp. L1006-16.
Praticò, D. (2008). Evidence of oxidative stress in Alzheimer's disease brain and antioxidant therapy: lights and shadows. *Ann N Y Acad Sci*, 1147, pp. 70-8.
Pryor, WA. (1994). Mechanisms of radical formation from reactions of ozone with target molecules in the lung. *Free Radic Biol Med*, 17, pp. 451–465.
Pryor, WA. Church DF. (1991). Aldehydes, hydrogen peroxide, and organic radicals as mediators of ozone toxicity. *Free Radic Biol Med*, 11, 1, pp. 41-6.
Pryor, WA. Squadrito, GL. (1995). The chemistry of peroxynitrite: a product from the reaction of nitric oxide with superoxide. *Am J Physiol*, 268, 5 Pt 1, pp. L699-722.
Rajendran, L. Schneider, A. Schlechtingen, G. Weidlich, S. Ries, J. Braxmeier, T. Schwille, P. Schulz, JB. Schroeder, C. Simons, M. Jennings, G. Knölker, HJ. Simons, K. (2008). Efficient inhibition of the Alzheimer's disease beta-secretase by membrane targeting. *Science*, 25,320,5875, pp. 520-3.
Rayman, MP. (2000). The importance of selenium in human health. *Lancet*, 356, pp. 233-41.
Ridker, PM. Stampfer, MJ. Rifai, N. (2001). Novel risk factors for systemic atherosclerosis: a comparison of C-reactive protein, fibrinogen, homocysteine, lipoprotein(a), and standard cholesterol screening as predictors of peripheral arterial disease. J Am Med Assoc, 285, pp. 2481-2485.
Rivas-Arancibia, S. Dorado-Martinez, C. Borgonio-Pérez, G. Hiriart-Urdanivia, M. Verdugo-Díaz, L. Durán-Vázquez, A. Colín-Barenque, L. Ávila-Costa, MR. (2000). Effects of taurine on ozone-induced memory déficits and lipid peroxidation levels in brain of young, mature and old rats. Environ. Res, 82, pp. 7-17.
Rivas-Arancibia, S. Dorado-Martinez, C. Colín-Barenque, L. Kendrick, K. M. de la Riva, C. Guevara-Guzmán, R. (2003). Effect of acute ozone exposure on locomotor behavior and striatal function. Pharm Biochem Beh, 74, pp. 891-900.
Rivas-Arancibia, S. Guevara-Guzmán, R. López-Vidal, Y. Rodríguez-Martínez, E. Zanardo-Gomes, M. Angoa-Pérez, M. Raisman-Vozari, R. (2010). Oxidative stress caused by ozone exposure induces loss of brain repair in the hippocampus of adult rats. *Toxicol Sci*, 113, 1, pp. 187-97.

Romero-Alvira, D. Calvo Rebollar, M. Villalba Martín, MP. Amiguet García, JA. Bueno Gómez, J. (1987). Radicales libres y especies activadasdeloxígeno. Química, Biología e implicaciones en patología médica. *I. An.Med. Intern.* 4, pp. 672-679.

Romieu, I. Meneses, F. Ramirez, M. Ruiz, S. Perez Padilla, R. Sienra, JJ. Gerber, M. Grievink, L. Dekker, R. Walda, I. Brunekreef, B. (1998). Antioxidant supplementation and respiratory functions among workers exposed to high levels of ozone. *Am J Respir Crit Care Med,* 158, 1. pp. 226-32.

Ryter, SW. Kim, HP. Hoetzel, A. Park, JW. Nakahira, K. Wang, X. Choi, AM. (2007). Mechanisms of cell death in oxidative stress. *Antiox Redox Signal,* 9, pp. 49-89.

Sáez, G. Tornalley, PJ. Hill, HA. O. Hems, R. Bannister, JV. (1982). The production of free radicals during the autoxidation of cysteine and their effecto on isolated Hepatocytes. *Biochem. Biophys. Acta,* 719, pp. 24-31.

Saintot, M. Bernard, N. Astre, C. Gerber, M. (1999). Ozone exposure and blood antioxidants: a study in a periurban area in Southern France. *Arch Environ Health,* 54, 1, pp. 34-9.

Salih, DA. Brunet, A. (2008). FoxO transcription factors in the maintenance of cellular homeostasis during aging. *Curr Opin Cell Biol,* 20, pp. 126-136.

Salminen, A. Kaarniranta, K. (2010). Genetics vs entropy: longevity factors suppress the NF-κB-driven entropic aging process. *Ageing Res Rev,* 9, pp. 298-314.

Santiago-López, JA. Bautista-Martínez, CI. Reyes-Hernandez, M. Aguilar-Martínez, S. Rivas-Arancibia. (2010). Oxidative stress, progressive damage in the substantia nigra and plasma dopamine oxidation, in rats chronically exposed to ozone, *Toxicol Lett,* 197, 3, pp. 193-200.

Schreck, R. Albermann, K. Baeuerle, PA. (1992). Nuclear factor kappa B: an oxidative stress-responsive transcription factor of eukaryotic cells. *Free Radic Res Commun,* 17, 4, pp. 221-37.

Schwela, D. (2000). Air pollution and health in urban areas. *Rev Environ Health,* 15,1-2, pp. 13-42.

Searing, DA. Rabinovitch N. (2011). Environmental pollution and lung effects in children. *Curr Opin Pediatr,* 23, 3, pp. 314-8.

Sevcsik, E. Trexler, AJ. Dunn, JM. Rhoades, E. (2011).Allostery in a disordered protein: oxidative modifications to α-synuclein act distally to regulate membrane binding. *J Am Chem Soc,* 133, 18, pp.7152-8.

Shite, J. Qin, F. Mao, W. Kawai, H. Stevens, SY. (2001). Antioxidant vitamins attenuate oxidative stress and cardiac dysfunction in tachycardia - induced cardiomiopathy. *J Am College Cardiol,* 38, 6, pp. 1734-40.

Silva, H. (2001). Mechanisms of action of mood stabilizers. Rev chil, neuropsiquiatr, 39, 3, pp. 219-230.

Smythies, JR. (1999). The neurochimical basis of learning and neurocomputation: the redox theory. *Behav Brain Res,* 99, pp. 17-25.

Soberman, RJ. (2003). The expanding network of redox signaling: new observations, complexities, and perspectives. *J Clin Invest,* 111, pp. 571–574.

Soffler, C. (2007). Oxidative stress. *Vet Clin North Am Equine Pract,* 23, pp. 135-157.

Somogyi, A. Rosta, K. Pusztai, P. Tulassay, Z. Nagy, G. (2007). Antioxidant measurements. *Physiol Meas,* 28, pp. R41-55.

Stepanik, T. Ewing, D. (1993). Isolation of Glutathione peroxidasa, Catalase and Superoxide dismutasa of human erythrocytes. *Journal of Biochemistry and Biophysics,* 20, pp. 157–169.

Stone, JR. Yang, S. (2006). Hydrogen peroxide: a signaling messenger. *Antioxidants & Redox Signaling*, 8, pp. 243–270.

Sugawara, T. Fujimura, M. Noshita, N. (2004). Neuronal death/survival signaling pathways in cerebral ischemia. *NeuroRx*, 1, pp. 17-25.

Sugaya, K. Chou, S. Xu, S. McKinney, M. (1998). Indicator of glial activation and brain oxidative stress after intraventricula infusion of an endotoxin. *Mol Brain Res*, 58, pp. 1-9.

Suzaki, Y. Yoshizumi, M. Kagami, S. Koyama, A. Taketani, Y. Houchi, H. Tsuchiya, K. Takeda, E. Tamaki, T. (2002). Hydrogen Peroxide Stimulates c-Src-mediated Big Mitogen- activated Protein Kinase 1 (BMK1) and the MEF2C Signaling Pathway in PC12 Cells. *The Journal of Biological Chemistry*, 277,11, pp. 9614–9621.

Tang, CH. Wei, W. Liu, L. (2011). Regulation of DNA repair by S-nitrosylation. *Biochim Biophys Acta*, May 5. [Epub ahead of print]

Thomas, DR. (2004). Vitamins in health and aging. *Clin Geriatric Med*, 20, 2, pp. 259-74.

Tillement, JP. Lecanu, L. Papadopoulos, V. (2010). Amyloidosis and neurodegenerative diseases: current treatments and new pharmacological options. *Pharmacology*, 85, 1, pp. 1-17.

Turrens, JF, Boveris, A. (1980). Generation of superoxide anion by NADHdehydrogenase of bovine heart mitochondria. *Biochem. J*, 191, pp. 421-424.

Turrens, JF. (2003). Mitochondrial formation of reactive oxygen species. *J. Physiol*, 552, pp. 335–344.

Tweedie, D. Frankola, KA. Luo, W. Li, Y. Greig, NH. (2011). Thalidomide Analogues Suppress Lipopolysaccharide-Induced Synthesis of TNF-α and Nitrite, an Intermediate of Nitric Oxide, in a Cellular Model of Inflammation. *Open Biochem J*, 5, pp. 37-44.

Valko, M. Leibfritz, D. Moncol, J. Cronin, MT. Mazur, M. Telser, J. (2007). Free radicals and antioxidants in normal physiological functions and human disease. *Int J Biochem Cell Biol*, 39, 1, PP. 44-84.

Van der Heide, LP. Hoekman, MF. Smidt, MP. (2004). The ins and outs of FoxO shuttling: mechanisms of FoxO translocation and transcriptional regulation. *Biochem J*, 380,Pt 2, pp. 297-309.

Wardman, P. Candeias, LP. (1996). Fenton chemistry: an introduction. Radiat Res, 145, 5, pp. 523-31.

Warner, DS. Sheng, SH. Batinic´-Haberle, I. (2004). Oxidants, antioxidants and the ischemic brain. The *Journal of Experimental Biology*, 207, pp. 3221-3231.

Willette, AA. Bendlin, BB. McLaren, DG. Canu, E. Kastman, EK. Kosmatka, KJ. (2010). Age-related changes in neural volume and microstructure associated with interleukin-6 are ameliorated by a calorie-restricted diet in old rhesus monkeys. *Neuroimage*, 51, pp. 987-994.

Willette, AA. Bendlin, BB. McLaren, DG. Canu, E. Kastman, EK. KosmatkaKJ. (2010). Age-related changes in neural volume and microstructure associated with interleukin-6 are ameliorated by a calorie-restricted diet in old rhesus monkeys. *Neuroimage*, 51, pp. 987-994.

Witherick, J. Wilkins, A. Scolding, N. Kemp, K. (2010). Mechanisms of oxidative damage in multiple sclerosis and a cell therapy approach to treatment. *Autoimmune Dis*, 15, pp. 164608.

Xinchun, P. Chen, Y. Bradford, C. (2004). Big Mitogen-Activated Protein Kinase (BMK1)/ERK5 Protects Endothelial Cells From Apoptosis. *Circulation Research*, 94, pp. 362-369.

Yan, C. Takahashi, M. Okuda, M. Lee, J. Berk, B. (1999). Fluid Shear Stress Stimulates Big Mitogen-activated Protein Kinase 1 (BMK1) Activity in Endothelial Cells. *The Journal of Biological Chemistry*, 274, 1, pp. 143–150.

Zawia, NH. Lahiri, DK. Cardozo-Pelaez, F. (2009) Epigenetics, oxidative stress, and Alzheimer disease. *Free Radic Biol Med*, 1,46,9, pp. 1241-9.

Zhao, W. Varghese, M. Yemul, S. Pan, Y. Cheng, A. Marano, P. Hassan, S. Vempati, P. Chen, F. Qian, X. Pasinetti, GM. (2011). Peroxisome proliferator activator receptor gamma coactivator-1alpha (PGC-1α) improves motor performance and survival in a mouse model of amyotrophic lateral sclerosis. *Mol Neurodegener*, 19, 6, 1, pp. 51.

Zhou, G. Bao, Z. Dixon, J. (1995). Components of a new human protein kinase signal ransduction pathway. *J. Biol. Chem*, 270, pp. 12665–12669.

4

Free Radicals in Neurodegenerative Diseases: Modulation by Palladium α-Lipoic Acid Complex

Chirakkal V. Krishnan[1,2], Merrill Garnett[1] and Frank Antonawich[1]
[1]*Garnett McKeen Laboratory, Inc, Bohemia;*
[2]*Department of Chemistry, Stony Brook University;*
USA

1. Introduction

Our research is based on the need for modern medicine to develop a safe and nontoxic product with a wide spectrum of uses. We strongly believe that one of the best ways to achieve this is to have a product that participates actively in most of the roles played by the mitochondria for optimal cellular function. Mitochondria are ubiquitous, and taking care of mitochondria is similar to taking care of all the parts leading to greater achievements than the sum of the parts [Krishnan et. al., 2011].

Oxidative stress is caused by the chemical imbalance between reactive oxygen species (ROS) production and their breakdown by antioxidants. Over-abundance of ROS has been found during neuronal development, as well as in numerous neuropathological conditions. A predominant feature of neuronal injury is the onset of oxidative stress.

Oxidative stress and mitochondrial dysfunction have been closely associated in many sub-cellular, cellular, animal, and human studies of both acute brain injury such as ischemia and stroke and neurodegenerative processes such as Parkinson's, Alzheimer's and Huntington's. While the oxidative stress occurs chronically in Alzheimer's disease, it is more acute in ischemic reperfusion injury. The consequences of mitochondrial dysfunction include DNA and protein damage, lipid peroxidation, disruption of the mitochondrial permeability transition, Ca^{2+} homeostasis, and triggering apoptosis. It is essential to have a healthy mitochondria contributing substantially to the physical, mental, and emotional elements needed to support the well being of patients suffering from brain injury or neurodegenerative diseases.

Energy metabolism, calcium regulation, and apoptosis-signaling pathways are the major roles of mitochondria. Energy requirements dictate the number of mitochondria in a cell [Beattie, 2002; Nagley et. al., 2010]. Cardiac and skeletal muscles, the brain, and the liver have the most mitochondria because of their high metabolic activities. These cells are also exposed to the most oxidative stress because the source of free radical production is also the mitochondria. Due to low levels of antioxidants in neurons, they are intrinsically ill-equipped to defend against an increase in oxidative stress. Glial cells including astrocytes play a supplementary role in antioxidant defense of neurons [Higgins et. al., 2010].

Our search for an extremely safe (up to 40 mL/day, 0.037 M aqueous solution) and nontoxic therapeutic agent resulted in the development of a novel redox molecule, "Palladium α-Lipoic Acid Complex" that is active in mitochondrial cellular metabolism and other functions. The selection of the naturally occurring coenzyme, α-lipoic acid, as our ligand was based on its safety as well as its redox, antioxidant, and fatty acid properties. After selecting the ligand that plays a critical role in biological energy metabolism and numerous other functions, we wanted to tweak the properties of the ligand by complexing it with a metal that is safe and has very high catalytic and electronic properties. After numerous investigations with a variety of metals, the final selection was made to use palladium.

The properties of the resulting palladium α-lipoic acid complex were remarkable in many ways and have been reviewed recently [Krishnan et. al., 2011]. Briefly, this complex enhances the enzymatic activities of Krebs cycle enzymes, isocitrate dehydrogenase, α-ketoglutarate dehydrogenase, succinate dehydrogenase, and malate dehydrogenase and mitochondrial respiratory enzymes, complex I, complex II, complex III, and complex IV. These enzymatic activity enhancements by the metal complex were, in general, much greater than that of the ligand, α-lipoic acid. Coupling this increase in the efficiency of the aerobic metabolic cascade with its powerful antioxidant properties, such as scavenging of free radicals, lowering lipid peroxidation, increasing the levels of glutathione, glutathione peroxidase, manganese superoxide dismutase, and catalase, gave us a powerful weapon to combat fatigue associated with numerous mitochondrial abnormalities. The complex also modulates mitochondrial dysfunction, acts as a prophylactic for neuronal protection from transient ischemic attack, repairs DNA damage resulting from radiation, acts as a prophylactic for protection from radiation, and improves the quality of life. The electronic properties corresponding to tunnel diode behavior and the therapeutic ability/potential of this complex may be exploited in its applications for combating brain injury resulting from transient ischemic attack, death of neurons and other progressive loss of structure or function of neurons associated with diseases such as Parkinson's and Alzheimer's.

2. Oxygen (the source of free radicals) and antioxidants

The appearance of oxygen in the atmosphere is associated with a great expansion of the varieties and numbers of higher living forms. Oxygen is the source for the emergence of respiratory metabolism and energy efficiency. It is also the source of free radicals such as hydroxyl and superoxide. Oxygen's imprint on earth's metabolic evolution, the effect of oxygen on biochemical networks, and the evolution of complex life have been reviewed [Falkowski, 2006; Raymond & Segré, 2006].

Oxygen is the most abundant element in the earth's mantle. Its limited solubility in water (48.9 mL of oxygen at 1 atm pressure in 1 liter water at 0°C) makes aquatic life possible [Pauling, 1970]. Ordinary oxygen consists of diatomic molecules with an unusual electronic structure. Instead of having a double bond between the two atoms in molecular oxygen in the ground state, only one shared pair is formed leaving two unshared electrons. This makes the molecule a diradical and paramagnetic. Liquid oxygen exhibits a pale blue color.

A free radical is a highly reactive species with an unpaired electron. It can be a neutral species such as hydroxyl, $HO^{\bullet}$, or a charged negative ion (anion) such as superoxide, $O_2^{\bullet-}$, or a charged positive ion (cation) such as the guanine radical. An unpaired electron is shown as a dot after the symbol (example: $HO^{\bullet}$). Being good oxidizing agents, free radicals can remove an electron from other materials and in that process get reduced with the pairing of the unpaired electron. They often participate in chain reactions producing new free radicals. Small fluctuations in the steady state concentrations of free radicals play a significant role in intracellular signaling. Uncontrolled increases in the production of these radicals lead to

chain reactions and damage to proteins, polysaccharides, and DNA. The steady state concentrations of $O_2^{\bullet-}$ and H_2O_2 are ~ 10^{-10} M and 5 x 10^{-9} M respectively [Dröge, 2002].
Another beneficial aspect of free radicals is that they participate with leukocytes in phagocytosis, the engulfing and destruction of particulate matter and bacteria. Leukocytes contain the enzymes of the hexose-monophosphate shunt, glycolysis, citric acid cycle, and respiratory enzymes. Phagocytosis requires a lot of energy, which is obtained from glucose by glycolysis and also by the hexose-monophosphate shunt. The role of this shunt is to produce hydrogen peroxide from superoxide free radical, which is used in the phagocytotic process. Thus the free radicals produced in this process are beneficial [Singh, 2006].
Oxidative damage to many biological molecules compromise the viability of cells. The results of this free radical mischief have been assessed [Sies, 1986].
Antioxidants or physiologic reducing agents get oxidized by donating electrons to free radicals. The relative abilities of antioxidants to donate electrons and free radicals to accept electrons are a function of their reduction or redox potentials, measured in volts.
The rate of a reaction cannot be predicted from redox potentials. However the direction of a reaction, decided by the free energy of the reaction, can be predicted from redox potentials. A positive voltage for the net reaction predicts the spontaneity of the reaction. Examples of one-electron and two-electron reduction potentials of reactions of biological interest are easily available [Buettner, 1993; Voet D. & Voet J. G., 1995; Krishnan et.al., 2011]. Positive voltage indicates that vitamin E is spontaneously regenerated by ascorbate or vitamin C.

$$\alpha\text{-Tocopheroxyl}^{\bullet} + \text{Ascorbate monoanion} \longrightarrow \alpha\text{-Tocopherol} + \text{Ascorbate}^{\bullet-},\ E = 218\ \text{mV} \quad (1)$$

The criteria often used to evaluate the antioxidant potential as well as preventive or therapeutic applications of a compound are 1) specificity of free radical quenching, 2) metal chelating ability, 3) interaction with other antioxidants, 4) effects on gene expression, 5) absorption and bioavailability, 6) concentration in tissues, cells, and extracellular fluid, and 7) location (in aqueous or membrane domains or in both) [Packer et. al., 1995].
ROS generation, which increases with increasing stress conditions, is characteristic for all tissues and cells. The interaction of molecular oxygen with biological molecules is not energetically favored because of the unique electronic configuration of molecular oxygen. Molecular oxygen, a diatomic molecule, in its normal or ground state is in its triplet state, $^3O_2$ [$^3\sum^-{}_g$]. It has two electrons of parallel spins singly occupied in its two π^* antibonding molecular orbitals. Most organic molecules cannot react with this spin-forbidden triplet oxygen because of their singlet configurations with antiparallel electron spins. By adding energy, the triplet oxygen can form two types of excited singlet oxygen, $^1O_2$, $^1\sum^+{}_g$ with the two electrons of opposite spins in two separate molecular orbitals or $^1\Delta_g$ with the two electrons of opposite spins occupying one molecular orbital leaving the other molecular orbital empty. The former is too short lived from a biological point of view. A two electron interaction with molecular oxygen is thus not possible without a spin inversion because it will result in parallel spins in the same orbital, which is spin-forbidden. Thus the preferable interaction is reduction of oxygen by addition of one electron at a time. This process leads to the production of oxygen radicals that can cause cellular damage. When one of the two unpaired electrons is excited and changes its spin, the resulting high energy singlet oxygen with two electrons and opposite spins in the two orbitals is capable of two-electron interactions. The initial step or one electron reduction of oxygen requires energy. The subsequent reduction reactions with appropriate electron donors can proceed spontaneously.

One must wonder at this stage whether nature has given this unique electron configuration for normal molecular oxygen purposefully or not, recognizing not the liability of free radicals but instead their usefulness.
Oxygen undergoes a series of progressive one electron reduction reactions, 2-5. The hydroxyl radical has a very short half life (10^{-9} s) with the highest rate constant with target molecules [Sies, 1993]. It reacts practically at the site of generation. It is one of the strongest oxidizing agents in nature (redox potential of 2310 mV). It is undoubtedly the most dangerous, with its well known involvement in lipid peroxidation of cell membranes and generation of other toxic radicals. The formation of $HO^{\bullet}$ is catalyzed by transition metals in a reduced state. The resulting oxidized metal is reduced back by $O_2^{\bullet-}$ and helps the formation of $HO^{\bullet}$ repeatedly.

$$O_2 + e^- \rightarrow O_2^{\bullet-} \text{ (superoxide anion)} \quad (2)$$

$$O_2^{\bullet-} + e^- + 2H^+ \rightarrow H_2O_2 \text{ (hydrogen peroxide)} \quad (3)$$

$$H_2O_2 + e^- \rightarrow OH^- + HO^{\bullet} \text{ (hydroxyl radical)} \quad (4)$$

$$HO^{\bullet} + e^- + H^+ \rightarrow H_2O \quad (5)$$

Superoxide ion is the precursor of most reactive oxygen species. It can act both as a reducing agent or reductant (for Fe^{3+}) and as an oxidizing agent or oxidant for catecholamines. To minimize production of free radical chain reactions such as reactions (6) and (7), metal ions are sequestered under physiological conditions by proteins.

$$O_2^{\bullet-} + Fe^{3+} \rightarrow O_2 + Fe^{2+} \quad (6)$$

$$H_2O_2 + Fe^{2+} + H^+ \rightarrow HO^{\bullet} + Fe^{3+} + H_2O \text{ (classical Fenton reaction)} \quad (7)$$

Adding reactions (6) and (7) gives the Haber-Weiss reaction (8) which is catalyzed by metal ions.

$$H_2O_2 + O_2^{\bullet-} + H^+ \rightarrow HO^{\bullet} + O_2 + H_2O \quad (8)$$

Damage to both mitochondrial DNA (mtDNA) and nuclear DNA (nDNA) may result in mutations. Nonspecific binding of Fe^{2+} to DNA may result in the formation of $HO^{\bullet}$ (reaction 7) that attack individual bases and cause strand breaks.
Strategies of antioxidant defense in terms of prevention, intervention, and repair have been elegantly summarized [Sies, 1993]. Cells employ enzymes such as superoxide dismutase (SOD), glutathione peroxidase (GSHPx), and catalase to scavenge free radicals. These enzymes are known as preventive antioxidants because they eliminate the species involved in the initiation of free radical chain reactions. SOD has three isoforms: Copper/Zinc SOD, Manganese SOD, and extracellular SOD. A very high rate of production of ~ 300 nmol superoxide/min/mg protein has been reported for a reaction of cyrtochromeb5 reductase using NADH as an electron donor [Starkov & Wallace, 2006]. The superoxide anion shown in reaction (2) and released by the mitochondria undergoes the dismutation reaction either spontaneously or catalytically(reaction 9) producing hydrogen peroxide and O_2. The role of

the SOD is to increase the rate of the reaction to that of a diffusion controlled process [Turrens, 2003].

$$2H^{+}+O_2^{\bullet-}+O_2^{\bullet-} \xrightarrow{SOD} H_2O_2+O_2 \tag{9}$$

The spontaneous decomposition of superoxide, but not the catalytic decomposition, produces singlet oxygen instead of the normal molecular oxygen [Klotz, 2002]. Singlet oxygen is produced by stimulated neutrophils in vivo. Superoxide produced by NADPH catalysis spontaneously dismutates to H_2O_2 and singlet O_2. Also the catalytic reaction of myeloperoxidase with H_2O_2 and Cl^- produces hypochlorite, which reacts with more H_2O_2 producing singlet O_2, H_2O and Cl^-.

Hydrogen peroxide is removed by GSHPx, at the expense of glutathione or γ-glutamylcysteinylglycine (GSH), and by catalase. Selenium (as selenocysteine) is a cofactor of GSHPx [Beattie, 2002]. GSHPx is located in both the mitochondrial and cytosolic compartments of the cell. Hydrogen peroxide and organic hydroperoxides in the cytosol are also destroyed by GSHPx. Catalase is highest in peroxisomes and it is less in cytosol and mitochondria [Beattie, 2002].

$$2GSH+H_2O_2 \xrightarrow{GSHPx} GSSG+2H_2O \tag{10}$$

$$2H_2O_2 \xrightarrow{Catalase} 2H_2O+O_2 \tag{11}$$

Glutathione or, GSH is a major nonenzymatic antioxidant. The aqueous compartments of cells and their organelles usually contain millimolar levels of GSH. It is the cell's primary preventative antioxidant. It can react with various highly oxidizing species such as $HO^{\bullet}$, $RO^{\bullet}$ or $ROO^{\bullet}$ and produce H_2O, ROH, or ROOH and $GS^{\bullet}$ (glutathiyl radical). Glutathiyl radical can react rapidly with GSH, most efficiently via GS^- to make $GSSG^{\bullet-}$, which is a very strong reducing species. It produces $O_2^{\bullet-}$ and glutathione disulfide, GSSG, by reaction with oxygen.

$$GSSG^{\bullet-}+O_2 \xrightarrow{GSHPx} O_2^{\bullet-}+GSSG \tag{12}$$

SOD and GSH provide an excellent natural combination for cellular antioxidant defense by removing $O_2^{\bullet-}$ and $HO^{\bullet}$ respectively. The intracellular concentration of GSH is about 1 mM while the mitochondrial respiration keeps O_2 about 0 to 10 μM in the cell. Therefore, 99% of $GS^{\bullet}$ formed should react with GSH to make GSSG and $O_2^{\bullet-}$. Thus the importance of SOD is obvious. The normal GSH to GSSG ratio in erythrocytes is 100:1 [Beattie, 2002].

Lipid (probably a polyunsaturated fatty acid) peroxidation is a free radical chain reaction process. Superoxide is a mediator in oxidative chain reactions. It is known to initiate as well as terminate this process. Overproduction of superoxide initiates the chain reaction by mobilizing iron from the tissue protein ferritin [McCord, 1998].

$$O_2^{\bullet-}+\text{Ferritin-}Fe^{3+} \rightarrow O_2+\text{Ferritin}+Fe^{2+} \tag{13}$$

$$Fe^{2+}+\text{lipid-OOH(lipidhydroperoxide)} \rightarrow \text{Lipid-O}^{\bullet}+OH^{-}+Fe^{3+} \tag{14}$$

$$\text{Lipid-O}^{\bullet}+\text{lipid-H} \rightarrow \text{Lipid}^{\bullet}+\text{lipid-OH} \tag{15}$$

$$O_2^{\bullet -} + Fe^{3+} \rightarrow O_2 + Fe^{2+} \quad (16)$$

Chain propagation reactions follow.

$$\text{Lipid}^{\bullet} + O_2 \rightarrow \text{Lipid-OO}^{\bullet} \quad (17)$$

$$\text{Lipid-OO}^{\bullet} + \text{Lipid-H} \rightarrow \text{Lipid-OOH+Lipid}^{\bullet} \quad (18)$$

If alkoyl (lipid-O$^{\bullet}$) or dioxyl (Lipid-OO$^{\bullet}$) radicals are scavenged by $O_2^{\bullet -}$, the chain reaction would be terminated.

$$\text{lipid-O}^{\bullet} + O_2^{\bullet -} + H^+ \rightarrow \text{Lipid-OH+}O_2 \quad (19)$$

$$\text{lipid-OO}^{\bullet} + O_2^{\bullet -} + H^+ \rightarrow \text{Lipid-OOH+}O_2 \quad (20)$$

Superoxide, in moderate concentrations, initiates lipid peroxidation as well as terminates. Over scavenging of $O_2^{\bullet -}$ by over expressed SOD limits the termination process. At intermediate concentrations, the SOD is able to suppress the lipid peroxidation process and $O_2^{\bullet -}$ concentration is sufficient enough to terminate the chain. Thus it has been found that for a certain level of oxidative stress there is an optimum concentration of SOD [McCord, 1998].

The rate constant values for the bis-allylic hydrogen atom abstraction from polyunsaturated lipids and for the addition to the double bond were found to be the same for hydroxyl radical (10^9), alkoxyl radical (10^6) and peroxyl radical (10^2) $M^{-1}s^{-1}$ [Takahashi & Niki, 1998].

Non-enzymatic antioxidants include water soluble vitamin C (ascorbic acid) and lipid soluble vitamin E. Ascorbic acid, or ascorbate anion at biological pH is also a cofactor in several biosynthetic pathways including the enzyme prolylhydroxylase, which modifies the polypeptide collagen precursor to facilitate the formation of collagen fibers.

Due to resonance, the ascorbate radical has a long half life of 1 second. Ascorbate can be oxidized in two successive one-electron steps to ascorbate free radical and dehydroascorbic acid respectively.

$$\text{Ascorbate anion - } e^- \longrightarrow \text{Ascorbate free radical} \quad (21)$$

$$\text{Ascorbate free radical - } e^- \longrightarrow \text{dehydroascorbic acid} \quad (22)$$

The oxidation of ascorbate to the radical and dehydroascorbic acid can easily be reversed by the enzyme systems that use NADH or NADPH.

$$\text{NADH} + 2\text{Ascorbate}^{\bullet -} \longrightarrow \text{NAD}^+ + 2\text{Ascorbate monoanion } [E = 597 \text{ mV}] \quad (23)$$

Vitamin E has eight different related homologues, the most abundant being α-tocopherol. The dynamics of this antioxidant, that acts only in lipid domains and quenches lipid peroxyl radicals as well as its numerous other functions, not related to its antioxidant property, such as inhibition of cell proliferation, platelet aggregation, and protein kinase C and 5-lipoxygenase inhibition have been reviewed, raising the possibility that the non-antioxidant mechanisms may contribute to many of the effects previously attributed to antioxidant functions [Ricciarelli et. al., 2002; Niki & Noguchi, 2004].

Vitamin E, and vitamin C, cooperate to protect lipids and lipid structures against peroxidation. Also vitamin C regenerates vitamin E (reaction 1), thereby permitting vitamin E to function again as a free radical chain breaking antioxidant. Other antioxidants such as ubiquinols and GSH also regenerate vitamin E and help to maintain its concentration (< 0.1 nmol/mg membrane) in spite of a very high lipid peroxyl radical generation rate of 1-5 nmol/mg membrane protein per minute [Packer et.al., 1995].

3. Hydrogen peroxide (H_2O_2)

H_2O_2 in its liquid state, is more strongly associated by hydrogen bonding than pure water. The dipole moment of hydrogen peroxide is 2.1 Debye units compared to 1.84 Debye units for water. This should make ion-dipole interactions stronger with H_2O_2 than with H_2O. The relative interactions of Na^+-H_2O and Na^+-H_2O_2 as well as Ca^{2+}-H_2O and Ca^{2+}-H_2O_2 and interactions of these ions with both the solvents depend on their relative concentrations.
A dilute aqueous solution of hydrogen peroxide is more acidic than water [Cotton & Wilkinson, 1972].

$$H_2O_2 = H^+ + HO_2^- \qquad K_{20^\circ C} = 1.5 \times 10^{-12} \tag{24}$$

The following equilibria suggest that H_2O_2 is a strong oxidizing agent in both acidic and basic solutions.

$$H_2O_2 + 2H^+ + 2e^- = 2H_2O \quad E^\circ = 1.77V \tag{25}$$

$$O_2 + 2H^+ + 2e^- = H_2O_2 \quad E^\circ = 0.68V \tag{26}$$

$$HO_2^- + H_2O + 2e^- = 3OH^- \quad E^\circ = 0.87V \tag{27}$$

The enzyme, monoamine oxidase, located in the outer mitochondrial membrane of mammalian tissues, catalyzes the oxidation of biogenic amines and produces H_2O_2. Other pro-oxidant enzymes include nitric oxide synthases, cyclooxygenases, xanthine dehydrogenase, xanthine oxidase, NADPH oxidase, and myeloperoxidase. Rodent heart and brain can produce H_2O_2 at a rate of 0.5-3 nmol/min/mg mitochondrial protein, which corresponds to about 5-20% of their total oxygen consumption [Starkov & Wallace, 2006].
Hydrogen peroxide and superoxide have been implicated as mediators of vascular and functional changes in hypertension [Tabet et. al., 2004]. They increase vascular contraction, stimulate vascular smooth muscle cell growth, and induce inflammatory responses that are characteristic features of small arteries in hypertension.
Hydrogen peroxide plays a dual role [Lázaro, 2007]. Cancer cells produce high amounts of H_2O_2. These increased levels of H_2O_2 result in DNA alterations, cell proliferation, apoptosis resistance, metastasis, angiogenesis, and hypoxia inducible factor 1(HIF-1) activation. Activation of HIF-1 plays crucial roles in apoptosis resistance, invasion/metastasis and angiogenesis. Many human cancers have over expressed HIF-1. On the other hand, hydrogen peroxide also induces apoptosis in cancer cells selectively and the activity of many anticancer drugs is mediated, at least in part by H_2O_2.
Hydrogen peroxide is less reactive than superoxide and is relatively more stable. It crosses the membrane lipid bilayer through aquaporins [Singh, 2006]. With increasing concentrations

of cellular H_2O_2, its function gradually changes from cell signaling, to cell malignant transformation, and to cell death [Lázaro, 2007]. The mystery surrounding the different roles of hydrogen peroxide may be solved, at least partially, by looking at its electronic properties. Our impedance data suggest that the electronic properties (and consequent circuits) of H_2O_2 are dependent on its concentration. Our data also suggest that one has to take a serious look at another important contribution of H_2O_2, the preferential solvation of ions and its biological consequences [Krishnan et.al., 2011] .

The beneficial aspect of H_2O_2 in cell signaling is emerging. Neurons and brain macrophages produce $O_2^{\bullet-}$ in pathological situations and the H_2O_2 produced from $O_2^{\bullet-}$ increases gap junctional communication in astrocytes [Rouach et. al., 2004]. Examples of signaling processes include the over-oxidation of the cysteine in peroxiredoxins from the cysteine sulfenic acid to cysteine sulfinic acid, and the over-oxidation of methionine residues in proteins to methionine sulfoxide [Sies, 1986; Wood et. al., 2003].

Embryonic and fetal growth are facilitated by a certain amount of redox imbalance or oxidative stress [Maiorino & Ursini, 2002; Dennery, 2010]. These investigations detail the level of oxygen and antioxidant status at the first, second and third trimester of pregnancy. Low levels of H_2O_2 and superoxide produced by human sperm are also crucial for the capacitation process that allows the sperm to penetrate the zona pellucida of the ovum. At low, moderate, and highly oxidative states, proliferation, differentiation, and apoptosis or necrosis respectively are favored suggesting the different functions of ROS depending on their concentrations.

4. Reactive nitrogen species

Nitric oxide, NO·, is a neutral free radical with a half life of the order of seconds [Beckman & Koppenol, 1996; Blokhina & Fagerstedt, 2006]. Three types of nitric oxide synthases have been described in mammalian cells: neuronal (nNOS), endothelial (eNOS) and an inducible (immunological) (iNOS). The first two are under the control of Ca^{2+}-calmodulin. The enzyme catalyzes oxygen dependent conversion of L-arginine to citrulline:

$$\text{L-arginine} + \text{NADPH} + O_2 \xrightarrow{\text{NOS}} \text{citrulline} + \text{NO}^{\cdot} + \text{NADP}^{+} \quad (28)$$

Mitochondrial NOS distinct from the ones given above has also been reported [Elfering et. al., 2002]. $NO^{\bullet}$ can be converted to other reactive nitrogen species such as nitrosonium cation (NO^{+}), nitroxyl anion (NO^{-}) or peroxynitrite, $ONOO^{-}$ with distinct chemical reactivity and physical properties. Some of the physiological effects may be mediated through the intermediate formation of S-nitroso-cysteine or S-nitroso-glutathione [Dröge, 2002].

ROS are produced at complex I and complex III during respiration. Superoxide ion produced at the mitochondria reacts with $NO^{\bullet}$ to produce peroxynitrite. The rate of this reaction is controlled by the rate of diffusion of the two reactants.

$$NO^{\bullet} + O_2^{\bullet-} \xrightarrow{\text{NOS}} ONOO^{-} \quad (29)$$

The reaction rate for the formation of $ONOO^{-}$ is $6.7 \times 10^{9}\ M^{-1}\ s^{-1}$. This is ~ 6 times faster than the scavenging of superoxide by copper, zinc superoxide dismutase. Inducible nitric oxide synthase, when expressed, can make substantial amounts of nitric oxide and this will out-

compete SOD for $O_2^{\bullet-}$. In aerobic metabolism about 1-5% of oxygen is reduced to superoxide. However its intracellular concentration is maintained at ~ 4-10 μM by superoxide dismutase. Copper, zinc superoxide dismutase is ~ 0.5% of total soluble proteins in brain.
Physiological levels of $NO^{\bullet}$ binds to cytochrome c oxidase leading to a competitive and reversible inhibition of mitochondrial respiration [Radi et. al., 2002]. Large levels of $NO^{\bullet}$ in mitochondria promote formation of more $O_2^{\bullet-}$ from complex I and the consequent formation of more $ONOO^-$.
The half-life of $ONOO^-$ is 0.05 - 1 s [Sies, 1993]. Mitochondrial scavenging systems for $ONOO^-$ and $ONOO^-$-derived radicals such as carbonate ($CO_3^{\bullet-}$) and nitrogen dioxide radicals ($NO_2^{\bullet}$) are cytochrome c oxidase, GSH and ubiquinol [Radi et. al., 2002]. Superoxide and $ONOO^-$ radicals significantly affect the mitochondrial integrity. Peroxynitrite is a very powerful oxidizing and nitrating agent. It reacts with tyrosine in proteins and produces nitrotyrosines. Nitration of the structural proteins, neurofilaments and actin disrupts the filament assembly leading to major pathological consequences in myocardial ischemia, distressed lung, and amyotropic lateral sclerosis.
The steady state concentrations of $NO^{\bullet}$ and $ONOO^-$ in liver are ~ 36 nM and 2.2 nM respectively based on the assumption of 20 μM intramitochondrial O_2 concentration. But there are claims that O_2 concentration is only 3 μM and not 20 μM [Turrens, 2003]. If this is true the steady state concentrations will be much lower. After cerebral ischemia, NO concentration increases 10-100-fold in a few minutes to 2-4 μM[Beckman & Koppenol, 1996]. Nitric oxide can penetrate the lipid bilayer and diffuse rapidly and isotropically through most tissues without any significant reaction or consumption. The rapid diffusion of nitric oxide between cells allows it to modulate, 1) synaptic plasticity in neurons, 2) the oscillatory behavior of neuronal networks, 3) blood flow, and 4) thrombosis [Beckman & Koppenol, 1996]. Since it reacts with oxy hemoglobin and is destroyed, it cannot be transported through the vasculature.
Nitric oxide diffuses and concentrates in the hydrophobic core of low density lipoprotein (LDL) and inhibits its oxidation [Rubbo et. al., 2002]. On the other hand peroxynitrite is involved in LDL oxidation. Since vascular cells are rich sources of superoxide, peroxynitrite formation is also facilitated. Thus the development of atherosclerosis may be intimately connected to the interactions of these two nitrogen species with LDL.
Both peroxynitrite and singlet oxygen are involved in activating mitogen-activated protein (MAP) kinases that respond to extracellular stimuli such as mitogen, osmotic stress, and proinflammatory cytokines and regulate various activities such as gene expression, mitosis, differentiation, proliferative cell survival, and apoptosis [Klotz, 2002].

5. Mitochondria

Mitochondria has unique roles; production of adenosine triphosphate (ATP) by cellular respiration, production of ROS, the distribution/redistribution of Ca^{2+} pools within cells, and control of apoptosis or programmed cell death.
In the absence of mitochondria, or with mitochondrial dysfunction, ATP is produced by an alternative pathway, anaerobic glycolysis. However, this conversion of glucose to pyruvate is not efficient and produces only 2 molecules of ATP compared to 36 molecules of ATP produced by normal glucose oxidation. The pyruvate and the fatty acids are transported into the mitochondrial matrix. There they are broken down into the acetyl group on acetyl coenzyme A (acetyl-CoA or acetyl-SCoA) and then fed into the Krebs cycle.

The ATP has a half-life of seconds to minutes depending on the cell where it is being continuously hydrolyzed and regenerated. Our average normal consumption and regeneration rate of ATP is ~3mol (1.5 kg) h^{-1}. During strenuous activity this rate increases by an order of magnitude [Voet D. & Voet J. G., 1995].

Oxygen deprivation rapidly deteriorates brain cells because ATP is available for only a few seconds [Voet D. & Voet J. G., 1995]. In muscles and nerve cells, ATP has high turnover rates and phosphocreatine acts as its reservoir.

$$\text{ATP} + \text{Creatine} = \text{Phosphocreatine} + \text{ADP} \tag{30}$$

This is an energy consuming reaction under standard conditions and is close to equilibrium under normal intracellular concentrations. At resting state, high ATP shifts the equilibrium to the right. High metabolic activity shifts the equilibrium to the left due to low ATP.

The breakdown of carbohydrates, lipids, and proteins produce the acetyl group of the common intermediate, acetyl-CoA. A series of consecutive enzymatic reactions of Krebs cycle, the electron transport chain (ETC), and oxidative phosphorylation then converts acetyl-CoA into CO_2 and H_2O. The net result is the transfer of electrons from the oxidative substrates to molecular oxygen to generate water, CO_2 and ATP.

In oxidative phosphorylation, a series of coupled reactions are involved in the transport of electrons through complexes 1-IV in the inner mitochondrial membrane. The entry point of electrons from the high energy molecules NADH and $FADH_2$ is at complex I and complex II respectively. With the help of a variety of enzymes, a series of coupled redox reactions drive the transport of electrons through these complexes. A proton gradient across the inner mitochondrial membrane is created during this process when protons are pumped out of the matrix at complexes I, III, and IV. The electrochemical gradient consisting of a pH gradient (ΔpH) and an electrical potential ($\Delta\psi$) drive the ATP synthesis from ADP as the protons re-enter the matrix through the ATP synthase (complex V).

Mitochondrial DNA (mtDNA) harboring their own genome with their own transcription, translation, and machinery for protein synthesis was discovered in the early 1960s. The codes for electron transport chain complexes, I, II, III, IV, and V for nuclear DNA (nDNA) are 36, 4, 10, 10, and 14 protein subunits and for mtDNA, 7, 0, 1, 3, and 2 subunits respectively [Carew & Huang, 2002]. Complex II is encoded by nDNA only. The mtDNA genome also encodes 22 mitochondrial tRNAs that are required for protein synthesis and 2 rRNAs that are essential for translation of mtDNA transcripts. The human mtDNA is a supercoiled, double-stranded molecule containing 16,569 base pairs [Chan, 2006; Carew & Huang, 2002].

A dynamic structural network consisting of about 70% stationary and 30% mobile mitochondria meets the energy demands of axons. The speed of the mobile mitochondria is ~ 1 μm/s [Kiryu-Seo et. al., 2010]. Mitochondrial fission and fusion, probable mitochondrial biogenesis within axons, and the transport of mitochondria to and from neuronal soma determine the content of mitochondria within axons.

Under highly reduced state of ETC, excess electrons at complex I produce $O_2^{\bullet-}$ in the mitochondrial matrix. This is reduced by the matrix MnSOD to H_2O_2. To a limited extent complex III also produces $O_2^{\bullet-}$ and is released into the mitochondrial intermembrane space where it is converted to H_2O_2 by Cu/ZnSOD. The presence of Fe^{2+} readily converts the H_2O_2 to the dangerous hydroxyl radical (reaction 7). The potential at the inner mitochondrial membrane, the pH in the matrix, local O_2 concentration and the nature of the substrates dictate the amount of $O_2^{\bullet-}$ production. When the mitochondria is actively producing ATP, both ΔpH and Δψ as well as NADH/NAD+ ratio are low and ROS production is also low.

Superoxide production occurs on the outer mitochondrial membrane, in the matrix, and on both sides of the innermitochondrial membrane [Turrens, 2003]. The highly reducing intra-mitochondrial environment has reduced coenzymes and prosthetic groups of flavoproteins, iron-sulfur clusters (in Complex I) and ubisemiquinones (Complex III) that thermodynamically favor one electron reduction of molecular oxygen to produce $O_2^{\bullet-}$. While the major source of $O_2^{\bullet-}$ in the heart and lung is Complex III, it seems to be Complex I in the brain [Turrens, 2003]. Also the production of $O_2^{\bullet-}$ varies depending on the organ and whether the mitochondria is respiring or not. For example, in the absence of ADP, the proton movement through ATP synthase stops, protons build up and cause a slowdown of electron flow and thus creating a more reduced State IV respiration state. This reduced state and increasing concentration of O_2 will increase the one electron reduction process of oxygen and the rate of $O_2^{\bullet-}$ production will increase.

Uptake of high concentrations of Ca^{2+} into mitochondria, declined ATP, and increased ROS production endanger the health of the mitochondria and the mitochondria resort into a destructive mode by opening the mitochondrial permeability transition pore and consequently releasing cytochrome c and initiating programmed cell death.

6. Mitochondrial dysfunction in neurodegenerative diseases

Since different organs can rely on mitochondrial energy to different extents, mitochondrial defects can cause organ-specific phenotypes. The organ system most reliant on mitochondrial energy is the central nervous system. The consequences of mitochondrial dysfunction are numerous and include oxidative stress, loss of cellular Ca^{2+} homeostasis, promotion of apoptosis, and metabolic failure. Hence, evidence continues to accrue implicating mitochondrial dysfunction in the etiology of a number of neurodegenerative conditions such as Parkinson's, Alzheimer's, and transient ischemia.

In transient ischemia, a lack of oxygen and glucose delivery compromise the integrity of aerobic metabolism, while reperfusion potentiates injury via the generation of free radicals. Superoxide, nitric oxide and peroxynitrite production in the brain is increased during reperfusion following 30 minutes of global ischemia. In patients with Parkinson's disease, excess Fe^{2+} can reduce peroxide and produce $HO^{\bullet}$. These radicals and their reactions cause oxidative stress and consequent mitochondrial damage resulting in mutations. Evidence for mitochondrial dysfunction in Alzheimer's disease pathogenesis comes from impaired activities of three key Krebs Cycle enzyme complexes and reduced respiratory chain complex I, III, and IV activity observed in postmortem Alzheimer's disease brain, and oxidative damage to both mtDNA and nDNA. It may be possible for mtDNA mutations to disrupt the normal electron flow and seriously affect energy production. Oxidative damage and the resulting serious consequences have been extensively reviewed recently [Singh, 2006]. Compared to nDNA, mtDNA is far more susceptible to mutations due to their being present in a highly oxidative environment, a lack of protective histones and limited repair capacity [Carew & Huang, 2002; Singh, 2006].

During the production of ATP in the cell, about 85% of oxygen is consumed by the mitochondria. Superoxide radical, $O_2^{\bullet-}$, may be produced from about 4% of all oxygen consumed [Singh, 2006]. Enzymes such as NADPH oxidases, xanthine oxidase, cyclooxygenases, and lipooxygenases also produce ROS. The iron-sulfur cluster in the aconitase enzyme, localized in the matrix space of mitochondria, is oxidized by superoxide and the exposed iron reacts with the peroxide to produce hydroxyl radicals [Singh, 2006]. Also the $NO^{\bullet}$ produced within mitochondria by mitochondrial NO synthase produces peroxynitrite [$ONOO^-$] by reaction with $O_2^{\bullet -}$. Superoxide radical and $ONOO^-$ contribute to substantial mitochondrial damage.

Enzymes such as SOD, GSHPx, catalase, peroxoredoxin, and thioredoxin can inactivate some of the ROS. MnSOD or Cu/ZnSOD converts the $O_2^{\bullet -}$ into H_2O_2. The active site of cytosolic and extracellular forms of SOD contains Cu/Zn and the mitochondrial form contains Mn [Beattie, 2002]. Oxidative damage is due to the inadequacy of these detoxifying processes.

In aging and neurodegenerative disorders, apart from inherited defects, mitochondrial DNA deletions and point mutations within neurons are well recognized.

Mitochondria is heavily involved in cell death. The various pathways involved in the cell death depend on the type of cellular injury or neurodegeneration. In the core region of stroke necrosis is observed. On the other hand in neurodegenerative diseases such as amyotropic lateral sclerosis, apoptosis markers are observed along with markers of endoplasmic reticulum(ER) stress and autophagy [Nagley et. al., 2010]. Mitochondria influences programmed cell death (type I-apoptotic as well as type III-necrotic). While autophagy routinely turns over various cellular constituents, it is involved in cell death (type II) in some stress conditions. Apart from changing the mitochondrial membrane potential and increasing the production of ROS, the elevation of intracellular and mitochondrial Ca^{2+} also modulates the process of programmed cell death. The involvement of mitochondria in the multifaceted neuronal death pathways is elegantly demonstrated in 4 steps in Fig. 1 [Nagley et. al., 2010]. Step A illustrates normal physiological conditions where equilibrium between homeostatic and deleterious factors is maintained. In this state of healthy functional neurons, cellular feedback mechanisms help maintain homeostasis. Step B is under conditions of minor stress. The deleterious factors such as reactive oxygen and nitrogen species (RONS) and misfolded proteins (MP) contribute to a decrease in energy production (ATP) and an increase in intracellular Ca^{2+}. Various channels and transporters elevate the Ca^{2+} in both cytoplasm and mitochondria. Neurons respond to this minor stress by activation of the unfolded protein response (UPR, in its initial, pro-survival phase), ubiquitin proteasome system (UPS), and chaperone-mediated autophagy (CMA). Step C indicates a much greater stress or imbalance due to substantial increases in RONS, MP, and Ca^{2+}. ATP production is substantially less. There is also a substantial decrease in mitochondrial membrane potential. The UPR switches to its destructive mode via induction of apoptotic effector proteins such as C/EBP homologous protein, caspase-12 and c-Jun N-terminal kinase. The UPS also becomes increasingly dysfunctional because of it s inability along with CMA to adequately handle the increased load of MP. This leads to the formation of intracellular aggregates of MP. Thus, deleterious factors overwhelm the cellular homeostatic processes. In spite of the chaperone mediated autophagic process switching to macroautophagy, it cannot adequately handle the load of MP leading to the final step D. There is a strong commitment to death at this level of stress and the cell advances to programmed cell death (type-I, type-II or type-III, or their combinations) [Nagley, 2010].

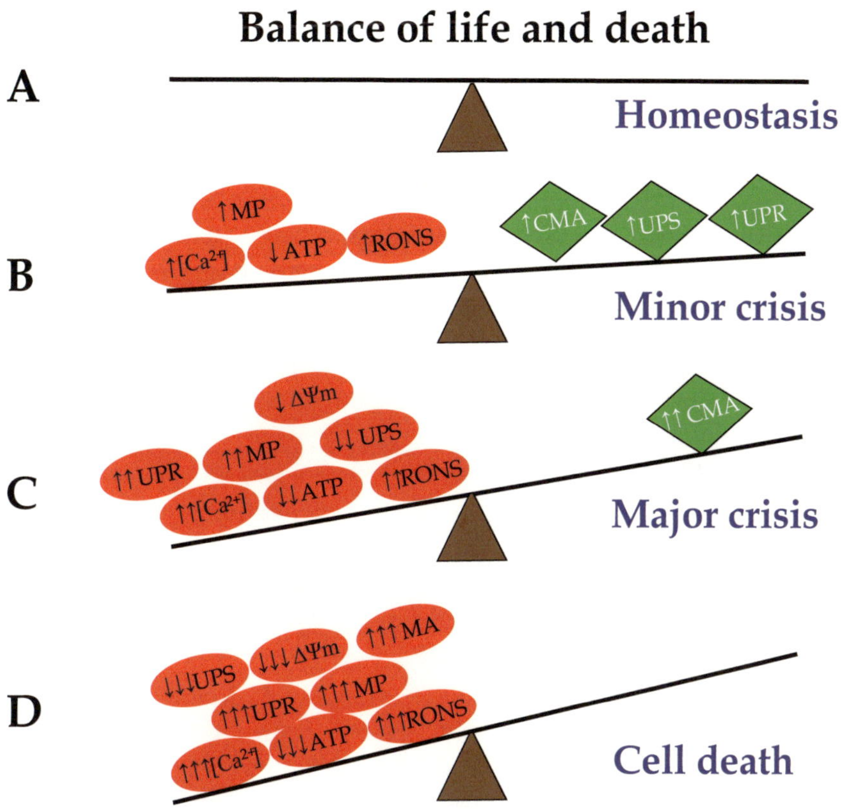

Fig. 1. Deleterious stress factors and restorative factors in neuronal homeostasis and neuronal death [Adpated from Nagley et. al., 2010]. $\Delta\Psi_m$, mitochondrial membrane potential; MP, misfolded proteins; RONS, reactive oxygen and nitrogen species; UPS, ubiquitin-proteasome system; UPR, unfolded protein response; CMA, chaperone mediated autophagy; MA, macroautophagy. Proteins failing to fold into native structure produces inactive and usually toxic proteins. Several neurodegenerative and other diseases are believed to result from misfolded proteins (MP). The unfolded protein response (UPR) is activated in response to a stress arising from an accumulation of unfolded or MP in the lumen of the endoplasmic reticulum. UPR attempts initially to restore the normal function of the cell by halting protein translation. They also activate the signaling pathways that lead to increasing the production of molecular chaperones involved in protein folding. If these efforts are not successful, then it induces apoptotic effector proteins. Proteasomes are very large protein complexes whose main function is to degrade unneeded or damaged proteins by proteolysis and thus helping cells to regulate proteins and MP. Ubiquitin, a small protein, is used to tag the proteins that need to be degraded. The overall system of ubiquitination and proteasomal degradation is known as the ubiquitin proteosome system (UPS). Autophagy, such as micro- and macro-autophagy, refers to the degradation of intracellular components via the lysosome. Chaperone mediated autophagy, CMA, can degrade only certain proteins and not organelles and thus very selective in what it degrades. Also the substrates are translocated across the membrane on a one on one basis instead of engulfing the substrate in bulk

7. Multiple sclerosis

Multiple sclerosis (MS) is a chronic inflammatory disease of the central nervous system. It is associated with demyelination and a variable degree of axonal and neuronal degeneration. Demyelination decreases nerve impulse conduction velocity. Also the axons become vulnerable to inflammatory conditions. The mechanisms of tissue injury and neurodegeneration in MS are still under active investigation. Most MS patients initially experience relapsing-remitting episodes of neurologic deficits that last for six to eight weeks. The initial relapse rate is about 0.3/year. This rate declines progressively with time [Siffrin et. al., 2010]. This is followed by a gradual progression of irreversible neurological impairment or secondary progressive multiple sclerosis (SPMS) [Campbell et. al., 2011]. With advancing disease the observed increase in gray matter atrophy, which is indicative of the loss of neurons and axons, correlates well with the corresponding clinical disability.

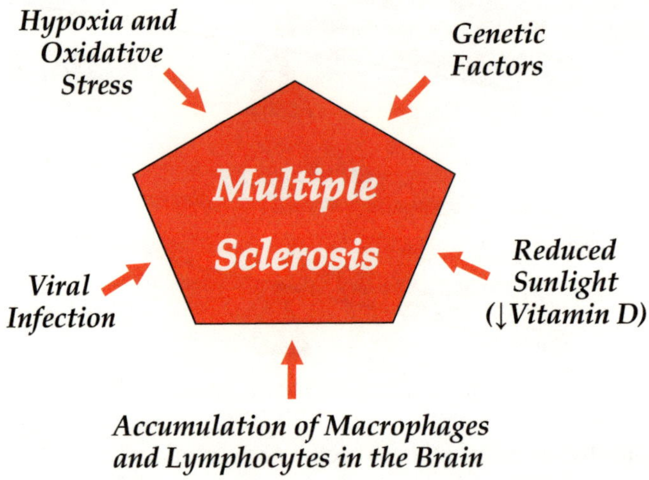

Fig. 2. Probable causal factors of multiple sclerosis [adapted from Mao & Reddy, 2010]

Apart from the consistent features, neuroaxonal injury and dysfunction in MS, the vascular aspects of MS, an increased risk for ischemic disease, global cerebral hypoperfusion, and a chronic state of impaired venous drainage are receiving a great deal of attention [D'haeseleer et. al., 2011; Filippi & Rocca, 2011].

The precise causal factors of multiple sclerosis are unknown. However, it is possible that multiple factors [Fig. 2] are involved in causing multiple sclerosis, including DNA defects in nuclear and mitochondrial genomes, viral infection, hypoxia and oxidative stress, lack of sunlight or sufficient levels of vitamin D, and increased macrophages and lymphocytes in the brain [Mao & Reddy, 2010].

Current research has shown that mitochondrial abnormalities are involved in the development and progression of multiple sclerosis [Fig. 3], including: mitochondrial DNA defects, abnormal mitochondrial gene expression, defective mitochondrial enzyme activities, abnormal or deficient mitochondrial DNA repair mechanisms, and mitochondrial dysfunction. Studies suggest that abnormal mitochondrial dynamics (imbalance in mitochondrial fission and fusion) plays a key role in tissues affected by multiple sclerosis. Furthermore, mitochondrial abnormalities and mitochondrial energy failure may impact other cellular pathways including increased demyelination and inflammation in neurons and tissues that are affected by multiple sclerosis [Mao & Reddy, 2010].

While remyelination is extensive in some MS lesions, it is absent or incomplete in others [Zambonin et. al. 2011]. Remyelination helps to restore conduction and helps protect the axons from further inflammation. As an adaptive process or compensatory mechanism, demyelination in the central nervous system causes an increase in the mitochondrial content within axons [Mahad et. al., 2009; Kiryu-Seo et. al., 2010]. This has been attributed to the axons from further inflammation. As an adaptive process or compensatory mechanism, response to the changes in energy needs of axons caused by redistribution of sodium channels. Demyelination compromises the ionic balance and structural integrity of the axons. It results in diffusely expressed Na^+ channels with persistent Na^+ leakage and forces the need for additional energy to operate the Na^+/K^+ ATPase pumps. The mitochondria were found to increase in the order of increased energy demand, myelinated, remyelinated and demyelinated axons [Mahad et. al., 2009; Kiryu-Seo et. al., 2010; Zambonin et.al., 2011]. The increase in mitochondrial content (mostly stationary) within remyelinated compared to myelinated axons was attributed to the increase in density of the porin elements. (Porin is a voltage gated anion channel located in the outer membrane of all mitochondria). This increase in mitochondrial content resulted in a corresponding increase in mitochondrial respiratory chain complex IV activity. The change in demyelinated axons was attributed to the change in size. While the number of mobile mitochondria in both remyelinated and myelinated axons were nearly the same, they were much less in demyelinated neurons. An approximately 4 fold increase in mitochondrial content has been observed in chronically demyelinated and non-degenerative axons [Zambonin et. al., 2011]. However, increased mitochondrial content does not necessarily mean more activity. It has been demonstrated that while the mass number may increase in amyloid precursor protein positive segments of demyelinated axons, they appear to harbor mitochondria with complex IV defects [Mahad et. al., 2009]. Within injured axons (non-phosphorylated neurofilaments: SMI32) mitochondrial depletion and decreased complex IV activity was evident, in contrast to chronically demyelinated SMI31 positive axons located in the relatively inactive areas of chronic multiple sclerosis lesions exhibiting a significant increase in complex IV activity and mass [Table 1].

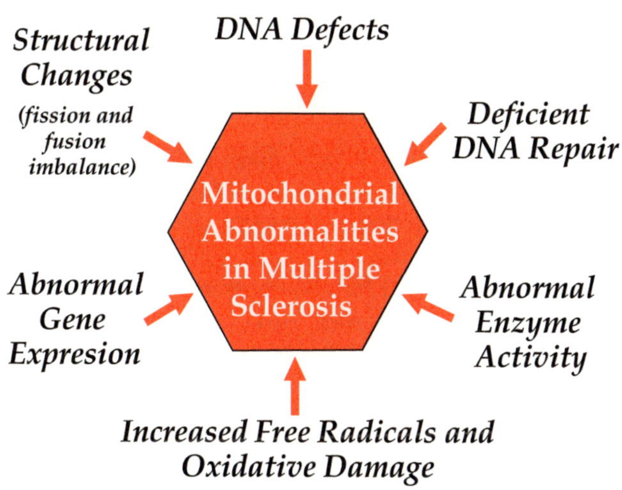

Fig. 3. Mitochondrial abnormalities in multiple sclerosis [adapted from Mao & Reddy, 2010]

	Control(SMI31)	NAWM(SMI31)	Lesion(APP)	Lesion(SMI32)	Lesion(SM131)
Complex IV					
Intensity					
Brian	17.93±5.89	16.14±6.54	9.85±6.94#	10.26±5.43#	20.10±7.38†, ‡
Spinal cord	16.99±15.49	16.87±12.44	9.01±11.16#	15.93±13.01	23.04±11.07*
Porin					
Percent Area					
Brian	6.74±.2.82	7.35±4.30	7.93±4.50	4.19±3.95†	11.15±5.23*
Spinal cord	5.93±4.38	3.46±3.92	8.26±7.40	1.64 ±1.39#	13.97±7.23*

Table 1. Quantification of the intensity of complex IV active elements and mitochondrial mass within axons [Mahad et. al., 2009]. The intensity of complex IV active elements represents the difference in densitometric value between background and complex IV active elements in inverted grey scale 100x brightfield images of cytochrome c oxidase or COX histochemistry. The percentage area of porin reactive elements within axons was calculated based on the total area of axonal porin reactive elements in triple labeled (porin, syntaphilin and axonal marker) and area of axons in confocal images. †P = 0.001 (versus NAWM) and ‡P = 0.002 (versus CON). #P<0.001 (versus SMI31 in CON, NAWM and lesion). *P<0.001 (versus SMI31 in NAWM and CON as well as SMI32 in lesion and APP in lesion). [For details, please see Mahad et. al., 2009]

Mitochondrial injury and subsequent energy failure have been implicated in the pathogenesis of MS [Lu et. al., 2000; Dutta et. al., 2006; Mahad et. al., 2008, 2009; Haider et. al., 2011; Campbell et. al., 2011]. Proteins and DNA in mitochondria are highly vulnerable to free radical damage and consequent mitochondrial injury in MS. The likely candidates involved in tissue injury in MS are the ROS and nitric oxide intermediates. These are produced by activated macrophages and microglia. In the brain tissue of patients with MS, oxidized DNA and oxidized lipids have been detected [Lu et. al., 2000]. Oxidized phospholipids and malondialdehyde (lipid peroxidation-derived structures) data from MS lesions of different activity of patients with acute, relapsing, remitting and progressive disease were found to be concentrated in active MS plaques, in areas known as initial demyelinating lesion or the "prephagocytic" stage of active MS lesions [Haider et. al., 2011]. There was good correlation between inflammation and the extent of DNA and lipid oxidation. Data in table 2 indicate up to a 5 fold increase in the extent of DNA damage (8-OHdG staining) and lipid oxidation (E06 and MDA-2 staining) in active lesions versus inactive lesions, normal white matter in MS patients, and white matter controls. The oxidation is predominantly seen in lesions with high T-cell and macrophage infiltrates and with profound microglial activation (HLA-D staining).

So far the efforts for complete restoration of axonal mitochondria following remyelination have not been successful. Thus the need for preservation of myelinated axons is exemplified by the fact that remyelinated axons have increased energy demand. This may also result in deficient neurons and reach detrimental levels in the long term. Mitochondrial DNA deletions have been found in the neurons in the progressive stage of MS [Campbell et. al., 2011]. The pathological features of MS lesions include demyelination and oligodendrocyte apoptosis, preferential destruction of small- caliber axons, differentiation arrest of oligodendrocyte progenitor cells and remyelination failure, and astrocyte dysfunction [Haider et. al., 2011].

	Active lesion	Slowly expanding Lesion	Inactive lesion	NAWM MS	White matter controls
	Median & (range)	Median & (range)	Median & (range)	Median & (range)	Median & (range)
Percentage of E06 positive area	3.1(26.5)	1.6 (16.7)	0.6 (9.2)	0.8 (17.1)	0.06 (2.9)
E06 axon spheroids	1.3 (18.2)	1.2 (121.2)	0.4 (2.3)	0.0 (1.2)	0.00 (0.0)
MDA-2 OG	1.6 (25.8)	0.9 (5.4)	0.9 (1.6)	0.4 (9.2)	0.00 (1.6)
8-OHdG nuclei	5.6 (78.1)	9.0 (19.0)	1.6 (6.8)	1.4 (12.0)	0.40 (10.4)
APP	44.3 (197.6)	16.1 (40.0)	0.3 (1.5)	0.0 (1.0)	0.00 (0.8)
CD3	73.6 (298.8)	51.2 (105.6)	10.0 (69.1)	4.8 (38.4)	9.60 (49.6)
HLA-D	324.8 (585.6)	148.3 (398.0)	29.0 (246.5)	99.3 (190.0)	43.10 (114.4)

Table 2. Quantification of oxidized lipids and oxidized DNA in different types of multiple sclerosis lesions in comparison with controls [Haider et. al., 2011]. Values represent medians and range (95th percentile range values); P-values are corrected by Bonferroni for multiple testing; all values represent counted cells/mm^2. Active lesions = classical actively demyelinating lesions; slowly expanding lesions = lesions with inactive lesion centre, surrounded by a small rim of activated microglia with recent myelin-degradation products; inactive lesions = lesions without any recent demyelinating activity; NAWM multiple sclerosis = normal-appearing white matter from patients with multiple sclerosis; white matter controls = normal white matter of all controls; APP = amyloid precursor protein reactive axonal spheroids or end bulbs; CD3 = T cells; percentage of E06 positive area = densitometric analysis of area covered by E06 immunoreactivity; E06 axon spheroids = axonal spheroids or end bulbs stained by E06 antibody; HLA-D = class II MHC-positive macrophages/microglia; MDA-2 OG = oligodendrocyte-like cells, immunoreactive for MDA-2; 8-OHdG nuclei = number of cell nuclei containing 8 hydroxy-D-guanosine immunoreactivity. Data show a highly significant accumulation of oxidized DNA and oxidized lipids in active multiple sclerosis lesions in comparison with controls. Oxidized DNA and lipids are predominantly seen in lesions with high T-cell and macrophage infiltrates and with profound microglia activation. (p values not included for brevity). [For details, please see Haider et. al., 2011]

A recent review details the current immunomodulatory treatments for MS. Other alternatives beyond immune-directed approaches are also speculated in this review [Aktas et. al., 2010]. Increased concentrations of reactive oxygen and nitrogen species found in MS, for example, lead to inhibition of ATP production within the axon. The ATP deficiency leads to loss of Na^+/K^+ ATPase and collapse of transmembrane ionic gradients. There is also an increase in intracellular Ca^{2+} levels and a decrease in mRNA levels of mitochondrial genes. At the same time immune -related demyelination also takes place. These results have prompted ion channel homeostasis as a potential therapeutic target to ameliorate the failed energy metabolism.

Peroxy nitrite formation at the site of inflammation has been measured using nitrotyrosine as a biochemical marker. Levels of nitrite and nitrate, the stable oxidation products of nitric oxide and peroxynitrite measured in cerebral fluid samples also revealed significantly higher levels of nitrate during clinical relapses of MS [Cross et. al., 1998].

In view of our data with palladium α-lipoic acid formulation (section 10) on the enhanced enzymatic activities of Krebs cycle and electron transport chain enzymes in animals, anti-oxidant activity and the ability of this formulation to repair DNA, we had decided, as a preliminary step, to investigate its usefulness in ameliorating the fatigue conditions in 15 MS patients. The study is expected to be completed soon.

8. Cerebral ischemia

An insufficient or reduced blood flow to the brain to meet the metabolic demand will result in cerebral or brain ischemia. The normal cerebral blood flow is ~ 50 to 60 mL/100g/min. Death of brain tissue is a consequence of poor oxygen supply or cerebral hypoxia resulting from the insufficient blood flow. A prototype of brain damage during cerebral ischemia is shown in Fig. 4. [adapted from Mehta et. al., 2007]. Maximum damage occurs as a result of ischemic necrosis (infarction) at the "core" or "focal" tissue region, where the blood flow is < 7 mL/100g/min. Since the cellular integrity is compromised during necrosis, cellular damage repair at the core is extremely hard. The blood flow in the surrounding less-severely ischemic boundary ("penumbral" or "perifocal" tissue) is ~ 7 to 17 mL/100g/min. The penumbra is metabolically active but electrically silent [Mehta et. al., 2007]. More moderate alterations develop in this region because of the near normal glucose use, but the oxidative metabolism is still impaired. Different mechanisms contribute to cell death in the core and penumbra due to differences in the severity of ischemia.

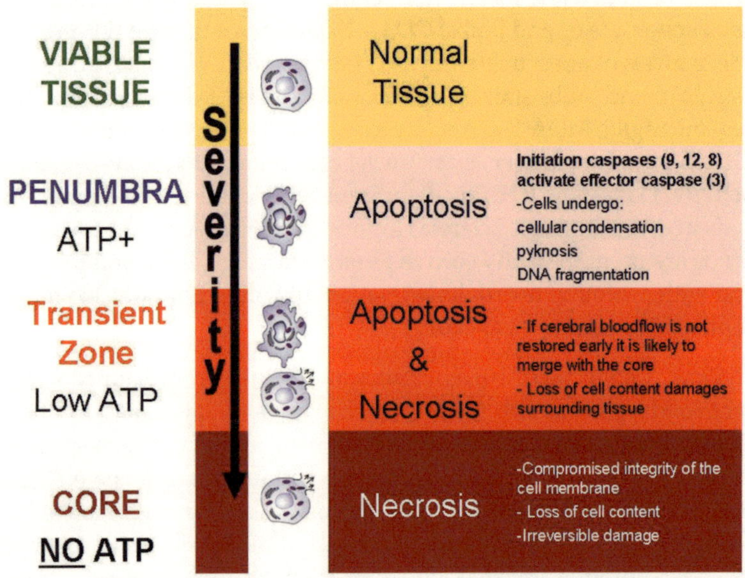

Fig. 4. A prototype brain damage during cerebral ischemia: core, a region where cells undergo necrosis. The region surrounding the core is called ischemic penumbra, a site of delayed mode of cell death (apoptosis) due to availability of ATP. Further, a transient zone in-between the core and penumbra is likely to merge to the core if the cerebral blood flow is not restored early. The penumbral region is surrounded by a region of viable tissue [adapted from Mehta et. al., 2007]

Therapeutic quick intervention may reduce the infarct volume in the penumbra because the irreversible damage occurs relatively slowly [Sims & Muyderman, 2010]. The only embolic or thrombolytic agent used to reverse arterial occlusion within the first 3 h is tissue plasminogen activator (tPA). As an enzyme, it catalyzes the conversion of plasminogen to the enzyme responsible for clot breakdown, plasmin. In ~17 % of ischemic stroke patients spontaneous reversal of occlusion takes place in 6 h and in 40-50% of patients in 4 days. Quick restoration of normal blood flow to this region can result in substantial recovery of energy- related metabolites. However, in the post ischemic tissue, energy requirements are low and the glucose oxidation is due to limitations on the mitochondrial oxidation of pyruvate. This results in a secondary impairment of mitochondrial function and consequent cell death. Normalcy of function can be maintained in the outermost viable tissue.

While focal ischemia is confined to a specific region of the brain, global ischemia encompasses wide areas of the brain tissue. Focal ischemia occurs in a region when a blood clot has occluded in a downstream region of artery in the brain (ischemic stroke). This occlusion or blockage may be caused by thrombosis (a blood clot formed locally obstructing the blood flow) or arterial embolism (obstruction of blood flow due to an embolus from elsewhere in the body). While ischemic strokes are caused by interruption of the blood supply, hemorrhagic strokes are the result of rupture of a blood vessel. Hemorrhagic strokes result in areas of friable tissue, containing areas of both viable and dead tissue. Transient global ischemia involves a brief interruption in blood flow usually in a larger cerebral vessel, e.g. middle cerebral artery, resulting in primarily apoptotic cell death.

More than 80% of all strokes are due to focal ischemia. Unless treated, the occlusion of an artery produces tissue infarction resulting in a loss of all cells including neurons, astrocytes, oligodendrocytes, microglia and endothelial cell [Sims & Muyderman, 2010]. The stroke results in mitochondrial impairment because the blood flow becomes < 20% of the normal and a consequent reduction in glucose and oxygen supplies ensue. This attenuates ATP and reactive oxygen species production as well as apoptosis. Lack of ATP production disrupts the ionic gradients across the plasma membrane. The net result is marked losses of intracellular K^+ and a large influx of Ca^{2+} into cells [Doyle et. al., 2008]. Thus there is heavy involvement of the impaired mitochondria in the development of the tissue injury after ischemic attack, due to modifications in ATP production and other mitochondrial changes leading to apoptosis and necrosis.

Further, a transient zone in-between the core and penumbra is likely to merge to the core if the cerebral blood flow is not restored early. The damage in this transient zone is a result of the release of cellular contents from those necrotic "core" cells, such as the oxidative enzymes of various organelles i.e. lysozomes and peroxisomes. Eventually this transient zone would contribute to the total infarct volume. The penumbral region is surrounded by a region of viable tissue [Mehta et. al., 2007]. Penumbra varies in size and can be rescued

Ischemic cell death is also attributed to abnormal activation of enzymes such as poly-ADP ribose polymerase (PARP) and the caspases. Oxidative stress, which produces free radical nitric oxide (NO·) and reactive peroxynitrite ($ONOO^-$), is implicated in both necrosis and apoptosis in focal ischemia. Peroxynitrite is formed by the reaction of NO· with superoxide. Mitochondria are targeted by peroxynitrite and the resulting mitochondrial dysfunction during severe hypoxia-ischemia increases generation of oxygen free radicals. This leads to dysfunction of cellular membrane causing necrosis [Mehta et. al. 2007]. An additional consequence of ischemia involves the dissociation of the electron transport chain within minutes of the insult. Ubiquinone and cytochrome C, which serve as electron shuttles,

translocate from the inner mitochondrial membrane. This is of particular consequence upon restoration of blood flow. While reperfusion limits some damage, oxidative stress is increased under these conditions. It has been found that over expression of Mn^{2+}-superoxide dismutase, which converts superoxide to hydrogen peroxide results in moderate reductions in the size of infarction in temporary ischemia [Sims & Muyderman, 2010]. Addition of the mitochondrial uncoupling agent, dinitrophenol, was found to modulate the Ca^{2+} content and production of free radicals in the mitochondria of penumbra [Korde et. al., 2005].
The reduced delivery of oxygen and glucose to the tissue in focal ischemia affects the function of the mitochondria. Mitochondrial properties undergo further changes depending on the severity and duration of ischemia and also following reperfusion. Development of cell death pathways depends on the impaired mitochondria's ability to generate ATP.

	Focal ischemia		**Reperfusion**	
	Core	Penumbra	Core	Penumbra
Metabolites				
ATP	↓↓↓	↓↓	↓↓	↓
Adenylate energy charge	↓↓	↓	↓/N.C.	N.C.
Total adenine nucleotides	↓↓	↓↓	↓↓	↓
Phosphocreatine	↓↓↓	↓	↓	N.C.
Lactate	↑↑	↑↑	↑↑	↑/N.C.
Glucose	↓↓↓	N.C.	N.C.	N.C.
Metabolic activity				
Glucose use	↓↓↓*	N.C.	↓↓	↓↓
Oxidative metabolism	↓↓↓*	↓↓↓	↓↓	↓↓

Table 3. The effects of focal ischemia for up to 2 h and of subsequent reperfusion for 1 h on the content of energy-related metabolites and pathways of energy metabolism [Sims & Muyderman, 2010]. Differences are shown compared to non-ischemic tissue. ↓: decreased to >65%; ↓↓: decreased to between 35% and 65% ; ↓↓↓: decreased to less than 35%; ↑: increased less than four-fold; ↑↑: increased greater than four-fold; N.C.: no significant change. Two symbols indicate findings that differ between published reports. *, direct evaluation of these properties in severely ischemic tissue may not give reliable information. The magnitude of these reductions is assumed from the large decrease in substrate delivery and large changes in ATP and phosphocreatine content [Sims & Muyderman, 2010]

The changes in energy-related metabolites and in the contributing metabolic pathways in brain tissue in the first 2 h of ischemia and reperfusion for 1 h are summarized in Table 3 [Sims & Muyderman, 2010]. In the core, the ATP and glucose content falls significantly in the first 5 min of occlusion and then ATP stabilizes to ~ 15-30% of normal for at least the first 2 h and then reaches about 50%. The initial rapid decrease is attributed to the major redistribution of ions across the plasma membrane of cells. In view of our admittance data on the H_2O_2-Ca^{2+}, H_2O_2-Na^+ interactions, we strongly believe that ion-peroxide interactions must also be playing a major part in this process. The adenylate energy charge, a measure of intracellular balance between ATP, ADP, and AMP, is given by:

$$\text{Adenylate energy charge} = \{[ATP] + 0.5\,[ADP]/\,[ATP] + [ADP] + [AMP]\} \qquad (31)$$

The adenylate energy charge decreases rapidly to ~ 0.4-0.5 during the initial hours and remains above 0.8 after 2 h compared to the normal value in the brain of ~ 0.93. While adenylate kinase catalyses the conversion of some ADP to AMP to meet short term energy needs of the brain, in ischemic tissue, the adenine nucleotide pool is depleted by the conversion of AMP to inosine and hypoxanthine. Phosphocreatine, the short term energy reserve of the brain falls quickly to <30% of normal during ischemia. Phosphocreatine stabilizes to about 70% of normal after ~ 2 h of ischemia. ATP regeneration from ADP is catalyzed by the enzyme creatine kinase. Lack of oxygen forces glucose to go the glycolytic pathway creating a 10-fold increase in lactate and consequent lowering of pH. Of course lack of removal of lactate due to limited blood flow may also be contributing to this accumulation. In addition, restricted blood flow appears to have a greater effect on the delivery of oxygen to the tissues versus glucose, since penumbral glucose levels are either the same or slightly higher, while lactate levels are much higher (but less than in the core).
During the first 2 h following reperfusion, phosphocreatine and adenylate energy charge are recovered to >90% of normal compared to ATP values of 50-70%. This resistance of ATP for restoration is attributed to the depletion of the adenine nucleotide pool. In the penumbral tissue, phosphocreatine and adenine nucleotide balance, but not ATP are recovered almost completely within 1 h of reperfusion for ischemic periods of 3 h or longer [Sims & Muyderman, 2010]. The glucose utilization is less in the penumbral region during the first hour of reperfusion. The lactate, on the other hand, is decreased during this period.
The reduction in ATP production in the ischemic brain may be associated with decreased neuronal activity of the post-ischemic brain as a result of the enzyme AMP-activated protein kinase enzyme [Sims & Muyderman, 2010].
It must be mentioned that there is a complete or near complete recovery of mitochondrial respiratory function in core and penumbral tissues within the first hour following reperfusion. This is followed by a secondary deterioration, indicative of the development of irreversible cell dysfunction.
Under normal physiological conditions, the channel within the N-methyl-D-aspartic acid (NMDA) glutamate receptor is blocked in a voltage dependent manner by Mg^{2+}. The triggering of energy deficits and neuronal depolarization are the results of decreased cerebral blood flow. The mild depolarization results in the dislodging of Mg^{2+} and glutamate, which are consequently released in large amounts to the extracellular space. This leads to an over-activation of the NMDA and AMPA glutamate receptors. Since these receptors regulate Ca^{2+} ion channels, a calcium ionic imbalance occurs in neurons. This influx of Ca^{2+}, is due to this increase in glutamate release from neurons and astrocytes induced by the ischemia. Apart from the traditional ionotropic glutamate receptors, the influx of Ca^{2+} is also attributed to some emerging metabotropic and channel mechanisms that include: sodium-calcium exchangers, hemi channels (unopposed half-gap junctions), acid sensing channels, volume-regulated anion channels, nonselective cation channels and signaling cascades that mediate crosstalk between redundant pathways of cell death [Besancon et al., 2008]. This abnormal intracellular accumulation of Ca^{2+} is involved in the triggering of cell death by up regulation of a wide range of cell death executioners that include ATPases that serve to further deplete energy stores, lipases that damage lipid membranes of organelles and the cell surface itself, proteases that dismantle the cytoarchitecture of the neuron, and DNAses that damage the nucleus [Besancon et. al. 2008].
Bioenergetics of cerebral ischemia (both focal and global) as well as gray and white matter ischemia were recently reviewed from a cellular perspective. A brief summary is given in

Table 4 [Hertz, 2008]. During the early stages of ischemia, fatal injury is observed for neurons and oligodendrocytes. They are very sensitive to the excitotoxicity of glutamate due to their cell process expression of NMDA receptors and cell body expression of AMPA/kinase receptors. Astrocytes and endothelial cells seem to survive longer. Neurons are damaged from lack of astrocyte support. Axonal injury is due to channel mediated Na^+ uptake followed by Na^+/Ca^{2+} exchange.

	Neurons	Axons	Oligodendrocytes	Astrocytes	Endothelial cells
Intracellular Na^+ increase	X	X	X	X	X
Increased metabolism	X	?	?	X	?
Intracellular Ca^{2+} increase	X	X	X	X	?
Mitochondrial damage	X		X	X	?
Formation of ROS	X		X	(X)	X

Table 4. Bioenergetic mechanisms involved in ischemic death of different cell types and constituents [Hertz, 2008]

Studies have demonstrated that ischemic damage may be reduced by blockade of ionotropic glutamate receptors using glutamate receptor antagonists [Mehta et. al., 2007; Besancon et. al., 2008; Doyle et. al., 2008; Sims & Muyderman, 2010]. The most extensively evaluated neuroprotectors that include calcium channel blockers, glutamate antagonists, GABA agonists, antioxidants and radical scavengers, and NO· signal down regulator, have been critically reviewed recently [Ginsberg, 2008].

Other neuroprotective approaches involve the use of anti-oxidants. As an example, α-lipoic acid reduced the mortality rate of male Sprague-Dawley rats from 78% to 26% during 24 hours of reperfusion. It was found effective in improving survival and protecting the rat brain against reperfusion injury following cerebral ischemia [Panigrahi et. al., 1996]. In another study rats that received subcutaneous treatment of R-or S-lipoic acid for 2 hours before ischemia significantly reduced the infarct volume [Wolz & Krieglstein, 1996]. Similar results with mice were obtained with 100 mg/kg of lipoic acid given subcutaneously 1.5 hours before ischemia [Clark et. al., 2001]. Transient global ischemia also benefits from pretreatment with α-lipoic acid. Administration of 40 mg/kg for 7 days protected from ischemic damage when gerbils were tested for locomotor behavior and morphological damage to the CA1 region of the hippocampus [Cao & Phillis, 1995].

Animal studies, using adult male Mongolian gerbils, used as controls or treatment group with palladium α-lipoic acid complex formulation (PdLA), demonstrated that acute, post ischemic and prophylactic administration of PdLA limits ischemic damage [Antonawich et. al., 2004]. Following bilateral carotid artery occlusion in the gerbil, the PdLA was administered intraperitoneally (IP) immediately after surgery, then once daily for 3 days. The control group received saline. PdLA treatment significantly protected hippocampal pyramidal cells (CA1) from transient global ischemia at 30, 50, and 70 mg/kg per 24 h.

While a delayed application of the palladium α-lipoic acid complex formulation after 48 hours of ischemic attack had no significant effect in protecting CA 1 cells, a delayed administration after 6 hours of ischemic attack was as good as giving it immediately after ischemic attack in minimizing cell death.

Five minutes of carotid artery occlusion was sufficient to hinder the characteristic nesting behavior of gerbils for ~ 3 days. Their nesting behavior was observed to improve significantly after treatment with palladium lipoic acid complex formulation (50 mg/kg every 24h and 30 mg/kg /24h at 24 and 72 hours after ischemia. The lack of nesting behavior at 70 mg/kg-treated animals was attributed to their excessive energy and consequent ignoring of the nesting material.

It was observed that preventive or prophylactic treatment with 10 mg/kg gerbil (or allometric scaling equivalent of 10 mL-human dosage) offered significant behavioral and morphological improvement from transient global ischemia.

Our studies demonstrate a greater protective effect of palladium α-lipoic acid complex versus α-lipoic acid alone (Cao & Phillis, 1995). Four times more α-lipoic acid and for a longer period of pre-treatment were necessary to obtain morphologiocal protection. Further more immediate administration of palladium α-lipoic acid complex formulation protected over 70%of the CA1 neurons, and administration delayed up to 24 hours after the TIA still offered significant protection (30% of the CA1 pyramidal cells) [Antonawich et. al., 2004].

9. The powerful super-antioxidant, α-lipoic acid

Alpha- lipoic acid is a very unique and simple biological molecule. It has a carboxylic acid group with a pK_a of 4.7. It is ionized at biological pH, and it has a cyclic disulfide or dithiolane ring [Baumgartner et. al., 1996; Patel & Packer, 2008]. It exists intracellularly as the reduced form, (±)-dihydrolipoic acid. Lipoic acid occurs naturally as a coenzyme in both prokaryotic and eukaryotic cells, as well as in plants, and animals including humans. It is enzymatically synthesized from octanoic acid in the mitochondrion.

α-Lipoic acid, absorbed intact from the diet, is readily converted into dihydrolipoic acid in many tissues. In the intracellular environment, two or more enzymes reduce the exogenous lipoic acid. The reversible reduction to dihydrolipoic acid is favored by the presence of the ring strain in the 1, 2-dithiolane ring of about 15-25 $kJmol^{-1}$ [Baumgartner et. al., 1996]. α-Lipoic acid exits as R(+)-and S(-)- enantiomers due to the presence of an asymmetric carbon. The biologically active enantiomer is mostly the former one. Since its first isolation in 1951, numerous investigations have been carried out to decipher the uniqueness of this simple but elegant molecule [Reed 2001; Patel & Packer, 2008].

Molecular mechanisms and therapeutic potential of α-lipoic acid, a dietary supplement, have been reviewed recently [Shay et. al., 2009]. Lipoic acid can cross the blood-brain barrier. The biological effects of lipoic acid are attributed to its redox property, the antioxidant capacity and the fatty acid properties. There is ample evidence indicating the usefulness of the lipoic acid/dihydrolipoic acid redox couple as a therapeutic agent for diabetes, ischemia-reperfusion injury, heavy metal poisoning, modulator of various inflammatory signaling pathways, age associated cardiovascular, cognitive, and neuromuscular deficits, protection from radiation damage, neurodegeneration, and HIV infection [Packer et. al., 1995; Patel & Packer, 2008; Shay et.al., 2009]. Dihydrolipoic acid can regenerate or recycle the antioxidants CoQ (ubiquinol), vitamins C and E (via glutathione), and glutathione without itself becoming one in the process. Dihydrolipoic acid also prevents lipid peroxidation by regenerating glutathione. [Packer et. al., 1995; Patel & Packer, 2008].

Lipoic acid and dihydrolipoic acid are efficiently transported in and out of both mitochondria and cells. Compared to this, the transport of disulfides such as cystine that is needed in modulating glutathione (GSH) levels in cells is very inefficient. The mitochondrial β-oxidation of lipoic acid has been attributed to its fatty acid properties, similar to that of octanoic acid [Patel & Packer, 2008]. Redox as well as biological antioxidant effects have been attributed to the β-oxidation products of lipoic acid, the oxidized and reduced forms of bisnorlipoic acid and tetranorlipoic acid [Patel & Packer, 2008].

Oxidant	Scavenged or not by LA and rate constant	Scavenged or not by DHLA and rate constant
Peroxynitrite	Yes, 1.4×10^3 M^{-1} S^{-1}	Yes, 2.5×10^2 M^{-1} S^{-1}
Nitric oxide	No	Yes, 3.19 M^{-1} S^{-1}
Hydroxyl radical	Yes, 4.7×10^{10} M^{-1} S^{-1}	No
	Yes	Yes
Superoxide	No	No
	Yes, 3.3×10^5 M^{-1} S^{-1}	
		Yes
Singlet oxygen	Yes, 1.3×10^8 M^{-1} S^{-1}	No
	Yes	
Peroxyl radical	Yes, 1.8×10^8 M^{-1} S^{-1}	Yes, 2.3×10^7 M^{-1} S^{-1}
	No	Yes
Hypochlorous acid	Yes	Yes
Hydrogen peroxide	No	No

Table 5. Antioxidant activities of lipoic acid (LA) and dihydrolipoic acid (DHLA) [detailed references in Shay et. al., 2009]

The α-lipoic acid/dihydrolipoic acid couple is called a "universal antioxidant" because it fulfills several criteria used to evaluate the antioxidant potential as well as preventive or therapeutic applications of a compound such as specificity of free radical quenching, metal chelating ability, interaction with other antioxidants, effects on gene expression, absorption and bioavailability, concentration in tissues, cells, and extracellular fluid, and location (in aqueous or membrane domains or in both) [Packer et.al., 1995].

The free radical scavenging activities of lipoic acid and dihydrolipoic acid are given in Table 5 [Shay et.al., 2009]. Both are capable of scavenging peroxynitrite, peroxyl radical and hypochlorous acid, but not hydrogen peroxide. There are conflicting data for singlet oxygen and radicals such as hydroxyl, superoxide, and peroxyl.

Questions have been raised regarding the direct-acting antioxidant status of LA/DHLA in vivo based on the invitro data [Shay et.al., 2009]. This is due to the large dosage, 200-600 mg, used for invivo studies and the amounts found in the plasma (both area under the curve and C_{max} are in the range of microgram to nanogram levels per mL). The administration of lipoic acid in acid form or salt form, oral or intravenous, with a meal or without meal also contributed to the fluctuations in the data. Also the invitro data cannot imitate the invivo clearance of 98% of LA excretion in the urine within 24 hours.

α-Lipoic acid was found to protect hematopoietic tissues in mice from radiation damage [Ramakrishnan et. al., 1992]. It was also found that α-lipoic acid offered protection from radiation for children affected by the Chernobyl nuclear accident [Korkina et al., 1993]. α-Lipoic acid scavenges hydroxyl radicals but is not effective against hydrogen peroxide and superoxide radical. The reduction potential for the α-lipoic acid/dihydrolipoic acid couple of -320 mV or -290 mV [Krishnan et. al., 2011] and the GSSG/GSH) couple of -240 mV indicate that dihydrolipoic acid can react with GSSG and regenerate GSH [Packer et. al., 1995]. Thus lipoic acid helps to maintain GSH/GSSG ratio (about 100 to 10,000 times greater than other redox couples such as NAD^+/NADH, and $NADP^+$/NADPH), an estimate of redox state, in cells [Patel & Packer, 2008].

Treatment with lipoic acid increases the GSH levels in human cell lines and primary cells including T cells, erythrocytes, lymphocytes, and glial and neuroblastoma cells.. This is explained by 1) facile transport of lipoic acid into cells, where it is reduced by NADH or NADPH dependent pathways to dihydrolipoic acid. 2) Dihydrolipoic acid is transported back into the extracellular media where it is oxidized by cysteine regenerating lipoic acid and producing cysteine, the limiting substrate on GSH synthesis. 3) Compared to cystine, cysteine is more easily transported into the cell and aids the synthesis of GSH [Patel & Packer, 2008].

Thus elevated levels of GSH and ascorbic acid, which in turn regenerates vitamin E, are all indicative of lipoic acid acting as an inducer of endogenous antioxidants. It has been reported that lipoic acid is also an effective regulator of signaling pathways and induces synthesis of GSH transcriptionally. Lipoic acid reverses the decline in transcriptional activity of Nrf2 caused by age-related loss of GSH [Suh et. al, 2004].

The pharmacokinetics of R-lipoic acid, reviewed recently [Patel & Packer, 2008; Shay et.al., 2009], revealed a plasma level concentration, C_{max}, of 1.154 μg/mL from 1 g R-lipoic acid compared to the proposed therapeutic range of 10-20 μg/mL or 50-100 μM (Carlson et al., 2008). A dose of 600-800 mg sodium R-lipoate gave plasma levels of 8-18 μg/mL, which is within the therapeutic range. The upper limit suggested for therapeutic action of 45 μg/mL or 225 μM is reached by a dose of about 1.2 g of racemic-α-lipoic acid. The no adverse observed effect level (NOAEL) of racemic lipoic acid is considered to be 60 mg/kg body mass/day. Therapeutic and energy production applications of this powerful antioxidant have been explored extensively [Patel & Packer, 2008].

Located within the mitochondrial matrix are lipoic acid requiring enzymes: three α-keto acid dehydrogenase complexes that catalyze the oxidative decarboxylation of α-keto acids such as pyruvate, α-ketoglutarate, and branched chain α-ketoacids [Voet D. and Voet J. G., 1995]. In organisms, hydrogen atom transfer and acyl group transfer take place in the oxidative decarboxylation of α-ketoacids with the aid of α-lipoic acid. The reversible redox reaction between α-lipoic acid and dihydrolipoic acid is thus a very important biochemical reaction. The reversible reduction to dihydrolipoic acid is favored by the presence of the ring strain in the 1,2-dithiolane ring of about 15-25 $kJmol^{-1}$ [Patel & Packer, 2008].

The multienzyme complex, pyruvate dehydrogenase, consists of three enzymes, pyruvate dehydrogenase (E1), dihydrolipoyl transacetylase (E2), and dihydrolipoyl dehydrogenase (E3) [Voet D. and Voet J. G., 1995]. This enzyme complex participates in five sequential reactions during the conversion of pyruvate to acetyl-CoA. The R- lipoic acid is covalently linked to a ε-amino group of lysine residue via an amide linkage. These lipoic acid containing enzymes participate in four out of the five reactions.

The multienzyme complex, α-ketoglutarate dehydrogenase, also consists of three enzymes, α-ketoglutarate dehydrogenase (E1), dihydrolipoyl transsuccinylase (E2), and dihydrolipoyl dehydrogenase (E3) [Voet D. and Voet J. G., 1995]. The branched chain α-ketoacid dehydrogenase is also a multienzyme complex resembling the other two enzymes mentioned above. These three enzymes have the same dihydrolipoyl dehydrogenase and employ the coenzymes thiamine pyrophosphate, lipoamide, FAD and the terminal oxidizing agent NAD^+ [Voet D. and Voet J. G., 1995]. The importance of lipoic acid in the energy metabolism is illustrated by these three enzymes.

Disulfide bonds in proteins are formed between the thiol groups of cysteine residues. The other sulfur-containing amino acid, methionine, cannot form disulfide bonds. More aggressive oxidants convert cysteine to the corresponding sulfinic acid and sulfonic acid. A variety of oxidants promote this reaction including air and hydrogen peroxide. Such reactions are thought to proceed via sulfenic acid intermediates.

The oxidized form α-lipoic acid can undergo further oxidation at sulfur or get reduced. This property, which is somewhat similar to an intermediate oxidation state in a transition metal or a nonmetal, makes this molecule very unique compared to other biological molecules. A biological oxidation product of α-lipoic acid (lipoic acid S-oxide or a thiolsulfinate) is known as β-lipoic acid or Protogen-B [Baumgartner et. al., 1996]. It has not been possible to conclusively prove which sulfur is oxidized [Stary et. al. 1975].

The oxidation of α-lipoic acid was found to be a one-electron charge transfer process, pH independent, and an irreversible process [Corduneanu et. al., 2009]. Most voltammetric studies were centered on the oxidation of α-lipoic acid and studies related to its reduction to dihydrolipoic acid were limited [Rogers & Mallett, 1983]. To understand the electrochemical behavior of α-lipoic acid, we had explored potential regions beyond the normal range of the mercury electrode, both on the cathodic side as well as on the anodic side. The advantage in using the mercury electrode is the ease with which we can obtain a fresh consistent surface and drop. We have not observed (visually) any passivation of mercury on the anodic side when lipoic acid was present without any background electrolyte. We had investigated the cathodic side, the normal potential region for mercury working electrode, in much greater detail.

The complexity of the redox process of α-lipoic acid is shown in the cyclic voltammograms in Fig. 5 [Krishnan & Garnett, 2011]. We had assigned the three cathodic peaks to 1) reduction of lipoic acid S-oxide, 2) reduction of lipoic acid to most probably dihydrolipoic acid, and 3) probable reduction of lipoic acid dimers or higher polymers. We have assigned the five anodic peaks to 4) the oxidation product of lipoic acid dimers or higher polymers, 5) oxidation product of dihydrolipoic acid, 6) formation of S-oxide of lipoic acid dimers or higher polymers, 7) formation of lipoic acid S-oxide, and 8) further oxidation of lipoic acid S-oxide/the formation of thiolsulfonates. The peak due to the formation of lipoic acid S-oxide (peak 7) is missing in Figure 3a because of the formation of S-oxide of lipoic acid dimers or higher polymers (peak 6). However, when the formation of lipoic acid polymers is minimized by restricting the scan to less cathodic potentials (to -0.5 V instead of -2.0 V) the formation of S-oxide of lipoic acid dimers or higher polymers is minimized and thus allowing the formation of lipoic acid S-oxide (peak 7) [Krishnan & Garnett, 2011]. Other complexities were expressed at differing scan rates, at higher concentrations and by the presence of electrolytes. The data shown in Fig. 5 are for 1mM α-lipoic acid where solute-solute interactions are minimized and in the absence of electrolytes so that the influence of ion-dipole interactions can be more readily investigated at the double layer.

The molecule, α-lipoic acid, is very unique because of its ability to form a variety of radicals, dimers and higher polymers as well as a variety of lipoic acid S-oxides. This complexity is reflected in its electrochemical redox behavior. Our data demonstrated that depending on the concentration of lipoic acid and the scanning potential, radicals and polymers are formed [Krishnan & Garnett 2011]. Also our data suggest the need for a revalidation of the reported redox potential of the lipoic acid/dihydrolipoic acid couple.

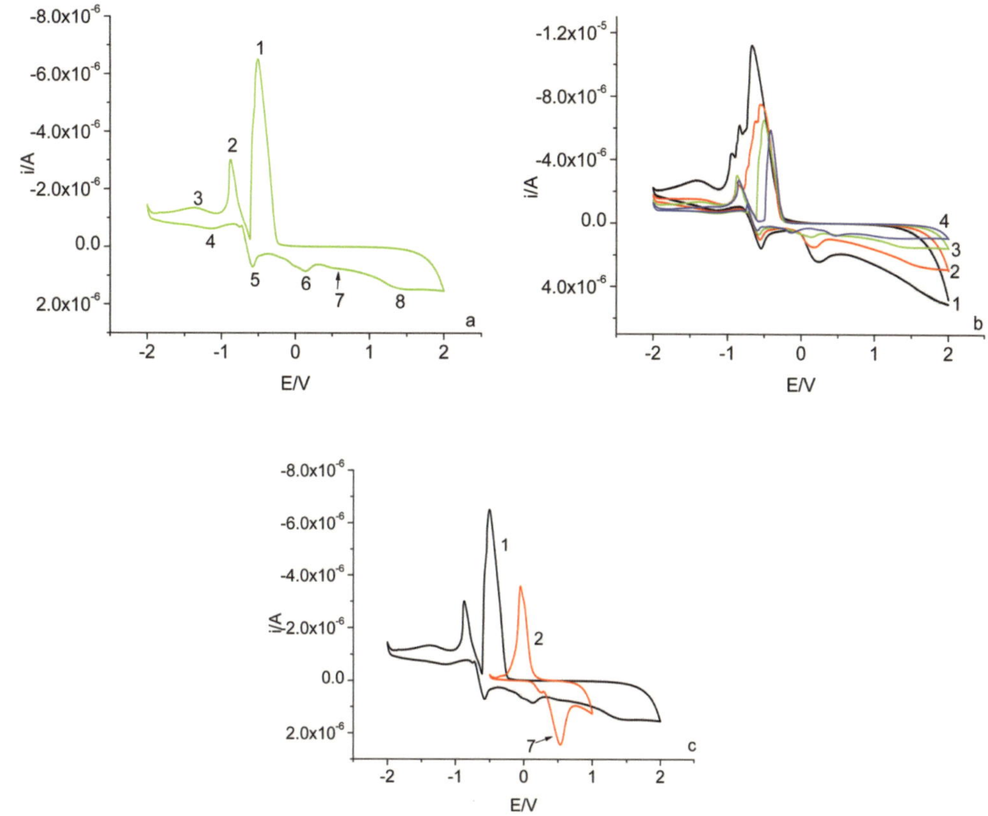

Fig. 5. Cyclic voltammogram of 1 mM α-lipoic acid (sodium salt), pH 7.2, scan 2.0 to -2.0 V and back, scan 3, scan rate a and c, 100mV/sec; b. scan rates 1) 400 2) 200 3) 100 4) 50 mV/sec; **c.** 1) scan 2.0 to -2.0 V and back, 2) scan 1.0 to -0.5V and back; peak 7 same as peak 7 in a. [Krishnan & Garnett 2011]

Our electrochemical data also suggested a caution in deciding on the dosage of oral supplements of lipoic acid because of its tendency to form dimers and higher polymers under reducing biological conditions. The pharmacokinetic data mentioned earlier is also subject to these complexities depending on the dosage chosen for the studies.

10. Catalytic, electronic, and therapeutic properties of palladium α-lipoic acid complex

The coordination chemistry of palladium complexes have recently been reviewed with an emphasis on cancer therapy[Gao et. al., 2009]. Even though there are many structural and thermodynamic similarities between the complexes of palladium and platinum, the palladium(II) complexes seem to exhibit biological action very different from those of the toxic platinum complexes. Copper, zinc, and arsenic complexes of α-lipoic acid and palladium α-lipoic acid complexes with 1:1 and 1:2 stoichiometry have been reported [Garnett, 1995a, 1995b; Strasdeit et. al., 1995; Baumgartner et. al., 1996].

Palladium α-lipoic acid complex has demonstrated numerous antitumor activities against various cell lines. Also it was found to halt the growth of glioblastoma in nude mice. Clinical veterinary studies indicated its effectiveness as a complimentary support to chemotherapy. A recent Phase I, dose escalation study, has revealed safety in humans up to 40 mL 0.037 M of this complex with no severe adverse events, and minor adverse events i.e. mild gastrointestinal irritation, and aversion to taste. Washout periods for palladium, monitored in blood serum and urine, ranged from three to seventeen weeks after cessation of the formulation [Krishnan et. al., 2011].

The electrochemical characteristics of α-lipoic acid and palladium α-lipoic acid complex have been explored using glassy carbon and highly oriented pyrolytic graphite electrodes [Corduneanu et al., 2007, 2009]. Palladium complex was found to dissociate at negative potentials with deposition of Pd(0) nanoparticles. The application of a positive potential induced the oxidation of the palladium complex and the formation of a mixed layer of lipoic acid and palladium oxides.

Superior free radical scavenging capacity, as measured by oxygen radical absorbance capacity or ORAC analysis, was observed for palladium α-lipoic acid complex formulation (5.65) compared to vitamin E (1.0, normalized value), vitamin A (1.6), vitamin C (1.12), and α-lipoic acid (1.4) [Krishnan et.al., 2011]. This may be compared to the superior antitumor activities observed for metal complexes compared to that of their ligands [Matesanz et. al., 1999; Maloň et. al., 2001].

The enhanced energy effects observed in gerbils during transient ischemia studies [Antonawich et. al., 2004] prompted us to investigate the influence of palladium α-lipoic acid complex on the activities of enzymes involved in mitochondrial energy production. The activities of four Krebs cycle enzymes, isocitrate dehydrogenase (ICDH), α-ketoglutarate dehydrogenase (α-KGDH), succinate dehydrogenase (SDH), and malate dehydrogenase (MDH) and mitochondrial complexes I, II, III, and IV in aged male albino rats were investigated [Sudheesh et. al., 2009]. The enhanced activity of the metal complex was superior to the activity of lipoic acid, the ligand.

The antioxidant status in the heart of aged male Albino Wistar rats, measured by MnSOD, CAT, and GSHPx, were higher with the palladium lipoic acid treated group than with the α-lipoic acid group [Sudheesh et al., 2010]. This was also true in alloxan induced diabetic rats [Sudheesh et. al. 2011]. Similarly the lipid peroxidation levels were lowered and the GSH levels were increased in the palladium α-lipoic acid treated group. It is not clear at this time whether scavenging some free radicals by either α-lipoic acid or palladium α-lipoic acid complex formulation is connected in any way to the enhanced activities of Krebs cycle and mitochondrial enzymes.

A specific example is illustrated here. The α-ketoglutarate dehydrogenase complex (KGDH) is a critical component of Krebs cycle and of glutamate metabolism. Glutamate is an excitotoxic neurotransmitter. Reactive oxygen species modify the activity of KGDH. It is also known that the activity of KGDH is lower than that of any other enzyme in the brain. Deficiencies in KGDH lead to brain neurological syndromes. Palladium α-lipoic acid complex increases the activity of KGDH and thus helps in the removal of the glutamate.

The antioxidant status in the liver, kidney and brain of mice after exposure to 2-6 Gy radiation were also measured recently [Menon et. al., 2009]. The results were similar to the ones observed in the heart of rats without radiation. Also an analysis of their blood leukocytes and bone marrow for DNA damage using alkaline single cell gel electrophoresis (alkaline comet assay) revealed DNA repair from the lowering of comet assay parameters, DNA in tail, tail length, tail moment, and olive tail moment. Administration of the complex also reduced the mortality of the mice and also aided recovery from the radiation induced weight loss [Ramachandran et. al., 2010]. DNA repair was also observed in human blood leukocytes with palladium α-lipoic acid complex treatment immediately after exposure to radiation [Menon & Nair, 2011].

The mechanism of the superiority of the metal complex compared to that of the ligand is still an unsolved puzzle. Compared to the high oral dose, the available plasma concentration of α-lipoic acid is very small. One possibility for the higher activity of the metal complex is probably due to its increased concentration in the plasma. This needs experimental verification. It is also known that 98% of α-lipoic acid is excreted in urine within 24 hours and since it takes 4-6 weeks for serum and urine clearance of palladium, the previous suggestion seems justified. Another possibility is the chemistry of the transition metal playing a dominant role in the enzymatic activity. The starting material in the synthesis of the palladium α-lipoic acid complex is palladium(II). The final complex is also palladium(II), based on preliminary ESR data. Palladium(II) complexes are diamagnetic. The complex concentration dependent electrochemical characteristics of α-lipoic acid suggest the possibility of free radical formation by one electron reduction under physiological conditions. In such a case the electron spin may be involved in the enzymatic process. The impedance characteristics of the palladium α-lipoic acid as well as that of the α-lipoic acid, described in this section, strongly suggest this possibility.

Another possibility for the superiority of the palladium α-lipoic acid complex compared to α-lipoic acid is its ability to form self-assembled structures, such as the one shown in Fig. 6. No self-assembly was observed for sodium lipoate. We want to point out that binding of a lysine residue in the protein to the lipoyl group of E2 in 2-oxoacid dehydrogenases results in a long flexible arm that can oscillate a distance of ~200 Å. This arm is utilized during the catalytic cycle [Patel & Packer, 2008]. It is obvious that the self assembled palladium α-lipoic acid complex can make this process more facile.

The physics and chemistry of non-equilibrium systems have been utilized to understand some of the spatial patterns and temporal patterning observed in biological processes such as bacterial colonies shaped by diffusive instabilities and calcium waves governed by nonlinear amplification during intracellular signaling [Levine & Jacob, 2004].

In homogeneous systems, spiral waves and spatiotemporal phenomena are formed from autocatalytic reactions and diffusion resulting from chemical instabilities. Our data suggest that the propagation of electrical signaling among the packing units and extending to long distances by global coupling is viable by such self-assembled systems.

We have utilized the technique of electrochemical impedance spectroscopy extensively to probe spatiotemporal phenomena in biological systems. This technique is routinely used to study corrosion and fuel cells. We have used admittance measurements for understanding solute-solvent interactions, "π -way" conduction, ion pair formation, water-structure enforced ion pair formation, potential induced and solvent mediated ion pair formation at the double layer, and semi conduction characteristics of simple biological molecules

[Krishnan & Garnett, 2006; 2011; Krishnan et al., 2007a,b; 2008a,b,c,d; 2009a,b; 2011]. Simple molecules such as arginine, histidine, lysine, flavin adenine dinucleotide, riboflavin, cysteine, lidocaine hydrochloride, α-lipoic acid, and hydrogen peroxide exhibit negative differential resistance, a characteristic of a tunnel diode.

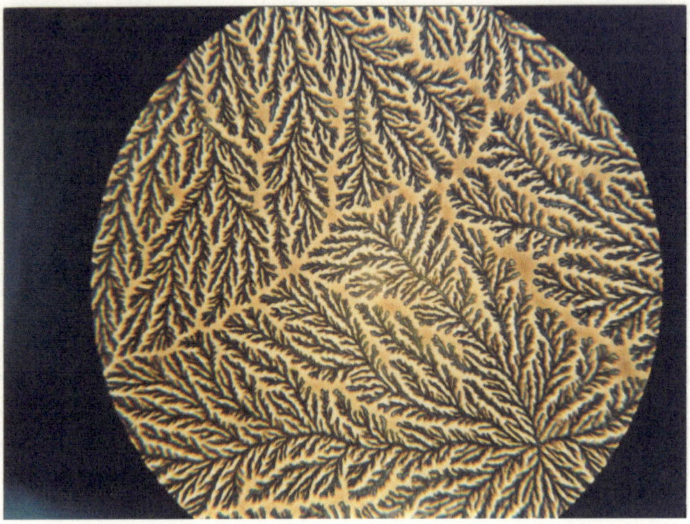

Fig. 6. Phase microscopy of palladium α-lipoic acid complex, 300X [Krishnan & Garnett, 2006]

In this technique a perturbing sinusoidal voltage $E = E_o\sin(\omega t)$ is applied at angular frequency ω (2πf, where f is the conventional frequency in Hz) to the electrode system consisting of a working electrode, counter electrode and reference electrode. The measurements reported in this chapter were made using and EG & G PARC Model 303A SMDE trielectrode system (mercury working electrode, platinum counter electrode and Ag/AgCl saturated KCl reference electrode) along with Autolab ecochemie. The measurements were carried out in the range 1000Hz to 30 mHz. The amplitude of the sinusoidal perturbation was 10 mV. The response of the applied sinusoidal voltage is analyzed in terms of the resultant current $I = I_o\sin(\omega t + \Phi)$, where Φ represents a characteristic phase angle shift. In the plane of Cartesian coordinates, an impedance is expressed by its real (Z′) and imaginary (Z″) parts. The modulus |Z| and phase angle Φ of **Z**(ω) can be obtained from $|Z| = [Z'^2 + Z''^2]^{1/2}$ and $\Phi = \tan^{-1}[Z''/Z']$, respectively [Macdonald & Johnson, 2005]. Admittance and impedance are interrelated:

$$Z'/Y' = Z''/Y'' = (Z')^2 + (Z'')^2 = 1/[(Y')^2 + (Y'')^2 \quad (32)$$

Over a frequency bandwidth of interest, there are various ways of representing the impedance spectrum. Most often, the well known Nyquist or Cole-Cole plot (Z″ as the Y-axis and Z′ as the X-axis for the range of frequencies explored at a fixed potential) and Bode plot (|Z| and Φ vs. logω) are employed to represent the data. In simple terms, impedance is like a frequency dependent generalized resistance and admittance is like a frequency dependent conductance. In electrochemistry, the imaginary impedance is almost always capacitive and therefore negative. Majority of impedance data require only the first quadrant in the plot. However, if there is inductance, the data will require the first and fourth quadrants. In corrosion studies, the oxides formed at passivation potentials exhibit, quite often, semiconduction characteristics and their impedance data will be in both first and second quadrants. The impedance in the second quadrant may be compared to the negative differential resistance (NDR) observed in the I-V curves of tunnel diodes and some enzymes. Impedance spectra spanning more than two quadrants and especially four quadrants are unusual and are often explained by nonequilibrium phenomena and compared to spatiotemporal oscillations in biological systems.

The impedance spectra for α-lipoic acid and its modulation by complexing with palladium are shown in Fig. 7. While α-lipoic acid exhibits NDR and shows impedance in only 3 quadrants (chaotic in quadrant 3), the spectra of the metal complex is extended to 4 quadrants and much more smoothly by complexation with palladium. Of course the NDR behavior can be optimized by slightly tweaking the applied potential. This enhancement in NDR behavior may be compared to the enhanced Krebs cycle and mitochondrial enzymatic activities of the palladium α-lipoic acid compared to that of the ligand.

We have reason to believe that the self-assembled structure of the complex, by providing a spatial extension of the membrane with much more surface area, may be catalyzing the electron transfer process by enhancing spin coupling. This may account, for example, the enhanced complex I and complex II activities activities of PdLA by 151% and 212% more than that of α-lipoic acid.

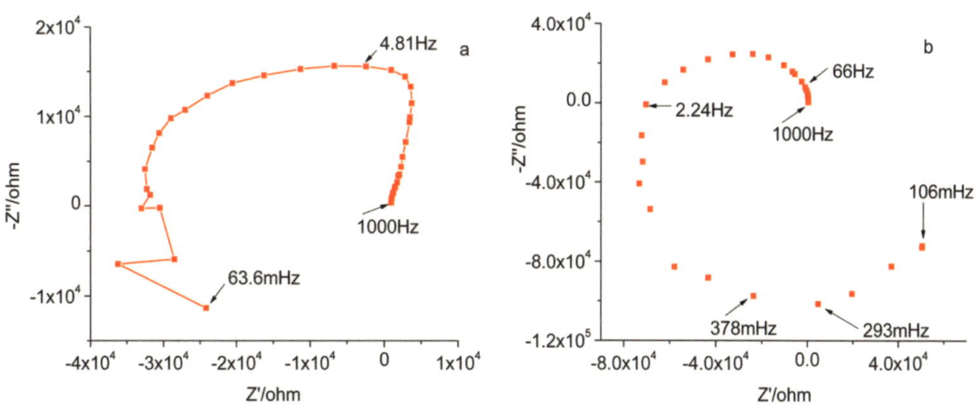

Fig. 7. a) Nyquist plot for 0.0373 M sodium lipoate, -1.15V, pH 7.79, NDR at 4.81Hz.
b) Modulation of lipoate impedance by palladium in 0.0373M palladium α-lipoic acid (1:1 complex) in 0.1792 M NaCl, -1.18V, pH 7.78, NDR at 66Hz [Krishnan et. al., 2011]

Another important aspect of this system is the fact α-lipoic acid is linked to lysine by an amide bond in the multienzyme complexes of pyruvate dehydrogenase, α-ketoglutarate dehydrogenase and branched chain α-ketoglutarate dehydrogenase. Thus both α-lipoic acid and lysine have heavy involvement in the electronic aspects of the enzymatic process.

11. Conclusions

Oxidative stress is caused by the chemical imbalance between ROS production and their breakdown by antioxidants. Over-abundance of ROS has been found during neuronal development, as well as in numerous neuropathological conditions. Oxidative stress and mitochondrial dysfunction have been closely associated in brain injury such as ischemia and stroke and neurodegenerative processes such as Multiple Sclerosis, Parkinson's, Alzheimer's, and Huntington's.

Lipoic acid was found to be effective in modulating many neurodegenerative disorders. The development of palladium α-lipoic acid complex was intended to augment the properties of this ligand by the catalytic properties of the transition metal. It is formulated to combat mitochondrial dysfunction. The unique electronic properties of palladium modulating the properties of α-lipoic acid appear to be a key to this physiological effectiveness. This is exemplified in our electrochemical impedance spectroscopic studies of α-lipoic acid and palladium α-lipoic acid complex.

Palladium α-lipoic acid complex facilitates aerobic metabolism much more than that of α-lipoic acid, by significantly enhancing the enzymatic activity of isocitrate dehydrogenase, α-ketoglutarate dehydrogenase, succinate dehydrogenase, and malate dehydrogenase at the Krebs cycle and mitochondrial complexes I, II, III, and IV of the electron transport chain. The electronic properties of palladium also appear to modulate the antioxidant properties of α-lipoic acid in that PdLA enhances the activities of catalase and glutathione peroxidase more than that of α-lipoic acid. The level of GSH also was significantly improved and the level of lipid peroxidation was decreased in the heart mitochondria of aged rats.

PdLA is similar to a multi-spectrum drug. Since it targets the mitochondria it is able to carry out several functions such as combating age-related as well as disease-associated fatigue, and minimizes the effects of ischemic injury. Being a powerful free radical scavenger, it may also be effective in combating death of neurons and other progressive loss of structure or function of neurons caused by free radicals.

PdLA is able to protect from radiation exposure and repair DNA. It also seems to ward off radiation exposure-associated weight loss in mice, possibly protecting susceptible gastrointestinal tract.

12. Acknowledgements

The area covered in this chapter is vast and warrants citation of numerous publications. The authors regret being unable to cite many publications due to space limitations. The authors wish to express their sincere thanks and gratitude for many fruitful discussions and collaborations in various aspects of the work presented in this chapter: B. Chu, K. K. Janardhanan, T.A. Ajith, C.K.K. Nair, N.P. Sudheesh, A. Menon, and L. Ramachandran.

13. References

Aktas O., Kieseier B. & Hartung, H. P. (2010). Neuroprotection, regeneration and immunomodulation: broadening the therapeutic repertoire in multiple sclerosis. *Trends in Neurosciences*, 33, 140-152.

Antonawich F. J., Fiore S. M., & Welicky L. M. (2004). Regulation of ischemic cell death by the lipoic acid-palladium complex, Poly MVA, in gerbils. *Experimental Neurology*, 189, 10-15.

Baumgartner M. R., Schmalle H. & Dubler E. (1996). The Interaction of transition metals with the coenzyme α-lipoic acid: synthesis, structure and characterization of copper and zinc complexes. *Inorg. Chim. Acta*, 252, 319-331.

Beattie D. S. (2002). Bioenergetics and Oxidative Metabolism. In: *Textbook of Biochemistry with Clinical Correlations*. Devlin T. M. (ed.) 5th edition, Wiley-Liss, A John Wiley & Sons, Inc., Publication, New York.

Beckman J. S., & Koppenol W. H. (1996). Nitric oxide, superoxide, and peroxynitrite: the good, the bad and the ugly, *Am. J. Physiol. 271 (Cell Physiol.* 40), C1424-1437

Besancon E., Guo S., Lok J., Tymianski M., & Lo E. H. (2008). Beyond NMDA and AMPA glutamate receptors: emerging mechanisms for ionic imbalance and cell death in stroke. *Trends in Pharmacological Sciences*, 29, 268-275.

Blokhina O., & Fagerstedt K. (2006). Oxidative Stress and Antioxidant Defenses in Plants, In: *Oxidative Stress, Disease and Cancer*, Singh K. K., Editor, Imperial College Press, London, WC2H 9HE.

Buettner G. R. (1993). The Pecking Order of Free Radicals and Antioxidants: Lipid Peroxidation, α-Tocopherol, and Ascorbate. *Arch. Biochem. Biophys*, 300, 535-543.

Campbell G. R., Res M., Ziabreva I., Reeve A. K., Krishnan K. J., Reynolds R., Howell O., Lassmann H., Turnbull D. M., & Mahad D. J. (2011). Mitochondrial DNA deletions and Neurodegeneration in MS. Ann. Neurol., 69, 481-491

Cao X., & Phillis J. W. (1995). The free radical scavenger, alpha-lipoic acid, protects against cerebral ischemia-reperfusion injury in gerbils. *Free Radic. Res*, 23, 365-70.

Carew J. S. & Huang P. (2002). Mitochondrial defects in cancer. *Molecular Cancer*, 1:9 (2002); http://www.molecular- cancer.com/content/1/1/9

Carlson D. A., Young K. L., Fischer S. J. & Ulrich H. (2008). An Evaluation of the Stability and Pharmacokinetics of R-Lipoic Acid and R-Dihydrolipoic Acid Dosage Forms in Human Plasma from Healthy Subjects. In: *Lipoic Acid: Energy Production Antioxidant Activity and Health Effects*, Patel M. S. and Packer L. (ed.), CRC press, Taylor & Francis Group, Florida, 255.

Chan D. C. (2006). Mitochondria: Dynamic Organelles in Disease, Aging, and Development. *Cell*, 125, 1241-1252

Clark W. M., Rinker L. G., Lessov N. S., Lowery S. L., Cipolla M. J. (2001). Efficacy of Antioxidant Therapies in Transient Focal Ischemia in Mice. *Stroke, Journal of the American Heart Association*, 32, 1000-1004

Corduneanu O., Garnett M., & Oliveira Brett A. M. (2007). Anodic oxidation of α-lipoic acid at a glassy carbon electrode and its determination in dietary supplements. *Anal Letters* 40, 1763-1778.

Corduneanu O., Paquim A. M. C., Garnett M., & Oliveira Brett A. M. (2009). Lipoic acid-palladium complex interaction with DNA, voltammetric and AFM characterization. *Talanta*, 77, 1843-1853.

Cotton F. A. & Wilkinson G. (1972). *Advanced Inorganic Chemistry*, 3rd edition, Interscience Publishers, New York, 415.

Cross A. H., Manning P. T., Keeling R. M., Schmidt R. E., & Misko T. P. (1998). Peroxynitrite formation within the central nervous system in active multiple sclerosis. *J. Neuroimmunology*, 88, 45-56.

Dennery P. A. (2010). Oxidative Stress in Development: Nature or nurture?. *Free radical Biology & Medicine*, 49, 1147-1151.

D'haeseleer M., Cambron M., Vanopdenbosch L., & De Keyser J. (2011). Vascular aspects of multiple sclerosis. *Lancet Neurol.*, 10, 657-666.

Doyle K. P., Simon R. P., & Stenzel-Poore M. P. (2008). Mechanisms of ischemic brain damage. *Neuropharmacol.*, 55, 310-318

Dröge W. (2002). Free radicals in the physiological control of cell function. *Physiol. Rev.* 82, 47-95

Dutta R., McDonough J., Yin X., Peterson J., Chang A., Torres T., Gudz T., Macklin W. B., Lewis D. A., Fox R. J., Rudick R., Mirnics K., & Trapp B. D. (2006). Mitochondrial Dysfunction as a Cause of Axonal Degeneration in Multiple Sclerosis Patients. *Ann. Neurol.*, 59, 478-489

Elfering S. L., Sarkela T. M., Giulivi C. (2002). Biochemistry of mitochondrial NOS. *J. Bio. Chem.*, 277, 38079-38086.

Falkowski P. G. (2006). Tracing Oxygen's Imprint on Earth's Metabolic Evolution. *Science*, 311, 1724-1725.

Filippi M. & Rocca M. A. (2011). The multiple sclerosis mystery: is there a vascular component? *Lancet Neurol.* 10, 597-598

Gao E., Liu C., Zhu M., Lin H., Wu Q., & Liu L. (2009). Current Development of Pd(II) Complexes as Potential Antitumor Agents. *Anti-Cancer Agents in Medicinal Chemistry*, 9(3), 356-368.

Garnett M. (1995 a). Synthetic DNA Reductase", Contents of 7th EBIC Conf. Abstracts Issue, C 48, *J. Inorg. Biochem*, 59, 231.

Garnett M. (1995 b). Palladium Complexes and Methods for Using the Same in the Treatment of Tumors or Psoriasis, *U.S.Patent, No. 5,463,093, Oct.31.*

Ginsberg M. D. (2008). Neuroprotection for ischemic stroke: Past, present and future. *Neuropharmacology*, 55, 363-389

Haider L., Fischer M. T., Frischer J. M., Bauer J., Hoftberger R., Botond G., Esterbauer H., Binder C. J., Witztum J. L. & Lassmann H. (2011). Oxidative damage in multiple sclerosis lesions. *Brain A Journal of Neurology*, 134, 1914-1924

Hertz L. (2008). Bioenergetics of cerebral ischemia: A cellular perspective. *Neuropharmacology*, 55, 289-309

Higgins G. C., Beart P. M., Shin Y. S., Chen M. J., Cheung N. S., & Nagley P. (2010). Oxidative Stress: Emerging Mitochondrial and Cellular Themes and Variations in Neuronal Injury. *Journal of Alzheimer's Disease*, 20, S453-S473.

Kiryu-Seo S., Ohno N., Kidd G. J., Komuro H., & Trap B. D. (2010). Demyelination Increases Axonal Stationary Mitochondrial Size and the Speed of Axonal Mitochondrial Transport. *The Journal of Neuroscience*, 30, 6658 – 6666

Klotz L. O. (2002). Oxidant-Induced Signaling: Effects of Peroxynitrite and Singlet Oxygen. *Biol. Chem*, 383, 443-456.

Korde A. S., Pettigrew L. C., Craddock S. D., & Maragos W. F. (2005). The mitochondrial uncoupler 2,4-dinitrophenol attenuates tissue damage and improves mitochondrial homeostasis following transient focal cerebral ischemia. J. Neurochem., 94, 1676-1684.

Korkina L. G., Afanas'ef I. B., & Diplock A. T. (1993). Antioxidant therapy in children affected by irradiation from the Chernobyl nuclear accident. *Biochemical Society Transactions*, 314S, 21.

Krishnan C. V. & Garnett M. (2006). Liquid crystal behavior in solutions, electrode passivation, and impedance loci in four quadrants. In: *Passivation of Metals and Semiconductors, and Properties of Thin Oxide Layers*, Marcus P. and Maurice V. (ed.), Elsevier, Amsterdam, 389-394.

Krishnan C. V., Garnett M., & B. Chu (2007 a). Spatiotemporal Oscillation in Peroxo-Molybdate Complexes in Acidic Solutions: 1. Impedance Measurements of $H_2Mo_2O_3(O\text{-}O)_4(H_2O)_2$. *Int. J. Electrochem Sci.*, 2, 444-461.

Krishnan C. V., Garnett M., & B. Chu (2007 b). Solute-Solvent Interactions from Admittance Measurements: Potential Induced and Water Structure-Enforced Ion-Pair Formation. *Int. J. Electrochem. Sci.*, 2, 958-972.

Krishnan C. V., Garnett M., & B. Chu (2008 a). Solute-solvent interactions in biological molecules: L-Cysteine. *Int. J. Electrochem. Sci.*, 3, 854-872.

Krishnan C. V., Garnett M., & B. Chu. (2008 b). Spatiotemporal oscillations in biological molecules: Molybdate-L-Cysteine. *Int. J. Electrochem. Sci.*, 3, 873-890.

Krishnan C. V., Garnett M., & Chu B. (2008 c). Oxidative Stress and Parkinson's Disease: Electrochemical Behavior of Hydrogen Peroxide in Aqueous Sodium Chloride, *Int. J. Electrochem. Sci.*, 3, 1348-1363.

Krishnan C. V., Garnett M., & B. Chu. (2008 d). Spatiotemporal oscillations in biological molecules: Hydrogen peroxide and Parkinson's disease. *Int. J. Electrochem. Sci.*, 3, 1364-1385.

Krishnan C. V., Garnett M., Hsiao B., & Chu B. (2009 a). Solute-Solvent Interactions from Impedance Measurements: 'π -way' Conduction and Water Structure-Enforced Ion Pair Formation in Aqueous Lidocaine Hydrochloride. *Int. J. Electrochem. Soc.*, 4, 1085-1099.

Krishnan C. V., Garnett M., & B. Chu (2009 b). Admittance as a useful tool for investigation of solute-solvent interactions at the double layer. *Electrochem. Communications* 11, 2229-2232.

Krishnan C. V. & Garnett M. (2011). Electrochemical Behavior of the Super Antioxidant, α-Lipoic Acid. *Int. J. Electrochem. Soc.*, 6, 3607-3630.

Krishnan C. V., Garnett M., & Antonawich F. (2011). Mitochondrial Dysfunction and Cancer: Modulation by Palladium α-Lipoic Acid Complex. In: *Recent Advances in Nanomedicine and Drug Delivery*, Apple Academics Inc, Canada

Lázaro M. L. (2007). Dual role of hydrogen peroxide in cancer: Possible relevance to cancer chemoprevention and therapy. *Cancer Letters*, 252, 1-8.

Levine H & Jacob E. B. (2004). Physical schemata underlying biological pattern formation-examples, issues and strategies. *Physical Biology*, 1(1-2), P14-P22.

Lu F., Selak M., O'Connor J., Croul S., Lorenzana C., Butunoi C., & Kalman B. (2000). Oxidative damage to mitochondrial DNA and activity of mitochondrial enzymes in chronic active lesions of multiple sclerosis, Journal of the Neurological Sciences 177, 95–103.

Macdonald J. R. & Johnson W. B. (2005). Fundamentals of Impedance Spectroscopy. In: *Impedance Spectroscopy: Theory, Experiment, and Applications*. 2nd Edition, Barsoukov E., Macdonald J. R. (ed.), 2nd edition, Wiley Interscience, New Jersey.

Mahad D, Ziabreva I., Lassmann H., & Turnbull D. (2008). Mitochondrial defects in acute multiple sclerosis lesions. *Brain A Journal of Neurology*, 131, 1722-1735

Mahad D. J., Ziabreva I., Campbell G., Lax N., White K., Hanson P. S., Lassmann H., & Turnbull D. M. (2009). Mitochondrial changes within axons in multiple sclerosis. *Brain A Journal of Neurology*, 132, 1161-1174

Maiorino M. & Ursini F. (2002). Oxidative Stress, Spermatogenesis and Fertility. Biol. Chem., 383, 591-597.

Maloň M., Trávníček Z., Maryško M., Zbořil R., Mašláň M., Marek J., Doležal K., Rolčík J., Kryštof V., & Strnad M. (2001). Metal complexes as anticancer agents 2. Iron(III) and copper(II) bio-active complexes with N6-benzylaminopurine derivatives. *Inorg. Chim. Acta*, 323, 119-129.

Mao P. & Reddy P. H. (2010). Is multiple sclerosis a mitochondrial disease. *Biochim. Biophys. Acta*, 1802, 66-79.

Matesanz A.I., Perez J. M., Navarro P., Moreno J. M., Colacio E., & Souza P. (1999). Synthesis and characterization of novel palladium (II) complexes of bis (thiosemicarbazone). Structure, cytotoxic activity and DNA biding of Pd (II)-benzyl bis (thiosemicarbazonate). *J. Inorg. Biochem.*, 76, 29-37.

McCord J. M. (1998). The Importance of Oxidant-Antioxidant Balance. In: *Oxidative Stress in Cancer, Aids, and Neurodegenerative Diseases*. Montagnier L., Olivier R., & Pasquier C. Editors, CRC Press, Taylor & Francis Group, New York.

Mehta S. L., Manhas N., & Raghubir R. (2007). Molecular targets in cerebral ischemia for developing novel therapeutics. *Brain Research reviews*, 54, 34-66.

Menon A., Krishnan C. V. & Nair C. K. K. (2009). Protection from gamma radiation insult to antioxidant defense and cellular DNA by POLY-MVA, a dietary supplement containing palladium lipoic acid formulation. *Int. J. Low Radiation*, 6, 248-262.

Menon A. & Nair C. K. K. (2011). POLY MVA - a dietary supplement containing α-lipoic acid palladium complex, enhances cellular DNA repair. *Int. J. Low Radiation,* 842-854

Nagley P., Higgins G. C., Atkin J. D., & Beart P. M. (2010). Multifaceted deaths orchestrated by mitochondria in neurons, *Biochim. Biophys. Acta.*, 1802, 167-185.

Niki E. & Noguchi N. (2004). Dynamics of Antioxidant Action of Vitamin E. *Acc. Chem. Res.*, 37, 45-51.

Packer L., Witt E. H., & Tritschler H. J. (1995). Alpha Lipoic Acid as a Biological Antioxidant. *Free Radical Biology and Medicine*, 19(2), 227-250.

Panigrahi M., Sadguna Y., Shivakumar B. R., Kolluri S. V. R., Roy S., Packer L., & Ravindranath V. (1996). α-Lipoic acid protects against reperfusion injury following cerebral ischemia in rats. *Brain Research*, 717, 184-188

Patel M. S. & Packer L. (ed.), (2008). *Lipoic Acid: Energy Production, Antioxidant Activity and Health Effects*. CRC Press, Taylor & Francis Group, New York.

Pauling L. (1970). *General Chemistry*, 3rd edition. , W.H. Freeman and Company, San Francisco, 215.

Radi R., Cassina A., & Hodara R. (2002). Nitric Oxide and Peroxynitrite Interactions with Mitochondria. *Biol. Chem.*, 383, 401-409

Ramachandran L., Krishnan C. V., & Nair C. K. K. (2010). Radioprotection by α-Lipoic Acid Palladium Complex Formulation (POLY-MVA) in Mice. *Cancer Biotherapy and Radiopharmaceuticals*, 25(4), 395-399.

Ramakrishnan N., Wolfe W. W., & Catravas G. N. (1992). Radioprotection of Hematopoietic Tissues in Mice by Lipoic Acid. *Radiation Research*, 130, 360-365.

Raymond J. & Segré D. (2006). The Effect of Oxygen on Biochemical Networks and the Evolution of Complex Life. *Science*, 311, 1764-1767

Reed L. J. (2001). A trail of research from lipoic acid to α-keto acid dehydrogenase complexes, *J. Biol. Chem.*, 276, 38329-38336

Ricciarelli R., Zingg J. M. & Azzi A. (2002). The 80th anniversary of vitamin E: beyond its antioxidant properties. *Biol. Chem.*, 383, 457-465

Rogers G. T., & D. N. Mallett D. N. (1983). Some electrode reactions of lipoic acid. *Bioelectrochem. and Bioenergetics*, 10, 269-277

Rouach N., Calvo C., Duquennoy H., Glowinski J., & Giaume C. (2004). Hydrogen Peroxide Increases Gap Junctional Communication and Induces Astrocyte Toxicity: Regulation by Brain Macrophages. *Glia*, 45, 28-38.

Rubbo H., Trostchansky A., Botti H., & Batthyany C. (2002). Interactions of Nitric Oxide and Peroxynitrite with Low-Density Lipoprotein. *Biol. Chem.*, 383, 547-552.

Shay K. P., Moreau R. F., Smith E. J., Smith A. R. & Hagen T. M. (2009). Alpha-lipoic acid as a dietary supplement: Molecular mechanisms and therapeutic potential, *Biochimica et Biophysica Acta, General Subjects*, 1790, 1149-1160.

Sies H. (1986). Biochemistry of Oxidative Stress. *Angew. Chem. Int. Ed. Engl.*, 25, 1058-1071

Sies H. (1993). Strategies of antioxidant defense. Eur. J. Biochem., 215, 213-219

Siffrin V., Vogt J., Radbruch H., Nitsch R. & Zipp F. (2010). Multiple sclerosis-candidate mechanisms underlying CNS atrophy. *Trends in Neurosciences*, 33, 202-210

Sims N. R. & Muyderman H. (2010). Mitochondria, oxidative metabolism and cell death in stroke. *Biochimica et Biophysica Acta*, 1802, 80–91

Singh K. K. (ed.), (2006). In: *Oxidative Stress, Disease and Cancer*. Imperial College Press, London, WC2H 9HE.

Starkov A. & Wallace W. K. (2006). Yin and Yang of Mitochondrial ROS. In: In: *Oxidative Stress, Disease and Cancer*. Singh K. K. (editor), Imperial College Press, London, WC2H 9HE.

Stary F. E., Jindal S. L., & Murray, R. W. (1975). Oxidation of α-Lipoic Acid, *J. Am. Chem. Soc.*, 40, 58-62

Strasdeit H., von Dollen A. & Duhme A. K. (1995). Metal Complexes of the Drug and Coenzyme α-Lipoic acid and Related Ligands. Contents of 7th EBIC Conference Abstracts Issue, C 45, *J. Inorg. Biochem*, 59, 228.

Sudheesh N. P., Ajith T. A., Janardhanan K. K. & Krishnan C. V. (2009). Palladium α-lipoic acid complex formulation enhances activities of Krebs cycle dehydrogenases and respiratory complexes I-IV in the heart of aged rats. *Food and Chemical Toxicology*, 47, 2124-2128.

Sudheesh N. P., Ajith T. A., Janardhanan K. K., & Krishnan C. V. (2010). Effect of POLY-MVA, a palladium α-lipoic acid complex formulation against declined mitochondrial antioxidant status in the myocardium of aged rats. *Food and Chemical Toxicology*, 48, 1858-1862.

Sudheesh N. P., Ajith T. A., Janardhanan K. K., & Krishnan C. V. (2011). Palladium-α-lipoic acid complex attenuates alloxan-induced hyperglycemia and enhances the declined blood antioxidant status in diabetic rats, J. Diabetes, in press

Suh J. H., Shenvi S. V., Dixon B. M., Liu H., Jaiswal A. K., Liu R. M., & Hagen T. M. (2004). Decline in transcriptional activity of Nrf2 causes age-related loss of glutathione synthesis, which is reversible with lipoic acid. Proc. Natl. Acad. Sci. USA, 101, 3381-3386

Tabet F., Savoia C., Schiffrin E. L., & Touyz R. M. (2004). Differential calcium regulation by hydrogen peroxide and superoxide in vascular smooth muscle cells from spontaneously hypertensive rats. *J. Cardiovasc. Pharmacol.* 44, 200-208.

Takahashi M., & Niki E. (1998). The Importance of Oxidant-Antioxidant Balance. In: *Oxidative Stress in Cancer, Aids, and Neurodegenerative Diseases*. Montagnier L., Olivier R., & Pasquier C. Editors, CRC Press, Taylor & Francis Group, New York.

Turrens J. F. (2003). Mitochondrial formation of reactive oxygen species. *J. Physiol*. 552, 335-344

Voet D. & Voet J. G. (1995). *Biochemistry*, 2nd edition, John Wiley & Sons, Inc., New York.

Wolz P. & Krieglstein J. (1996). Neuroprotective Effects of α-Lipoic Acid and its Enantiomers Demonstrated in Rodent Models of Focal Cerebral Ischemia. *Neuropharmacology*, 35, 369-375

Wood Z. A., Poole L. B., & Karplus P. A. (2003). Peroxoredoxin Evolution and the Regulation of Hydrogen Peroxide. *Science*, 300, 650-653.

Zambonin J. L., Zhao C., Ohno N., Campbell G. R., Engeham S., Ziabreva I., Schwarz N., Lee S. E., Frischer J. M.,Turnbull D. M., Trapp B. D., Lassmann H., Robin J. M. Franklin R. J. M., & Don J. Mahad D. J. (2011). Increased mitochondrial content in remyelinated axons: implications for multiple sclerosis. *Brain A Journal of Neurology*, 134, 1901-1913

5

Docosahexaenoic Acid (DHA), in the Prevention and Treatment of Neurodegenerative Diseases

Rodrigo Valenzuela B.[1] and Alfonso Valenzuela B.[2]
[1]*University of Chile, Faculty of Medicine, Nutrition and Dietetic School*
[2]*University of Chile, Institute of Nutrition and Food Technology (INTA), Lipid Center and University of Los Andes, Faculty of Medicine; Santiago, Chile*

1. Introduction

The scientific and technological development observed since the late nineteenth century until nowadays has caused a significant increase in the life expectancy of the population, being people over 65 a significant and yearly increasing 15% of the population (Szymański et al., 2010). As result, the increase in the life expectancy has also increased the prevalence of diseases associated to ageing, especially neurodegenerative diseases such as Alzheimer's disease, Multiple sclerosis and Parkinson's disease (Habeck et al., 2010). These diseases, besides its increasing with age, are also associated to the socioeconomic status, work and physical activity, family history and genetic, and in the last two decades, the nutrition has also aroused as a relevant factor (Stampfer, 2006). In this sense, there is general consensus that a healthy diet may prevent the development of many diseases such as obesity, hypertension, diabetes mellitus, stroke, certain kinds of cancers and now neurodegenerative diseases (Massaro et al., 2010). Epidemiological evidences suggest that populations having a significant consumption of fish, a food rich in n-3 long-chain polyunsaturated fatty acids (n-3 LCPUFA), show lower incidence of neurodegenerative diseases (Tully et al, 2003). n-3 LCPUFA, especially docosahexaenoic acid (DHA, C22: 6 Δ 4, 7, 10, 13, 16, 19; n-3), play a fundamental role in the development and preservation of the nervous system, and in the recent years solid evidences of their involvement in the prevention and/or eventually in the treatment of neurodegenerative diseases have appeared (Ikemoto et al., 2001). In neuronal tissue DHA is found in high concentrations, especially in the phospholipids of neuronal and glial membranes. However, as ageing progress and during the development of neurodegenerative diseases, a significant reduction in the DHA content of the brain is produced (Tully et al., 2003), especially in the cortex, cerebellum and hypothalamus, which result in a considerable reduction in the fluidity of neuronal membranes and an alteration of the neuronal homeostasis (Sodeberg et al., 1991; Kalminj et al., 2004). Beyond the effect of DHA at the neuronal membranes, the fatty acid also exerts other protective effects which are mediated by a metabolic derivative named neuroprotectin D-1 (NPD-1) which may protect neurons against oxidative stress, inflammation, disruption of the cytoskeleton and from the activation of apoptotic signaling pathways (Bazan, 2009). NPD-1, formed from DHA, is normally present in the nervous system, especially in the brain, but it is especially relevant in states and/or situations that may compromise the activity, integrity and neuronal viability, as it is the case of neurodegenerative diseases, brain injury by ischemia - reperfusion, leukocyte infiltration and activation of proapoptotic signaling pathways (Bazan, 2009; Belayev et al., 2009). In this context, NPD-1 has anti-inflammatory, antiapoptotic and even neuroregenerative effects, which would help to preserve in general, both the neuronal functioning and the nervous system (Reinoso et al 2008). A significant reduction of the neuronal DHA content is produced during the developing of neurodegenerative diseases. This reduction, which is not only produced by dietary factors, (i.e. low intake), it is also produced by metabolic process such as increased DHA metabolism and/or oxidation (Tully et al., 2003). The greatest evidence about the neuroprotective effect of DHA has been observed in Alzheimer's disease. DHA may suppress the cytotoxic effects of the accumulation of the β-amyloid peptide, being the main mechanism associated to the neuroprotective action of the fatty acid (Bazan, 2009; Reinoso et al., 2008). Facing this evidence, it is reasonable to consider the beneficial effect of increasing the consumption of DHA by eating foods rich in the fatty acid, such as fatty fish or DHA containing supplements. This chapter reviews the neuroprotective effects of DHA in the context of the brain ageing and some neurodegenerative diseases. It is also suggested to promote the consumption of food and/or supplements rich in DHA, as an effective strategy for preserving the brain function during ageing and especially to prevent the incidence, or to delay the onset of neurodegenerative diseases.

2. DHA and brain physiology

DHA is a LCPUFA with six double bonds, which belong to the series or family of the n-3 polyunsaturated fatty acids (Figure 1). It is relevant that DHA is the most unsaturated fatty acid in our organism and is found specifically concentrated in the brain, retina and sperms of higher animals (Uauy et al., 2001). DHA, when provided by the diet, comes mainly from marine organisms such as fish (fatty or blue species), shellfish, and algae (Horrocks et al., 2004). The first report of a deficiency of n-3 fatty acids was documented in 1982, which described the case of a six years girl, who received parenteral nutrition without the addition of n-3 fatty acids for five months after intestinal surgery (Holman et al., 1982). After the nutritional intervention, the girl presented low plasma DHA levels, dermatitis associated with neurological symptoms including neuropathy, blurred vision and psychological disturbances, which suggested an important role of n-3 LCPUFA, especially DHA, in the nervous system functions. In fact, it is now accepted that DHA is the most important n-3 LCPUFA in the formation of neuronal plasma and synaptosomal membranes (synaptic vesicles), especially in the brain (McNamara & Carlson, 2006). DHA amounts approximately 30-40% of fatty acids of the phospholipids forming the gray matter of the cerebral cortex and retinal photoreceptors (Carlson, 2002). The most important growing of the brain in humans is produced during the third trimester of fetal development and in the first two years of life. It is during these periods that the requirements of n-3 and n-6 LCPUFA are roused considerably, especially the requirements of DHA and arachidonic acid (AA, C20: 4 Δ 5, 8, 11, 14; n-6). Animal studies have shown that the reduced availability of DHA during the perinatal period is associated with deficits in the establishing of neuronal networks, and also with multiple expressions of synaptic pathologies, including deficits in serotonin neurotransmission and alterations in the mesocorticolimbic dopamine pathway, neurocognitive deficits, and a greater anxious behavior, aggression, depression and decreased visual acuity (McNamara & Carlson, 2006). Similar problems have been observed in preterm primates and humans, which may be reversed after n-3 LCPUFA supplementation. DHA intake remains also essential after the end of the brain development. It is required to maintain the normal brain functions, including synaptic plasticity, neurotransmission and visual function (McCann & Ames, 2005).

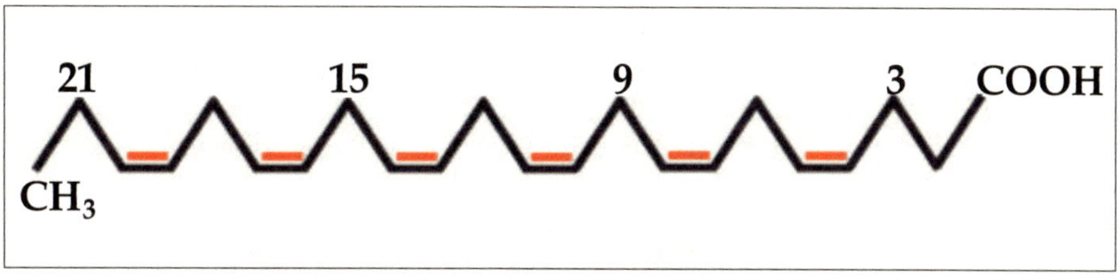

Fig. 1. Molecular structure of docosahexaenoic acid (DHA)

3. DHA and brain metabolism

Due to lack of enzymes necessary for neuronal de novo synthesis of DHA and AA, these fatty acids must be obtained preformed directly from the diet, or be synthesized from their precursors, α-linolenic acid (ALN, C18: 3 Δ 9, 12, 15; n-3) for DHA, and linoleic acid (LA, C18: 2 Δ 9, 12, n-6) for AA (Williard et al., 2001). This synthesis is carried out mainly in the liver and to a lesser extent in the cerebral endothelium by the astrocytes, which may export these fatty acids to the neurons (Lesaet al., 2003, Kalant & Cianflone, 2004). Although is still under discussion how these fatty acids (ALN, LA) can cross the blood-brain barrier, it has been demonstrated that may diffuse through the phospholipids of neuronal membranes (McCann & Ames, 2005). Other evidences suggest that some membrane proteins may facilitate the transport of ALN and/or DHA through the hematoencephalic barrier. One of these transporters has been identified as a caveolin binding protein type or CD36 (Williard et al., 2001 ; Lesa et al., 2003). However, plasma levels of LCPUFA are poorly correlated with the dietary intake of the precursors (Kalant & Cianflone, 2004). In fact, in healthy individuals, Δ5-and Δ6-desaturases, the key enzymes in the conversion process of LA to AA and ALN to DHA, are only induced in the absence of precursors and suppressed when the intake of the precursors (LA and ALN) is sufficient (Kalant & Cianflone, 2004). In contrast, the Δ6-desaturase activity appears to decrease with age, as has been demonstrated in rodent models (Cho et al, 1999; Hrelia et al., 1990). The reduction of the activity of this enzyme could be significantly important during ageing, considering that the elderly shows low tissue levels of DHA, especially when the intake of ALN is chronically low (Strokin et al., 2006; Kalmijn et al., 1997). This situation could lead to profound alterations in the metabolism of the nervous system, especially in the density of the synaptosomes and/or in the release of neurotransmitters, as suggested from studies carried-out in the nematode *Caenorhabditis elegans* deficient for the enzyme Δ6-desaturase (Lesa et al., 2003). DHA is present in the phospholipids of neuronal membrane predominantly at the sn-2 position; therefore the incorporation of DHA in membrane phospholipids depends of the cycle deacylation - reacylation which occurs at the sn-2 position (Serhan et al., 2008). In rodent brains, this cycle has significant activity (Rapoport et al., 2001) and is dependent directly on the specific activities of the enzymes acyl-CoA synthetase (ACS) and phospholipase A2 (PLA2). ACS performs the activation process by binding the fatty acid to CoA, which is an

ATP-dependent reaction. Once activated, the fatty acids can be incorporated into phospholipids. ACS isoenzymes 3, 4 and 6 are specific to LCPUFA, and in the brain the ACS 6 isoform is specific for the acylation of DHA (Marszalek et al., 2005). At present, there is not sufficient background about the type of phospholipase that participate in the release of DHA from phospholipids. However, it has been established that in astrocytes the release of DHA involve a mechanism dependent of $^{2+}$Ca but independent of PLA2 (Strokin et al., 2003). The role of PLA2 in neurons has not been clearly demonstrated, but a study in the hippocampus of rats, indicated that the enzyme may be of fundamental importance in the release of DHA in neuronal tissue (Strokin et al., 2006). Figure 2 shows a proposal of how DHA may be incorporated into the phospholipids of neuronal membranes.

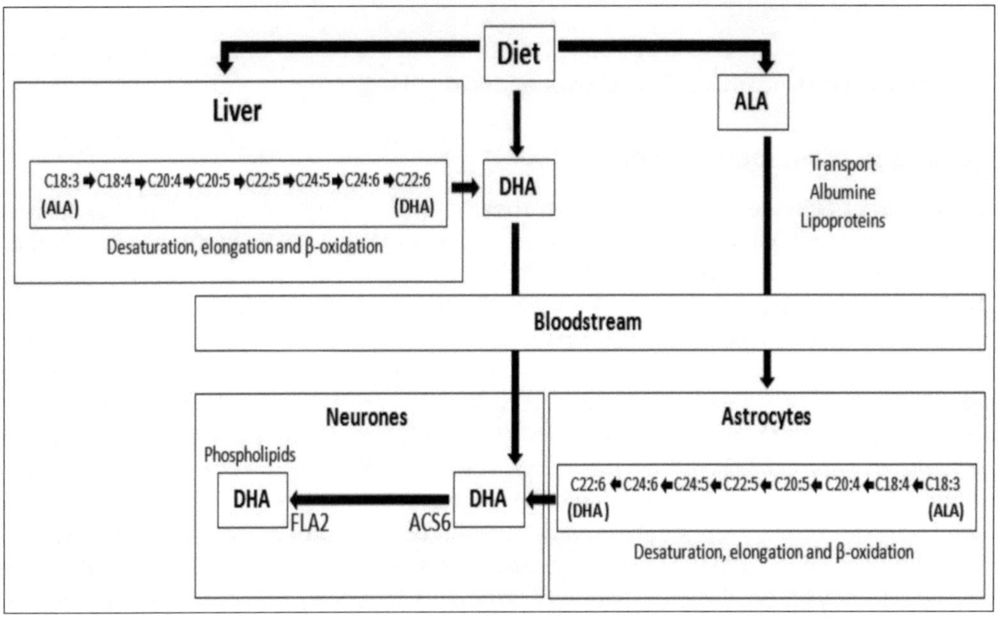

Fig. 2. Incorporation of DHA into the phospholipids of neuronal membranes

4. DHA and brain ageing

The presence of high concentrations of DHA, especially in the phospholipids of neuronal membranes, has been encouraged for more than 30 years the research about the roles of DHA in the nervous system. The evidence has demonstrated that during the embryonic stage and the first years of life, DHA plays a key role in the growth and development of the nervous and visual systems, actively participating in the processes of neurogenesis, neuronal migration, myelination and synaptogenesis (Uauy et al., 2001), thus directly impacting on cognitive development, visual, auditory, and in the memory and learning capabilities (McNamara & Carlson, 2006). As result of these observations, it is now strongly recommended to increase the consumption DHA during the pregnancy and childhood, in order to ensure the proper development of the nervous and visual systems (Uauy et al., 2001). The close relationship between DHA and the developing of the nervous system, encouraged investigators to study what happens with this fatty acid during ageing. It was observed that as the individual ages, the content of DHA in neural tissue is significantly reduced, being even greater this decrease in the population that develops neurodegenerative diseases (Sodeberg et al., 1991). This significant reduction may be caused either, by a lower intake of the fatty acid or of its metabolic precursor and/or by an increased in the cellular utilization of DHA (Jicha & Markesbery, 2010). DHA plays a relevant role in the preservation of both the histology and physiology of the neuronal tissue as the individual ages, by preserving the nervous system functions among which memory and learning are the most remarkable (Lukiw & Bazan, 2008). Several epidemiological studies have strongly established that a higher intake of foods rich in DHA (fatty fish and/or nutritional supplements based on fish oils or microalgae) is highly correlated with a lower risk of developing neurodegenerative diseases (Kalminj et al., 2004; Kalmijn et al., 1997), which is also associated with a clinical history indicating that patients with neurodegenerative disease have significantly lower levels of DHA in plasma and brain (Tully et al., 2003; Sodeberg et al., 1991).

5. Neuroprotectin D-1 and neuroprotection

A relevant question about the attributed neuroprotective effects of DHA in ageing and especially against neurodegenerative diseases is referred as how this fatty acid exerts these effects at the molecular level. Their role in the fluidity of the neuronal membrane appears as one of the most relevant attributes (Saiz & Klein, 2001). In fact, up to day the classification of membrane fluidity is based on the level of DHA present in the phospholipids that form the membrane matrix (Stillwell et al., 2005). However, the higher fluidity that confers DHA to neuronal membrane is not sufficient to explain the neuroprotective effects attributed to the fatty acid. As result of multiple investigations, it has been established that acylation of DHA at the sn-2 position in the membrane phospholipids and the activity of PLA-2, are additional features of DHA, by itself, to achieve an additional neuroprotective action of the fatty acid against certain cytotoxic situations, as are neurodegenerative diseases (Stillwell et al., 2005; Brown & London, 2000). It is no casual that DHA is present mainly at the sn-2 position in the phospholipids of neuronal membranes (48% in phosphatidylcholine, 52% in fosfatidilserine and 20% in phosphatidylethanolamine) (Aveldano & Bazan, 1983). It was the discovery of a number of bioactive compounds derived from DHA, called protectins and resolvins, which show cytoprotective properties that open the way to a better understanding of how DHA may exert at the molecular level its neuroprotective actions (Mukherjee et al., 2004). Among these bioactive DHA-derivatives, NPD-1 (protectin D1 or D1 neuroprotectin: 10R, 17S-dihydroxy-docosa-4Z, 7Z, 11E, 13E, 15Z, 19Z-hexaenoic acid), appears the most relevant neuroprotective agent (Serhan et al., 2008). NPD-1 is generated once DHA is released from the phospholipids by the hydrolytic action of PLA-2, where the enzyme 15 lipoxygenase initiate a complex process of lipooxidation, epoxidation and hydrolysis resulting in the formation of NPD-1 (Serhan, 2005). Figure 3 shows a diagram of the formation of NPD-1. NPD-1 may exert its neuroprotective function either through a receptor (as yet unidentified), which may act in an autocrine form and/or NPD-1, once formed, may be diffused to other neurons. The mechanisms involved in the neuroprotection afforded by NPD-1 may include: (i) inhibition of the expression of proinflammatory cytokines (TNFα and IL1β), (ii) inhibition of the generation and neurotoxicity of β-amyloid peptides and Ab42 (iii) increased gene expression of antiapoptotic molecules (Bcl-2 and Bcl-xL), (iv) reduction in the gene expression of proapoptotic molecules (Bax and Bad) and (v) increased neuronal antioxidant potential (Chu Chen & Bazan, 2005). Moreover, inflammatory cytokines and oxidative stress may activate the synthesis of NPD-1 (Aksenov & Markesbery, 2001).

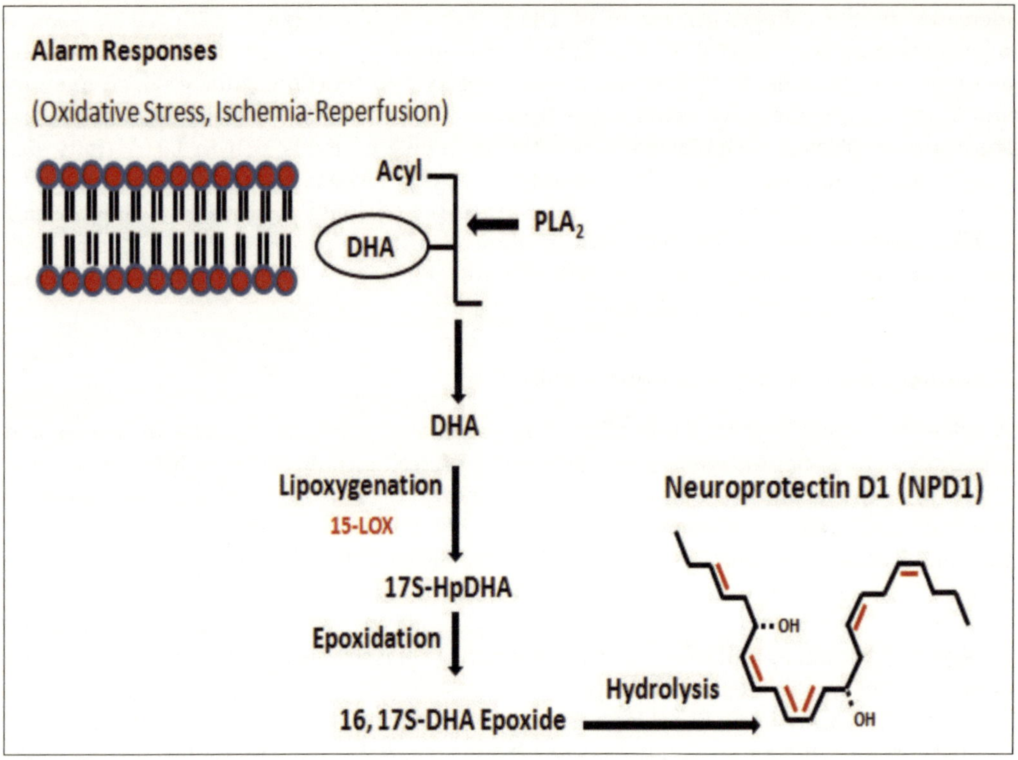

Fig. 3. Biosynthesis of Neuroprotectin D-1 (NPD-1)

6. DHA and neurodegenerative diseases

Several epidemiological, clinical and basic-experimental studies have demonstrated the beneficial effects of n-3 LCPUFA against various diseases, among which; cardiovascular disease (Hamer and Steptoe., 2006), some cancers (Gillet et al., 2011), inflammatory diseases such as rheumatoid arthritis (Kremer et al., 1990) and asthma (Yokoyama et al., 2000), neurological disorders such as schizophrenia (Laugharne et al., 1996), depression (Hibbeln & Salem, 1995), migraine (Wagner & Nootbaar-Wagner, 1997) and neurodegenerative diseases such as Alzheimer's disease (Morley & Banks, 2010), Multiple sclerosis (Mehta et al., 2009) and Parkinson's disease (Calon & Cole, 2007). The evidence of the beneficial effect of DHA has been clearly demonstrated mainly in neurodegenerative diseases.

6.1 DHA and Alzheimer´s disease

Alzheimer's disease (AD) is a progressive dementia that is early manifested by the loss of synaptic function and memory capacity of the individual. The number of patients who are diagnosed the neuropathological disorder has increased substantially in all countries, mainly in those where has been produced an increase in the life expectancy. In fact, it is estimated that about 5% of the population that borders 65 is affected by AD. The prevalence of the disease doubles every 5 years over 65 years (Cummings, 2004), and many studies suggest that almost half the population up to 85 years show symptoms related to the disease (Nussbaum & Ellis, 2003; Forsyth & Ritzline, 1998).The presence of the β-amyloid peptide, which is associated with neurotoxic effects, is one of the characteristic expression of the molecular damage observed in patients (Hardy & Higgins, 1992; Yankner, 1996). Its origin occurs from the degradation (altered or incomplete) of the β-amyloid peptide precursor (APP) (Selkoe, 1994). A significant reduction in DHA levels, both in erythrocytes and in the brain, is observed in AD, specifically in the frontal lobe, and occipital and temporal cortex (Guan et al., 1994). It is also produced a replacement of DHA in phospholipids by saturated fatty acids (SFA) among which myristic acid (14:0), palmitic (16:0) and stearic acid (18:0) are the most frequent (Skinner et al., 1993). Thus, it is likely that changes in the ratio AGS/n-3 and n-6 LCPUFA could alter the neuronal function, especially at the membrane phospholipids, which in turn could result in neurological deficits. The altered fatty acid composition observed in the brains of AD patients could be caused by a deficiency in the LCPUFA transport from blood to the brain. It is remarkable that in patients with certain types of dementia or cognitive impairment it is observed the same reduction in the levels of n-3 LCPUFA, especially DHA (Kyle et al., 1999; Conquer et al., 2000). Interestingly, a decrease of DHA in plasma does not appear to be unique to AD, it is also common in the general cognitive impairment observed in ageing (Catalán et al., 2002). Many studies have demonstrated that a high intake of DHA is associated with a lower risk of AD, and in individuals diagnosed the disease, consumption of DHA result in a decrease in the progression of the characteristic symptoms, especially in relation to the cognitive impairment (Barberger-Gateau et al., 2002).

6.2 DHA and multiple sclerosis

In the case of multiple sclerosis (MS), the benefits associated with n-3 LCPUFA, especially DHA, have been shown in both the mental and physical disabilities. Evaluation of patients that has been supplemented with DHA indicates a significant improvement in the symptoms characteristic of the disease (Nussbaum & Ellis, 2003; Shinto et al., 2009). Some of these beneficial effects have been observed even in patients who consume a diet low in fat, but supplemented with n-3 LCPUFA of marine origin (fish oil). However, the evidence regarding a benefic in the progression of MS is not yet fully conclusive (Weinstock-Guttman et al., 2005). Considering the information currently available, it is not yet possible to establish a direct association between the consumption of n-3 LCPUFA and a lower incidence of MS, more studies are required on the issue (Weinstock-Guttman et al., 2005; Marcheselli et al., 2003). A study showed a relationship between reduced risk of this disease and the consumption of fish, but only among women (Nordvik et al., 2000). Currently, most hypotheses about MS suggest that n-3 LCPUFA would provide the molecules needed to rebuild the myelin sheath, which is severely affected in patients with this pathology. Dietary supplementation with n-3 LCPUFA helps to reduce the severity of MS in patients recently diagnosed the pathology and may delay the onset of symptoms. This is especially effective when supplementation is from marine oils along with vitamins and dietary professional counseling (Kelley, 2001). Perhaps the severity of the MS disease can be also reduced by modulating the immune response. Several studies have shown that a reduction in the dietary fat intake and changes in the relationship n-6/n-3 produce changes in the immune response (Kew et al., 2003). The use of nutritional supplements rich in n-3 LCPUFA is associated with a reduced activity and plasma levels of circulating immune cells (lymphocytes, polymorph nuclear neutrophils and monocytes), including the reduction in the production of inflammatory mediators (Weinstock-Guttman et al., 2005; Nordvik et al., 2000). Moreover, a reduction in the intake of n-3 LCPUFA improves a number of indexes associated with the immune response, including lymphocyte proliferation, increased macrophage activity and cytokine production (Serhan et al., 2000). These records allow the suggestion of a protective role of n-3 LCPUFA in MS, which would lead to establish the potential of the use of n-3 LCPUFA as anti-inflammatory and neuroprotective in MS, although it remains a topic for further research.

6.3 DHA and Parkinson´s disease

In contrast to AD, the relationship of fat intake and the risk of developing Parkinson's disease (PD) is very limited. Two studies have only established an association between high consumption of saturated fatty acids, low intake of n-3 LCPUFA and the increased of the risk to develop PD (Chen et al., 2003; de Lau et al., 2005). To date researchers have not been able to establish a direct association between low intake of n-3 LCPUFA and increased risk of developing PD. However, as in patients with AD, in the brains of people with PD it is also observed a significant decrease in the levels of n-3 LCPUFA, especially DHA (Johnson et al., 1999). Research in primates allow to observe a significant reduction in the extent of levodopa-induced dyskinesia (a damage model for the PD) in animals supplemented with DHA, which suggests that these effects would be mediated by the activation of retinoid X receptors (RXR) (Samadi et al., 2006). In addition, data from these investigations show a drastic drop in neural DHA levels (Julien et al., 2006; Breckenridge et al., 1973). Also, the dietary supplementation with DHA of animals reduced the neuronal damage produced by a characteristic PD-inducer agent, the neurotoxin 1-methyl-4-phenyl-1,2,3,6-tetrahydropyridine (MPTP) (Bousquet et al., 2008). Currently, the available information is not sufficient to establish a neuroprotective effect of DHA in the development of PD, being necessary to carry out more studies on the subject.

7. Dietary sources and intake of DHA

The metabolic precursor of n-3 LCPUFA, ALA, is found almost exclusively in land-based plant foods, such as nuts (walnuts 6%), chia seeds (*Salvia hispanica*) and flax seeds (*Linum usitatissimum*) and in some edible oils, such as soy (7 %), canola (11%), evening primrose (27%), chia (58%) and clary sage (60%). While, the already-formed DHA is found exclusively in marine foods, either of animal or vegetal origin, especially in fatty fish such as tuna, mackerel, menhaden, salmon, and some algae and microalgae. Unfortunately, the western consumption of ALA and DHA is very low, which has forced the development of nutritional supplements rich in DHA either from fish oils or microalgae, and also to add this fatty acid to foods such as vegetable oils, milk and derivatives. In this regard, in addition to the capsules containing fish oil or DHA concentrates which are very popular and available DHA can be also added to various foods such as dairy, dairy products, juices, beverages, bakery products, etc. The fatty acid may be provided in the form of triglycerides, phospholipids, and in pure form as ethyl esters (Valenzuela et al., 2006). Today, a wide variety of foods containing DHA are available from the retail and nutraceutical market.

8. Conclusion and perspectives

Neurodegenerative diseases may significantly alter the functioning of the nervous system, reducing both the number and function of neurons, which seriously affects the quality of life for those suffering these diseases. New strategies aiming to the prevention and/or the treatment of these diseases are of high priority. In this context DHA and its derivative NPD-1, emerged as a new perspective for the prevention and/or therapeutic management of these diseases, especially considering the social and economic devastation that neurological diseases may produce to the individual and the family. Future clinical research and nutritional interventions should be planned directly to establish the necessary doses of DHA needed to achieve significant beneficial effects, as well as to encourage the development and consumption of foods and/or supplements rich in this fatty acid. In this regard, the development of functional foods and/or nutraceuticals containing DHA at different concentrations is an alternative that the pharmaceutical and the food industries should consider very seriously (Valenzuela et al., 2009). To day the increase of the consumption of fish or seafood appear as not entirely feasible, due to the massive depredation of the resource, which has decreased its availability and consequently has increased the price of the products from the sea. Perhaps, in the future the increasing activity of the aquaculture may offer a viable alternative to improve the general consumption of n-3 LCPUFA to the western population and helping to prevent the early onset of neurodegenerative diseases.

9. Acknowledgment

The authors are grateful from FONDECYT and INNOVA-Chile the support of their research.

10. References

Aksenov, M.Y. & Markesbery, W.R., (2001). Changes in thiol content and expression of glutathione redox system genes in the hippocampus and cerebellum in Alzheimer's disease. *Neurosci Lett*, Vol. 302, pp. 141-145

Aveldano, M.I. & Bazan, N.G., (1983). Molecular species of phosphatidylcholine, -ethanolamine, -serine, and -inositol in microsomal and photoreceptor membranes of bovine retina. *J. Lipid Res*, Vol. 24, pp. 620–627

Barberger-Gateau, P., Letenneur, L., Deschamps, V., et al. (2002). Fish, meat, and risk of dementia: cohort study. *BMJ*, Vol. 325, pp. 932-933

Bazan, N.G., (2009). Neuroprotectin D1-mediated anti-inflammatory and survival signaling in stroke, retinal degenerations, and Alzheimer's disease. *J Lipid Res*, Vol. 50 (Suppl), pp. 400-405

Belayev, L., Khoutorova, L., Atkins, K.D., et al. (2009). Robust docosahexaenoic acid-mediated neuroprotection in a rat model of transient, focal cerebral ischemia. *Stroke*, Vol. 40, pp. 3121-3126

Bousquet, M., Saint-Pierre, M., Julien, C., et al. (2008). Beneficial effects of dietary omega-3 polyunsaturated fatty acid on toxin-induced neuronal degeneration in an animal model of Parkinson's disease. *FASEB J*, Vol. 22, pp. 1213-1225

Brown, D.A. & London, E., (2000). Structure and function of sphingolipid and cholesterol-rich membrane rafts. *J Biol Chem*, Vol. 275, pp. 17221-17224

Breckenridge, W.C., Morgan, I.G., Zanetta, J.P., et al. (1973). Adult rat brain synaptic vesicles. II. Lipid composition, *Biochim Biophys Acta*, Vol. 320, pp. 681-686

Calon, F. & Cole, G., (2007). Neuroprotective action of omega-3 polyunsaturated fatty acids against neurodegenerative diseases: evidence from animal studies. *Prostaglandins Leukot Essent Fatty Acids*, Vol. 77, pp. 287-93

Carlson, S.E., (2002). Docosahexaenoic acid and arachidonic acid in infant development. *Seminars Neonatol*, Vol. 6, pp. 437-449

Catalán, J., Moriguchi, T., Slotnick, B., et al. (2002). Cognitive deficits in docosahexaenoic acid-deficient rats. *Behav Neurosci*, Vol. 116, pp. 1022-1031

Conquer, J.A., Tierney, M.C., Zecevic, J., et al. (2000). Fatty acid analysis of blood plasma of patients with Alzheimer's disease, other types of dementia, and cognitive impairment. *Lipids*, Vol. 35, pp. 1305-1312

Cummings, J.L., (2004). Alzheimer's disease. *N Engl J Med*, Vol. 351, pp. 56-67

Chen, C. & Bazan, N.G., (2005). Lipid signaling: Sleep, synaptic plasticity, and neuroprotection. *Prostaglandins & Other Lipid Mediators*, Vol. 77, pp. 65-76

Chen, H., Zhang, S.M., Hernan, M.A., et al. (2003). Dietary intakes of fat and risk of Parkinson's disease. *Am J Epidemiol*, Vol. 157, pp. 1007-1014

Cho, H.P., Nakamura, M.T., and Clarke, S.D., (1999). Cloning, expression, and nutritional regulation of the mammalian Δ6-desaturase. *J Biol Chem*, Vol. 274, pp. 471-477

de Lau, L.M., Bornebroek, M., Witteman, J.C., et al. (2005). Dietary fatty acids and the risk of Parkinson disease: the Rotterdam study. *Neurology*, Vol. 64, pp. 2040-2045

Forsyth, E. & Ritzline, P.D., (1998). An overview of the etiology, diagnosis, and treatment of Alzheimer disease. *Phys Ther*, Vol. 78, pp. 1325-31

Gillet, L., Roger, S., Bougnoux, P., et al. (2011). Beneficial effects of omega-3 long-chain fatty acids in breast cancer and cardiovascular diseases: voltage-gated sodium channels as a common feature?. *Biochimie*, Vol. 93, pp. 4-6

Guan, Z.Z., Söderberg, M., Sindelar, P., et al. (1994). Content and fatty acid composition of cardiolipin in the brain of patients with Alzheimer's disease. *Neurochem Int*, Vol. 25, pp. 295-300

Habeck, C. & Stern, Y. (2010). Alzheimer's Disease Neuroimaging Initiative. Multivariate data analysis for neuroimaging data: overview and application to Alzheimer's disease. *Cell Biochem Biophys*, Vol. 58, pp. 53-67

Hardy, J.A. & Higgins, G.A., (1992). Alzheimer's disease: the amyloid cascade hypothesis. *Science*, Vol. 256, pp. 184-185

Hamer, M. & Steptoe, A., (2006). Influence of specific nutrients on progression of atherosclerosis, vascular function, haemostasis and inflammation in coronary heart disease patients: a systematic review. *Br J Nutr*, Vol. 95, pp. 849-859

Hibbeln, J.R. & Salem, Jr N. (1995). Dietary polyunsaturated fatty acids and depression: when cholesterol does not satisfy. *Am J Clin Nutr*, Vol. 62, pp. 1-9

Holman, R.T., Johnson, S.B., and Hatch, T.F., (1092). A case of human linolenic acid deficiency involving neurological abnormalities. *Am J Clin Nutr*, Vol. 35, pp. 617-23

Horrocks, L.A. & Farooqui, A.A., .Docosahexaenoic acid in the diet: its importance in maintenance and restoration of neural membrane function. (2004). *Prostaglandins Leukot Essent Fatty Acids*, Vol. 70, pp. 361-72

Hrelia, S., Celadon, M., Rossi, C.A., et al. (1990). Δ6-Desaturation of linoleic and α-linolenic acids in aged rats: a kinetic analysis. *Biochem Int*, Vol. 22, pp. 659–667

Ikemoto, A., Ohishi, M., Sato, Y., et al. (2001). Reversibility of n-3 fatty acid deficiency - induced alterations of learning behavior in the rat: level of n-6 fatty acids as another critical factors. *J Lipid Res*, Vol. 42, pp.1655-1663

Jicha, G.A. & Markesbery, W.R., (2010). Omega-3 fatty acids: potential role in the management of early Alzheimer's disease. *Clin Interv Aging*, Vol. 5, pp.45-61

Johnson, C.C., Gorell, J.M., Rybicki, B.A., et al. (1999). Adult nutrient intake as a risk factor for Parkinson's disease. *Int J Epidemiol*, Vol. 28, pp. 1102-1109

Julien, C., Berthiaume, L., Hadj-Tahar, A., et al. (2006). Postmortem brain fatty acid profile of levodopa-treated Parkinson disease patients and parkinsonian monkeys. *Neurochem Int*, Vol. 48, pp. 404-414

Kalant, D. & Cianflone, K., (2004). Regulation of fatty acid transport. *Curr Opin Lipidol*, Vol 15, pp. 309-314

Kalmijn, S., Launer, L.J., Ott, A, Witteman, J.C., et al. (1997). Dietary fat intake and the risk of incident dementia in the Rotterdam Study. *Ann Neurol*, Vol. 42, pp. 776-782

Kalminj, S., van Boxtel, M.P.J., Ocke, M., et al. (2004). Dietary intake of fatty acid and fish in relation to cognitive performance at middle age. *Neurology*, Vol. 62, pp. 275-280

Kelley, D.S. (2001). Modulation of human immune and inflammatory responses by dietary fatty acids. *Nutrition*, Vol. 17, pp. 669-73

Kew, S., Banerjee, T., Minihane, A.M., et al. (2003). Lack of effect of foods enriched with plant- or marine -derived n-3 fatty acids on human immune function. *Am J Clin Nutr*, Vol. 77, pp. 1287-95

Kremer, J.M., Lawrence, D.A., Jubiz, W., et al. (1990). Dietary fish oil and olive oil supplementation in patients with rheumatoid arthritis. Clinical and inmmunologic effects. *Arthritis Rheum*, Vol. 33, pp. 810-820

Kyle DJ, Schaefer E, Patton G, et al. (1999). Low serum docosahexaenoic acid is a significant risk factor for Alzheimer's dementia. *Lipids*, Vol. 34, Suppl: S245

Laugharne, J.D., Mellor, J.E., and Peet, M. (1996). Fatty acids and schizophrenia. *Lipids*, Vol. 31, pp. 163-165

Lesa, G.M., Palfreyman, M., Hall, D.H., et al. (2003). Long chain polyunsaturated fatty acids are required for efficient neurotransmission in C. elegans. *J Cell Sci*, Vol. 116, pp. 4965-4975

Lukiw, W.J. & Bazan, N.G., (2008) Docosahexaenoic acid and the aging brain. *J Nutr*, Vol. 138, pp. 2510-2514

Marcheselli, V.L., Hong, S., Lukiw, W.J., et al. (2003). Novel docosanoids inhibit brain ischemia-reperfusion-mediated leukocyte infiltration and pro-inflammatory gene expression. *J Biol Chem*, Vol. 31, pp. 43807-43817

Marszalek, J.R., Kitidis, C., Dirusso, C.C., et al. (2005). Long-chain acyl-CoA synthetase 6 preferentially promotes DHA metabolism. *J Biol Chem*, Vol. 280, pp. 10817-10826

Massaro, M., Scoditti, E., Carluccio M.A., et al. (2010). Nutraceuticals and prevention of atherosclerosis: focus on omega-3 polyunsaturated fatty acids and Mediterranean diet polyphenols. *Cardiovasc Ther*, Vol. 28, pp. 13-9

McCann, J.C. & Ames, B.N., (2005). Is docosahexaenoic acid, an n-3 long-chain polyunsaturated fatty acid, required for development of normal brain function? An overview of evidence from cognitive and behavioral tests in humans and animals. Am J Clin Nutr, Vol. 82, pp. 281-295

McNamara, R.K. & Carlson, S.E., (2006). Role of omega-3 fatty acids in brain development and function: potential implications for the pathogenesis and prevention of psychopathology. *Prostaglandins Leukot Essent Fatty Acids*, Vol. 75, pp. 329-349

Mehta, L.R., Dworkin, R.H., and Schwid, S.R., (2009). Polyunsaturated fatty acids and their potential therapeutic role in multiple sclerosis. *Nat Clin Pract Neurol*, Vol. 5, pp. 82-92

Morley, J.E. & Banks, W.A., (2010). Lipids and cognition. *J Alzheimers Dis*, Vol. 20, pp. 737-747

Mukherjee, P.K., Marcheselli, V.L., Serhan, C.N., et al. (2004). Neuroprotectin D1: a docosahexaenoic acid-derived docosatriene protects human retinal pigment epithelial cells from oxidative stress. *Proc. Natl. Acad. Sci. USA*, Vol. 101, pp. 8491–8496

Nordvik, I., Myhr, K.M., Nyland, H., et al. (2000). Effect of dietary advice and n-3 supplementation in newly diagnosed MS patients. *Acta Neurol Scand*, Vol. 102, pp. 143-149

Nussbaum, R.L., & Ellis, C.E., (2003). Alzheimer's disease and Parkinson's disease. *N Engl J Med*, Vol. 348, pp. 1356–64

Rapoport, S.I., Chang, M.C., and Spector, A.A., (2001). Delivery and turnover of plasma-derived essential PUFAs in mammalian brain. *J Lipid Res*, Vol. 42, pp. 678-685

Reinoso, M.A., Mukherjee, P., Marcheselli, V., et al. (2008). PEDF Promotes Biosynthesis of a Novel Anti-inflammatory and Anti-apoptotic Mediator NPD1 in Retinal Pigment Epithelial Cells. *Ochsner J*, Vol. 8, pp. 39-43

Saiz, L. & Klein., M.L., (2001). Structural properties of a highly polyunsaturated lipid bilayer from molecular dynamics simulations. *Biophys J*, Vol. 81, pp. 204-216

Samadi, P., Gregoire, L., Rouillard, C., et al. (2006). Docosahexaenoic acid reduces levodopa-induced dyskinesias in 1-methyl-4-phenyl-1,2,3,6-tetrahydropyridine monkeys. Ann. Neurol, Vol. 59, pp. 282–288.

Selkoe, D.J. (1994). Alzheimer's disease: a central role for amyloid. *J Neuropathol Exp Neurol*, Vol. 53, pp.438-447

Serhan, C.N., Clish, C.B., Brannon, J., et al. (2000). Novel functional sets of lipid-derived mediators with antiinflammatory actions generated from omega-3 fatty acids via cyclooxygenase 2-non-steroidal antiinflammatory drugs and transcellular processing. *J Exp Med*, Vol. 192, pp. 1197-204

Serhan, C.N., (2005). Special Issue on Lipoxins and Aspirin-Triggered Lipoxins. *Prostaglandins Leukot Essent Fatty Acids*, Vol. 73, pp.139–321

Serhan, C.N., Chiang, N., and Van Dyke, T.E., (2008). Resolving inflammation: dual anti-inflammatory and pro-resolution lipid mediators. *Nat Rev Immunol*, Vol. 8, pp. 349-361

Shinto, L., Marracci, G., Baldauf-Wagner, S., et al. (2009). Omega-3 fatty acid supplementation decreases matrix metalloproteinase-9 production in relapsing-remitting multiple sclerosis. *Prostaglandins Leukot Essent Fatty Acids*, Vol. 80, pp. 131-136

Skinner, E.R., Watt, C., Besson, J.A., et al. (1993). Differences in the fatty acid composition of the grey and white matter of different regions of the brains of patients with Alzheimer's disease and control subjects. *Brain*, Vol. 116, pp. 717-725

Sodeberg, M., Edlund, C., Kristensson, K., et al. (1991). Fatty acid composition of brain phospholipids in aging and in Alzheimr´s disease. *Lipids*, Vol. 26, pp. 421-425

Stampfer, M.J., (2006). Cardiovascular disease and Alzheimer´s: common links. *J Inter Med*, Vol. 260, pp. 211-223

Stillwell, W., Shaikh, S.R., Zerouga, M., et al. (2005) Docosahexaenoic acid affects cell signalling by altering lipid rafts. *Reprod Nutr Dev*, Vol. 45, pp. 559-579

Strokin, M., Sergeeva, M. and Reiser, G., (2003). Docosahexaenoic acid and arachidonic acid release in rat brain astrocytes is mediated by two separate isoforms of phospholipase A2 and is differently regulated by cyclic AMP and Ca2+. *Br J Pharmacol*, Vol. 139, pp. 1014-1022

Strokin, M., Chechneva, O., Reymann, K.G., et al. (2006). Neuroprotection of rat hippocampal slices exposed to oxygen-glucose deprivation by enrichment with docosahexaenoic acid and by inhibition of hydrolysis of docosahexaenoic acid-containing phospholipids by calcium independent phospholipase A2. *Neuroscience*, Vol. 140, pp. 547-553

Szymański, P., Markowicz, M., Janik, A., et al. (2010). Neuroimaging diagnosis in neurodegenerative diseases. *Nucl Med Rev Cent East Eur*, Vol. 13, pp. 23-31

Tully, A.M., Roche, H.M., Doyle, R., et al. (2003). Low serum colesterol ester-docosahexaenoic acid levels in Alzheimer´s disease: a case - control study. *Br J Nutr*, Vol. 89, pp. 483-489

Uauy, R., Hoffman, D.R., Peirano, P., et al. (2001). Essential fatty acids on visual and brain development. Lipids, Vol. 36, pp. 885-895

Valenzuela, A., Sanhueza, J., and Nieto, S., (2006). Docosahexaenoic acid (DHA), essentiality and requirements: why and how to provide supplementation. *Grasas & Aceites*. Vol. 57, pp. 229-237

Valenzuela, A. (2009). Docosahexaenoic acid (DHA), an essential fatty acid for the proper function of neuronal cells: Their role in mood disorders. *Grasas & Aceites*, Vol. 60, pp. 203-22

Wagner, W. & Nootbaar-Wagner, U,. (1997). Prophylactic treatment of migraine with gamma-linolenic and alpha linolenic acids. *Cephalalgia*, Vol. 17, pp. 127-130

Weinstock-Guttman, B., Baier, M., Park, Y., et al. (2005). Low fat dietary intervention with omega-3 fatty acid supplementation in múltiple sclerosis patients. *Prostaglandins Leukot Essent Fatty Acids*, Vol. 73, pp. 397-404

Williard, D.E., Harmon, S.D., Preuss, M.A., et al. (2001). Production and release of docosahexaenoic acid by differentiated rat brain astrocytes. *World Rev Nutr Diet*, Vol. 88, pp. 168-172

Yankner, B.A., (1996). Mechanisms of neuronal degeneration in Alzheimer's disease. *Neuron*, Vol. 16, pp. 921-32

Yokoyama, A., Hamazaki, T., Ohshita, A., et al. (2000). Effects of aerosolized docosahexaenoic acid in mouse model of atopic asthma. *Int Arch Allergy Immunol*, Vol 123, pp. 327-332

6

Effect of Zinc and DHA on Expression Levels and Post-Translational Modifications of Histones H3 and H4 in Human Neuronal Cells

Nadia Sadli[1], Nayyar Ahmed[1], M. Leigh Ackland[2], Andrew Sinclair[3], Colin J. Barrow[4] and Cenk Suphioglu[1]
[1]*NeuroAllergy Research Laboratory (NARL),*
[1,2,4]*School of Life and Environmental Sciences,*
[3]*School of Medicine, Deakin University,*
Australia

1. Introduction

Docosahexaenoic acid (DHA) is an important omega-3 fatty acid required for the development of the human central nervous system and the continuous maintenance of neuronal cell function. The DHA composition of the brain decreases with age possibly as a result of increased oxidative damage to the lipid membranes (Schaefer, Bongard et al. 2006). Epidemiological studies have shown that patients with Alzheimer's disease (AD) have significantly lower levels of omega-3 fatty acids in their plasma phospholipids (Moriguchi, Greiner et al. 2000; Friedland 2003).

There is an association between DHA levels in the brain and zinc homeostasis, which is particularly interesting as both are involved in neuroprotection. A reduction of DHA levels in the brain causes over expression of ZnT3, a transmembrane proteins that is associated with sequestration of cytoplasmic Zn^{2+} into synaptic vesicles (Jayasooriya, Ackland et al. 2005), resulting in zinc toxicity and neuronal cell death in cultured neuronal cells (Suphioglu, De Mel et al. 2010a; Naganska and Matyja 2006). Mice that lacked a zinc-transporting gene ZnT3 were shown to develop fewer and smaller plaques than Alzheimer's-prone mice with the gene (Lee, Cole et al. 2002), suggesting that altered zinc homeostasis may contribute to the plaque formation in AD. DHA, on the other hand, has neuroprotective properties against neurodegenerative diseases. Dietary supplement of omega-3 fatty acid may protect against Alzheimer's disease, through inhibiting amyloid plague formation (Calon, Lim et al. 2004; Oksman, Iivonen et al. 2006; Florent-Bechard, Malaplate-Armand et al. 2007). DHA was also observed to significantly increase neuronal survival by preventing cytoskeleton perturbations, caspase activation and apoptosis (Florent-Bechard, Malaplate-Armand et al. 2007).

Our recent data has shown that histone gene and protein expression were affected by both zinc and DHA. The expression levels of histones H3 and H4, in human neuronal cells, were down-regulated by zinc and up-regulated by DHA (Suphioglu, Sadli et al. 2010b), suggesting a possible interaction between the two nutrients. Further investigations into the effects of zinc and DHA on histone post-translational modifications (PTMs) were carried out. Zinc was found to reduce acetylation, while increasing histone deacetylase (HDACs) expression levels. This is consistent with dysfunctional acetylation-deacetylation apparatus seen in neurodegenerative diseases (Saha and Pahan 2006). DHA, however, showed an increase in acetylation of histones while it reduced the HDACs to the basal level, indicating that zinc and DHA have distinct epigenetic patterns. Both may be involved in neurodegenerative process possibly mediated by histone post-translational modification. Epigenetic mechanisms, including DNA methylation and histone modifications are critically important in mediating precise neural gene regulation. Studies reported that abnormal epigenetic regulation was associated with mental retardation and neurodegenerative symptoms (Al-Gazali, Padmanabhan et al. 2001).

Although it is still unclear that the change in DHA levels, which result in an alteration in zinc homeostasis, could contribute to the beta amyloid formation (Koh 2001) and neuronal cell death, a growing number of studies do in fact indicate this altered molecular interaction between zinc and DHA as a trigger of the pathology (Jomova, Vondrakova et al., 2010; Tougu, Tiiman et al., 2011).

In this chapter, we will summarize the current findings regarding molecular interactions between zinc and DHA that may provide a potential molecular mechanism to explain the beneficial effects of dietary DHA in neuroprotection.

1.1 Neurodegenerative diseases

As life expectancies are increasing and populations are ageing, neurodegenerative diseases have become a global issue (Nepal, Brown et al. 2008; Nepal, Ranmuthugala et al. 2008). Neurodegenerative diseases such as Alzheimer's disease is the leading cause of dementia in the elderly, which is characterized by molecular changes in nerve cells that result in nerve cell degeneration and ultimately nerve dysfunction and cell death (Dong, Wang et al. 2009). In 1995, Australia had a population of 18 million and 13,000 people were estimated to have dementia. It is predicted that Australia will have 25 million people in 2041, and 460,000 of these will have dementia (Jorm 2001). In other words, while our total population will increase by 40%, our population with dementia will increase by more than three-fold (Jorm 2001).

The expected human lifespan is now longer than ever due to improved hygiene, the discovery of medicines such as antibiotics, and economic welfare. The consequences for this aging population are the increased incidence of age-related diseases. Therefore, treatments to prevent age related neurodegeneration will have economic benefits as well as major impact on the quality of life of the patients (Karasek 2004). A great deal is already known about the pathology of neuronal diseases, but the molecular mechanisms underlying many of these diseases remain unknown. Thus, more research is needed to find the cause and to improve the treatment methods for these significant mental health problems.

1.1.1 Risk factors associated with neurodegeneration

The most consistent risk factor for developing neurodegenerative disease is aging (Pardon and Rattray 2008; Yankner, Lu et al. 2008; Fratiglioni and Qiu 2009). While it is possible to develop dementia early in life, the chances of developing it increases dramatically as people get older (Rocca, van Duijn et al. 1991). Although AD can strike people in their 30s, 40s, or 50s, the vast majority of cases of AD are diagnosed in people older than 65

(Breteler, van den Ouweland et al. 1992; Launer, Brayne et al. 1992; McDowell 2001). A family history of dementia, gender (women are more likely to develop dementia than men), a head injury in the past (Plassman, Havlik et al. 2000), atherosclerosis, high cholesterol, hypertension, diabetes and high homocysteine levels, excessive alcohol and tobacco consumption, exposure to environmental substances and non-healthy diets are some of the factors likely to increase risk of dementia (Larrieu, Letenneur et al. 2004; Letenneur 2004).

While there are some risk factors that cannot be controlled, such as genetics or age, many risk factors can be managed through lifestyle changes or appropriate dietary intakes. These dietary and lifestyle interventions cannot stop people from developing dementia but they may reduce the risk (Simopoulos 1999; Simopoulos, Leaf et al. 1999; Crawford, Bazinet et al. 2009). The adequate omega-3 fatty acid and zinc intake are examples of dietary factors associated with a substantially reduced risk of neurodegenerative diseases (Simopoulos 1991; Crawford, Bazinet et al. 2009; Devore, Grodstein et al. 2009).

1.2 The importance of zinc and DHA in neuronal cells

1.2.1 Zinc in the brain

Zinc is the second most prevalent trace element in the body and is present in particularly high concentrations in the mammalian brain (Weiss, Sensi et al. 2000), including synaptic vesicles where it is tightly bound to intracellular proteins and zinc finger-containing transcription factors (Frederickson, Hernandez et al. 1989). The concentration of intracellular free zinc in the brain is thought to be very low under physiological conditions (Frederickson, Hernandez et al. 1989; Outten and O'Halloran 2001). However, it can rise to >300 nM in response to injurious stimuli (Canzoniero, Turetsky et al. 1999).

Zinc plays an important role in growth and development, the immune response, neurological function and reproduction (Stefanidou, Maravelias et al. 2006). Zinc is also a constituent of many enzymes and is essential for the proper function of various enzymes including carbonic anhydrase (Lukaski 2005), RNA polymerase, and superoxide dismutase (Paik, Joung et al. 1999).

The role of zinc in cognitive function has been studied extensively in both children (Sandstead, Penland et al. 1998) and the elderly (Bertoni-Freddari, Mocchegiani et al. 2006). Zinc deficiency during fetal life is associated with developmental delays and low serum zinc levels in elderly is linked with poor global cognitive function (Golub, Keen et al. 1995), particularly verbal function, and also increases stress (Mocchegiani, Bertoni-Freddari et al. 2005; Mocchegiani, Malavolta et al. 2006). Zinc deficiency most often occurs when zinc intake is inadequate or poorly absorbed (Hambidge, Goodall et al. 1989; Golub, Keen et al. 1995; Paik, Joung et al. 1999), when there are increased losses of zinc from the body or when the body's requirement for zinc increases (Hambidge, Goodall et al. 1989). Nonetheless, despite its importance, recent studies have revealed that excess zinc release in the pathological condition is toxic to the central nervous system. Moreover, disruption of zinc homeostasis has been implicated in several neurodegenerative diseases, such as AD (Huang, Cuajungco et al. 2000; Watt and Hooper 2003) where excess extracellular synaptic zinc was found to induce the formation of amyloid plaques, the characteristic feature of AD brains (Linkous, Adlard et al. 2009; Zatta, Drago et al. 2009). These studies suggest the link between an altered neuronal zinc homeostasis and neurodegenerative disease progression.

1.2.2 Omega-3 fatty acids in the brain

Docosahexaenoic acid (DHA) is the predominant omega-3 fatty acid in the brain of mammals which comprises up to 15% of the concentration of fatty acids in the nervous system (Calderon and Kim 2004). It is found in the neuronal phospholipids in high concentrations in synapses (Bazan 2003). Epidemiological studies suggest that dietary DHA, which is commonly found in fish (Kalmijn, Launer et al. 1997), may modify the risk for certain neurodegenerative disorders (Hibbeln and Salem 1995). As evidence, decreased blood levels of omega-3 fatty acids have been associated with several neurodegenerative conditions, including Alzheimer's disease, schizophrenia and depression (Fenton, Hibbeln et al. 2000; Young and Conquer 2005). Communities with regular consumption of fish have shown to possess reduced prevalence of neurodegenerative disease and cognitive decline in general (Fenton, Hibbeln et al. 2000; He, Song et al. 2004; van Gelder, Tijhuis et al. 2007).

DHA can be linked with many aspects of neural function, including neurotransmission, membrane fluidity (Lauritzen, Hansen et al. 2001), ion channel (Lai, Wang et al. 2009), enzyme regulation (Strokin, Sergeeva et al. 2003) and gene expression (Qi, Seo et al. 2006). DHA is found in breast milk, and may be required for early visual (Bazan 2009) and brain development in children (Willatts 2002; Simmer and Patole 2004). Furthermore, studies in animal models have provided support for the protective role of omega-3 fatty acid. For example, mice fed on diets high in omega-3 fatty acids were shown to improve in neurological function, such as better regulation of nerve cell membrane excitability (Xiao and Li 1999), increased levels of neurotransmitters and higher density of neurotransmitter membrane receptors (Innis 2000). Hossain et al (1998) found that administration of DHA led to improvement in memory function and reduction in free radical levels while maintaining high level of antioxidant enzyme, suggesting a role of DHA in antioxidant defense (Hossain, Hashimoto et al. 1998). Study by Calon et al (2004) has reported that dietary DHA protects the cells against apoptosis by decreasing caspase activity (Calon, Lim et al. 2004). While others have supported this finding by showing that the enrichment of dietary DHA prevents apoptosis under damaging conditions (Gomez de Segura, Valderrabano et al. 2004). DHA also increases phosphotidylserine levels (PS) in neuronal membrane, which result in Akt translocation (Akbar, Calderon et al. 2005) and contributes to survival signaling by suppression of caspase-3 (Akbar, Baick et al. 2006).

1.2.3 Molecular link between DHA and zinc in neuronal cells: DHA decreases neuronal cell death in association with altered zinc transport

The alteration in both DHA and zinc homeostasis are key features of neurodegenerative disorders (Lukiw, Cui et al. 2005) (Cuajungco and Lees 1997). A study by Jayasooriya et al (2005) has demonstrated the link between an altered zinc homeostasis in the brain of rats fed on an omega 3-deficient diet (Jayasooriya, Ackland et al. 2005); this diet lead to a significant decrease in brain DHA levels. Though these data have shown a relationship between DHA and zinc homeostasis, the basis of a molecular mechanism has not been elucidated. We therefore used this fundamental idea to investigate the molecular mechanisms underlying the zinc and DHA interaction. With the use of human neuroblastoma cell line M17, we have shown that DHA reduces cellular zinc uptake, possibly mediated by the zinc transporter ZnT3 followed by a significant reduction in pro-apoptotic marker, caspase-3 (Suphioglu, De Mel et al. 2010a). This indicates the effect of DHA deficiency in the progression of neurodegenerative disease, which is partly mediated by altered zinc fluxes.

Zinc homeostasis in the brain is regulated and tightly controlled by Zn transporters, which are divided into two gene families; the ZnT proteins [solute-linked carrier 30 (SLC30)] and the Zip family [solute-linked carrier 39 (SLC39)](Overbeck, Uciechowski et al. 2008; Lichten and Cousins 2009). ZnT and Zip proteins appear to have opposite roles in cellular zinc homeostasis, where ZnT transporters reduce intracellular cytoplasmic zinc by promoting zinc efflux from cells or into intracellular vesicles, while Zip transporters increase intracellular cytoplasmic zinc by promoting extracellular and, perhaps, vesicular zinc transport into cytoplasm (Murakami and Hirano 2008). In M17 cells, we detected the expression of these two zinc transporter families, including Zip1, Zip2, Zip3, Zip4, Znt1, ZnT2, ZnT3, ZnT4, ZnT5, ZnT6 and ZnT7 (Suphioglu, De Mel et al. 2010a). ZnT3 has been the focus of our studies, as it is associated with brain zinc accumulation, as well as Alzheimer's disease, the condition where the expression was found to be up-regulated (Zhang, Wang et al. 2008).

Progressive neuronal cell loss is a pathological hallmark of neurodegenerative diseases. Apoptosis or alternative pathways of neuronal death have been discussed in Alzheimer's disease and other disorders (Culmsee and Landshamer 2006). We propose that the alteration of zinc metabolism may play a significant role in cellular apoptosis, which is a key feature in the pathology of neurodegenerative disorders such as Alzheimer's disease (Mattson and Duan 1999). Using western blot analysis of human neuroblastoma M17 cell line, we observed a link between DHA treatment and inhibition of apoptosis, where more than 66% reduction in active caspase-3 protein levels was detected in cells treated with 20μg/ml DHA, compared with the untreated control (Suphioglu, De Mel et al. 2010a). The suppression of activated caspase-3 might be mediated by phosphatidylinositol 3-kinase-dependent pathway resulting in the phosphorylation of Akt and DHA may act through this pathway. Akbar et al. (2005) reported the beneficial effect of DHA in neurosurvival through an increase in phosphatidylserine concentration, which resulted in translocation and phosphorylation of Akt suppressing the activation of caspase-3 (Akbar, Calderon et al. 2005). Zinc on the other hand directly activates Akt by phosphorylation at Ser-473/Thr-308 in H1907 embryonic hippocampal cells, leading to activation of GSK-3beta and cell death (Min, Lee et al. 2007). Therefore, we hypothesize that DHA inhibits apoptosis through decreasing intracellular zinc ion concentration, which leads to an increase in Akt activity and neuronal survival.

In summary, dietary DHA deficiency is associated with neurodegenerative condition, which has shown to be a factor in zinc toxicity. DHA also inhibits cellular apoptosis in M17 cells through decreasing cellular zinc uptake and reduction of ZnT3 mRNA and protein levels. Therefore, zinc homeostasis plays an important role in neuronal cell survival and altered zinc homeostasis may contribute to the development of neurodegenerative diseases such as Alzheimer's disease.

1.3 Zinc and DHA affect neuronal histone levels

The connection between zinc homeostasis and DHA metabolism contributes significantly towards neuronal survival and neurodegenerative diseases. A greater understanding of the fundamental basis by which dietary DHA plays an important role in regulating zinc homeostasis, may lead to the development of effective strategies for the prevention and treatment of neurodegenerative diseases. In recent years, our research has been focusing on the key proteins that are regulated by both zinc and DHA and we have also studied how zinc and DHA, alone and in combination might affect the expression levels of these novel proteins.

Two-dimensional gel electrophoresis and mass spectrometry were applied to identify the major protein changes in the protein lysates of M17 human neuronal cells that had been grown in the presence and absence of zinc and DHA. Four protein spots were selected for mass spectrometry analysis to reveal their identity as human histone variants H3 and H4. In order to investigate the change in the expression levels of the histones, proteomic findings were further investigated using western blot and real-time PCR analyses. Our results have revealed the differential expression of histones, particularly histone H3 and H4 in response to DHA and zinc supplementation (Suphioglu, Sadli et al. 2010b). In this study, we reported for the first time that both H3 and H4 were significantly down-regulated by zinc in the absence of DHA (zinc effect) and up-regulated following DHA treatment at the physiological zinc level (DHA effect), suggesting the interrelationship between zinc and DHA in neuroprotection, which is mediated by histones (Suphioglu, Sadli et al. 2010b).

1.3.1 Histones

Histones are a group of conserved, highly basic proteins that are rich in lysine (K) and arginine (R) (Kinkade and Cole 1966; DeLange and Smith 1971; Elgin and Weintraub 1975; Munishkina, Fink et al. 2004) (Table 1). Histones are the nuclear protein that are involved in the assembly of chromatin through electrostatic interaction between the highly negatively charged polymeric DNA and the positively charged histones, which play a determining role in stabilizing the nucleosomes at physiological conditions (Korolev, Lyubartsev et al. 2004). About 85% of the DNA in chromatin is represented by uniform units, the nucleosomes, which are the complexes of DNA double helix with five histone proteins (H2A, H2B, H3, H4, and H1) (Luger, Rechsteiner et al. 1997). The central part of the nucleosome is called the nucleosome core particle and consists of 147 bp DNA wrapped around the histone octamer, which is formed from one $(H3/H4)_2$ tetramer and two H2A/H2B dimers (Luger, Rechsteiner et al. 1997; Woodcock and Dimitrov 2001). The four core histones have similar isoelectric points (pI) and share a common structural motif called the histone fold, which facilitates the interactions between the individual core histones (Arents and Moudrianakis 1995). Flanking the core domains are the relatively unstructured *N*-terminal tail domains. The histone tails extend out from the face of the nucleosome and through the gyres of DNA

Histone type	Class (amino acid distribution)	M.W. (Da)	Sequence length	Isoelectric point (pI)
H1	Very lysine rich	~ 21,500	~215	
H2A	Lysine rich	14,004	129	10.9
H2B	Lysine rich	13,774	125	10.3
H3	Arginine rich	15,324	135	11.1
H4	Arginine rich	11,282	102	11.4

Table 1. Characteristics of histones. Molecular weight (MW) is given in Daltons (Da) and isoelectric points (pI) are shown

superhelix into the area surrounding the nucleosome (Luger, Rechsteiner et al. 1997). In contrast to the structural core histone proteins, histone H1 is associated into linker DNA, which connects the nucleosomes together, resulting in the formation of "beads-on-a-string" chromatin structure (Davie and Chadee 1998).

1.3.2 Possible mechanism of the effect of zinc and DHA on H3 and H4 expression

We observed a significant reduction in both mRNA and protein levels of histones H3 and H4 following zinc treatment suggesting that zinc may inhibit the transcription of histones H3 and H4 in M17 human neuronal cells (Suphioglu, Sadli et al. 2010b). Histones H3 and H4 possess multiple metal response elements upstream of their start codon, which indicates the possible involvement of zinc in their transcription. Previous studies showed that inhibition of DNA synthesis triggers a concerted repression of histone synthesis, indicating that sustained histone synthesis depends on continued DNA synthesis. We proposed that the termination of H3 and H4 synthesis may possibly be caused by the effect of zinc in inhibiting DNA synthesis (Suphioglu, Sadli et al. 2010b). Conversely, DHA was found to up-regulate H3 and H4 expression levels and abolished the effect of zinc, suggesting the potential contribution of DHA in increasing DNA synthesis, which result in the increase of histone protein levels. Our results are supported by previous studies, by which zinc regulates a variety of transcription and translation related factors, including the H3 histone family 3A protein (Barcelo-Coblijn, Hogyes et al. 2003). Since there's association between alteration in histone subunit expression and DNA replication, the condition may then alter the expression of many other genes.

From this study, we propose that DHA may contribute positively to minimizing the onset of neurodegenerative disease through maintaining the integrity of DNA and histones H3 and H4 synthesis. The inhibition of DNA synthesis, which subsequently lead to the loss of neurons, however, is a pathological process of neurodegenerative disorders and potentially cause the death of the cells.

1.4 Histone post-translational modifications (PTMs) and gene activities

In addition to nucleosome assembly, studies have found that histones are potentially important carriers of epigenetic information. They, therefore, play significant role in regulating gene activities, such as DNA damage repair, replication and transcription through post-translational modifications (PTMs) (Hasan and Hottiger 2002). Core histones are characterized by the presence of fold domain (Alva, Ammelburg et al. 2007) and *N*-terminal tails which are exposed to nucleosomal surface (Ausio, Dong et al. 1989). These *N*-terminal tails of core histones are subjected to extensive post-translational modifications in many cellular processes (Ausio, Dong et al. 1989), which play pivotal roles in the epigenetic control of chromatin structure necessary for DNA accessibility during gene expression (Iizuka and Smith 2003). Some PTMs, including acetylation and phosphorylation, are reversible and are often associated with increase in gene expression. Other PTMs, such as lysine methylation, are often found to be more stable and participate in long term epigenetic maintenance (Bernstein and Allis 2005).

One of the best-studied post-translational modifications is the acetylation of lysine residues, which is a reversible process that is catalyzed by either histone acetyltransferases (HATs) or histone deacetylases (HDACs). The main acetylation sites in histone H3 of most species are at lysine 9, -14, -18 and -23 (Thorne, Kmiciek et al. 1990). Histone acetylation is a hallmark of transcriptionally active regions, whereas hypoacetylated histones are associated with tightly compacted nucleosomes, resulting in transcriptional repression due to restricted access of transcriptional factors to their targeted DNA (Oliva, Bazett-Jones et al. 1990). The addition of an acetyl group by a member of HAT family create appropriate 'histone code' for chromatin modification and decrease the interaction between the negatively charged DNA backbone and the positively charged histone tail enhancing DNA accessibility to transcription factors (TFs), which therefore increase gene transcription. Conversely, HDAC removes the acetyl group and potentially leads to general repression of gene transcription (Dangond, Henriksson et al. 2001).

So far, in humans, 18 HDACs enzymes have been identified on the basis of similarity to yeast counterparts and classified based on sequence identity and domain organization as well as cofactor dependency (Heltweg, Dequiedt et al. 2003). The classic HDACs (Class I, II and IV) require Zn^{2+} for their activity, whereas the sir2-related HDACs (sirtuins) require (nicotinamide adenine dinucleotide) NAD+ as cofactor (Koyama, Adachi et al. 2000). Class I HDACs (HDAC1, 2, 3 and 8), which are homologs of the yeast histone deacetylase RPD3, are found primarily in the nucleus of most cell lines and tissue types (Fischle, Emiliani et al. 1999; Fischle, Kiermer et al. 2001), whereas Class II HDACs (HDAC 4, 5, 6, 7 9 and 10) share a significant degree of homology with the yeast Hda1 and are able to shuttle in and out of the nucleus depending on different signals (Fischle, Emiliani et al. 1999; Fischle, Kiermer et al. 2001), suggesting a potential extranuclear functions by regulating the acetylation status of nonhistone substrates (Grozinger, Hassig et al. 1999; Heltweg, Dequiedt et al. 2003). Class III HDACs are composed of the Sirtuins (SIRT) proteins 1–7 and require NAD+ for deacetylase activity in contrast to the zinc-catalyzed mechanism used by class I and II HDACs (Koyama, Adachi et al. 2000; Lo, Trievel et al. 2000; Blander and Guarente 2004). The most recently described HDACs are Class IV, which is represented by HDAC11. This enzyme is phylogenetically different from class I and II HDACs and is therefore classified separately (Gao, Cueto et al. 2002). So far, very little is known about its function and regulation (Yang and Seto 2008).

In addition to acetylation, important progress has also been made in the studies of other types of covalent modifications including methylation and phosphorylation of histones H3. It has long been known that histone H3 is methylated at a number of lysine (Lys) and arginine (Arg) residues. The major sites of Lys-methylation on histones identified so far are: Lys4, Lys9, Lys27, Lys36, Lys79 and arginine methylation takes place at R2, R17 and R26 (Sims, Nishioka et al. 2003; Lee, Teyssier et al. 2005). The addition of methyl-group on histone tail residues is catalyzed by histone methyltransferases (HMTs). These enzymes can catalyze mono-, di-, or trimethylation on lysine residues and this differential methylation provides further functional diversity to each site of lysine methylation. Similar to histone acetylation, histone methylation can also modulate histone interaction with DNA, which result in an alteration of nucleosome structures and functions and therefore contribute to different cellular process (Rice and Allis 2001). The specific methylation of histone tails such as H3(K4), H3(K36), and H3(K79) have been associated with active transcriptional activity (Strahl, Ohba et al. 1999; Berger 2007), whereas methylation of H3(K9), H3(K27) and H4(K20) have been correlated with gene silencing (Lee, Teyssier et al. 2005).

Histone phosphorylation have also been shown to occur on all histones, and are located within the highly conserved amino acid residues alanine, arginine, lysine and serine (Clayton and Mahadevan 2003). For histone H3, phosphorylation takes place specifically at Thr3, -11 and at Ser10, -28 (Hendzel, Wei et al. 1997; Hsu, Sun et al. 2000; Dai, Sultan et al.

2005). Studies have reported the involvement of H3 phosphorylation in transcriptional activation (Mizzen, Kuo et al. 1998; Clayton, Rose et al. 2000; Nowak and Corces 2000), chromatin fiber decondensation, and chromosomes compaction during cell division (Hendzel, Wei et al. 1997; Hsu, Sun et al. 2000). Histone H3 is phosphorylated during both mitosis and meiosis and initiated at different phase of the cell division in different organisms (Hans and Dimitrov 2001). The phosphorylation of Thr(T)3 of histone H3, which is catalyzed by kinase haspin occurs during mitosis and it plays an essential role in facilitating condensation and resolution of sister chromatids in the late G2 and prophase (Dai, Sultan et al. 2005). To ensure this orderly cell cycle progression, the regulation of chromatin structure and spindle activity must be precisely integrated. The inappropriate H3(T3) phosphorylation causes defects in chromatin structure which might hinder chromosome alignment in mitosis (Enomoto, Koyamazaki et al. 2001), leading to genomic instability (Dai, Sultan et al. 2005). Threonine-3 residue is found in histone H3 of all eukaryotes, suggesting a highly conserved and critical function for this residue (Dai, Sultan et al. 2005).

1.4.1 Histone post-translational modifications (PTMs) and neurodegenerative disease

As previously discussed, histone post-translational modifications (PTMs) play significant role in regulating gene activities. Therefore, aberrant pattern of epigenetic regulation has been linked to the development of neurodegenerative diseases such as Alzheimer's disease.

During normal neuronal condition, HATs and HDACs remain in a state of balance, which they counteract each other to ensure neurophysiological homeostasis. Such equilibrium (Figure 1A) is responsible for regulating gene expression leading to normal function of neuronal cell activity and memory formation (Saha and Pahan 2006). During neurodegenerative diseases, the acetylation homeostasis is altered when histone acetylation significantly decreases (Rouaux, Jokic et al. 2003), reflecting dysfunctional acetylation-deacetylation apparatus (Figure 1B). General loss of acetylating agent would cause excessive increase in HDAC activity, which is then associated with transcriptional repression (Figure 1B). Studies have reported that reduction in histone acetylation followed by the increase in HDAC activity or DNA methylation is common in many neurodegenerative and neuropsychiatric disorders (Faraco, Pancani et al. 2006; Fischer, Sananbenesi et al. 2007).

In recent years, the increasing numbers of structurally diverse HDAC inhibitors have been identified with the potential to target specific brain regions and in cell-specific manner to reverse disorder-specific epigenetic dysregulation (Abel and Zukin 2008). The HDAC inhibitors include: short-chain fatty acid (i.e. valproic acid) (Kothari, Joshi et al. 2009), hydroxamic acid (i.e. SAHA, TSA, oxamflatin) (Archin, Espeseth et al. 2009), cyclic tetrapeptides (i.e trapoxin, apicidin) (Masuoka, Shindoh et al. 2008) and benzamide (i.e MS-275) (Gahr, Peter et al. 2008). These HDACs inhibitors are aimed to inhibit its enzymatic activity and to remove the repressive blocks from promoters of essential genes and therefore induce active gene transcription (Saha and Pahan 2006). The X-ray crystallographic studies showed that this type of HDAC inhibitor act as a chelator of zinc ion in the catalytic site of HDACs which therefore block the substrate access to the active zinc ion and subsequently inhibit the deacetylation ativity (Ficner 2009). However, it is still uncertain whether certain neurodegenerative disorders are mediated by a specific HDAC.

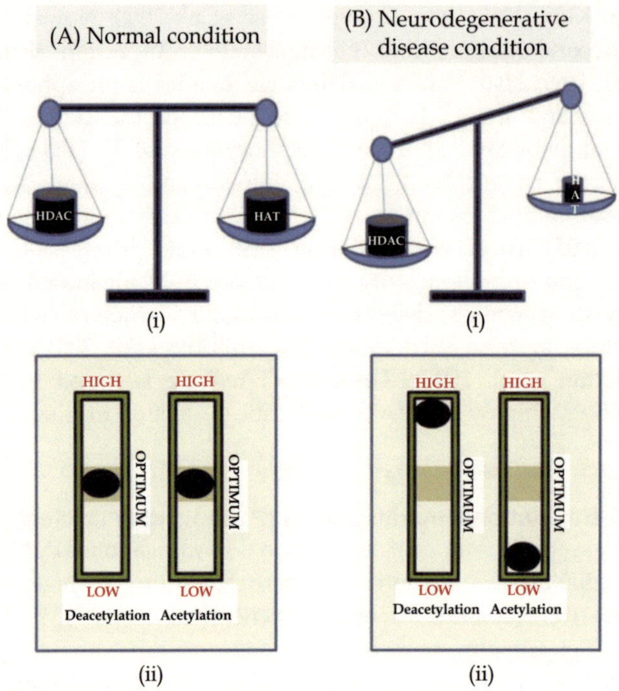

Fig. 1. Neuronal acetylation homeostasis. (i) Weights on the balance represent the protein level of HATs and HDACs. (ii) Enzymatic activity scale represents the activity and dark grey areas are physiologically optimal. (A) Under normal neuronal conditions, the level and activity of both HATs and HDACs are within their point of balance where they counteract each other to maintain internal equilibrium (homeostasis). (B) During neurodegenerative disease condition, acetylation homeostasis is altered resulting in the loss of HATs level and activity which balance towards an excessive production of HDACs and subsequent increase in deacetylation

Aging is also considered as the greatest risk factor for the development of the neurodegenerative diseases, such as Alzheimer's disease where neuronal function declination and gene expression alternation could be detected in the aging human brain (Giovacchini, Chang et al. 2002). Studies have found the altered pattern of histone modification in aging cells, such as, trimethylation of histone H4 at lysine 20, which was increased in kidneys and liver of the old-aged rat (Sarg, Koutzamani et al. 2002), and the level of H4 acetylation, which was decreased in the rat brain cortical neurons with age (Pina, Martinez et al. 1988). Several new methylated sites, such as H3(K24), H3(K128) and H2A(R89) were also detected in the study of aged mouse brain, however, no functional studies on these three sites had been reported (Wang, Tsai et al. 2009). It has been reported that in aging brains, most PTMs sites were found on histone H3 which has the longest N-terminal tails amongst other core histones (Wang, Tsai et al. 2009). These studies suggest the importance of proper epigenetic modification in biological activities and neuronal cell development, while the altered epigenetic regulation leads to neurodegenerative diseases.

1.5 Importance of zinc and DHA in epigenetics of human neuronal cells

1.5.1 Effect of zinc and DHA on acetylation levels of Histone H3(K9)

Proper regulation of gene expression in the nervous system is not only controlled by the transcriptional machinery but is also subject to modulation by epigenetic mechanisms such as histone modifications. Following our histone expression study, for the first time, we have also investigated the effect of zinc and DHA on post-translational modifications of histones, in particular histone H3 in human neuronal cells.

One-dimensional electrophoresis and western immunoblot analysis were used to investigate the change in post-translational modified histones of human neuronal cells that had been grown in the presence and absence of zinc and DHA. Our results showed that zinc decreased acetylation of H3(K9), whereas DHA increase H3(K9) acetylation. This suggests the potential involvement of zinc in the progress of neurodegenerative disease through an altered acetylation homeostasis in neuronal cells. During the acetylation dyshomeostasis, transcriptional regulation may be affected which has been reported to be one of the prime causes of neurodegenerative diseases (Saha and Pahan 2006). This altered gene transcription then caused opposite effects from normal gene regulation pattern in neuronal cells. This attributed to degenerative fate of neurons that subsequently reduced the expression of survival-associated genes by altered acetylation and at the same time, stimulated the expression of death-inducing genes (Saha and Pahan 2006).

The increase in Histone H3(K9) acetylation in response to DHA, however, indicates the ability of DHA to normalize the histone H3(K9) acetylation to the basal level (control) and abolishes the effect of zinc (Sadli et al., 2011, *unpublished results*). Therefore, DHA may contribute to neuroprotection through reinstating the altered acetylation dyshomeostasis caused by zinc toxicity, which would possibly up-regulate the expression of neuroprotective genes (Saha and Pahan 2006).

1.5.2 Effect of zinc and DHA on histone deacetylases (HDACs) 1, 2, 3

We performed western immunoblotting to investigate the change in the expression levels of histone deacetylase (HDACs) 1, 2, 3 using anti-HDAC1, 2 and 3 antibodies, where we found that zinc significantly up-regulated HDAC1, 2 and 3 expression levels compared with the control, while DHA significantly down-regulated HDAC1, 2 and 3 (Sadli et al., 2011, *unpublished results*). It's been reported that the activity of HDACs were increased in dying neurons, due to the loss of counterbalancing effect of HATs activity (Saha and Pahan 2006). From our results, we propose that the increase in zinc can also contribute to the neurodegenerative process through up-regulating HDACs enzyme expression levels, and therefore increasing the activity of histone deacetylation.

The HDACs catalytic domain contains a Zn^{2+} ion, in the active site, which contributes significantly to its catalytic activity (Vannini, Volpari et al. 2004; Ficner 2009). *In vitro,* the deacetylase activity of the purified HDAC homologue was observed only after incubation with zinc chloride (Finnin, Donigian et al. 1999), which suggests that HDAC activity requires a metal cofactor (Hassig, Tong et al. 1998). X-ray crystallographic studies have shown that HDAC inhibitors could chelate zinc ions in the catalytic sites of HDACs and therefore block substrate access to the active zinc ions and inhibit the deacetylation reaction (Marks, Richon et al. 2000; Ficner 2009).

It has been established in the scientific literature that the isotopic selective inhibition of HDAC enzyme may be the potential treatment for neurodegenerative diseases. It has also been demonstrated that the transcriptional dysregulation by HDACs may play significant role in causing neurodegenerative disease and that HDACs therapy may prevent or slow down the neurodegenerative disease process. So far, the HDAC inhibitors investigated in treating neurodegenerative diseases are very limited and mainly focused on the well-establish experimental drug trichostatin A (member of hydroxamic acid group) and the clinically used HDAC inhibitors sodium butyrate, valproic acid, phenylbutyrate and vorinostat, which belong to short chain fatty acid group that are known to be able to penetrate the blood-brain barrier (Butler and Bates 2006). From our observation, DHA, being a long chain n-3 fatty acid that is selectively allowed to cross the blood-brain barrier, is likely to have neuroprotective characteristic that mimic the behavior of HDACs inhibitors. This significantly down-regulates the HDACs expression levels and therefore induces histone acetylation, which then allow the transcription and expression of genes, in what had been a too tightly packaged chromatin structure in which certain genes do not get transcribed.

Generally, increase in HDACs during neurodegenerative disease is associated with increase in gene repression and transcriptional dysfunction of certain transcription factors (TFs) such as CREB, which is important in regulating the expression of pro-survival elements such as Bcl-2 (Freeland, Boxer et al. 2001; Saha and Pahan 2006). In our study, we show how zinc contributes to dysfunctional acetylation homesostasis in M17 cells by up-regulating HDACs, which influence the reduction of HATs and consequently histone acetylation levels. DHA, however, is shown to reestablish the imbalance of acetylation homesostasis and therefore capable of correcting the down-regulation of specific genes caused by reduction in histone acetylation (Sadli et al., 2011, *unpublished results*). The mechanism by which DHA inhibits the HDACs expression is unclear, whether DHA directly chelates zinc ion from the catalytic sites of HDACs or hinder the zinc ion binding to the enzymes.

1.6 Link between cellular apoptosis and neurodegenerative diseases

A characteristic of many neurodegenerative diseases, such as Alzheimer's disease, Parkinson's disease and stroke - is neuronal cell death (Cavallucci and D'Amelio, 2011; Calissano, Matrone et al. 2009). Central nervous system tissue has very limited regenerative capacity and therefore it is important to limit the damage caused by neuronal cell death (Rossi and Cattaneo 2002) (Kuhn, Palmer et al. 2001). In recent years, the investigation regarding the contribution of caspases and neuronal apoptosis to neurodegenerative diseases has gained increasing attention. This evidence has been generated by using a variety of complementary approaches, including evaluating human tissue and using transgenic mouse and *in vitro* models (Kuhn, Palmer et al. 2001).

Studies have shown the imbalance level of pro-apoptotic (Bax, Bak and Bad) and anti-apoptotic Bcl-2 protein (Su, Deng et al. 1997; Kitamura, Shimohama et al. 1998), as well as caspase-3 and -6 in post-mortem brains of AD patients (Stadelmann, Deckwerth et al. 1999). In addition, immunohistochemical and biochemical studies reported the presence of active caspases and caspase-cleaved substrates around senile plague and neurofibrillary tangles in neuron (Gastard, Troncoso et al. 2003). There's also a marked co-localization of hyperphosphorylated tau, caspase-3 and caspase-6 in TUNEL-positive neurons in the brainstem of AD patients (Wai, Liang et al. 2009), suggesting the potential involvement of apoptotic death in the etiology of AD.

Caspase-mediated apoptotic pathways have specifically been linked to the progression of AD, especially toward the formation of amyloid precursor protein (APP) and Aβ peptide production. Caspase-3-mediated APP stabilizes BACE1 (the β-secretase enzyme that is responsible for the cleavage of APP and the associated creation of beta-amyloid), which lead to an increase in Aβ production (Tesco, Koh et al. 2007). Studies also indicate that caspases have been implicated in the mechanism of tau-mediated neurodegeneration of AD (Garcia-Sierra, Mondragon-Rodriguez et al. 2008) (Dickson 2004). According to this hypothesis, Aβ peptide was reported to promote neuronal pathological tau filament assembly by triggering caspase activation leading to tau cleavage, which in turn generate more tau pathological filaments (Tesco, Koh et al. 2007) that further contribute to increase of cellular dysfunction in AD (Fasulo, Ugolini et al. 2000).

1.6.1 Effect of zinc and DHA on Bcl-2 (anti-apoptotic marker) and caspase-3 (pro-apoptotic marker) expression levels

As mentioned previously, zinc toxicity is one of the important causes of cell death in neurodegenerative disease, including Alzheimer's disease (Naganska and Matyja 2006). It has been reported that intracellular zinc release, as a result of altered zinc metabolism, leads to the activation of caspase-3, which then subsequently trigger neuronal cell apoptosis (Zhang, Wang et al. 2004). In our study, we aimed to determine whether anti-apoptotic Bcl-2 and pro-apoptotic caspase-3 were involved in the cellular pathway affected by zinc and DHA interactions in M17 cells by investigating their expression levels using western blot analysis.

Both zinc and DHA have been shown to opposingly modulate the levels of Bcl-2 and caspase-3 in M17 cells (Sadli et al., 2011, *unpublished results*). An increase in zinc levels causes up-regulation of caspase-3 and down-regulation of Bcl-2 expression, suggesting the potential occurrence of apoptosis of zinc-induced M17 cells, which is representative of neurodegenerative conditions such as AD where intracellular zinc ion is elevated while DHA level is reduced. Conversely, DHA treatment of M17 cells increased expression levels of Bcl-2 and reduced caspase-3, which suggest that DHA exclusively activates the extracellular signal regulated kinase/mitogen-activated protein kinases (ERK/MPK) pathway to promote cell survival that lead to the up-regulation of Bcl-2 and inhibition of caspase-3 activation (German, Insua et al. 2006). Our observation was supported by Akbar et al. (2006), which showed the involvement of DHA in neuronal cell survival by driving Akt translocation resulting in activation of Bcl-2 and subsequent suppression of caspase-3 activity leading to inhibition of apoptosis in neuronal cells (Akbar, Baick et al. 2006).

Our findings with Bcl-2 and caspase-3 highlight the importance of DHA in neuroprotection and zinc toxicity in apoptosis. The blockage of caspase-3 activity by DHA might protect against the apoptotic cell death following zinc toxicity, which may offer a useful and alternative therapeutic strategy to delay neuronal loss associated with neurodegenerative diseases. Further investigations on the role of DHA in neuroprotection through inhibition of caspase needs to be done, which will provide additional insights into this cascade activity pathway. This in return will establish the idea whether cascade-induced zinc toxicity is a direct cause of apoptosis or a downstream consequence, which will eventually lead to cell death in neurodegenerative diseases.

1.7 M17 cell line as a model

Neurodegeneration is very difficult to study *in vivo*. Neuronal cells do not regenerate and cannot be observed or manipulated without removing them from the patients. For these reasons, *in vitro* models are very important options. An ideal cell line would possess similar characteristic as the *in vivo* neurons, while having the advantage of immortalization to ensure continuous supply of cells. Immortalized cells are also convenient to handle and experiments can be performed during continuous conditions in which biochemical process can easily be studied.

Throughout our studies, M17, a neuronal-derived cell line was used. M17 cells are originally isolated from the bone marrow of a two year old male suffering from disseminated neuroblastoma (Global Bio-resource Center, 2007). Microscopic analysis shows that the cell type indicates a neuronal characteristic; being morphologically small in size and dense with triangular-shaped cell bodies. The advantage of this cell line is that it is of human origin, and by now, M17 cells constitute a well studied and defined cellular system. Our in-house results suggest that M17 cell line is a suitable model for studying the effects of DHA and zinc supplementation on the gene and protein expression profiles of neuronal cells throughout this study.

1.8 Application of proteomic and molecular analysis in neurodegenerative disease research

The need for protein-level analysis arises because the phenotype of human neuronal cells in relation to neurodegeneration corresponds to the functions of expressed and modified protein networks. Unlike the genome that is relatively static, the proteome is extremely dynamic and constantly adjusted in response to changing internal (e.g aging) and external events (e.g toxic exposure, drugs).

Proteins are composed of a variety of combinations of amino acids, and are subject to co- as well as post-translational modification, such as deletion of amino acid sequences and chemical modification of specific amino acids (e.g oxidation and phosphorylation) (Anderson, Matheson et al. 2001). These modifications will influence the activity state, function and interactions of proteins.

The word "*proteome*" is derived from proteins expressed by a genome, and it refers to all the proteins produced by an organism, first coined by Wilkins et al. in 1996 (Wilkins, Sanchez et al. 1996). In its wider sense, proteomic research assesses protein expression, modification, interaction and localization. By studying global patterns of proteins and their changes dynamically, proteomic research can improve our understanding of system-level cellular behavior. Although proteomics as an entity is relatively new, the methodological and theoretical foundations have been under development for more than three decades (Campostrini, Pascali et al. 2004). Two-dimensional protein electrophoresis, coupled with peptide mass fingerprinting analysis by mass spectrometry (MS), has become the most powerful techniques for proteome analysis (Binz, Muller et al. 1999).

In the future, downstream steps after genomics and proteomics will aim at understanding functional consequences of biomolecule interactions in different biological pathways in a system. Comparative studies to quantitate, identify and characterize the proteins expressed in normal neuronal cells and diseased cells will give insight into the mechanisms of neurodegenerative disease. This will allow the identification of novel diagnostic and treatment reagents for Alzheimer's disease.

Proteomic analysis data has become an important resource in the investigation of neurodegenerative diseases. Proteomic profiling, in particular, has enabled researchers to investigate a vast number of proteins at once. Such principles have been utilized in order to detect specific alterations in the protein expression levels in various regions of the neuro-degenerated brain compared to control brain. This may, in turn, facilitate the construction of hypotheses on the mechanisms by which the disease progresses.

When considering neurological disorders, one good example for the usability of two-dimensional gel electrophoresis (2-DE) in exploring new biomarkers, was the discovery of two unknown protein isoforms p130 and p131 that were suggested to be able to discriminate Creutzfeldt-Jakob disease from other type of dementia (Harrington, Merril et al. 1986). Most efforts in understanding the pathogenesis using 2-DE-based expression proteomics have been made by comparing brain proteomes of AD patients and controls. Some of the first 2-DE studies examined the levels of AD brain proteins where they revealed alterations in the levels of a number of proteins, such as GFAP, tubulin, and creatine kinase (Smirnov, Shevtsov et al. 1991; Burbaeva 1992). Subsequently, the number of 2-DE studies has multiplied and at present, changes in the levels of more than 100 brain protein isoforms have been identified in neurodegenerative disorders (Fountoulakis, Juranville et al. 2002; Butterfield and Castegna 2003; Vlahou and Fountoulakis 2005). Despite the multiplicity of isoform specific protein changes, the findings still remain rather fragmented and novel hypothesis related to the pathogenesis of AD still remains to be revealed.
Proteomic methods were also successfully applied in the study of tau protein phosphorylation in AD where tau become phosphorylated and accumulated to form neurofibrillary tangles (Ksiezak-Reding, Binder et al. 1990). The increased phosphorylation of elongation factor II has also been demonstrated in AD brain by the 2-D approach (Johnson, Gotlib et al. 1992). As a consequence of rapid demographic aging, AD has become one of the most devastating socioeconomical challenges of the present-day. Now, the new hope of unraveling the secrets of AD is done by the so-called "new technologies" (i.e. proteomics) which have been suggested to represent a breakthrough in improving our understanding, diagnosis and treatment of AD.

1.9 Conclusions and future perspectives

We characterized the effect of zinc and DHA in modulating gene and protein expression in M17 human neuronal cells. This idea was based on the fact that both zinc and DHA play significant roles in neuroprotection and are known to interact biochemically. DHA treatment of M7 cells results in lower zinc transporter ZnT3 protein levels and reduction in pro-apoptotic marker caspase-3 indicates the involvement of zinc in pathways that regulate brain cell survival and that alteration in zinc homeostasis may contribute to the development of neurodegenerative diseases.
Both zinc and DHA may possibly be involved in the signaling mechanism that regulates histone expression levels in M17 human neuronal cells. Here we hypothesize that DHA may play a protective role by up-regulating histones H3 and H4, which accounts for the positive effect of DHA in minimizing the onset of neurodegenerative disease through facilitating DNA synthesis and therefore increasing histone protein levels.
Following our previous study, we also investigated the effect of zinc and DHA in regulating gene expression through histones post-translational modifications. Zinc was found to reduce histone acetylation and increase HDACs, which represent a critical step commonly underlying catastrophic neuronal dysfunction, whereas, DHA reinstated the imbalance of acetylation homeostasis indicating its potential neuroprotective ability to ameliorate neurodegenerative diseases. Reduction in acetylation along with parallel gain of HDAC levels represents the crux of the altered situation and we propose that DHA could possibly mimic the action of a HDAC inhibitors and therefore, reverses the zinc-mediated altered acetylation homeostasis.

Currently, the acetylation homesostasis system in neuronal cells is still in its infancy, so more research needs to be done in this field, especially in relation to neurodegenerative diseases. However, evidence provides us with some insights into the distinct epigenetic pattern and activity between zinc and DHA, which suggest their opposing role in the progression of neurodegenerative diseases. Our study highlights the functional mechanism in relation to beneficial effect of DHA in a number of ways and the involvement of zinc toxicity in cellular apoptosis (Figure 2).

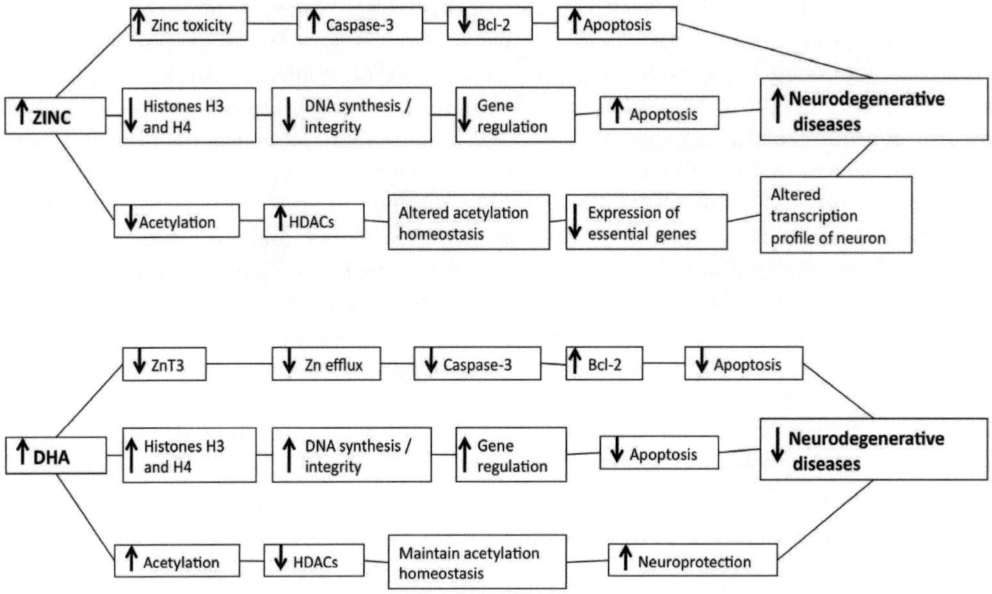

Fig. 2. Proposed model depicting the role of zinc and DHA in progression of neurodegenerative diseases. Various models representing neurodegenerative diseases are marked by irregular gene expression, altered epigenetic patterns as well as apoptosis. Cellular zinc toxicity contributes to neurodegenerative condition through a number of different pathways, which seem to be reversed by the presence of DHA. Zinc and DHA may share common pathways in the progression of neurodegenerative disease where DHA play a significant role in restoring the condition caused by altered zinc homeostasis

2. References

Abel, T. and R. S. Zukin (2008). "Epigenetic targets of HDAC inhibition in neurodegenerative and psychiatric disorders." *Curr Opin Pharmacol* 8(1): 57-64.

Akbar, M., J. Baick, et al. (2006). "Ethanol promotes neuronal apoptosis by inhibiting phosphatidylserine accumulation." *J Neurosci Res* 83(3): 432-40.

Akbar, M., F. Calderon, et al. (2005). "Docosahexaenoic acid: a positive modulator of Akt signaling in neuronal survival." *Proc Natl Acad Sci U S A* 102(31): 10858-63.

Al-Gazali, L. I., R. Padmanabhan, et al. (2001). "Abnormal folate metabolism and genetic polymorphism of the folate pathway in a child with Down syndrome and neural tube defect." *Am J Med Genet* 103(2): 128-32.

Alva, V., M. Ammelburg, et al. (2007). "On the origin of the histone fold." *BMC Struct Biol* 7: 17.

Anderson, N. G., A. Matheson, et al. (2001). "Back to the future: the human protein index (HPI) and the agenda for post-proteomic biology." *Proteomics* 1(1): 3-12.

Archin, N. M., A. Espeseth, et al. (2009). "Expression of latent HIV induced by the potent HDAC inhibitor suberoylanilide hydroxamic acid." *AIDS Res Hum Retroviruses* 25(2): 207-12.

Arents, G. and E. N. Moudrianakis (1995). "The histone fold: a ubiquitous architectural motif utilized in DNA compaction and protein dimerization." *Proc Natl Acad Sci U S A* 92(24): 11170-4.

Ausio, J., F. Dong, et al. (1989). "Use of selectively trypsinized nucleosome core particles to analyze the role of the histone "tails" in the stabilization of the nucleosome." *J Mol Biol* 206(3): 451-63.

Barcelo-Coblijn, G., E. Hogyes, et al. (2003). "Modification by docosahexaenoic acid of age-induced alterations in gene expression and molecular composition of rat brain phospholipids." *Proc Natl Acad Sci U S A* 100(20): 11321-6.

Bazan, N. G. (2003). "Synaptic lipid signaling: significance of polyunsaturated fatty acids and platelet-activating factor." *J Lipid Res* 44(12): 2221-33.

Bazan, N. G. (2009). "Cellular and molecular events mediated by docosahexaenoic acid-derived neuroprotectin D1 signaling in photoreceptor cell survival and brain protection." *Prostaglandins Leukot Essent Fatty Acids.*

Berger, S. L. (2007). "The complex language of chromatin regulation during transcription." *Nature* 447(7143): 407-12.

Bernstein, E. and C. D. Allis (2005). "RNA meets chromatin." *Genes Dev* 19(14): 1635-55.

Bertoni-Freddari, C., E. Mocchegiani, et al. (2006). "Synaptic and mitochondrial physiopathologic changes in the aging nervous system and the role of zinc ion homeostasis." *Mech Ageing Dev* 127(6): 590-6.

Binz, P. A., M. Muller, et al. (1999). "A molecular scanner to automate proteomic research and to display proteome images." *Anal Chem* 71(21): 4981-8.

Blander, G. and L. Guarente (2004). "The Sir2 family of protein deacetylases." *Annu Rev Biochem* 73: 417-35.

Breteler, M. M., F. A. van den Ouweland, et al. (1992). "A community-based study of dementia: the Rotterdam Elderly Study." *Neuroepidemiology* 11 Suppl 1: 23-8.

Burbaeva, G. (1992). "[Physiologically active brain proteins as possible markers of mental diseases]." *Vestn Ross Akad Med Nauk*(7): 51-4.

Butler, R. and G. P. Bates (2006). "Histone deacetylase inhibitors as therapeutics for polyglutamine disorders." *Nat Rev Neurosci* 7(10): 784-96.

Butterfield, D. A. and A. Castegna (2003). "Proteomics for the identification of specifically oxidized proteins in brain: technology and application to the study of neurodegenerative disorders." *Amino Acids* 25(3-4): 419-25.

Calderon, F. and H. Y. Kim (2004). "Docosahexaenoic acid promotes neurite growth in hippocampal neurons." *J Neurochem* 90(4): 979-88.

Calissano, P., C. Matrone, et al. (2009). "Apoptosis and in vitro Alzheimer disease neuronal models." *Commun Integr Biol* 2(2): 163-9.

Calon, F., G. P. Lim, et al. (2004). "Docosahexaenoic acid protects from dendritic pathology in an Alzheimer's disease mouse model." *Neuron* 43(5): 633-45.

Campostrini, N., J. Pascali, et al. (2004). "Proteomic analysis of an orthotopic neuroblastoma xenograft animal model." *J Chromatogr B Analyt Technol Biomed Life Sci* 808(2): 279-86.

Canzoniero, L. M., D. M. Turetsky, et al. (1999). "Measurement of intracellular free zinc concentrations accompanying zinc-induced neuronal death." *J Neurosci* 19(19): RC31.

Cavallucci, V. and M. D'Amelio (2011). "Matter of life and death: the pharmacological approaches targeting apoptosis in brain diseases." *Curr Pharm Des* 17(3): 215-29.
Clayton, A. L. and L. C. Mahadevan (2003). "MAP kinase-mediated phosphoacetylation of histone H3 and inducible gene regulation." *FEBS Lett* 546(1): 51-8.
Clayton, A. L., S. Rose, et al. (2000). "Phosphoacetylation of histone H3 on c-fos- and c-jun-associated nucleosomes upon gene activation." *EMBO J* 19(14): 3714-26.
Crawford, M. A., R. P. Bazinet, et al. (2009). "Fat intake and CNS functioning: ageing and disease." *Ann Nutr Metab* 55(1-3): 202-28.
Cuajungco, M. P. and G. J. Lees (1997). "Zinc metabolism in the brain: relevance to human neurodegenerative disorders." *Neurobiol Dis* 4(3-4): 137-69.
Culmsee, C. and S. Landshamer (2006). "Molecular insights into mechanisms of the cell death program: role in the progression of neurodegenerative disorders." *Curr Alzheimer Res* 3(4): 269-83.
Dai, J., S. Sultan, et al. (2005). "The kinase haspin is required for mitotic histone H3 Thr 3 phosphorylation and normal metaphase chromosome alignment." *Genes Dev* 19(4): 472-88.
Dangond, F., M. Henriksson, et al. (2001). "Differential expression of class I HDACs: roles of cell density and cell cycle." *Int J Oncol* 19(4): 773-7.
Davie, J. R. and D. N. Chadee (1998). "Regulation and regulatory parameters of histone modifications." *J Cell Biochem Suppl* 30-31: 203-13.
DeLange, R. J. and E. L. Smith (1971). "Histones: structure and function." *Annu Rev Biochem* 40: 279-314.
Devore, E. E., F. Grodstein, et al. (2009). "Dietary intake of fish and omega-3 fatty acids in relation to long-term dementia risk." *Am J Clin Nutr* 90(1): 170-6.
Dickson, D. W. (2004). "Apoptotic mechanisms in Alzheimer neurofibrillary degeneration: cause or effect?" *J Clin Invest* 114(1): 23-7.
Dong, X. X., Y. Wang, et al. (2009). "Molecular mechanisms of excitotoxicity and their relevance to pathogenesis of neurodegenerative diseases." *Acta Pharmacol Sin* 30(4): 379-87.
Elgin, S. C. and H. Weintraub (1975). "Chromosomal proteins and chromatin structure." *Annu Rev Biochem* 44: 725-74.
Enomoto, R., R. Koyamazaki, et al. (2001). "Phosphorylation of histones triggers DNA fragmentation in thymocyte undergoing apoptosis induced by protein phosphatase inhibitors." *Mol Cell Biol Res Commun* 4(5): 276-81.
Faraco, G., T. Pancani, et al. (2006). "Pharmacological inhibition of histone deacetylases by suberoylanilide hydroxamic acid specifically alters gene expression and reduces ischemic injury in the mouse brain." *Mol Pharmacol* 70(6): 1876-84.
Fasulo, L., G. Ugolini, et al. (2000). "The neuronal microtubule-associated protein tau is a substrate for caspase-3 and an effector of apoptosis." *J Neurochem* 75(2): 624-33.
Fenton, W. S., J. Hibbeln, et al. (2000). "Essential fatty acids, lipid membrane abnormalities, and the diagnosis and treatment of schizophrenia." *Biol Psychiatry* 47(1): 8-21.
Ficner, R. (2009). "Novel structural insights into class I and II histone deacetylases." *Curr Top Med Chem* 9(3): 235-40.
Finnin, M. S., J. R. Donigian, et al. (1999). "Structures of a histone deacetylase homologue bound to the TSA and SAHA inhibitors." *Nature* 401(6749): 188-93.
Fischer, A., F. Sananbenesi, et al. (2007). "Recovery of learning and memory is associated with chromatin remodelling." *Nature* 447(7141): 178-82.
Fischle, W., S. Emiliani, et al. (1999). "A new family of human histone deacetylases related to Saccharomyces cerevisiae HDA1p." *J Biol Chem* 274(17): 11713-20.

Fischle, W., V. Kiermer, et al. (2001). "The emerging role of class II histone deacetylases." *Biochem Cell Biol* 79(3): 337-48.
Florent-Bechard, S., C. Malaplate-Armand, et al. (2007). "Towards a nutritional approach for prevention of Alzheimer's disease: biochemical and cellular aspects." *J Neurol Sci* 262(1-2): 27-36.
Fountoulakis, M., J. F. Juranville, et al. (2002). "Proteomic analysis of the fetal brain." *Proteomics* 2(11): 1547-76.
Fratiglioni, L. and C. Qiu (2009). "Prevention of common neurodegenerative disorders in the elderly." *Exp Gerontol* 44(1-2): 46-50.
Frederickson, C. J., M. D. Hernandez, et al. (1989). "Translocation of zinc may contribute to seizure-induced death of neurons." *Brain Res* 480(1-2): 317-21.
Freeland, K., L. M. Boxer, et al. (2001). "The cyclic AMP response element in the Bcl-2 promoter confers inducibility by hypoxia in neuronal cells." *Brain Res Mol Brain Res* 92(1-2): 98-106.
Friedland, R. P. (2003). "Fish consumption and the risk of Alzheimer disease: is it time to make dietary recommendations?" *Arch Neurol* 60(7): 923-4.
Gahr, S., G. Peter, et al. (2008). "The histone-deacetylase inhibitor MS-275 and the CDK-inhibitor CYC-202 promote anti-tumor effects in hepatoma cell lines." *Oncol Rep* 20(5): 1249-56.
Gao, L., M. A. Cueto, et al. (2002). "Cloning and functional characterization of HDAC11, a novel member of the human histone deacetylase family." *J Biol Chem* 277(28): 25748-55.
Garcia-Sierra, F., S. Mondragon-Rodriguez, et al. (2008). "Truncation of tau protein and its pathological significance in Alzheimer's disease." *J Alzheimers Dis* 14(4): 401-9.
Gastard, M. C., J. C. Troncoso, et al. (2003). "Caspase activation in the limbic cortex of subjects with early Alzheimer's disease." *Ann Neurol* 54(3): 393-8.
German, O. L., M. F. Insua, et al. (2006). "Docosahexaenoic acid prevents apoptosis of retina photoreceptors by activating the ERK/MAPK pathway." *J Neurochem* 98(5): 1507-20.
Giovacchini, G., M. C. Chang, et al. (2002). "Brain incorporation of [11C]arachidonic acid in young healthy humans measured with positron emission tomography." *J Cereb Blood Flow Metab* 22(12): 1453-62.
Golub, M. S., C. L. Keen, et al. (1995). "Developmental zinc deficiency and behavior." *J Nutr* 125(8 Suppl): 2263S-2271S.
Gomez de Segura, I. A., S. Valderrabano, et al. (2004). "Protective effects of dietary enrichment with docosahexaenoic acid plus protein in 5-fluorouracil-induced intestinal injury in the rat." *Eur J Gastroenterol Hepatol* 16(5): 479-85.
Grozinger, C. M., C. A. Hassig, et al. (1999). "Three proteins define a class of human histone deacetylases related to yeast Hda1p." *Proc Natl Acad Sci U S A* 96(9): 4868-73.
Hambidge, K. M., M. J. Goodall, et al. (1989). "Post-prandial and daily changes in plasma zinc." *J Trace Elem Electrolytes Health Dis* 3(1): 55-7.
Hans, F. and S. Dimitrov (2001). "Histone H3 phosphorylation and cell division." *Oncogene* 20(24): 3021-7.
Harrington, M. G., C. R. Merril, et al. (1986). "Abnormal proteins in the cerebrospinal fluid of patients with Creutzfeldt-Jakob disease." *N Engl J Med* 315(5): 279-83.
Hasan, S. and M. O. Hottiger (2002). "Histone acetyl transferases: a role in DNA repair and DNA replication." *J Mol Med* 80(8): 463-74.
Hassig, C. A., J. K. Tong, et al. (1998). "A role for histone deacetylase activity in HDAC1-mediated transcriptional repression." *Proc Natl Acad Sci U S A* 95(7): 3519-24.

He, K., Y. Song, et al. (2004). "Fish consumption and incidence of stroke: a meta-analysis of cohort studies." *Stroke* 35(7): 1538-42.

Heltweg, B., F. Dequiedt, et al. (2003). "Nonisotopic substrate for assaying both human zinc and NAD+-dependent histone deacetylases." *Anal Biochem* 319(1): 42-8.

Hendzel, M. J., Y. Wei, et al. (1997). "Mitosis-specific phosphorylation of histone H3 initiates primarily within pericentromeric heterochromatin during G2 and spreads in an ordered fashion coincident with mitotic chromosome condensation." *Chromosoma* 106(6): 348-60.

Hibbeln, J. R. and N. Salem, Jr. (1995). "Dietary polyunsaturated fatty acids and depression: when cholesterol does not satisfy." *Am J Clin Nutr* 62(1): 1-9.

Hossain, M. S., M. Hashimoto, et al. (1998). "Influence of docosahexaenoic acid on cerebral lipid peroxide level in aged rats with and without hypercholesterolemia." *Neurosci Lett* 244(3): 157-60.

Hsu, J. Y., Z. W. Sun, et al. (2000). "Mitotic phosphorylation of histone H3 is governed by Ipl1/aurora kinase and Glc7/PP1 phosphatase in budding yeast and nematodes." *Cell* 102(3): 279-91.

Huang, X., M. P. Cuajungco, et al. (2000). "Alzheimer's disease, beta-amyloid protein and zinc." *J Nutr* 130(5S Suppl): 1488S-92S.

Iizuka, M. and M. M. Smith (2003). "Functional consequences of histone modifications." *Curr Opin Genet Dev* 13(2): 154-60.

Innis, S. M. (2000). "The role of dietary n-6 and n-3 fatty acids in the developing brain." *Dev Neurosci* 22(5-6): 474-80.

Jayasooriya, A. P., M. L. Ackland, et al. (2005). "Perinatal omega-3 polyunsaturated fatty acid supply modifies brain zinc homeostasis during adulthood." *Proc Natl Acad Sci U S A* 102(20): 7133-8.

Johnson, G., J. Gotlib, et al. (1992). "Increased phosphorylation of elongation factor 2 in Alzheimer's disease." *Brain Res Mol Brain Res* 15(3-4): 319-26.

Jomova, K., D. Vondrakova, et al. (2010). "Metals, oxidative stress and neurodegenerative disorders." *Mol Cell Biochem* 345(1-2): 91-104.

Jorm, A. F. (2001). "History of depression as a risk factor for dementia: an updated review." *Aust N Z J Psychiatry* 35(6): 776-81.

Kalmijn, S., L. J. Launer, et al. (1997). "Dietary fat intake and the risk of incident dementia in the Rotterdam Study." *Ann Neurol* 42(5): 776-82.

Karasek, M. (2004). "Melatonin, human aging, and age-related diseases." *Exp Gerontol* 39(11-12): 1723-9.

Kinkade, J. M., Jr. and R. D. Cole (1966). "A structural comparison of different lysine-rich histones of calf thymus." *J Biol Chem* 241(24): 5798-805.

Kitamura, Y., S. Shimohama, et al. (1998). "Alteration of proteins regulating apoptosis, Bcl-2, Bcl-x, Bax, Bak, Bad, ICH-1 and CPP32, in Alzheimer's disease." *Brain Res* 780(2): 260-9.

Koh, J. Y. (2001). "Zinc and disease of the brain." *Mol Neurobiol* 24(1-3): 99-106.

Korolev, N., A. P. Lyubartsev, et al. (2004). "Electrostatic background of chromatin fiber stretching." *J Biomol Struct Dyn* 22(2): 215-26.

Kothari, V., G. Joshi, et al. (2009). "HDAC inhibitor valproic acid enhances tumour cell kill in adenovirus-HSVtk mediated suicide gene therapy in HNSCC xenograft mouse model." *Int J Cancer*.

Koyama, Y., M. Adachi, et al. (2000). "Histone deacetylase inhibitors suppress IL-2-mediated gene expression prior to induction of apoptosis." *Blood* 96(4): 1490-5.

Ksiezak-Reding, H., L. I. Binder, et al. (1990). "Alzheimer disease proteins (A68) share epitopes with tau but show distinct biochemical properties." *J Neurosci Res* 25(3): 420-30.

Kuhn, H. G., T. D. Palmer, et al. (2001). "Adult neurogenesis: a compensatory mechanism for neuronal damage." *Eur Arch Psychiatry Clin Neurosci* 251(4): 152-8.

Lai, L. H., R. X. Wang, et al. (2009). "Effects of docosahexaenoic acid on large-conductance Ca2+-activated K+ channels and voltage-dependent K+ channels in rat coronary artery smooth muscle cells." *Acta Pharmacol Sin* 30(3): 314-20.

Larrieu, S., L. Letenneur, et al. (2004). "Nutritional factors and risk of incident dementia in the PAQUID longitudinal cohort." *J Nutr Health Aging* 8(3): 150-4.

Launer, L. J., C. Brayne, et al. (1992). "Epidemiologic approach to the study of dementing diseases: a nested case-control study in European incidence studies of dementia." *Neuroepidemiology* 11 Suppl 1: 114-8.

Lauritzen, L., H. S. Hansen, et al. (2001). "The essentiality of long chain n-3 fatty acids in relation to development and function of the brain and retina." *Prog Lipid Res* 40(1-2): 1-94.

Lee, D. Y., C. Teyssier, et al. (2005). "Role of protein methylation in regulation of transcription." *Endocr Rev* 26(2): 147-70.

Lee, J. Y., T. B. Cole, et al. (2002). "Contribution by synaptic zinc to the gender-disparate plaque formation in human Swedish mutant APP transgenic mice." *Proc Natl Acad Sci U S A* 99(11): 7705-10.

Letenneur, L. (2004). "Risk of dementia and alcohol and wine consumption: a review of recent results." *Biol Res* 37(2): 189-93.

Lichten, L. A. and R. J. Cousins (2009). "Mammalian zinc transporters: nutritional and physiologic regulation." *Annu Rev Nutr* 29: 153-76.

Linkous, D. H., P. A. Adlard, et al. (2009). "The Effects of Enhanced Zinc on Spatial Memory and Plaque Formation in Transgenic Mice." *J Alzheimers Dis.*

Lo, W. S., R. C. Trievel, et al. (2000). "Phosphorylation of serine 10 in histone H3 is functionally linked in vitro and in vivo to Gcn5-mediated acetylation at lysine 14." *Mol Cell* 5(6): 917-26.

Luger, K., T. J. Rechsteiner, et al. (1997). "Characterization of nucleosome core particles containing histone proteins made in bacteria." *J Mol Biol* 272(3): 301-11.

Lukaski, H. C. (2005). "Low dietary zinc decreases erythrocyte carbonic anhydrase activities and impairs cardiorespiratory function in men during exercise." *Am J Clin Nutr* 81(5): 1045-51.

Lukiw, W. J., J. G. Cui, et al. (2005). "A role for docosahexaenoic acid-derived neuroprotectin D1 in neural cell survival and Alzheimer disease." *J Clin Invest* 115(10): 2774-83.

Marks, P. A., V. M. Richon, et al. (2000). "Histone deacetylase inhibitors: inducers of differentiation or apoptosis of transformed cells." *J Natl Cancer Inst* 92(15): 1210-6.

Masuoka, Y., N. Shindoh, et al. (2008). "Histone deacetylase inhibitors from microorganisms: the Astellas experience." *Prog Drug Res* 66: 335, 337-59.

Mattson, M. P. and W. Duan (1999). ""Apoptotic" biochemical cascades in synaptic compartments: roles in adaptive plasticity and neurodegenerative disorders." *J Neurosci Res* 58(1): 152-66.

McDowell, I. (2001). "Alzheimer's disease: insights from epidemiology." *Aging (Milano)* 13(3): 143-62.

Min, Y. K., J. E. Lee, et al. (2007). "Zinc induces cell death in immortalized embryonic hippocampal cells via activation of Akt-GSK-3beta signaling." *Exp Cell Res* 313(2): 312-21.

Mizzen, C., M. H. Kuo, et al. (1998). "Signaling to chromatin through histone modifications: how clear is the signal?" *Cold Spring Harb Symp Quant Biol* 63: 469-81.

Mocchegiani, E., C. Bertoni-Freddari, et al. (2005). "Brain, aging and neurodegeneration: role of zinc ion availability." *Prog Neurobiol* 75(6): 367-90.

Mocchegiani, E., M. Malavolta, et al. (2006). "Zinc, oxidative stress, genetic background and immunosenescence: implications for healthy ageing." *Immun Ageing* 3: 6.

Moriguchi, T., R. S. Greiner, et al. (2000). "Behavioral deficits associated with dietary induction of decreased brain docosahexaenoic acid concentration." *J Neurochem* 75(6): 2563-73.

Munishkina, L. A., A. L. Fink, et al. (2004). "Conformational prerequisites for formation of amyloid fibrils from histones." *J Mol Biol* 342(4): 1305-24.

Murakami, M. and T. Hirano (2008). "Intracellular zinc homeostasis and zinc signaling." *Cancer Sci* 99(8): 1515-22.

Naganska, E. and E. Matyja (2006). "Apoptotic neuronal changes enhanced by zinc chelator--TPEN in organotypic rat hippocampal cultures exposed to anoxia." *Folia Neuropathol* 44(2): 125-32.

Nepal, B., L. Brown, et al. (2008). "Years of life lived with and without dementia in Australia, 2004-2006: a population health measure." *Aust N Z J Public Health* 32(6): 565-8.

Nepal, B., G. Ranmuthugala, et al. (2008). "Modelling costs of dementia in Australia: evidence, gaps, and needs." *Aust Health Rev* 32(3): 479-87.

Nowak, S. J. and V. G. Corces (2000). "Phosphorylation of histone H3 correlates with transcriptionally active loci." *Genes Dev* 14(23): 3003-13.

Oksman, M., H. Iivonen, et al. (2006). "Impact of different saturated fatty acid, polyunsaturated fatty acid and cholesterol containing diets on beta-amyloid accumulation in APP/PS1 transgenic mice." *Neurobiol Dis* 23(3): 563-72.

Oliva, R., D. P. Bazett-Jones, et al. (1990). "Histone hyperacetylation can induce unfolding of the nucleosome core particle." *Nucleic Acids Res* 18(9): 2739-47.

Outten, C. E. and T. V. O'Halloran (2001). "Femtomolar sensitivity of metalloregulatory proteins controlling zinc homeostasis." *Science* 292(5526): 2488-92.

Overbeck, S., P. Uciechowski, et al. (2008). "Intracellular zinc homeostasis in leukocyte subsets is regulated by different expression of zinc exporters ZnT-1 to ZnT-9." *J Leukoc Biol* 83(2): 368-80.

Paik, H. Y., H. Joung, et al. (1999). "Serum extracellular superoxide dismutase activity as an indicator of zinc status in humans." *Biol Trace Elem Res* 69(1): 45-57.

Pardon, M. C. and I. Rattray (2008). "What do we know about the long-term consequences of stress on ageing and the progression of age-related neurodegenerative disorders?" *Neurosci Biobehav Rev* 32(6): 1103-20.

Pina, B., P. Martinez, et al. (1988). "Differential acetylation of core histones in rat cerebral cortex neurons during development and aging." *Eur J Biochem* 174(2): 311-5.

Plassman, B. L., R. J. Havlik, et al. (2000). "Documented head injury in early adulthood and risk of Alzheimer's disease and other dementias." *Neurology* 55(8): 1158-66.

Qi, K., T. Seo, et al. (2006). "Triglycerides in fish oil affect the blood clearance of lipid emulsions containing long- and medium-chain triglycerides in mice." *J Nutr* 136(11): 2766-72.

Rice, J. C. and C. D. Allis (2001). "Histone methylation versus histone acetylation: new insights into epigenetic regulation." *Curr Opin Cell Biol* 13(3): 263-73.

Rocca, W. A., C. M. van Duijn, et al. (1991). "Maternal age and Alzheimer's disease: a collaborative re-analysis of case-control studies. EURODEM Risk Factors Research Group." *Int J Epidemiol* 20 Suppl 2: S21-7.

Rossi, F. and E. Cattaneo (2002). "Opinion: neural stem cell therapy for neurological diseases: dreams and reality." *Nat Rev Neurosci* 3(5): 401-9.

Rouaux, C., N. Jokic, et al. (2003). "Critical loss of CBP/p300 histone acetylase activity by caspase-6 during neurodegeneration." *EMBO J* 22(24): 6537-49.

Saha, R. N. and K. Pahan (2006). "HATs and HDACs in neurodegeneration: a tale of disconcerted acetylation homeostasis." *Cell Death Differ* 13(4): 539-50.

Sandstead, H. H., J. G. Penland, et al. (1998). "Effects of repletion with zinc and other micronutrients on neuropsychologic performance and growth of Chinese children." *Am J Clin Nutr* 68(2 Suppl): 470S-475S.

Sarg, B., E. Koutzamani, et al. (2002). "Postsynthetic trimethylation of histone H4 at lysine 20 in mammalian tissues is associated with aging." *J Biol Chem* 277(42): 39195-201.

Schaefer, E. J., V. Bongard, et al. (2006). "Plasma phosphatidylcholine docosahexaenoic acid content and risk of dementia and Alzheimer disease: the Framingham Heart Study." *Arch Neurol* 63(11): 1545-50.

Simmer, K. and S. Patole (2004). "Longchain polyunsaturated fatty acid supplementation in preterm infants." *Cochrane Database Syst Rev*(1): CD000375.

Simopoulos, A. P. (1991). "Omega-3 fatty acids in health and disease and in growth and development." *Am J Clin Nutr* 54(3): 438-63.

Simopoulos, A. P. (1999). "Genetic variation and nutrition." *World Rev Nutr Diet* 84: 118-40.

Simopoulos, A. P., A. Leaf, et al. (1999). "Workshop on the Essentiality of and Recommended Dietary Intakes for Omega-6 and Omega-3 Fatty Acids." *J Am Coll Nutr* 18(5): 487-9.

Sims, R. J., 3rd, K. Nishioka, et al. (2003). "Histone lysine methylation: a signature for chromatin function." *Trends Genet* 19(11): 629-39.

Smirnov, A. V., P. N. Shevtsov, et al. (1991). "[Two-dimensional electrophoretic analysis of the protein spectrum of human brain structures in schizophrenia and senile dementia of the Alzheimer type]." *Zh Nevropatol Psikhiatr Im S S Korsakova* 91(10): 34-6.

Stadelmann, C., T. L. Deckwerth, et al. (1999). "Activation of caspase-3 in single neurons and autophagic granules of granulovacuolar degeneration in Alzheimer's disease. Evidence for apoptotic cell death." *Am J Pathol* 155(5): 1459-66.

Stefanidou, M., C. Maravelias, et al. (2006). "Zinc: a multipurpose trace element." *Arch Toxicol* 80(1): 1-9.

Strahl, B. D., R. Ohba, et al. (1999). "Methylation of histone H3 at lysine 4 is highly conserved and correlates with transcriptionally active nuclei in Tetrahymena." *Proc Natl Acad Sci U S A* 96(26): 14967-72.

Strokin, M., M. Sergeeva, et al. (2003). "Docosahexaenoic acid and arachidonic acid release in rat brain astrocytes is mediated by two separate isoforms of phospholipase A2 and is differently regulated by cyclic AMP and Ca2+." *Br J Pharmacol* 139(5): 1014-22.

Su, J. H., G. Deng, et al. (1997). "Bax protein expression is increased in Alzheimer's brain: correlations with DNA damage, Bcl-2 expression, and brain pathology." *J Neuropathol Exp Neurol* 56(1): 86-93.

Suphioglu, C., D. De Mel, et al. (2010a). "The omega-3 fatty acid, DHA, decreases neuronal cell death in association with altered zinc transport." *FEBS Lett* 584(3): 612-8.

Suphioglu, C., N. Sadli, et al. (2010b). "Zinc and DHA have opposing effects on the expression levels of histones H3 and H4 in human neuronal cells." *Br J Nutr* 103(3): 344-51.

Tesco, G., Y. H. Koh, et al. (2007). "Depletion of GGA3 stabilizes BACE and enhances beta-secretase activity." *Neuron* 54(5): 721-37.

Thorne, A. W., D. Kmiciek, et al. (1990). "Patterns of histone acetylation." *Eur J Biochem* 193(3): 701-13.
Tougu, V., A. Tiiman, et al. (2011). "Interactions of Zn(II) and Cu(II) ions with Alzheimer's amyloid-beta peptide. Metal ion binding, contribution to fibrillization and toxicity." *Metallomics* 3(3): 250-61.
van Gelder, B. M., M. Tijhuis, et al. (2007). "Fish consumption, n-3 fatty acids, and subsequent 5-y cognitive decline in elderly men: the Zutphen Elderly Study." *Am J Clin Nutr* 85(4): 1142-7.
Vannini, A., C. Volpari, et al. (2004). "Crystal structure of a eukaryotic zinc-dependent histone deacetylase, human HDAC8, complexed with a hydroxamic acid inhibitor." *Proc Natl Acad Sci U S A* 101(42): 15064-9.
Vlahou, A. and M. Fountoulakis (2005). "Proteomic approaches in the search for disease biomarkers." *J Chromatogr B Analyt Technol Biomed Life Sci* 814(1): 11-9.
Wai, M. S., Y. Liang, et al. (2009). "Co-localization of hyperphosphorylated tau and caspases in the brainstem of Alzheimer's disease patients." *Biogerontology* 10(4): 457-69.
Wang, C. M., S. N. Tsai, et al. (2009). "Identification of histone methylation multiplicities patterns in the brain of senescence-accelerated prone mouse 8." *Biogerontology*.
Watt, N. T. and N. M. Hooper (2003). "The prion protein and neuronal zinc homeostasis." *Trends Biochem Sci* 28(8): 406-10.
Weiss, J. H., S. L. Sensi, et al. (2000). "Zn(2+): a novel ionic mediator of neural injury in brain disease." *Trends Pharmacol Sci* 21(10): 395-401.
Wilkins, M. R., J. C. Sanchez, et al. (1996). "Progress with proteome projects: why all proteins expressed by a genome should be identified and how to do it." *Biotechnol Genet Eng Rev* 13: 19-50.
Willatts, P. (2002). "Long chain polyunsaturated fatty acids improve cognitive development." *J Fam Health Care* 12(6 Suppl): 5.
Woodcock, C. L. and S. Dimitrov (2001). "Higher-order structure of chromatin and chromosomes." *Curr Opin Genet Dev* 11(2): 130-5.
Xiao, Y. and X. Li (1999). "Polyunsaturated fatty acids modify mouse hippocampal neuronal excitability during excitotoxic or convulsant stimulation." *Brain Res* 846(1): 112-21.
Yang, X. J. and E. Seto (2008). "Lysine acetylation: codified crosstalk with other posttranslational modifications." *Mol Cell* 31(4): 449-61.
Yankner, B. A., T. Lu, et al. (2008). "The aging brain." *Annu Rev Pathol* 3: 41-66.
Young, G. and J. Conquer (2005). "Omega-3 fatty acids and neuropsychiatric disorders." *Reprod Nutr Dev* 45(1): 1-28.
Zatta, P., D. Drago, et al. (2009). "Alzheimer's disease, metal ions and metal homeostatic therapy." *Trends Pharmacol Sci* 30(7): 346-55.
Zhang, L. H., X. Wang, et al. (2008). "Abundant expression of zinc transporters in the amyloid plaques of Alzheimer's disease brain." *Brain Res Bull* 77(1): 55-60.
Zhang, Y., H. Wang, et al. (2004). "Peroxynitrite-induced neuronal apoptosis is mediated by intracellular zinc release and 12-lipoxygenase activation." *J Neurosci* 24(47): 10616-27.

7

Free Radicals, Neuronal Death and Neuroprotection

Diana Gallego, Manuel Rojas and Camilo Orozco
Departamento de Ciencias para La Salud Animal
Facultad de Medicina Veterinaria y de Zootecnia
Universidad Nacional de Colombia, Sede Bogotá
Colombia

1. Introduction

The Reactive Oxygen Species (ROS) and the Reactive Nitrogen Species (RNS) are highly reactive molecules participating as mediators in biological processes such as metabolic cellular respiration, neurotransmission, translation and transcription gene, and inflammatory-type reactions among others (D. Almaguer & L.E. Almaguer, 2006; Boots et al., 2008; Uttara, 2009). Additionally, these molecules have the capacity to interact with nucleophilic centers of biomolecules by modulating their activity or by irreversibly modifying them in order to generate different kind of radicals (D. Almaguer & L.E. Almaguer, 2006).
The main oxygen radicals are the hydroxyl (-OH), the superoxide anion (O2-), and the hydrogen peroxide (H2O2), while the main nitrogen radical is the nitric oxide (•NO), but also, it is known that the ROS can interact with -NO generating new species with high oxidizing power (Martinez et al., 2010). In aerobic systems most of the ROS come from the mitochondrial oxidative metabolism, where 1-2% of the oxygen is converted into free radicals (Uttara et al., 2009). Other less important sources of ROS are the autoxidation of catecholamines and hemoproteins that occurs in the cytoplasm, nuclear membrane, endoplasmic reticulum and peroxisomes (Boots et al., 2008; Martínez et al, 2010). The concentration of ROS or RNS in organisms is determined by the balance between the rate of production of reactive species and the elimination rate of these compounds by the action of enzymes and antioxidants (AO) (Dorado et al., 2003). Thus, under conditions of physiological homeostasis, a balance exists between the cellular processes that contribute to the production of ROS / RNS, and those factors such as superoxide dismutase (SOD), catalase (Cat) and glutathione peroxidase (GPx), which contribute to their elimination (Dorado et al., 2003; Martínez et al., 2010). Thus, alterations in the balance between these systems, pro-oxidants and antioxidants can lead to intracellular accumulation of free radicals (FR), causing oxidative stress states (Dorado et al., 2003; Kelsey, et al , 2010; Uttara, 2009).
Specifically, oxidative stress and redox imbalance is the combined result of excessive formation of oxidant species (ROS/RNS) and/or a decreasing in the efficiency of endogenous antioxidant systems. Thus, the combination of these factors converge in damaging to biomolecules such as DNA, RNA, proteins, carbohydrates and lipids. This probably initiate processes of mitochondrial dysfunction and excitotoxicity (Kelsey, et al.,

2010; Dorado et al., 2003), which in turn results in structural and functional alterations of organic macromolecules, leading the affected cells to degenerative processes and cell death by necrosis or apoptosis (D. Almaguer & L.E. Almaguer, 2006; Gonzalez et al. 1999; Martinez et al., 2010). The deleterious effects of ROS on cell integrity, eventually may drive or participate in the development of diseases or pathological processes such as atherosclerosis, cancer, diabetes, rheumatoid arthritis, ischemia-reperfusion syndrome, cardiovascular disease, chronic inflammatory processes, shock Blackwater and other degenerative diseases in humans and animals (Freidovich, 1999; Fang et al., 2002). However, is hard to establish whether these reactive species represent a primary etiologic factor or product from the damaged tissue (Gonzalez et al., 1999).

The biochemical composition of the brain tissue makes it especially susceptible to the action of ROS/RNS, as it contains a pool of unsaturated lipids which are suitable to oxidative modification and lipid peroxidation. The double chains of unsaturated fatty acids are targeted for attack by free radicals, which initiate a cascade or chain reaction that damages these acids (Butterfield et al, 2002). Several researchers consider the brain as an organ highly susceptible to oxidative damage, and several studies have demonstrated how easy occurs the peroxidation of brain cell membranes (Chance, 1979). Also, the brain seems to be more susceptible than other organs to peroxidation, this is probably due to its high oxygen requirements, it uses 20% of the total oxygen intake, while weighing only 2% of the total body weight. Neuronal cells are considered the most susceptible cells to oxidative damage, owing to their low antioxidant activity in comparison to other tissues , as well as the high content of methyl ions in certain brain regions (Floyd, 1992). In this regard, some authors have suggested that the continuous state of oxidative stress may produce specific structural alterations of proteins, leading to abnormal protein aggregate formation, which is responsible for perpetuating oxidative damage. In fact, these abnormal proteins are considered as molecular markers of neurodegenerative diseases such as Alzheimer, Parkinson, and Cognitive Dysfunction Syndrome in geriatric dogs (Gallego et, al., 2010a, 2010b).

There are several risk factors involved in the development of these neuropathologies, one of them is the aging process "per se". In this regard, when the production of ROS / RNS has an exaggerated and prolonged increasing, and the antioxidant response is not enough, the system reach a different point of equilibrium (homeoresis, rather than homeostasis). This equilibrium is accompanied by high concentrations of free amino acids and differences in gene expression patterns, allowing survival but causing irreversible neuronal damage in the long term (Rivas et al., 2001). The original hypothesis of the free radicals in aging was proposed by Harman Gerschman and Harman in the 50´s (Sohal, 1993). The central dogma of this theory is that during the aerobic metabolism there is an incidental and uncontrollable production of oxygen radical species. Then, these species promote reactions damaging the macromolecules. This irreversible damage accumulates over time and results in a gradual loss of functional capacity of the cells (Hayflick, 1993). According to recent studies this might be related to neuronal processes of senescence (Passos, et al, 2010).

2. Oxidative stress (OS) and neurodegenerative diseases (ND)

There are plenty scientific evidence that considers the brain tissue as a preferential target for the accumulation of ROS and RNS, thereby triggering oxidative stress chronic conditions, which lead to injury and degeneration of neuronal cells (Contestabile, 2001). It has been reported that the nervous system is rich in iron (Fe3 +) and unsaturated fatty acids (Halliwell, 2001), this is one of the main features that make this organ particularly sensitive to oxidative stress. Thus, the high lipid content of nervous tissue and its high metabolic activity make it particularly vulnerable to oxidative damage (T.M. Dawson & V.L. Dawson, 1996). It has been reported that iron is essential in the brain, particularly during development, but high amounts can lead to the generation of damage to brain cells, because Fe 3 + can lead to oxidative stress by catalyzing the formation processes of ROS (Butterfield et al, 2002; Gerlach et al, 1994). In addition, the brain consumes a high proportion of the total oxygen, since the energy it uses comes almost exclusively from oxidative metabolism which occurs in the mitochondrial respiratory chain located in the bodies, dendrites, axons and synaptic buttons of cells neural, where the ATPase maintains the ionic gradient across the neuronal membrane (Pavón et al., 1998). Another reason that explains why ROS are particularly active in the brain is that in this tissue, the metabolism of the aminoacids and neurotransmitters acts as an important source of these highly reactive molecules (Uttara et al., 2009). Thus, considering that this organ contains low levels of protective enzymes and other enzymatic antioxidants, it is easy to understand why their susceptibility (Contestabile, 2001).

Although oxidative stress is not the direct cause or the etiological factor responsible for the neuropathologies, it is known that it induces toxic effects by oxidizing lipids, proteins, carbohydrates and nucleotides. This causes accumulation of intracellular aggregates, mitochondrial dysfunction, excitotoxicity and apoptosis. Formation of modified lipids by oxidation can cause cellular dysfunction and death in postmitotic cells. Likewise, the peroxidation of polyunsaturated fatty acids in cell membranes, initiates a cumulative deterioration of membrane functions and causes a decrease in flow, reduction in the electrochemical potential and increased permeability of the membrane. Similarly, oxidation causes changes in the structure of some proteins and the formation of protein aggregates. These abnormal proteins induce oxidative damage that has been observed in neurodegenerative diseases as AD and PD. On another hand, ROS also can affect both glial cells and neuronal cells, which exhibit a particular sensitivity to free radicals and therefore are prone to cell degeneration processes (Gilgun-Sherki et al., 2001). For example, there is a biological phenomenon known as "selective neuronal vulnerability", which is involved in the response of different neuronal populations against neurodegenerative conditions. For example, neurons in the entorhinal cortex, the CA1 region of hippocampus, frontal cortex and amygdala, are highly susceptible populations to neurodegeneration associated with oxidative stress in Alzheimer's disease (AD) (Braak et al., 1991; Hyman et al, 1984; Terry et al, 2001).

The relationship between aging and neurodegenerative diseases is more than evident. This is supported by recent investigations that have observed that during the aging process there is an increase in the formation of H2O2 that alters the conditions of the electrons flow in the transport chain, facilitating their 'escape' of normal stream flow. This leads the neurons to suffer the harmful effect of free radicals. Moreover, studies performed by Sohal, et al., 1993, Benzi & Mareti, 1995, and others, have postulated that ROS can inflict damage to the mitochondrial inner membrane, the components of the electron transport chain or the mitochondrial DNA (mtDNA). Oxidative stress further increases ROS production and, consequently, damage to the mitochondria, creating a cycle that perpetuates the effects of ROS (González et al., 1999). Thus, it is obvious because aging itself is a key factor in diseases such as AD or PD; since the increase of oxidative damage, the progressive mitochondrial failure accumulated with aging, and coupled with the characteristics of brain, make aging itself a common risk factor in neurodegeneration. Another fact that may explain the relationship between neurodegeneration and aging is that during aging can occurs certain level of iron accumulation, which increases oxidative stress. This occurs mainly through the Fenton reaction, where the production of highly reactive hydroxyl radicals ends up causing damage to DNA, lipids and proteins (Ang et al., 2010; González et al., 1999; Uttara et al., 2009).

In addition to the accumulation of free radicals that can occurs in the brain of individuals with ND, it is also clear that the antioxidant systems decrease during the aging process. Then, the action of ROS turns up in a process even more damaging to neuronal tissue. Scientific data suggest that all this deleterious effect seems to be magnified by pathological proteins such as beta-amyloid in AD and alpha-synuclein in PD, which act as initiators and perpetuators of the intraneuronal oxidative stress, generating injuries and disease-specific symptoms.

2.1 Alzheimer disease

According to some authors, the ROS in AD induce a prolonged increase pro-oxidant state (Benzi & Mareti, 1995). This statement is supported by clinical and experimental evidence (for example, high concentrations of Fe and Cu identified in the brains of some patients with AD), showing that ROS cause neuronal death and other neuropathological changes associated with this disease (González et al., 1999; Ramesh et al., 2010). However, the role of oxidative processes in AD is still a matter of debate, with conflicting and divergent data in the literature, which could be related to the difficulty of directly measuring the activity of ROS in biological systems due to their short half-life and its high reactivity (Gonzalez et al., 1999).

Several studies have identified the capacity of the protein βA as a chelating agent for transition metals (Cu2, Zn2 and Fe3). Regarding this, it is important to note that the binding of Cu2 and Fe3 provides free radicals OH ˙, and toxic chemical reactions, due to the altered state of oxidation of these two metals, causing the appearance of catalytic H2O2 in the presence transition metal (Uttara et al., 2009). Additionally, the Fe3 in AD neurofibrillary plaque accumulates (NFT) and depots βA, which probably explains the evidence that suggests increased levels of Zn (II), Fe (III) and Cu (II) in the neuropil and senile plaques (Ramesh et al., 2010). Moreover, it appears that the Fe3 directly involved in plaque formation βA, and thus indirectly in the formation of ROS, as it promotes amyloidosis by modulating the ability of the α-secretase to cleave the amyloid precursor protein (APP), or to facilitate the aggregation of Aβ.

In 1994, Behl C. and colleagues showed that toxicity in AD is associated with the Aβ protein, which causes increased production of H2O2. These authors also showed that catalase blocks the toxicity of Aβ, which allows us to understand how the H2O2 and its derivatives such as OH-radical, cause lipid peroxidation leading to neuronal cell death in this disease (González et al., 1999). In addition, hemoxigenasa1 the Cu\ZnSOD and MnSOD, have been identified in neurofibrillary tangles of human brains with AD, suggesting a close interaction between ROS and the products from these enzimes. It has also been suggested that cellular toxicity of βA that is specifically related to damage by ROS or its products, generates insoluble protein aggregates, as is known, is a crucial event in AD (González et al., 1999).

Moreover, there is indirect evidence that ROS can relate to AD. For example, some dietary factors such as saturated fatty acids, high calories and heavy drinking have been reported as factors that may increase the risk of dementia and AD. In contrast, consumption of foods with antioxidants such as fruits, proteins rich in methionine and vitamins have been identified as protective factors against the disease. In this sense, it is possible that the variation in the diets may be associated with the prevalence of AD by geographic area, as several studies have suggested a link between nutrients of each diet and the presence of cognitive changes. However, it is necessary to confirm this experimentally (Ramesh et al., 2010).

2.2 Parkinson disease

Experimental data suggest a relationship between the PD and two mitochondrial-specific conditions, dysfunction and oxidative damage to neuronal mitochondria. This assertion is supported by research suggesting mitochondrial dysfunction and impairment of mitochondrial complex I activity in the neurons of the substantia nigra and frontal cortex in PD patients. In addition, several genes whose mutations or polymorphisms increase the risk of developing PD are related to mitochondrial function. In this regard, dysfunction of mitochondrial complex I, becomes important, since its inhibition creates a biochemical environment that increases the production of FMNH semiquinone flavin, which increases the generation of O2 and in turn, the latter promotes lipid peroxidation, damage oxidative protein and protein nitration mediated by peroxynitrite (ONOO-) and nitrosylation. This is a process leading neurons to apoptosis and α-synuclein aggregation with subsequent death of dopaminergic neurons. (Navarro & Boveris, 2008, 2010).

According to Dorado et al., 2003, the substantia nigra has characteristics that tend to make it more vulnerable to attack by ROS. These features include low levels of glutathione and vitamin E, high levels of free iron (prooxidant), mono amine oxidase (MAO generates ROS), •NO (radical neurotoxic pro-oxidant) and neuromelanin. The neuromelanin is a black pigment found in certain subpopulations of monoaminergic neurons, and is the result of auto-oxidation, condensation and polymerization of dopamine and its oxidation products. Neuromelanin binds to any neutralizing reactive species, but can become a reservoir of toxic under certain conditions (oxidative attack, low levels of glutathione) releases these reactive species. Thus, neurons that contain greater amounts of neuromelanin in the substantia nigra pars compacta die more easily.

Glutathione (GSH) which is the most important intracellular molecule for the removal of hydroperoxides in the brain, is decreased in Parkinsonian patients. This could be related to the increased concentration of MDA (a marker of lipid oxidation). One of the facts that suggests the role of ROS in this disease is that they have identified high levels of glycosylation end products (AGE resulting from impaired glucose oxidation and cause irreversible oxidation of protein) in the substantia nigra and cortex. Also, it appears that a factor associated with oxidative damage is that the distribution of transition metals in the brain shows large regional differences, so that regions with large amounts of iron (which is easily oxidized) as the substantia nigra are at risk of suffer a more aggressive oxidative attack (Dorado et al., 2003). However, this is not the only mechanism to explain why dopaminergic neurons are especially sensitive to oxidative stress, because its high metabolic rate and the oxidation of dopamine, either by autoxidation or by the metabolic pathway by means of the MAO (Dorado et al., 2003), they represent a major source of ROS. Likewise, dopamine may act as metal chelator electron donors, and owing to its tendency towards reduction can initiate the Fenton reaction to generate H2O2. Some evidence suggests that mutations in the protein α-synuclein play a crucial role in modulating the activity of dopamine, but negatively, initiating neuronal cytoplasmic accumulation and interaction of dopamine with iron to cause the production of ROS (Uttara et al., 2009).

3. Cellular defense systems against oxidative stress (OE)

ROS and RNS molecules are well known for their deleterious effects on cellular integrity and their relation to different neurodegenerative diseases such as described in the previous section. However, it is important to note that these molecules also play a physiological role, quite distant from the aforementioned pathological role. In homeostatic physiological conditions their responses participate in cell signaling systems such as in the defense response against infectious agents and induction of mitogenic responses (Valko et al., 2007). These cellular responses bring the intra and extracellular environments to a continuous exposure to FR (González et al., 1999). Owing to this condition, aerobic organisms have evolved specific defense mechanisms, programmed to form cell protective barriers, which allow them to restrict the harmful effects of free radicals and neutralize the damage caused by the action of these reactive species (D. Almaguer & L.E. Almaguer, 2006; Cadenas, 1997; Contestabile, 2001; Perez et al., 2008; Valko et al., 2007; Vian et al., 1999). These mechanisms refer to antioxidants. These are molecules of different weights whose function is basically delay or inhibit oxidation. The mechanism is to transfer electrons to the reactive species to saturate its electron affinity, and thus, maintain ROS at a level compatible with metabolic processes and cellular functions (D. Almaguer & L.E. Almaguer, 2006; Contestabile, 2001; Viant, 1999).

3.1 Classification of the main antioxidant systems

Taking into account specific aspects of antioxidants, such as their chemical nature, mechanism of action or origin, several strategies have been proposed for classification. According to Gilgun-Sherki et al.2008, these compounds can be classified into two major groups: antioxidant enzymes and low molecular weight antioxidants. To the first group belong some antioxidant enzyme systems derived from enzymes as cytochrome oxidase, superoxide dismutase (Cu-ZnSOD and MnSOD), catalases and peroxidases such as glutathione peroxidase and glutathione reductase (Dorado et al., 2003). The group of low molecular weight antioxidants involves a variety of antioxidants, so some authors have sub-classified this group into two: indirect antioxidants (eg, chelating agents) and direct antioxidants. The latter group is of great importance in combating oxidative stress and contains hundreds of components, however, only a minority of these molecules such as glutathione and NADPH are synthesized by the cell itself.

Another classification for antioxidant systems, refers to its source. In this sense, we can identify endogenous antioxidants and antioxidant of exogenous origin. The first group are vitamins such as ascorbic acid, tocopherol and retinoic acid also found glutathione in its reduced form, coenzyme Q10, melatonin, uric acid and lipoic acid. Also are included some isoforms of the enzyme superoxide dismutase (copper/zinc SOD, manganese SOD, extracellular SOD), catalase and glutathione peroxidase (Gilgun-Sherki et al.,2008; Chan, 2001; Contestabile, 2001). With respect to the group of antioxidants of exogenous origin, ie those that can only be obtained from external sources, we should mention some substances such as acetyl cysteine and carotenoids, which act as precursors of endogenous antioxidant type (Gilgun-Sherki et al.,2008; Chan, 2001; Contestabille, 2001).

Due to this variety in the classification of antioxidants, a new classification has been proposed recently, which seeks to involve the full range of antioxidants based on aspects such as chemical nature and mechanism of action (Cui et al., 2004; Pérez, A. et al., 2008). Such a classification sets these compounds into the following groups:

1. Antioxidant enzymes: They act on specific ROS, in order to change them into less harmful molecules. Examples of such enzymes are SOD, CAT, and GPx.
2. Preventive Antioxidants: These bind to promoters of oxidation and sequester transition metal ions such as iron and copper, which contain unpaired electrons and greatly accelerate the formation of free radicals. Examples of such antioxidants are transferrin and lactoferrin (Pauls & Thompson, 1980). Also, ceruloplasmin Cu hijacking to prevent the formation of free radicals from peroxides, catalyzes the oxidation of ferrous ions to ferric ions due to its ferroxidase activity, and increases the binding of iron to transferrin. In addition, the haptoglobins that bind to hemoglobin, hemopexin that binds heme groups and albumin binds to heme and Cu (Benedetti et al., 1988).
3. Antioxidant ROS sequestrant: These inhibit the initiation of chain reactions of free radicals or break the chain of spreading it. The main intracellular sequesters are vitamin E, carotene and coenzyme Q (Murthy, 2001), while extracellular sequesters include protein systems, and water-soluble compounds such as ascorbic acid, uric acid and bilirubin (Cui et al, 2004; Frei et al., 1988; Pérez, A. et al., 2008;).
4. Nutritional Antioxidants: Diet is the major source of substances with antioxidant properties or elements for the synthesis of antioxidant enzymes. Several metals (copper, zinc, selenium, manganese, iron) are involved as components or cofactors of numerous enzymes antioxidants, and certain vitamins (ascorbic acid, α-tocopherol and β-carotene, folic acid) act as a sequestrant of ROS (Pérez, A. et al., 2008).

3.2 Mechanisms of neutralization of ROS

The different antioxidant systems work in a coordinated manner, following a series of metabolic processes where •O2-metabolized by superoxide dismutase SOD generates H2O2, and this in turn is metabolized to H2O and O2 by a catalase or glutathione peroxidase, which act as coupled with glutathione reductase (Dorado et al, 2003). However, it is difficult to think of a single molecular mechanism that acts as a regulator of the generation and the effects of FR, so some authors, for instance, Cadenas, 1997, propouse at least three types of molecular mechanisms that underlie the activities of various antioxidants. Such mechanisms are: (a) a process involving the transfer of the radical nature of ROS, together with the formation of a reactive radical, an antioxidant derived previously, (b) a similar process in which the transfer of the radical, and the formation of a stable or inert radical is carried out through enzymatic activity, and (c) mechanisms of action of small molecules that mimic the activity of enzymes such as SOD and GPx. These mechanisms describe to some extent the action of a variety of molecules with antioxidant properties, for example, enzymes such as SOD, CAT and GPx, which are responsible for initiating the process of neutralization of ROS by the dismutation of O•2 to H2O2 (D. Almaguer & L.E. Almaguer, 2006). Other defense mechanisms used by different antioxidants include, recycling of ROS/RNS or their precursors, inhibition of ROS formation, binding of metal ions required for catalysis of ROS generation and activation of endogenous antioxidant defenses (Gilgun-Sherki et al.,2008).

According to some researchers (Halliwell, B., 1994, 1997; Cadenas, 1997; Dorado et al, 2003), the protective efficiency of this variety of antioxidants, is somewhat dependent on the type of ROS generated, the place where they are produced (physical barriers like the blood-brain barrier permeability reduce many antioxidants) and the severity of cell damage.

4. Antioxidants and neurodegeneration

During the last decades in many populations around the world there has been a notable increase in the number of adults over 60´s (United Nations [ONU], 2009). Consequently, there has been an increase in the incidence and prevalence of various diseases affecting the elders. Among this group of diseases, the neurodegenerative type have become very important, especially in industrialized countries, which are listed as the third leading cause of death after cardiovascular diseases and cancer (Boyd, 2000; Gallego et, al., 2010a; United Nations [ONU], 2009; Segura, 2003; Troenes B, et al 2003). However, the ND related to aging, not only represent a problem for human health because there are substantial data showing that aging also predisposes other species to suffer dementia syndromes. For example, some old dogs can develop neuropathology similar to AD, known as Cognitive Dysfunction Syndrome in Senior Dogs (CDS) or "dog´s Alzheimer". This disease affects dogs over 7 years old and due to its clinical and pathophysiological similarities with AD has been proposed as a model for doing research in the field of neurodegeneration, especially in the study of AD (Adams B, et al., 2000; Gallego, 2010b; Overall, 2001; Ruehl et al., 1995).

As already mentioned, the incidence of ND increases with age, however, we must clarify that the risk of having them can be determined, partially, by factors such as lifestyle, obesity, metabolic syndrome, genetic susceptibility, predisposing medical factors and increased oxidative stress, among others, but the last one is the main factor related to the presentation of these diseases (Contestabile, 2001; James et al., 2009; Kelsey et al., 2010; Uttara et al., 2009;). In this sense, today it seems clear the role of oxidative stress during the onset and course of ND associated with aging (Meydani et al., 1998; Passos et al., 2010). So, recognizing this fact has allowed us to identify therapeutic targets where the activation of cellular mechanisms of antioxidant type appear to be a suitable option for the treatment of neurodegenerative diseases such as AD, PD and CDS (Casetta et al., 2005; James et al., 2009, Contestabile, 2001). In general terms, the main goal of the antioxidant therapy for these diseases is to interrupt or modulate the interaction of pathological neuronal protein (Aβ protein and Tau protein) with redox metals. This is in order to prevent damage or decomposition of metalloenzymes, and innate antioxidant systems by promoting homeostasis of metals and minimizing the OE and its effects (Uttara et al., 2009). Additionally, several studies suggest that increasing cellular protection through the use of antioxidants could be beneficial for maintaining or reducing the rate of neuronal death during the course of certain ND, such as PD (Casseta et al., 2005; Kelsey et al., 2010).

Thus, taking into account the growing interest in antioxidant therapy for the treatment and/or prevention of ND, and considering that diet is a main source of natural Anti-Oxidants (AO), then we present a systematic review of scientific evidence showing the action and effect of some food products on the course or the beginning of the characteristic lesions of this type of pathology.

4.1 The role of diet as a preventive factor against the development of ND

Given that the lifestyle and the type of diet can act as important risk factors for the emergence of various diseases (Kalaria et al., 2008), the relationship between a particular diet and its effects long-term research center have been some authors who seek through diet and antioxidant compounds, mechanisms to develop or enhance protective responses against a constant state of oxidative stress. In addition, people generally consider that there are several advantages to the use of antioxidants, in fact, there are a consumer culture around these compounds, where people attempt to consume diets rich in antioxidants and/or supplement their diet with one or more of these substances to "improve living conditions for the geriatric stage" (Mullie et al., 2009). Several studies have shown that diet has a long-term effect on general health (Leibson et al., 1997; Uttara et al., 2009; Vermeer, et al., 2003), acting as a principal source of natural antioxidants due to its ability to provide a variety of molecules that activate or enhancer the action of some endogenous antioxidants (Sun et al., 2008). In this sense, it is important to consider the effect of these molecules on processes of neuroprotection, since according to some reports, the diet also has the ability to extend human cognitive longevity (Peter, et al, 2004; Casseta, 2005, Glade, 2010; Ramesh et al., 2010). There are several antioxidant research in the field of ND, such as AD and PD, but despite the variability of results and poor clinical trials, diets rich in vitamins and other natural antioxidants still seem to be publicly recognized for their action as useful supplements in reducing risk of suffering some types of dementia (Kamphuisa & Scheltensb, 2010).

Evidence of this can be seen in some studies indicating that Indian diets, which contain spices like red chilli, coriander and turmeric (plant widely used as food preservative and medicinal), apparently reduced the prevalence of patients with AD in India, since its incidence is 4.4 times lower compared to countries like the U.S. (James et al., 2009; Ramesh et al., 2010). Additionally, some reports indicate supplementing diets high in fat that usually lead to the development of cardiovascular diseases with a high intake of dietary antioxidants, such as polyphenols, may reduce the risk of disease. Likewise, consumption of nutritional substances such as berries, nuts or fish oil can dramatically impact on the aging brain, possibly leading to improved motor and cognitive skills (James, et al, 2009). In this context, the interest in finding low-cost therapeutic alternatives that improve living conditions and reduce the risk of age-related diseases has led to the identification of a growing list of antioxidant supplements as Vitamins C and E, β-carotene, coenzyme Q, ascorbate and polyphenols, among others (Burton & Ingold, 1989, 1990; Kelsey et al., 2010).

4.2 Scientific evidence of AO supplementation in the treatment of ND

Natural antioxidants can act as a therapeutic tool against excess ROS, because several of them have a high ability to cross the blood brain barrier (Uttara et al., 2009), and can activate various antioxidant mechanisms in the brain in order to create conditions to achieve and maintain the neuronal homeostasis (Gilgun-Sherki et al., 2001). However, an antioxidant substance that has some use in preventing the ND must have some additional capabilities to its ability to sequester free radicals. For example, one of the main AO found in mammalian cells is glutathione (GSH), however, this substance, despite its large capacity anti FR can´t be directly used for supplementation, due to their inability to cross the blood-brain barrier and reach the brain tissue (Witschi et al., 1992). Despite this, some of its precursors or analogs have been tested in various animal models (Contestabile, 2001). Thus, studies such as Martinez, et al., 2000, suggest that long-term supplementation with GSH precursors such as N-acetylcysteine can partially restore the impaired memory and decreased mitochondrial lipid peroxidation, characteristic of aging process. (Contestabile, 2001; Prasad et al., 1999).

The use of AO decreases oxidative damage and also reduce the cognitive decline associated with age, this in both human and animal models (Joseph et al., 1998; Milgram et al., 2002). Examples are the studies conducted in geriatric dogs, which indicate that oxidative damage may be related to cognitive dysfunction and that long-term treatment with AO, with a behavioral enrichment program, reduce cognitive decline in dogs CDS (Cotman et al., 2002; Gallego et al, 2010a; Head E, 2002; Landsberg, 2005). Also, some authors argue that the intake of fruits and vegetables may reduce the risk of cognitive decline associated with aging in rodents, dogs and even humans, attributing that property to the capabilities of some antioxidants and anti-inflammatory compounds found in these foods (Araujo et al., 2005; Gallego et al., 2010; Landsberg, 2005; Opii et al., 2008).

With regard to vitamins, their results seem contradictory. Studies conducted with various vitamins have suggested these compounds as potential protective factors against states of neurodegeneration. Thus, recently demonstrated that supplementation of Vitamin E 500UI long term in the rats diet can protect against cognitive decline associated with aging (Morris, et al., 2005; Peterson et al., 2005). However, other studies in this category showed contrasting results, for example, a research conducted by Young KW, et, al, 2005, which included subjects with mild cognitive impairment, who were given a daily dose of 2.000UI of Vitamin E and 10 mg of donepezil (compound with anticholinergic activity) or a placebo for a period of three years. The results of this study showed that the overall rate of progression from mild cognitive impairment to clinical expression of AD was 16% per year, and no difference was found between the subjects who were administered placebo, and subjects who received vitamin E, suggesting a disagreement over the validity of vitamin supplements to patients with AD (Kelsey et al., 2010).

With respect to the PD, some of the AO compounds that have been suggested as protective factors include vitamins A, C (3000 mg/d) and E (3200 mg/d) (Fahn, 1991). Several epidemiological studies have shown that consumption of these vitamins may improve cognition and reduce the risk of developing clinical symptoms characteristic of this disease (Masaki et al., 1994). Likewise, the study by Chen et al, 1997, showed that administration of coenzyme Q10 improved clinical symptoms in patients with mitochondrial encephalopathy. Similarly, Birkmayer, et al, 1990, in a study of 415 patients with PD showed that administration of a dose of 1.4 mg/kg NADH can be an effective therapeutic tool in the treatment of PD. According to some authors, the efficiency of AO such as vitamins E and C, is the most convincing evidence of the involvement of free radicals in PD. However, in order to determine the efficacy of an antioxidant treatment, it is necessary to perform additional studies including high doses of vitamin E (3200 mg/d) in combination with vitamin C (3000 mg/d), before the administration of levodopa in patients with early PD (Fahn, 1991; Rao & Balachandran, 2002).

Acetyl-L-carnitine as a metabolite of vitamins involved in the process of synaptic transmission and has a potent neuroprotective effect can reduce the structural damage caused by states of oxidative stress in neurons. Neuroprotective capacity of this metabolite is evidenced through the increase in resistance to oxidation of cellular components such as mitochondrial RNA, and various proteins (Sharman et al., 2002; Poon et al., 2006). Previous research has shown that the brains of old rats respond positively to the diets supplemented with acetyl-L-carnitine in the long term. This effect is generated by activating the expression of intracellular enzymes such as GSH and SOD, which leads to a reduction in the formation of 4-hydroxynonenal in the mitochondria, and thus decreases the degree of carboxylation and oxidative nitrosylation mitochondrial protein (Calabrese, et al., 2006; Poon et al., 2006).

Additionally, some authors suggest that the severity of demyelination and neuronal necrosis is reduced in brain areas such as cortex, hippocampus, cerebellar cortex and optic nerve of rats consuming acetyl-L-carnitine (Ramacci et al., 1998; Glade, 2010). Likewise, the use of acetyl-L-carnitine as a dietary supplement to improve cognitive longevity has been demonstrated by the results of a study by Passeri et al., 1990, in which two parallel groups and assessed homogeneous subjects of both sexes aged 65 years and with mild cognitive functions. One group was supplemented with 2 gr/day of acetyl-L-carnitine for three months, while the other group was treated with a placebo. The group of patients treated with acetyl-L-carnitine showed a significant improvement in learning abilities, and long-term memory skills, suggesting the therapeutic importance of this metabolite for the treatment of geriatric patients with mental disfunction.
Besides the natural AO, there is also a growing list of synthetic AO that have been widely studied, for example, conjugated forms of the enzymes SOD and CAT (Greenwald, 1990) and supplements of selenium (Parnham et al., 1991). Similarly, there is growing evidence that give, some drugs with different therapeutic uses to neuroprotection such as probucol (hypocholesterolemic) and salicylates, a certain capacity as recycler of free radicals under experimental conditions (Cui et al., 2004; Juliano et al., 1995; Zhao et al., 1995).
However, despite the existing literature suggesting beneficial effects of AO, there are several questions regarding the therapeutic value that some natural AO may have compared to pathological processes such as AD and PD. There are conflicting data emerging from research on in vitro and in vivo neurodegeneration models, and some authors argue that the fact that one type of antioxidant molecule is produced physiologically or is taken normally from the diet is not a guarantee that this supplementation can be safe and advantageous therapeutic standpoint, since it must be took into account the physiological regulation of the redox state of the cell (Contestabile, 2001). In conclusion, experimental data are converging in terms of the therapeutic benefits of various natural antioxidants with neuroprotective capabilities, however, according to some authors, there are very few clinical data to demonstrate a clear and lasting effect of this type of treatments. Some possible reasons for such a disadvantage might be specific criteria such as dose, stability, duration of treatment, side effects and ability to cross the blood brain barrier, among others (Contestabile, 2001; James, 2009; Meydani et al., 1998). Because of this, it is essential to expand research on the use of AO diet supplements compared to the onset and development of ND as AD and PD.

4.3 Dietary supplements with antioxidant used in the management of ND

Considering the cascade of degenerative events of diseases such as AD and PD (degradation and abnormal folding of proteins, inadequate energy production in CNS degeneration by oxidative damage, excitotoxicity and inflammation), there is interest in whether the AO, or changes in eating habits can prevent and/or block one or more of these pathways of neurodegeneration in slowing the progression of the disease (Mazzio, et al., 2011). In this regard, several studies have suggested some properties of antioxidants as protective factors against the risk of diseases such as AD and PD. In addition, it is considered that changes in the concentration of AO in states of neurodegeneration may be a primary event or secondary to the ingestion of a particular type of diet (Kedar, 2003). Therefore, considering the usefulness of certain AO and its possible uses in therapy of ND, the following describes some of the main AO that are consumed in the diet or supplemented in order to treat or prevent the onset of neurodegenerative conditions such as AD or PD.

4.3.1 Vitamins

4.3.1.1 Vitamin E

Vitamin E or tocopherol is a powerful antioxidant capable of stopping the spread of the chain reaction of free radicals in the lipid portion of cell membranes, inhibiting lipid peroxidation in plasma membrane phospholipids (Mandel et al., 2003; McCay, 1985; Gilgun-Sherki et al., 2001). There are eight tocopherols with vitamin E activity, and α-tocopherol is

Use	Results	Reference
The individual or combined action of tocopherols are protective factors against the incidence of AD and cognitive dysfunction	The different forms of tocopherol that make vitamin E exert greater protective effect associated with AD, compared with α-tocopherol alone	Morris et al. 2005
Supplementation with vitamins E and C to reduce lipid peroxidation in patients with AD.	Increases in plasma levels of vitamin E does not affect the oxidation resistance of lipoproteins, it is necessary to use combinations of the two vitamins.	Kontush et al. [281],
Supplementation with 3000 IU / day vitamin E and C can delay the onset of symptoms associated with dopamine deficiency in PD patients	Increase the time interval between the onset of the disease and the need for treatment with L-dopa in 75% of patients.	Fahns A, 1998
Combination of supplements of vitamins C and E affect the prevalence and incidence of AD.	The combined use of vitamin supplements showed a decrease in the incidence and prevalence of AD in a population of 5092 individuals	Zandi et al., 2004
Supplementation with 2000 IU / day vitamin E reduces the EO implicated in the pathogenesis of AD.	Treatment delays functional impairment in patients with mild Alzheimer's disease.	Sano et al., 1997
High doses of α-tocopherol and ascorbate can delay the time of administration of L-dopa in PD patients	The combination of these natural antioxidants delayed by 2.5 years, the time for the start of the administration of L-dopa in PD patients.	Fahn S, 1991
Long-term supplementation with vitamin E may provide cognitive benefits.	No differences were found between groups treated with vitamin E and placebo groups	Jae Hee Kang, 2006
The intake of high doses of vitamin E (400-4000 IU / day) can slow the progression of PD by inhibiting nigral cell death	No increased levels of vitamin E in the cerebrospinal fluid of patients with PD. However, the subjects had clinical symptoms of the disease when vitamin E was administered.	Pappert, E.J

Table 1. Vitamin E or Tocopherol starring in several studies evaluating the antioxidant supplementation and its effects on cognitive deficits related with ND

the most active and widely distributed (Elejalde, 2001); it is found naturally in foods such as vegetable oils, fats, vegetables, egg yolks, nuts, seeds, fruits and green vegetables (Berman & Brodaty, 2004). In addition to its antioxidant properties, also has capabilities such as specific enzymes regulating agent, anti-inflammatory and neuroprotective (Martin et al., 1999). Due to its neuroprotective properties, researchers worldwide have taken a particular interest in elucidating their protective mechanisms, as opposed to development of cognitive dysfunction related to aging and various ND (Table 1) (Ramesh et al, 2010).

The neuroprotective effect of vitamin E was first described in 1992 in an in vitro study using neuronal cells cultures (Behl C, et al, 1992). However, in order to know whether dietary supplementation with antioxidants can increase their brain levels, it is essential to investigate the effect of such molecules in animal models of ND like the EP (Prasad et al., 1999). In this regard, previous studies suggest that long-term feeding of rats (6 to 15 months of age) with a dietary supplement of 500 IU of vitamin E, induces protective effects against cognitive deficit related to age (Morris et al., 2005; Peterson et al., 2005). Similarly, it has been reported that supplementation with vitamin E in combination with vitamin C, increases the concentration of these vitamins in plasma and cerebrospinal fluid, where the resistance of lipoproteins to oxidation in in vitro studies is increased (Kontush et al, 2001; Casetta et al., 2005). It has also been reported that dietary supplementation with α-tocopherol (1000 IU/day) for four months increases brain levels of vitamin E in rats (Vatassery et al., 1988), as in the brain and cerebrospinal fluid of dogs treated during two years (SR Pillai, 1993). These results suggest that dietary supplementation with vitamin E may be valuable in animal models of PD (Prasad et al., 1999).

On the other hand, one of the largest studies with antioxidants as a treatment for AD, included 341 patients with moderate dementia who were given 4 different treatments: 10mg/day of selegiline (a selective MAO inhibitor), 2000 IU daily α-tocopherol, a combination of selegiline and-tocopherol, or placebo. The effect of the treatments was assessed through the presentation of clinical signs such as loss of ability to perform basic activities of daily living, severe dementia or death. After the treatments the authors observed a significant delay in the time of presentation of clinical signs in patients treated with selegiline, alpha-tocopherol, or in combination compared with placebo (Sano, 1996, 1997). However, there was no additive effect of selegiline and vitamin E, possibly due to a common mechanism of action in which lower levels of free radicals, and prevents its formation through inhibition of oxidative metabolism of catecholamines (Casetta et al., 2005). Similarly, studies by Behl, C., 2000, suggest a neuroprotective activity of both, the natural tocopherol and the synthetic. In addition, the effect appears to be superior to that described for estradiol (powerful antioxidant), in terms of the ability of neuronal protection against oxidative damage generated by β-amyloid protein in AD. Additionally, there are studies that seek to enhance the antioxidant effect of tocopherol, in combination with other vitamins such as Vitamin C. For example, in a prospective study in the Netherlands (Engelhart et al., 2002), they used a population of 5395 subjects at least 55 years, where the high intake of vitamin C and E was associated with a lower risk of developing AD after a follow up of 6.5 years. The relative risk was 0. for vitamin E, and 0.82 for vitamin C (Casetta et al., 2005).

With respect to the source, the vitamin E supplements do not appear to offer better results than those obtained by eating foods rich in this vitamin (Kontush & Schekatolina, 2004). This may be due to the cumulative and synergistic, as the bioavailability of vitamins is

concerned. However, not be ruled out that the apparent protection provided by the supplementation of vitamins E and C, is the result of the synergy of these vitamins and other substances in fruits and vegetables such as flavonoids, which have both anti-inflammatory properties as antioxidants (Ramesh et al., 2010; Seshadri & Wolf, 2003). It has also been suggested that vitamin E supplements can reduce levels of β-amyloid in a transgenic model of AD. However, this effect was only observed in young mice but not in older animals. These results may suggest that antioxidant therapy may be beneficial only if given at an early stage of the disease (Sung et al., 2004; Casetta et al., 2005).
The inconsistencies found between the results of these and other studies of vitamin E, lead to consider that most supplements used are composed exclusively of α-tocopherol, leaving aside the action of other forms of tocopherol that make this vitamin. Therefore, it has been suggested that the protective effect of vitamin E in the brain is the result of the combined intake of all forms of tocopherol (Farrell & Roberts, 1994).

4.3.1.2 Vitamin C

Vitamin C or ascorbic acid is a soluble molecule that has a variety of functions, which include the recycling of oxidized forms of vitamin E and the activation of certain enzymes (McCay, 1985; Chan, 1993; Elejalde, 2001). Importantly, in vivo there are interactions between vitamin E and vitamin C, where the role of antioxidant vitamin E has proven to be improved by supplementation of vitamin C. This interaction, however, involves the two vitamins, whose levels are not regulated by metabolism, but depend on consumption in the diet (Kagan, & Tyurina, 1998). Humans and other primates are unable to synthesize this vitamin, while most mammals, including rats and mice produce the endogenous form of this molecule in the liver (Chatterjee et al., 1975).
Vitamin C is found at high levels in a variety of cells, including neurons, where it participates in the biosynthesis of catecholamines and plays an important role as a cofactor of dopamine-hydroxylase. Vitamine C and vitamin E inhibit peroxidation of membrane phospholipids and act as free radicals scavenger (Gilgun-Sherki et al., 2001). Some authors report that ascorbic acid protects low density lipoprotein from oxidation and reduces oxidizing molecules that damage the integrity of the Central Nervous System (Sales et al., 2009). Given these properties, the scientific interest in this vitamin is to know about their effects on neuronal damage induced by agents such as pilocarpine, where has been found that antioxidant treatment significantly reduces the level of lipid peroxidation and nitrite content, and also potentiates the activity of SOD and CAT in the hippocampus of adult rats after pilocarpine-induced seizures. (Sales et al., 2009).
With respect to the ND, Hellenbrand et al., 1996, found that vitamin C has a protective effect against PD, with statistically significant trend. Several studies in populations aged 65 or older focused their interest on the combined effect of vitamin C and other antioxidants such as vitamin E, beta-carotene, or flavonoids, and these could be associated with reduction of dementia / incidence of AD or reduction of cognitive decline (Esposito et al, 2002; Coley et al., 2008). Zandi et al., 2004 reported that using the combination of high doses of vitamins E and C are associated with reduced prevalence and incidence of AD, even, once initiated the disease.

4.3.1.3 Vitamin B

B complex vitamins such as thiamin (vitamin B1), lipoic acid, biotin, vitamin B6, folic acid, vitamin B12, pantothenate, symbiotically work together to boost the pyruvate dehydrogenase complex, and the contribution of gluconeogenesis oxygen to the brain. In addition, due to the critical role that these nutrients play in the metabolism of glucose and mitochondrial respiration justifies the use of B vitamins for patients with PD (Mazzio et al., 2011). Some authors argue that a relationship exists between the PD, vitamin B6, vitamin B12 and folic acid. This relationship refers to the role played by these molecules in the regulation of homocysteine, since they are responsible for their cleavage to methionine and tetrahydrofolate. Such effects may attenuate the neurotoxicity associated with a condition known as hyperhomocysteinemia, which is associated with PD and cytotoxicity related Mitochondrial Transitory Permeability Pore (Mazzio et al., 2011). Additionally, it has been suggested that elevated levels of homocysteine may increase the severity of PD, since this amino acid could mediate neuronal toxicity through NMDA receptors, precipitating oxidative stress, calcium overload and apoptosis (Mazzio et al., 2011). Homocysteine has also been associated with states of oxidative stress related with AD. In fact, there are some reports of an increased intake of vitamin B6 (Tucker et al., 2005; Corrada et al., 2005), vitamin B12 or folate (Wang et al., 2001; Morris et al., 2005), in middle-aged or advanced age people, with the belief of obtaining a beneficial effect on the incidence of AD or cognitive impairment (Coley et al, 2008).

In this regard, several studies seeking to assess the impact of high doses of vitamin supplements on plasma homocysteine levels in patients with AD (Aisen et al., 2003). For example, a study in patients with AD evaluated the effects of supplementation of these individuals over a period of 18 months. The results indicated that the groups treated with high doses of folic acid, vitamin B6 and B12 reduced by 20-30% peripheral levels of homocysteine, however, the study showed no cognitive differences between individuals treated with antioxidants and individuals treated with placebo (Aisen et al., 2003).

4.4 Polyphenols

As mentioned above, the use of vitamin supplements may promote the biological integrity of systems, however, the combined use of vitamins and plant-derived polyphenolic compounds, seems to have good recognition as antioxidants (Mazzio et al., 2011). The use of supplements from plants to improve health is an issue that is gaining popularity among most people because it is considered that the use of natural products is safe and produces fewer side effects, compared to synthetic drug, in fact, to date over 50 different species of plants, and more than 8000 phenolic compounds have been identified with beneficial effects on health (Sun et al., 2008).

Polyphenols can be divided into different groups depending on the number of rings of phenol and the chemical group attached to these rings. The most representative of this group of substances are the flavonoids, which are subdivided into flavonoids (catechin, epicatechin), flavonols (quercetin, myricetin, kaempferol), flavanones (hesperetin, naringenin), flavones (apigenin, luteolin), isoflavones (genistein, daidzein) and anthocyanins (cyanide, malvidin) (Ramassamy, 2006; Sun, et al., 2008). These molecules are found in a wide variety of food products from plants. One of the most important aspects of the polyphenols current research is their neuroprotective capacity. This section will define and describe in detail the neuroprotective mechanisms of these macromolecules, and also, will discuss recent evidence regarding their potentially antioxidant effect to prevent or to control the development of neuropathology as AD or PD.

4.4.1 Plant polyphenols

Polyphenols are a class of phytoalexins found in a wide range of plants, fruits and vegetables (Bastianetto & Quirion, 2002; Brannon et al., 2010; Ramassamy, 2006; Ramesh et al., 2010). When ingested they are transported from the circulatory system to various body organs including the brain (Sun et al., 2008). It has also been found to be potent recyclers of superoxide radicals, hydrogen peroxide and oxygen (Morel et al., 1993; Nanjo et al., 1996; Ramassamy, 2006), mechanisms that together with the anti-inflammatory activity have been extensively studied in order to know their beneficial effects against aging-related processes (Table 2) (Brannon & Trygve, 2010; James et al., 2009).
The ability of polyphenols to act as antioxidants is given by its ability to chelate metal ions, which is achieved by suppressing reactive species that contribute to oxidative damage (Brannon & Trygve, 2010). This antioxidant capacity depends on the molecular structure of each polyphenol, the position of hydroxyl groups, and other substitutions in their chemical structure (Sun et al., 2008). In addition to the antioxidant capacities, several polyphenols exhibit multiple biological properties among which are the anti-inflammatory, anticancer, antiviral, antimicrobial, vasodilator and anti-coagulant (Rahman et al., 2007). Additionally, *in vitro* studies demonstrate that polyphenols may possess the ability to activate or inhibit several signaling pathways such as NF-κβ, SIRT1, MAPK's, heat shock proteins and other regulatory molecules, which may play an important role in basic functions such as senescence, apoptosis and the activation or production of transcription factors (Brannon & Trygve, 2010).
Furthermore, polyphenols are natural antioxidants that after consumption tend to produce an increase in plasma antioxidant capacity, and also can inhibit the oxidation of low density

Polyphenol	Effect	Result
Resveratrol	Activation of SIRT1 driving to deacetylation of p53, NF-κβ, HSF-1, FOXO1/3/4 y PGC-1α. Activation of SIRT1 can mimic caloric restriction It binds to receptors in the brain to stimulate the production of transthyretin (TTR)	Influence on senescence, inflammation, apoptosis, resistance to stress and metabolism Increment of half life TTR sequesters beta-amyloid fibrils
EGCG	Regulates NO production in endothelial cells Regulates NO production in carcinoma cells Blocks EGF receptor in cervical cancer cells	Prevents inflammation associated with atherosclerosis Prevention of metastasis Prevention of tumor growing
Quercetine	Regulates production of TNF-α	Anti-inflammatory properties that reduce development of atherosclerosis.

Table 2. Attenuation of diseases associated to aging by action de polyphenols (Brannon & Trygve, 2010)

lipoprotein. These features have drawn public attention, since several of these substances have therapeutic potential against diseases such as cancer, ischemia, heart, liver, and neurodegenerative diseases (Mandel et al., 2003). Thus, numerous studies in different models of neurodegeneration *in vitro* and *in vivo* have shown that polyphenols can prevent and/or reduce oxidative damage by free radicals generated (Mandel & Youdim, 2004; Scalbert et al., 2005). Numerous epidemiological estudies have shown neuroprotective effects of polyphenols and have established a clear relationship between these effects and decreased risk of neurological dysfunction associated with aging (Mandel et al., 2003). However, the nature of these protective effects, is not limited to the antioxidant properties, since recent evidence derived from *in vitro* cellular models, suggest that polyphenols such as resveratrol and EGCG, besides having the ability to recycle free radicals directly, also may regulate the cytotoxic effects of oligomers of βA via phosphorylation of phosphokinase C. In addition, polyphenols such as EGCG and resveratrol possess the ability to activate the enzyme transmembrane α-secretase, which catalyzes the formation of a soluble and amyloidogenic (no plaque-forming) from the amyloid precursor protein (APP). Through this pathway, APP is formed and therefore do not allow the formation of neuritic plaques, a hallmark of AD. This information indicates that polyphenols may be used in therapies to exert control over the APP related molecules, and may suggest avenues for the development of new treatments that reduce the risk of developing AD according to the aging process. (Brannon & Trygve, 2010).

Additionally, studies such as James et al., 1999, showed the extracts of blueberry or strawberry (high in polyphenols) as substances that can significantly attenuate cognitive and motor deficits related to aging in rodents. In this study, rodents of all treatments showed improvement in short-term memory according to the Morris water test. However, while these diets were supplemented based on an equal antioxidant capacity (determined by absorbance capacity test the oxygen radical, ORAC) was not found equal effectiveness in the prevention or reversal of the changes associated with aging. Additionally, the antioxidant capacity alone was not predictive in evaluating the potential of these compounds against certain age-related disorders. In fact, markers of oxidative stress (DCF fluorescence, and glutathione peroxidase level in the brain) were slightly reduced by the diets, suggesting that the polyphenols from berries can have multiple actions in addition to the antioxidant.

Other possible mechanisms for the beneficial effects of these foods are: direct effects on signaling to enhance neuronal communication, the ability to act as a buffer against excess calcium, enhancement of neuroprotective proteins and reduction of signs of stress such as NF -κβ. (Calabrese et al., 2010). According to studies in cell cultures and animal models, there is a cascade of signaling between the molecules and effects of eating berries. For example, treatment with berries to COS-7 cells exposed to dopamine or to hippocampal primary neurons, significantly increased the expression of MAPK mitogen. Additionally, mice supplemented with berries APP/PS1, exhibited high levels of hippocampal extracellular signaling regulated by ERK, such as protein kinase C (PKC) α, compared with transgenic mice maintained on control diets. In addition, Brannon & Trygve, 2010, suggests that treatment with berries is effective protection against the toxic effect of βA and against the decline in the induction of dopamine in the regulation of intracellular calcium in COS-7 cells transfected hippocampal neurons. This protection suggests an increase in phosphorylated MAPK and decreased PKCγ.

4.4.1.1 Epigallocatechin 3-Gallate (EGCG)

EGCG is a polyphenol flavonoid type found in large quantities in green tea. According to some authors, this compound has exerts significant neuroprotective effects against a wide range of oxidative insults in a multitude of neuronal cell models (Calabrese et al., 2010; Kelsey et al., 2010). In one study, CGNs incubated cells with an inhibitor of Bcl-2 known as HA14-1, which generates oxidation and mitochondrial intrinsic apoptosis (Zimmermann et al., 2007), applying the co-treatment with EGCG, was found that the microtubule network of CGNs exposed to HA14-1 was significantly preserved, and so, was prevented the apoptotic nuclear morphology (Kelsey et al., 2010). In fact, studies like that of Weinreb et al., 2004, showed that treatment of neuronal cells with EGCG affects the expression levels of various proteins, including proteins related to components of the cytoskeleton, metabolism, and binding proteins (Calabrese et al., 2010; Izumi et al., 2005). EGCG similarly protects human neuroblastoma cells (SH-SY5Y) against the cytotoxicity associated with the amyloid precursor protein (APP), and the 6-hydroxydopamine (6-OHDA) (Avramovich et al., 2007), thus, rescues PC12 cells from serum deprivation-induced apoptosis or paraquat (Hou et al., 2008; Kelsey et al., 2010; Mandel et al., 2003). Also, supplementation of transgenic mice over expressing APP (APPsw) substantially reduced amyloid plaque burden and reduced cognitive impairment (Rezai-Zadeh et al., 2005, Kelsey et al., 2010). Similarly, in murine N2A cells transfected with a mutant form of human APP (Rezai-Zadeh et al., 2005) was found that EGCG reduced the generation of β-amyloid (Ramassamy, 2006).
In addition to the neuroprotective effects of EGCG observed in *in vitro* studies, this antioxidant also preserved neuronal survival and function in several *in vivo* models of neurodegeneration. For example, supplementation to mice with EGCG protected dopaminergic neurons in the substantia nigra pars compacta from toxicity induced MPTP, therefore it could preserve the levels of dopamine in the striatum (Levites et al., 2001). Similarly, the acute and chronic administration of EGCG has been evaluated in various cell and animal models of AD, where it has been suggested that EGCG significantly reduced the toxicity induced by β-amyloid (Kelsey et al., 2010). With respect to PD, Sung et al, 2010, used models *in vitro* and *in vivo* to investigate the modulation of the effects of EGCG on L-dopa and induced neuronal damage. The results indicated that oral supplementation with this antioxidant initiated potential beneficial effects in patients with PD treated with L-dopa as moderately inhibits methylation of this molecule. Similarly, Levitas et al., 2001, using mice as animal model of PD which were given a pre-treatment with green tea extract (0.5 *and* 1 mg / kg) or EGCG (2 and 10 mg / kg) prevented the damage generated by the neurotoxin (MPTP) on dopaminergic neurons in the nigrostriatal pathway.
Another type of molecular mechanism involved in neuroprotection by EGCG is mediated gene activation in apoptosis. Evidence of this assertion is found in studies such as that by Levites et al., 2002, which results in neuroblastoma cells SH-SY5Y showed that EGCG decreased the gene expression of pro-apoptotic such as Bax, Bad, Fas ligand and TRAIL (tumor necrosis factor-related apoptosis-inducingligand), however, the expression of Bcl-2 and Bcl-x was not affected (Levites et al., 2002). These results suggest that the neuroprotective effects of EGCG may involve the inactivation of proapoptotic genes, rather than the action of anti-apoptotic mitochondrial proteins (Ramassamy, 2006). Taken together, these findings indicate that EGCG may be a therapeutic candidate for chronic neurodegenerative diseases like AD and PD (Weinreb et al.,2004; Frank & Gupta, 2005), and may be beneficial in acute episodes of neuronal damage, such as spinal cord trauma.

4.4.1.2 Quercetin

Quercetin is a flavonoid found in different types of food such as apples, capers, onions, broccoli, tea and wine (Boots et al., 2008; Esposito et al., 2002; Kelsey et al, 2010). As EGCG, quercetin has been widely studied in *in vitro* and *in vivo* assays in neural models (Ossola et al., 2009). Thus, PC12 cell studies showed that quercetin enhances cell survival in the presence of hydrogen peroxide (Dajas et al., 2003; Heo & Lee, 2004), linoleic acid (Sasaki, et al., 2003), and tert-butyl (Silva et al., 2008). Furthermore, in human neuroblastoma cells SH-SY5Y used as experimental models for PD, this substance has shown to have protective ability against toxicity by 6-OHDA (Kelsey et al., 2010). Also, other study about neurodegeneration in animal models have suggested that the neuroprotective capacity of quercetin could be related to increased blood-brain barrier permeability, thus facilitating the penetration of the substance in the brain (Ossola et al., 2009).

Taken together, these studies indicate that quercetin has the potential, such as EGCG, to block the starting of the enzymatic oxidation of dopamine (Tamura et al., 1994), and this could means a new therapy against neurodegenerative diseases such as PD (Kelsey et al., 2010). However, Ossola, et al., 2009 states that despite the fact that quercetin has not shown significant toxicity in several animal studies, the risk of neurotoxicity is not negligible due to its narrow therapeutic dose range in *in vitro* experiments, also the effectiveness of quercetin in ND is quite low.

4.4.1.3 Resveratrol

Resveratrol (trans-3, 4 ',5-trihydroxystilbene) is a polyphenol found abundantly in grapes and red wine, it is known for its antioxidant and neuroprotective properties in several experiments, therefore, consumption of wine has been proposed as a possible benefit in neurodegenerative processes (Calabrese et al., 2010; Esposito et al., 2002; Kiziltepe et al., 2004; Ramasamy, 2006). The main biological activities attributed to resveratrol include: inhibition of lipid peroxidation and free radicals in cell cultures and rat brains (Virgili & Contestabile, 2000, Casetta et al., 2005), vasodilator, anti-inflammatory and anticancer. Also, It has been shown that mice fed with daily dose of resveratrol for 45 days, had resveratrol or its metabolites in the brain, indicating its bioavailability to neuronal cells (Casseta et al., 2005; Contestabile, 2001; Karuppagounder et al., 2008; Ramesh et al., 2010).

In the field of ND has been suggested that resveratrol not only attenuated the cytotoxicity induced by β-amyloid, but also blocks the accumulation of intracellular reactive oxygen species typical of apoptosis (Casetta et al., 2005; Jang & Surh, 2003). In addition, partial neuroprotection was demonstrated in rats with chronic supplementation of resveratrol in *in vivo* studies of excitotoxicity related to the administration of agonists for glutamate and kainic acid receptors, (Contestabille, 2001; Virgili & Contestabile, 2000). The consumption of about 8 mg/kg/day of resveratrol for 45 days decreased excitotoxic damage measured on the basis of the reduction of certain neuromarcador of GABAergic neurons, from 38% to 14% in the olfactory cortex and 27 % to 12% in the hippocampus. This was the first report of neuroprotection by long-term administration of resveratrol in an *in vivo* model of neurodegeneration (Contestabille, 2001). Similarly, Han, 2003, showed that cell death induced by administration of β-amyloid peptide (20μM), decreased significantly, and protein concentration-dependent by treatment with resveratrol administered 2 hours later. Also, in two different transfected cell lines (HEK293 and N2A), Marambaud et al., 2005, showed that resveratrol may reduce the secretion of β-amyloid peptide, perhaps through the activation of proteosomal degradation of the peptide. This effect of resveratrol occurred

without the direct involvement of the β and γ-secretase, but, Brannon & Trygve, 2010, argues that resveratrol can activate transmembrane protein α-secretase. However, it is still unclear the effect of resveratrol on the mechanism of degradation of ß-amyloid levels in neurons, although it is suggested that may have a key effect on the route of clearance of beta-amyloid (Marambaud et al., 2005; Ramesh et al., 2010).
With respect to cell signaling pathways related to the effects of resveratrol has been shown that its protective activity is related to the PCK phosphorylation, leading to its activation, and the activation of no amyloidogenic cleavage pathways of APP, decreasing the release of β-amyloid (Han, 2003; Ramesh et al., 2010). Similarly, studies in neuroblastoma cells SH-SY5Y by Miloso et al.,1999, argue that resveratrol can induce activation of MAP kinases ERK1 and ERK2. In addition to these signaling pathways, resveratrol can also induce the expression of the response of the transcription early growth factor (Egr1) (Della Ragione et al., 2002), which could regulate some aspects of synaptic plasticity related to learning and memory (Li et al., 2005). Additionally, resveratrol may interact with other proteins, including members of the sirtuins family. Deacetylases sirtuins are related to mechanisms of cellular longevity (Guarente, 2001), resveratrol acts as a potent activator of these molecules, thus related to neuroprotective pathways (Araki et al., 2004; Ramesh et al., 2010). Other intracellular signaling mechanisms that may be implicated with the neuroprotective effect of resveratrol against β-amyloid peptide include the modulation of NF-kB pathways or NF-κB/SIRT1, where resveratrol can inhibit the activity of NF-kB induced β-amyloid peptide through the activation of SIRT1 (Ramassamy, 2006).
With respect to the high amounts of resveratrol contained in red wine, investigations that assess moderate alcohol consumption show that this practice was significantly associated with lower risk of acquiring dementia and AD, compared to non-consumption (Casseta et al., 2005). Similarly, several epidemiological studies indicate that moderate wine consumption may be associated with a lower incidence of AD (Lindsay et al., 2002; Orgogozo et al., 1997; Truelsen et al., 2002), and additionally, different studies *in vitro* and *in vivo* have investigated the basis for this association. For example, doses from 10 microM of resveratrol in PC12 cells have demonstrated protective ability against the cytotoxicity induced by amyloid β (Jang & Surh, 2003). It has also been reported that the combination of resveratrol with other flavonoids such as catechin, may exert synergistic protection against the toxicity of amyloid β peptide in PC12 cells (Conte et al., 2003). However, there has not been demonstrated the relevance of these findings *in vivo* models (Ramassamy et al., 2010). Moreover, it is difficult to reconcile the therapeutic potential of resveratrol with the well known toxic effects of ethanol (Calabrese et al., 2010), because it does not seem reasonable to recommend alcohol consumption to those with tendency to addiction (Ramesh et al, 2010; Resnick & Junlapeeya, 2004).

4.4.1.4 Ginkgo biloba

The extract of Ginkgo biloba EGb 761 is a substance from the green leaves of Ginkgo biloba (Drieu, 1986). This extract was patented in 1990 and has a wide range of biochemical and pharmacological activities, including the antioxidant activity (Marcocci et al., 1994), the neurotrophic capacity in the hippocampal formation (Barkats et al., 1995; Bastianetto & Quirion, 2002), and the neuroprotective ability against neurotoxicity induced by β-amyloid peptide (Casseta, et al., 2005; Luo et al., 2002; Yao et al., 2001;).
The therapeutic use of Ginkgo biloba has been proposed due to its high content of flavonoids and terpenoids, and is widely used in Europe to alleviate symptoms associated

with the progression of cognitive impairment, in fact, several studies argue that extracts of Ginkgo biloba may be effective in delaying the clinical deterioration of patients with dementia (Ernst & Pittler, 1999; Casseta et al., 2005). The effects of EGb 761 may be explained, at least in part, based on their protective actions in animal models of hypoxia and ischemia (Droy-Lefaix et al., 1995) and *in vitro* models of toxicity (Ni et al., 1996; Oyama et al., 1996; Xin et al., 2000), also a prospective placebo-controlled study demonstrated the therapeutic efficacy of oral administration of EGb 761 in dementia patients and healthy adults showed improved memory and attention (Bastianetto & Quirion, 2002; Maurer et al., 1997; Mix et al., 2000). A case-control study that used a cohort of 1,462 women aged 75 years was conducted to test the effectiveness of the prevention of AD using EGb761, the conclusion is that the small number of women who developed dementia were prescribed with the supplement at least for two years. These results suggest that EGb 761 treatment may reduce the risk of developing Alzheimer's dementia in older women (Andrieu et al, 2003; Casseta, et al., 2005).

Additionally, Bastianetto & Quirion, in 2002, conducted a study *in vitro* with embryonic mouse hippocampal cells on which were used two different protocols of citotoxididad, one with β-amyloid (A_25-35 (25_M) A_1-40 (5_M) A_1-42 or (25_M)), and the other with sodium nitroprusside (SNP) to assess whether the components of red wine were able to reduce cell death caused by β-amyloid and oxidative stress. We found that EGb 761, possibly through the antioxidant properties of its flavonoids was able to protect hippocampal cells against the toxic effects previously described.

The mechanisms of action underlying the protective effects of EGb 761, have been evaluated in different studies. For example Bastianetto& Quirion, in 2002, noted in his study that the treatment with EGb 761 were able to inhibit the injury induced by βA 25-35, and NO. In addition, the extract showed protective effect against the harmful effects of H2O2, a supposed mediator of the toxicity caused by β-amyloid (Behl et al., 1994). These data suggest that the scavenging properties of hydroxyl radical of the EGb 761, may be part of the protection against β-amyloid toxicity (Oyama et al., 1996; Bastianetto & Quirion, 2002). Finally, it has been reported that EGb 761 inhibits a number of apoptotic events induced by βA 25-35, a process that may be relevant to the neuro-degeneration that occurs in AD (Johnson, 1994). In addition, these anti-apoptotic effects of EGb 761 are apparently related to the ability to inhibit the toxicity induced by H2O2, and that this natural extract has been reported as an effective tool to the apoptosis hydroxyl radical-induced in cultured neurons (Bastianetto & Quirion, 2002; Ni et al., 1996, Xin et al., 2000).

4.4.1.5 Curcuminoides

The curcuminoids are the active component of turmeric, which have been attributed to have capacity as an inhibitor of lipid peroxidation, and free radical scavenger, it is a potent anti-inflammatory and anticancer, and is also traditionally used in Asia (Aggarwal et al., 2007; James, et al., 2009; Ramesh et al., 2010). In light of its antioxidant, anti-inflammatory and anti-amyloid actions, curcumin is being investigated as a candidate compound for the prevention or treatment of diseases such as multiple myeloma, pancreatic cancer, myelodysplastic syndromes, colon cancer, psoriasis and AD (Calabrese et al., 2010; Goel, et al., 2008).

The curcumin reduces pro-inflammatory cytokines, oxidative damage, the Aβ42 and cognitive deficits in models of AD (Frautschy et al., 2001). Also, has been told that it is a direct inhibitor of βA aggregation and fibril formation (Cole et al., 2003; James et al., 2009).

Similarly, curcumin has anti-AD activities, including, limitation of the kinase JNK (c-Jun N-terminal protein kinase) and stimulation of neurogenesis (Cole et al., 2007; James et al., 2009). Moreover, previous research has shown that turmeric reduces inflammation and oxidative damage in Tg2576 transgenic mouse brain AβPPSw (Kumar & Singh, 2008; Lim et al., 2001,), and that curcumin reduces the level of soluble and insoluble βA in several brain regions. Therefore, it has been suggested that this substance could prevent the onset of AD, not only by scavenging reactive oxygen species, but also by inhibiting the aggregation of βA in the brain (Ramesh et al., 2010). Similarly, Lim et al., 2001, studied the effects of the curcumin in transgenic mice carrying a human mutation of the amyloid precursor protein (APPsw) that causes AD (Lim et al., 2001) and found a reduction in brain level of oxidized proteins, and a decrease in both the level of soluble and insoluble βA, and the plaque burden (Lim et al., 2001). However, more studies are needed to test the potential therapeutic use of curcumin for the treatment or prevention of AD in humans (Calabrese et al., 2010).

The benefits of curcumin derive from its complex chemical structure and its ability to influence multiple signaling pathways, for instance, survival pathways such as those regulated by NF-kB, the Nrf2-dependent cytoprotective pathways, and routes of metastasis and angiogenesis (Calabrese et al., 2010; Goel et al.,2008; Ramsewak et al., 2000).

Because curcumin is highly toxic and has a limited bioavailability, the assessment of their impact on clinical practice has not been easy, however, using lipid formulations, this obstacle has been largely mitigated (Begum et al., 2008; James et al., 2009; Calabrese et al., 2010).

5. Dietary recommendations for patients with ND as AD and PD

Some evidence suggest that high intake of dietary antioxidants or fruits and vegetables provides nutritional compounds with antioxidant properties that may contribute to improving the quality of life, due to the decreased risk of degenerative diseases associated with aging and the accumulation of free radicals (Meydani et al.,1998). Therefore, although it is important to consider that dietary supplementation with AO may enhance cognitive longevity, and to some extent, reduces the risk of developing these diseases, it is also important to do some additional considerations. For example, the use of a single antioxidant, is not the best option, since the oxidation of individual antioxidants may promote oxidative stress, therefore, we recommend using combinations of antioxidants at the appropriate doses. Also, as mentioned previously, it has been found that diets rich in vitamin E may reduce the risk of EP, and has also been suggested that moderate wine consumption may reduce the risk to suffer from AD. However, there is still controversy about the epidemiological data related to these hypotheses, which could be due partially to the intrinsic difficulties of epidemiological surveys on the eating habits in large populations (Esposito, et al., 2002).

However, nutritional factors remain a very relevant topic when setting up a comprehensive treatment in patients with dementia. In addition, the formulation of a specific diet for people with AD or PD, requires a prior careful review of the patient, in order to identify their nutritional deficiencies, and thus design a healthy diet to ensure good physical health. For example, certain vitamins such as B12 and folic acid must be replaced to ensure that AD dementia is not due in part to this deficiency (Ramesh et al, 2010).

Finally, some authors argue that there is a lack of knowledge on these issues among medical professionals and clinicians, so they overlooked some dietary recommendations that could be used in conjunction with the approach of Neurogerontology (James et al, 2009), so, it is necessary to continue investigating the potential benefits of various AO against the prevention and/or treatment of ND as AD and PD.

6. Conclusions

As described earlier in this chapter, a variety of scientific evidence that describes the importance of different oxidative mechanisms which are part of the dynamic biological relevance of the ND as AD, PD or the CDS. Such approaches have led to a series of theories on the therapeutic use of antioxidants to slow down the chain reaction of oxidative events and thus to reduce its cytotoxic effects. Thus, consumption of antioxidants such as vitamin E and C, polyphenols and other antioxidants has became very important because they provide a series of defense mechanisms that promote longevity, reduce the risk of developing certain neuropathologies, and also can be consumed in a daily diet.

However, there are some data that are incompatible with these theories, leading to various disputes regarding antioxidant supplementation and its possible beneficial effects on the body. In this sense, it is important to consider factors that may limit somewhat the research in this field. Among these factors: choosing an appropriate dose, long-term monitoring of a large cohort study, the inclusion or exclusion of different environmental factors, and *in vivo* application of the results obtained in *in vitro* studies.

Occasionally, the start of antioxidant therapy for ND, is given when there may be a significant number of injured neurons, giving rise to specific clinical symptoms. In this case, antioxidants act on viable neurons, but do not recover the population of dead neurons. Therefore, in several studies of neuroprotection, supplying long-term supplements at the onset of the disease or even earlier is recommended; these results provide a valid evidence of the therapeutic effects of these substances and are a guarantee of further trials.

7. References

Aisen P.S., Egelko S., Andrews H., Diaz-Arrastia R., Weiner, M. DeCarli, C., Jagust, W.; Miller, J.W.; Green, R K. Bell & Sano, M. (2003). A pilot study of vitamins to lower plasma homocysteine levels in Alzheimer disease, *Am J Geriatr Psychiatry,* Vol.11, pp.246–249.

Aggarwal BB, Sundaram C, Malani N, Ichikawa H (2007). Curcumin: the Indian solid gold. *Adv Exp Med Biol,* Vol.595, pp.1–75.

Andrieu S, Gillette S, Amouyal K, Nourhashemi F, Reynish E, Ousset PJ, et al. (2003). EPIDOS study. Association of Alzheimer's disease onset with ginkgo biloba and other symptomatic cognitive treatments in a population of women aged 75 years and older from the EPIDOS study. *J Gerontol A Biol Sci Med Sci,* Vol.58, pp. 372-7.

Araki T, Sasaki Y, Milbrandt J. (2004). Increased nuclear NAD biosynthesis and SIRT1 activation prevent axonal degeneration. *Science,* Vol.13, pp.1010–1013.

Araujo, J.A.; Studzinski, C.M. & Milgram, N.W. (2005). Further evidence for the cholinergic hypothesis of aging and dementia from the canine model of aging. *Prog. Neuropsychopharm. Biol. Psychiat,* Vol.29, pp.411-422.

Avramovich-Tirosh, Y.; Reznichenko, L.; Mit, T.; Zheng, H.; Fridkin, M.; Weinreb, O.; Mandel, S. & Youdim, M.B. (2007). Neurorescue activity, APP regulation and amyloid-beta peptide reduction by novel multi-functional brain permeable iron-chelating- antioxidants, M-30 and green tea polyphenol, EGCG. *Curr. Alzheimer. Res*, Vol.4, pp. 403-411.

Barkats M, Venault P, Christen Y, Cohen-Salmon C. (1995). Effect of longterm treatment with EGb 761 on age-dependent structural changes in the hippocampi of three inbred mouse strains. *Life Sci*, Vol.121, pp. 213–222.

Bastianetto, S. & Quirion, R. (2002). Natural extracts as possible protective agents of brain aging. *Neurobiology of Aging*, Vol.23, pp.891–897.

Begum AN, Jones MR, Lim GP, Morihara T, Kim P, Heath DD, Rock CL, Pruitt MA, Yang F, Hudspeth B, Hu S, Faull KF, Teter B, Cole GM, Frautschy SA (2008). Curcumin structure-function, bioavailability, and efficacy in models of neuroinflammation and Alzheimer's disease. *J Pharmacol Exp Ther* , Vol.326, pp.196 –208.

Behl, C.; Davis, J.B.; Cole, G.M. & Schubert, D. (1992). Vitamin E protects nerve cells from amyloid _ protein toxicity. *Biochem Biophys Res Commun*, Vol.186, pp.944–50

Behl, C.; Davis, J.B.; Lesley, R. & Schubert, D. (1994). Hydrogen peroxide mediates amyloid b protein toxicity. *Cell*, Vol.77, No.6, pp817-827, ISSN: 0092-8674.

Behl, C. (2000). Vitamin E protects neurons against oxidative cell death in vitro more effectively than 17-beta estradiol and induces the activity of the transcription factor NF-kappaB. *J Neural Transm*, Vol.107, No.4, pp. 393-407.

Benedetti, A.; Ferretti, G.; Curatola, G.; Jezequel, A.M. & Orlandi, F. (1988). Age and sex related changes of plasma membrane fluidity in isolated rat hepatocytes. *Biochemical and Biophysical Research Communications*, Vol.156, No2, pp. 840-845, ISSN 0006-291X.

Berman, K. & Brodaty, H. (2004). Tocopherol (Vitamin E) in Alzheimer's Disease and Other Neurodegenerative Disorders. *CNS Drugs*, Vol.18, No.12, pp. 807-825.

Birkmayer, W.; Birkmayer, J.; Vrecko, C.; Paletta, B.; Reschenhofer, E. & Ott, E. (1990). Nicotnamide adenine dinucleotide (NADH) as medication for Parkinson's disease: Experience with 415 patients. *Trends Clin Neuropharmacol* , Vol.4, pp.7–24.

Boots, A.; Haenen, G. & Bast, A. (2008). Health effects of quercetin: from antioxidant to nutraceutical. *European Journal of Pharmacology*, Vol.585, No.2-3, pp. 325-337, ISSN 0014-2999.

Braak, H. & Braak, E. (1991). Neuropathological stageing of Alzheimer-related changes. *Acta Neuropathologica*, Vol.82, No.4, pp. 239–259, ISSN 0001-6322.

Brannon, L. & Trygve O. (2010). Polyphenols and Aging. *Curr Aging Sci*, Vol.3, No.1, pp.34–42.

Burton, G.W. & Ingold, K.U. (1989) Vitamin E as an *in vitro* and *in vivo* antioxidant. *Annals of the New York Academy of Sciences*, Vol. 570, pp.7-22, ISSN 1749-6632.

Burton, G.W. & Ingold, K.U. (1990). Mechanisms of antioxidant action: preventive and chain-breaking antioxidants. In: *CRC Handbook of Free Radicals and Antioxidants in Biomedicin,* Miguel, A., Quintanilha, A.T., Weber, H. (Eds.). Vol. II, CRC Press Inc. Boca Raton, FL. pp 29-43.

Butterfield, D.A.; Castegna, A; Lauderback, C.M. & Drake, J. (2002) Evidence that amyloid beta-peptide induced lipid peroxidation and its sequelae in Alzheimer's disease brain contribute to neuronal death. *Neurobiology of Aging*, Vol.23, No.5, pp.655-664, ISSN 0197-4580.

Cadenas, E. (1997). Basic mechanism of antioxidant activity. *Biofactors*, Vol.6, No.4, pp.391-397, ISSN 1872-8081

Calabrese, V.; Calvani, M. & Butterfield, D.A. (2006). Acetyl-L-carnitineinduced up-regulation of heat shock proteins protects cortical neurons against amyloid-beta peptide 1-42-mediated oxidative stress and neurotoxicity: implications for Alzheimer's disease. *J Neurosci Res*, Vol.84, pp. 398-408.

Calabrese, V.; Cornelius, C.; Trovato-Salinaro, A.; Cambria, M.T.; Locascio, M.S.; Di Rienzo, L.; Condorelli. D.F.; Mancuso, C.; De Lorenzo, A. & Calabrese, E.J. (2010). The Hormetic Role of Dietary Antioxidants in Free Radical-Related Diseases. *Current Pharmaceutical Design*, Vol.16, pp.877-883.

Casetta, I.; Govoni, V. & Granieri, E. (2005). Oxidative Stress, Antioxidants and Neurodegenerative Diseases. *Current Pharmaceutical Design*, Vol.11, pp. 2033-2052, ISSN 1381-6128.

Chan, A.C. (1993). Partners in defense. Vitamin E and vitamin C. *Canadian Journal of Physiology and Pharmacology*, Vol.71, No.9, pp.725–731

Chan, P.H. Reactive oxygen radicals in signaling and damage in the ischemic brain. (2001). *Journal of Cerebral Blood Flow & Metabolism*, Vol. 21, No.1, pp.2-14, ISSN 0271-678X.

Chance, B.; Sies, H. & Boveris, A. (1979) Hydroperoxide metabolism in mammalian organs. *Physiological. Reviews*, Vol. 59, No.3, pp. 527-605, ISNN 0031-9333.

Chatterjee, I.B., Majunder, A.L., Nandi, B.K., Subramanian, N. (1975). Synthesis and some major functions of vitamin C in animals. *Annals of the New York Academy of Sciences*, Vol.258, pp.24–47.

Chen, R.S.; Huang, C.C. & Chu, N.S. (1997). Coenzyme Q10 treatment in mitochondrial encephalomyopathies. Short-term double-blind, crossover study. *Eur Neurol*, Vol.37, pp.212–218.

Cole G, Yang F, Lim G, Cummings J, Masterman D, Frautschy S (2003). A rationale for curcuminoids for the prevention or treatment of Alzheimer's disease. *Curr Med Chem Immun Endoc Metab Agents*, Vol.3, pp.15–25.

Cole GM, Teter B, Frautschy SA. (2007) Neuroprotective effects of curcumin.*Adv Exp Med Biol*, Vol.595, pp.197–212.

Coley, N.; Andrieul, S.; Gardette, V.; Gillette-Guyonnet, S.; Sanz, C.; Vellas, B. & Grand, A. (2008). Dementia Prevention: ethodological Explanations for Inconsistent Results. *Epidemiol Rev*, Vol.30, pp.35–66.

Conte, A., Pellegrini, S. & Tagliazucchi, D. (2003). Synergistic protection of PC12 cells from beta-amyloid toxicity by resveratrol and catechin. *Brain Res. Bull*, Vol.62, pp.29–38.

Contestabile, A. (2001). Oxidative Stress in Neurodegeneration: Mechanisms and Therapeutic Perspectives. *Current Topics in Medicinal Chemistry*, Vol.1, No.6, pp.553-568, ISNN 1862-2461.

Corrada M, Kawas C, Hallfrisch J, et al. (2005). Reduced risk of Alzheimer's disease with high folate intake: the Baltimore Longitudinal Study of Aging. *Alzheimers Dement*, Vol.1, pp.11–18.

Cotman, C.W.; Head, E.; Muggenburg, B.A.; Zicker, S. & Milgram, N.W. (2002). Brain aging in the canine: a diet enriched in antioxidants reduces cognitive dysfunction. *Neurobiology Aging*, Vol.23, No.5, pp.809–18.

Cui, K.; Luo, X.; Xu, K. & Ven, M.R. (2004). Role of oxidative stress in neurodegeneration: recent dvelopments in assay methods for oxidative stress and nutraceutical antioxidants. *Progress in Neuro-Psychopharmacology & Biological Psychiatry*, Vol. 28, No.5, pp. 771- 799, ISSN 0278-5846.

Dajas, F.; Rivera, F.; Blasina, F.; Arredondo, F.; Echeverry, C.; Lafon, L.; Morquio, A. & Heizen, H. (2003). Cell culture protection and in vivo neuroprotective capacity of flavonoids. *Neurotox. Res*, Vol.5, pp. 425-432.

Dawson, T.M. & Dawson, V.L. (1996). Free radical and neuronal cell death. *Cell Death & Differentiation*, Vol.3, No1, pp. 71-78, ISNN 1350-9047.

Della Ragione, F., Cucciolla, V., Criniti, V., Indaco, S., Borriello, A., Zappia, V. (2002). Antioxidants induce different phenotypes by a distinct modulation of signal transduction. *FEBS Lett*, Vol.532, pp. 289–294.

Dreosti, I.; Meydani, M. & Joseph, J. (1998). Annals of the New York Academy of Sciences (1998, 854:463-76).

Drieu, K. (1986). Preparation and definition of *G. biloba* extract. *Press Med*, Vol.15, pp.1455–7.

Droy-Lefaix MT, Menerath JM, Szabo-Tosaki E, Guillaumin D, Doly M. (1995). Protective effect of EGb 761 on ischemia-reperfusion damage in the rat retina. *Transplantation Proc* , Vol.27, pp.2861–2862.

Elejalde, R. (2001). Estrés oxidativo, enfermedades y tratamientos antioxidantes. *Ann. Med. Interna*, Vol.18, No. 6, pp. 326-335.

Ernst E & Pittler MH. (1999). Ginkgo Biloba for dementia: a systematic review of double-blind placebo-controlled trials. *Clinical Drug Investigation*, Vol.17, pp. 301-308.

Engelhart M.J., Geerlings MI, Ruitenberg A, van Swieten JC, Hofman A, Witteman JC, *et al*.(2002). Dietary intake of antioxidants and risk of Alzheimer disease. *JAMA*, Vol. 287, pp.3223-3229.

Esposito, E.; Rotilio, D.; Di Matteo, V.; Di Giulio, C.; Cacchio, C. & Algeri, S. (2002). A review of specific dietary antioxidants and the effects on biochemical mechanisms related to neurodegenerative processes. *Neurobiology of Aging* Vol.23, pp. 719–735.

Fahn, S. (1991) An open trial of high-dosage antioxidants in early Parkinson's disease. *American Journal of Clinical Nutrition*, Vol.53 pp.380–382.

Fang, Y.; Yanq, S. & Wu, G. (2002) Free radicals, antioxidants, and nutrition. *Nutrition*, Vol.18, No.10, pp. 872- 879, ISSN 0899-9007.

Farrell, P.M. & Roberts, R.J. (1994) Vitamin E. In: Modern nutrition in health and disease, Shils ME, Olson JA, Shike M, eds, pp.326–341. Philadelphia.

Floyd, R.A & Carney, J.M. (1992) Free radical damage to protein and DNA: Mechanism involved and relevant observations on brain undergoing oxidative stress. *Annals of Neurology*, Vol.32, Suppl.S22-27

Frank, B. & Gupta, S. (2005). A review of antioxidants and Alzheimer's disease. *Ann. Clin. Psychiatry*, Vol.17, pp. 269-286.

Frautschy SA, Hu W, Kim P, Miller SA, Chu T, Harris-White ME, Cole GM (2001) Phenolic anti-inflammatory antioxidant reversal of Abetainduced cognitive deficits and neuropathology. *Neurobiol Aging*, Vol.22, pp.993–1005.

Frei, B., Stocker, R., Ames, B.N., (1988). Antioxidant defenses and lipid peroxidation in human blood plasma. *National Academy of Sciences of the United States of America*, Vol. 85, No.24, pp. 9748– 9752, ISSN 0027-8424.

Freidovich, I. (1999). Fundamental aspects of reactive oxygen species, or what's the matter with oxygen? *Annals of the New York Academy of Sciences*, Vol.893, No.1, pp. 13-18, ISSN 0077-8923.

Gallego, D.Y; Figueroa, J. & Orozco, C.A. (2010a). Síndrome de disfunción cognitiva del perro como modelo de investigación de las enfermedades neurodegenerativas del humano. *Revista de la Facultad de Medicina*, Vol.58, No.2, pp.142-154, ISSN 0120-0011.

Gallego, D.Y.; Figueroa, J. & Orozco, C. (2010b) Síndrome de Disfunción Cognitiva de Perros geriátricos. *Revista MVZ Córdoba,* Vol.15, No.3, pp.2252-2262, ISSN 0122-0268.

Gerlach, M., Ben-Shachar, D., Riederer, P. & Youdim, M.B. (1994). Altered brain metabolism of iron as a cause of neurodegenerative diseases. *Journal of Neurochemistry,* Vol.63, No.3, pp. 793-807, ISNN 1471-4159

Gilgun-Sherki, Y.; Melamed, E. & Offen, D. (2001) Oxidative stress induced-neurodegenerative diseases: the need for antioxidants that penetrate the blood brain barrier. *Neuropharmacology,* Vol.40, No.8, pp. 959-975, ISNN 0028-3908.

Glade, M. (2010). Oxidative stress and cognitive longevity. *Nutrition,* Vol.26, pp. 595–603.

Goel A, Kunnumakkara AB, Aggarwal BB. (2008). Curcumin as "Curecumin": from kitchen to clinic. *Biochem Pharmacol,* Vol.75, pp. 787-809.

Greenwald, R.A. (1990). Superoxide dismutase and catalase as therapeutic agents for human diseases: a critical review. *Free Radic. Biol. Med.* Vol.8, pp.201- 209.

Guarente, L. (2001). SIR2 and aging--the exception that proves the rule. *Trend Genet,* Vol.17, pp.391–392.

Halliwell, B. (1994). Free radicals, antioxidants, and human disease: curiosity, cause or consequence? *The Lancet,* Vol.344, No. 8924, pp. 721–724, ISSN 0140-6736.

Halliwell, B. (1997). Antioxidants: the basics — what they are and how to evaluate them. *Advances in Pharmacology,* Vol.38, pp. 3–20, ISSN ISSN: 0568-0123.

Halliwell, B. (2001). Role of free radical in the neurodegenerative diseases. *Drugs & Aging,* Vol. 18, 685-716, ISNN 1170-229X.

Han, M.K., 2003. Epigallocatechin gallate, a constituent of green tea, suppresses cytokine-induced pancreatic beta-cell damage. Exp. Mol. Med. 35, 136–139.

Hayflick, L. (1993). Theories biological Aging. *Experimental Gerontology,* Vol.20, pp.145-159, ISSN 0531-5565.

Head, E.; Liu, J.; Hagen, T.M.; Muggenburg, B.A.; Milgram, N.W. et al. (2002). Oxidative damage increases with age in a canine model of; human brain aging. Journal of Neurochemistry, Vol.82, No.2, pp.375–81.

Hellenbrand W, Boeing H, Robra B-P, Seidler A, Vieregge P, Nischan P, et al. (1996). Diet and Parkinson's disease II: a possible role for the past intake of specific nutrients. *Neurology,* Vol.47, pp.644–50.

Heo, H.J. & Lee, C.Y. (2004). Protective effects of quercetin and vitamin C against oxidative stress-induced neurodegeneration. *J. Agric. Food Chem,* Vol.52, pp.7514-7517.

Hou, R.R.; Chen, J.Z.; Chen, H.; Kang, X.G.; Li, M.G. & Wang, B.R. (2008). Neuroprotective effects of (-)-epigallocatechin-3-gallate (EGCG) on paraquat-induced apoptosis in PC12 cells. *Cell Biol.Int,* Vol.32, pp. 22-30.

Hyman, B.T.; Van Horsen, G.W.; Damasio, A. R. & Barnes, C.L. (1984). Alzheimer's disease: cell-specific pathology isolates the hippocampal formation. *Science,* Vol.225, No.4667, pp.168–1170, ISSN 1095-9203.

Izumi, Y.; Sawada, H.; Sakka, N.; Yamamoto, N.; Kume, T.; Katsuki, H.; Shimohama, S. & Akaike, A. (2005). p-Quinone mediates 6-hydroxydopamine-induced dopaminergic neuronal death and ferrous iron accelerates the conversion of p-quinone into melanin extracellularly. *J. Neurosci. Res,* Vol.79, pp.849-860.

James JA, Shukitt-Hale B, Denisova NA, Bielinski D, Martin A, McEwen JJ. & Bickford PC. (1999). Reversals of age-related declines in neuronal signal transduction, cognitive, and motor behavioral deficits with blueberry, spinach, or strawberry dietary supplementation. *J Neurosci,* Vol.19, pp.8114 - 8121.

Jang, J.H. & Surh, Y.J. (2003). Protective effect of resveratrol on beta-amyloidinduced oxidative PC12 cell death. *Free Radic. Biol. Med*, Vol.34, pp. 1100–1110.

Johnson, E.M. (1994).Possible role of neuronal apoptosis in Alzheimer's disease. *Neurobiol Aging*, Vol.2, pp.S187–189.

Joseph, J.A.; Denisova, N.; Fisher, D.; Bickford, P.; Prior, R. & Cao, G. (1998). Agerelated neurodegeneration and oxidative stress: putative nutritional intervention. *Neurology Clinical*, Vol.16, No.3, pp.747–755.

Juliano, L., Pedersen, J.Z., Rotilio, G., Ferro, D., Violi, F. (1995). A potent chain-breaking antioxidant activity of the cardiovascular drug dipyridamole. *Free Radic. Biol. Med.*, Vol.18, pp. 239- 247.

Kagan, V.E. & Tyurina, Y. (1998). Recycling and Redox Cycling of phenolic Antioxidants. Ann N Y Acad Sci., Vol.20, No.854, pp.425-34.

Kalaria, R.N.; Maestre, G.E.; Arizaga, R.; Friedland, R.P.; Galasko, D.; Hall, K.; Luchsinger, J.A.; Ogunniyi, A.; Perry, E.K.; Potocnik, F.; Prince, M.; Stewart, R.; Wimo, A.; Zhang, Z.X. & Antuono, P. (2008). Alzheimer's disease and vascular dementia in developing countries: prevalence, management, and risk factors. *Lancet Neurol*ogy, Vol.7, pp.812–826.

Kamphuisa, J. & Scheltensb, P. (2010). Can Nutrients Prevent or Delay Onset of Alzheimer's Disease?. *Journal of Alzheimer's Disease*, Vol.20, pp.765–775, ISSN 1387-2877

Karuppagounder SS, Pinto JT, Xu H, Chen HL, Beal MF & Gibson GE. (2008). Dietary supplementation with resveratrol reduces plaque pathology in a transgenic model of Alzheimer's disease. *Neurochem Int,* Vol.54, pp.111–118.

Kedar, N.P. (2003). Can we prevent Parkinson's and Alzheimer's disease. *J Postgrad Med,* Vol.49, pp.236–245.

Kelsey, N.; Wilkins, H. & Linseman, D. (2010). Nutraceutical Antioxidants as Novel Neuroprotective Agents. Molecules, Vol.15, No.11, pp. 7792-7814, ISSN 1420-3049.

Kiziltepe U, Turan NN, Han U, Ulus AT. & Akar F. (2004). Resveratrol, a red wine polyphenol, protects spinal cord from ischemia-reperfusion injury. *J Vasc Surg* , Vol.40, pp.138-45.

Kontush A.; Mann U, Arlt S, Ujeyl A, Luhrs C, Muller-Thomsen T, *et al.* (2001). Influence of vitamin E and C supplementation on lipoprotein oxidation in patients with Alzheimer's disease. *Free Radic Biol Med*, Vol.31, pp.345-354.

Kontush, K. & Schekatolina, S. (2004). Vitamin E in neurodegenerative disorders: Alzheimer's disease. *Ann N Y Acad Sci*, Vol.1031, pp.249–262.

Kumar A & Singh A. (2008). Possible nitric oxide modulation in protective effect of Curcumin (*Curcuminlonga,* Zingiberaceae) against sleep pdeprivation induced behavioural alterations and oxidative damage in mice. *Phytomedicine,* Vol.15, pp.577–586.

Landsberg, G. (2005). Therapeutic agents for the treatmen of cognitive dusfunction syndrome in senior dogs. *Prog Neuropsychopharmacol Biol Psychiatry,* Vol.29, No.3, pp.471-479.

Leibson, C.L.; Rocca, W.A.; Hanson, A.; Cha, R.; Kokmen, E.; O'Brien, P.C. & Palumbo PJ. (1997). The risk of dementia among persons with diabetes mellitus: a population-based cohort study. *Annals of the New York Academy of Sciences, Vol.*826, pp.422–427.

Levites, Y., Weinreb, O., Maor, G., Youdim, M.B. & Mandel, S. (2001). Green tea polyphenol (−)-epigallocatechin-3-gallate prevents N-methyl-4-phenyl-1,2,3,6-

tetrahydropyridine-induced dopaminergic neurodegeneration. *J. Neurochem*, Vol.78, pp.1073–1082.

Levites, Y., Amit, T., Youdim, M.B. & Mandel, S. (2002). Involvement of protein kinase C activation and cell survival/cell cycle genes in green tea polyphenol (−)-epigallocatechin 3-gallate neuroprotective action. *J. Biol. Chem*, Vol. 277, pp.30574–30580.

Li, L., Carter, J., Gao, X., Whitehead, J., Tourtellotte, W.G. (2005). The neuroplasticity-associated arc gene is a direct transcriptional target of early growth response (Egr) transcription factors. *Mol. Cell Biol*, Vol.25, pp. 10286–10300.

Lim GP, Chu T, Yang F, Beech W, Frautschy SA, Cole GM. (2001).The curry spice curcumin reduces oxidative damage and amyloid pathology in an Alzheimer transgenic mouse. *J Neurosci*, Vol.21, pp.8370-8377.

Lindsay, J., Laurin, D., Verreault, R., Hebert, R., Helliwell, B., Hill, G.B., McDowell, I. (2002). Risk factors for Alzheimer's disease: a prospective analysis from the Canadian Study of Health and Aging. *Am. J. Epidemiol*, Vol.156, pp. 445–453.

Luo Y, Smith JV, Paramasivam V, Burdick A, Curry KJ, Buford JP, et al. (2002). Inhibition of amyloid-beta aggregation and caspase-3 activation by the Ginkgo biloba extract EGb761. *Proc Natl Acad Sci USA*, Vol.99, pp.12197-202.

Mandel, S.; Gr ¨ unblatt, E.; Riederer, P.; Gerlach, M.; Levites, Y. & Youdim, M. (2003). Neuroprotective Strategies in Parkinson's Disease An Update on Progress. *CNS Drugs*, Vol.17, No10, pp.729-762.

Mandel, S. & Youdim, M.B. (2004). Catechin polyphenols: neurodegeneration and neuroprotection in neurodegenerative diseases. *Free Radic Biol Med*, Vol.37, pp.304-17.

Marambaud, P.; Zhao, H. & Davies, P. (2005). Resveratrol promotes clearance of Alzheimer's disease amyloid-beta peptides. *J Biol Chem*, Vol.280, No.45, pp.37377-82.

Marcocci L, Maguire JJ, Droy-Lefaix MT. & Packer L. (1994). The nitric oxide-scavenging properties of *G. biloba* extract EGb 761. *Biochem Biophys Res Commun*, Vol.201, pp.748–55.

Martin, A.; Janigian, D.; Shukitt-Hale, B., et al. Effect of vitamin E intake on levels of vitamins E and C in the central nervous system and peripheral tissues: implications for health recommendations. *Brain Res*, Vol.845, No.1, pp.50-59

Martínez, J.; Boll-Woehrlen, C.; Hernández, A.; Rubio, M.; Sánchez, M.; Ríos, C. & Pérez, F. (2010). Radicales libres y estrés oxidativo en las enfermedades neurodegenerativas. *Mensaje Bioquímico*, Vol.34, pp. 43-59, ISSN -0188-137X.

Martinez, M.; Hernandez, A.I. & Martinez. (2000). N-acetylcysteine delays age-associated memory impairment in mice: role in synaptic mitochondria. *Brain Research, Vol.855, No.1, pp.* 100-106, ISSN 00068993

Masaki, K.H., White, L.R. & Petrovich, H. (1994) The influence of prior and concurrent use of aspirin and vitamins on cognitive function scores in elderly Japanese-American men. Fourth International Conference on Alzheimer's disease and Related disorders", Neurobiology of Aging 15, S1, Fourth International Conference on Alzheimer's disease and Related disorders.

Maurer K, Ihl R, Dierks T, Frölich L. (1997). Clinical efficacy of *G. biloba* special extract EGb 761 in dementia of the Alzheimer type. *J Psychiat Res*, Vol.31, pp.645–55.

Mazzio, E.; Close, F. & Soliman K. (2011). The Biochemical and Cellular Basis for Nutraceutical Strategies to Attenuate Neurodegeneration in Parkinson's Disease *Int. J. Mol. Sci*, Vol.12, pp.506-569

McCaddon, Homocysteine and cognitive impairment; a case series in a General Practice setting, Nutr J 5 (2006), 6.

McCay, P.B. (1985). Vitamin E: interactions with free radicals and ascorbate. *Annu Rev Nutr*, Vol.5, pp. 322-40.

Meydani, M.; Lipman, R.D.; Han, S.N.; Wu, D.; Eharka, A.; Martin, K.R.; Brosnson, R.L., Cao, G.; Smith, D. & Meydani, S.N. (1998). The Effect of Long-term Dietary Supplementation with Antioxidant. *Annals of the New York Academy of Science*, Vol.854, pp. 352–360.

Milgram, N.W.; Zicker, S.C.; Head, E.; Muggenburg, B.A.; Murphey, H.; Ikeda-Douglas, C et al. (2002). Dietary enrichment counteracts age-associated cognitive dysfunction in canines. *Neurobiology Aging*, Vol.23, pp.737–745.

Miloso, M., Bertelli, A.A., Nicolini, G. & Tredici, G. (1999). Resveratrol-induced activation of the mitogen-activated protein kinases, ERK1 and ERK2, in human neuroblastoma SH-SY5Y cells. *Neurosci. Lett*, Vol.264, pp.141–144.

Mix JA & Crews Jr WD. (2000). An examination of the efficacy of *G. biloba* extract EGb 761 on the neuropsychologic functioning of cognitively intact older adults. *J Altern Comp Med*, Vol.6, pp.219–29.

Morel, I., Lescoat, G., Cogrel, P., Sergent,O., Pasdeloup, N., Brissot, P., Cillard, P. & Cillard, J. (1993). Antioxidant and iron-chelating activities of the flavonoids catechin, quercetin and diosmetin on iron-loaded rat hepatocyte cultures. *Biochem. Pharmacol*, Vol. 45, pp.13–19.

Morris MC, Evans DA, Bienias JL, et al. (2005). Dietary folate and vitamin B12 intake and cognitive decline among communitydwelling older persons. *Arch Neurol*, Vol.62, pp.641–645.

Morris, M.C.; Evans, D.A.; Tangney, C.C.; Bienias, J.L.; Wilson, R.S.; Aggarwal, N.T. & Scherr, P.A. (2005). Relation of the tocopherol forms to incident Alzheimer disease and to cognitive change. *Am J Clin Nutr, Vol.*81, pp.508–514.

Mullie, P.; Guelinckx1, I.; Clarys, P.; Degrave, E.; Hulens, M.& Vansant1 G.(2009). Cultural, socioeconomic and nutritional determinants of functional food consumption patterns. *European Journal of Clinical Nutrition, Vol.* 63, No.11, pp.1290-1296.

Murthy, M.R.V. (2001). Coenzyme-Q and related isoprenoid compounds: biosynthesis, regulation, functions and biomedical implications. In: *Mitochondrial Ubiquinone (Coenzyme Q-10): Biochemical, Functional, Medical, and Therapeutic Aspects in Human Health and Diseases*, Chopra, R. (Eds.), Prominent Press, pp. 231– 346, Arizona.

Nanjo, F., Goto, K., Seto, R., Suzuki, M., Sakai, M. & Hara, Y. (1996). Scavenging effects of tea catechins and their derivatives on 1,1-diphenyl-2-picrylhydrazyl radical. *Free Radic. Biol. Med*, Vol.21, pp. 895–902.

Navarro, A. & Boveris, A. (2008). Brain mitochondrial dysfunction in aging. *IUBMB Life*, Vol.60, No.5, pp.308–314, ISSN 1521-6551.

Navarro, A. & Boveris, A. (2010). Brain mitochondrial dysfunction in aging, neurodegeneration, and Parkinson's disease. *Frontiers in Aging neuroscience*, Vol.2, No.34, pp.1-11, ISSN 1663-4365.

Ni Y, Zhao B, Hou J, Xin W. (1996). Preventive effect of G. *biloba* extract on apoptosis in rat cerebellar neuronal cells induced by hydroxyl radicals. *Neurosci Lett*, Vol.214, pp.115-118.

Opii, O.; Joshi, G; Head, E.; Milgram, W; Bruce, C.; Muggenburg, A.; Klein, J.; Cotmanb, c. & Butterfield, A. (2008). Proteomic identification of brain proteins in the canine model of human aging following a long-term treatment with antioxidants and a program of behavioral enrichment: Relevance to Alzheimer's disease. *Neurobiology of Aging*, Vol.29, pp. 51–70.

Orgogozo, J.M., Dartigues, J.F., Lafont, S., Letenneur, L., Commenges, D., Salamon, R., Renaud, S., Breteler, M.B. (1997). Wine consumption and dementia in the elderly: a prospective community study in the Bordeaux area. *Rev. Neurol*, Vol.153, pp. 185–192.

Ossola B, Kääriäinen TM. & Männistö, P.T. (2009). The multiple faces of quercetin in neuroprotection. *Expert Opin Drug Saf*, Vol.8, No.4, pp.397-409

Oyama Y, Chikahisa L, Ueha T, Kanemaru K, Noda K. (1996). *G. biloba* extract protects brain neurons against oxidative stress induced by hydrogen peroxide. *Brain Re*, Vol.712, pp.349-52.

Parnham, M.J.; Leyck, S. & Graf, E.E.A. (1991). The pharmacology of ebselen. *Agents Actions*, Vol.32, pp.4- 9.

Passeri, M.; Cucinotta, D.; Bonati, P.A.; Iannuccelli, M.; Parnetti, L. & Senin, U. (1990). Acetyl-L-carnitine in the treatment of mildly demented elderly patients. *Int J Clin Pharmacol Res*, Vol.10, No.1-2, pp.75-79.

Passos, J.; Nelson, G.; Wang, C.; Richter, T.; Simillion, C.; Proctor, C.; Miwa, S.; Olijslagers, S.; Hallinan, J.; Wipat, A.; Saretzki, G.; Kirkwood, T. & von Zglinicki, T. (2010). Feedback between p21 and reactive oxygen production is necessary for cell senescence. *Molecular Systems Biology*, Vol.6, No. 347, pp. 1-14, ISSN 1744-4292.

Pauls, K.P. & Thompson, J.E. (1980). In vitro simulation of senescente-related membrana damage by ozone-induced lipid peroxidation. *Nature*, Vol.283, pp. 504-6, ISSN 0028-0836.

Pav6n, N.; Vidal, L.; Blanco, L.; Á, P.; Torres A.; Lorigados, L.; Álvarez, L.; Macías, R. (1998). Factores que desencadenan la muerte neuronal en enfermedades neurodegenerativas. *Revista de Neurología*, Vol.26, No.152, pp.554-560, ISSN 0210-0010.

Pérez, A.; Abilés, J & Castaño, J. (2008). Estrés oxidativo y su implicaci6n en distintas patologías. *Nutrición clínica en Medicina*, Vol.2, No.2, pp. 45-64, ISSN 1889-1332

Peter, P.Z.; James, C.; Anthon, A.; Khachaturian, S.; Stone, V.; Deborah, G.; JoAnn, T.; Tschanz, M.C.: Norton, K.A. & John C.S.(2004) Reduced risk of Alzheimer disease in users of antioxidant vitamin supplements-The Cache County Study. *Archives of Neuroogy*, Vol.61, pp.82-88, ISSN 0375-8540.

Peterson, R.C.; Ronaldhomas, G.; Grundman, M.; Bennett, D.; Doody, R.; Ferris, S.; Galasko, D.; Jin, S.; Kaye, J.; Levey, A.; Pfeiffer, E.; Sano, M.; Christopher, H.; Dyck, V. & Thal, L.J. (2005). Vitamin E and Donepezil for the treatment of mild cognitive impairment. *The N Eng J Med*, Vol.353, pp. 2379–2388.

Pillai SR, Traber MG, Steiss JE, Kayden HJ & Cox NR (1993). Alphatocopherol concentrations of the nervous system and selected tissues of adult dogs fed three levels of vitamin E. *Lipids*, Vol. 28, pp.1101–1105.

Poon, H.F.; Calabrese, V.; Calvani, M. & Butterfield, D.A. (2006). Proteomics analyses of specific protein oxidation and protein expression in aged rat brain and its modulation by L-acetylcarnitine: Insights into the mechanisms of action of this proposed therapeutic agent for CNS disorders associated with oxidative stress. *Antioxid Redox Signal*, Vol.8, pp.381–94.

Poon, H.F.; Calabrese, V.; Calvani, M.& Butterfield, D.A.(2006). Proteomics analyses of specific protein oxidation and protein expression in aged rat brain and its modulation by L-acetylcarnitine: Insights into the mechanisms of action of this proposed therapeutic agent for CNS disorders associated with oxidative stress. *Antioxid Redox Signal*, Vol.8, pp.381–94.

Prasad, K.N.; Cole, W.C. & Kumar, B. (1999). Multiple Antioxidants in the Prevention and Treatment of Parkinson's Disease. *Journal of the American College of Nutrition*, Vol.18, No.5, pp.413–423, ISSN 0731-5724

Rahman M, Riaz M. & Desai U.R. (2001). Synthesis of biologically relevant biflavanoids--a review. *Chem Biodivers*, Vol.4, pp.2495–2527.

Rao, A.V. & Balachandran, A. (2002). Role of Oxidative Stress and Antioxidants in Neurodegenerative Diseases. *Nutritional Neuroscience*, Vol.5, No.5, pp. 291–309.

Ramacci, M.T.; De Rossi, M.; Lucreziotti, M.R.; Mione, M.C. & Amenta, F. (1998). Effect of long-term treatment with acetyl-L-carnitine on structural changes of ageing rat brain. *Drugs Exp Clin Res*, Vol.14, pp.593–601.

Ramassamy, C. (2006). Emerging role of polyphenolic compounds in the treatment of neurodegenerative diseases: A review of their intracellular targets. *European Journal of Pharmacology* , Vol.545, pp.51–64

Ramassamy, C.; Doggui, S.; Arseneault, M. & Dao, L. (2010). Towards a nutritional approach for the prevention of Alzheimer's disease: Promise of polyphenolic components. Recent Advances on Nutrition and the Prevention of Alzheimer's Disease, Ramassamy, C & Bastianetto, S (Ed), pp.1-18, ISBN: 978-81-7895-470-7

Ramsewak RS, DeWitt DL, Nair MG.(2000). Cytotoxicity, antioxidant and anti-inflammatory activities of curcumins I-III from Curcuma longa. *Phytomedicine*, Vol.7, pp.303-308

Resnick B & Junlapeeya P. (2004). Falls in a community of older adults: findings and implications for practice. *Application of Nursing Research*, Vol.17, pp.81–91.

Rezai-Zadeh, K.; Arendash, G.W.; Hou, H.; Fernandez, F.; Jensen, M.; Runfeldt, M.; Shytle, R.D. & Tan, J.(2008). Green tea epigallocatechin-3-gallate (EGCG) reduces beta-amyloid mediated cognitive impairment and modulates tau pathology in Alzheimer transgenic mice. *Brain Res*, Vol.1214, pp.177-187.

Rivas, A.S.; Colín, L.; Dorado, C. & Fortoul, T. (2001). Estrés oxidativo y neurodegeneración, In: *temas selectos de neurociencias* II, J. Velázquez (Ed.), UNAM-PUIS, México, ISBN 970-654-850-5.

Sales, I.; Rocha, A.; Barros, G.; Pinheiro, P. Ferreira, P. & Mendes, R. (2009). Oxidative stress in the hippocampus during experimental seizures can be ameliorated with the antioxidant ascorbic acid. *Oxidative Medicine and Cellular Longevity*, Vol.2, No.4, pp.214-221.

Sano M, Ernesto C, Klauber MR, Schafer K, Woodbury P, Thomas R, *et al* . (1996). Rationale and design of a multicenter study of selegilina and alpha-tocopherol in the treatment of Alzheimer disease using novel clinical outcomes. Alzheimer's Disease Cooperative Study. *Alzheimer Dis Assoc Disord*, Vol.10, pp.132-140.

Sano M, Ernesto C, Thomas RG, Klauber MR, Schafer K, Grundman M, *et al.* (1997). A controlled trial of selegiline, alphatocopherol, or both as treatment for Alzheimer's disease. The Alzheimer's Disease Cooperative Study. *N Engl J Med,* Vol.336, pp.1216-1222.

Sasaki, N.; Toda, T.; Kaneko, T.; Baba, N. & Matsuo, M. (2003). Protective effects of flavonoids on the cytotoxicity of linoleic acid hydroperoxide toward rat pheochromocytoma PC12 cells. *Chem. Biol. Interact.* Vol.145, pp.101-116.

Scalbert A, Johnson IT & Saltmarsh, M. (2005). Polyphenols: antioxidants and beyond. *Am J Clin Nutr,* Vol.81, pp.215S-7S.

Seshadri, S. & Wolf, P.A. (2003). Homocysteine and the brain: vascular risk factor or neurotoxin? *Lancet Neurol,* Vol.2, No.11

Sharman, E.H.; Vaziri, N.D.; Ni, Z.; Sharman, K.G. & Bondy, S.C. (2002). Reversal of biochemical and behavioral parameters of brain aging by melatonin and acetyl L-carnitine. *Brain Res,* Vol.957, pp. 223–30.

Silva, J.P.; Gomes, A.C. & Coutinho, O.P. (2008). Oxidative DNA damage protection and repair by polyphenolic compounds in PC12 cells. *Eur. J. Pharmacol,* Vol.601, pp.50-60.

Sohal, R.S. (1993). The free radical hypothesis of aging: an appraisal of the current status. *Aging Clinical and Experimental Research,* Vol.5, No.1, pp.3-17, ISSN 1594-0667.

Sun, A.; Wang, Q.; Simonyi, A.. & Sun, G. (2008). Botanical phenolics and brain health. *Neuromolecular Medicine,* Vol.10, No.4, pp, 259–274.

Sung S, Yao Y, Uryu K, Yang H, Lee VM, Trojanowski JQ, *et al.* (2004). Early vitamin E supplementation in young but not aged mice reduces Abeta levelsand amyloid deposition in a transgenic model of Alzheimer's disease. *FASEB J,* Vol.18, pp.323-5.

Tamura, M.; Kagawa, S.; Tsuruo, Y.; Ishimura, K.& Morita, K. (1994). Effects of flavonoid compounds on the activity of NADPH diaphorase prepared from the mouse brain. *Jpn. J. Pharmacol,* Vol.65, pp. 371–373.

Terry, R.D.; Masliah, E.; Salmon, D.P.; Butters, N.; DeTeresa, R.; Hill, R.; Hansen, L.A. & Katzman, R. (1991). Physical basis of cognitive alterations in Alzheimer's disease: synapse loss is the major correlate of cognitive impairment. *Annals of Neurolology,* Vol.30, No.4, pp. 572–580, ISSN 0364-5134.

Truelsen, T., Thudium, D., Gronbaek, M. (2002). Amount and type of alcohol and risk of dementia: the Copenhagen City Heart Study. *Neurology,* Vol.59, pp.1313–1319.

Tucker KL, Qiao N, Scott T, et al. (2005). High homocysteine and low B vitamins predict cognitive decline in aging men: the Veterans Affairs Normative Aging Study. *Am J Clin Nutr,* Vol.82, pp.627–35.

Valko, M.; Leibfritz, D.; Moncola, J.; Cronin, M.; Mazura, M. & Telser, J. (2007). Free radicals and antioxidants in normal physiological functions and human disease. *The International Journal of Biochemistry & Cell Biology, Vol.* 39, No.1, pp.44–84, ISSN 1357-2725.

Vatassery GT, Brin MF, Fahn S, Kayden HJ &Traber MG. (1988). Effect of high doses of dietary vitamin E on the concentrations of vitamin E in several brain regions, plasma, liver, and adipose tissue of rats. *J Neurochem,* Vol.51, pp.621–623.

Vermeer, S.E.; Prins, N.D.; denHeijer, T.; Hofman, A.; Koudstaal, P.J. & Breteler, M.M. (2003). Silent brain infarcts and the risk of dementia and cognitive decline. *New England Journal of Medicine,* Vol.3, No.348, pp.1215–1222, ISSN 1533-4406.

Viant, D.; Fonseca, C. & Ileana, C. (1999). Radicales libres y su papel en la homeostasia neuronal. *MEDISAN*, Vol.3, No3, pp. 5-11, ISSN 1029-3019

Virgili M & Contestabile A. (2000). Partial neuroprotection of in vivo excitotoxic brain damage by chronic administration of the red wine antioxidant agent, trans-resveratrol in rats. *Neurosci Lett*, Vol.281, pp.123-6.

Wang HX, Wahlin A, Basun H, et al. (2001). Vitamin B(12) and folate in relation to the development of Alzheimer's disease. *Neurology*, Vol.56, pp.1188–94.

Weinreb, O.; Mandel, S.; Amit, T. & Youdim, M.B. (2004). Neurological mechanisms of green tea polyphenols in Alzheimer's and Parkinson's diseases. *J. Nutr. Biochem*, Vol.15, pp.506-516.

Witschi. A.; Reddy, S.; Stofer, B. & Lauterburg, B.H. (1992). The systemic availability of oral glutathione. European Journal of Clinical Pharmacology, Vol.43, pp.667–669.

Xin W, Wei T, Chen C, Ni Y, Zhao B, Hou J. (2000). Mechanisms of apoptosis in rat cerebellar granule cells induced by hydroxyl radicals and the effects of EGb 761 and its constituents. *Toxicology*, Vol.148, pp.103–10.

Yao Z, Drieu K & Papadopoulos V. (2001). The Ginkgo biloba extract EGb 761 rescues the PC12 neuronal cells from beta-amyloid-induced cell death by inhibiting the formation of beta-amyloid-derived diffusible neurotoxic ligands. *Brain Res*, Vol.889, pp.181-90.

Zandi PP, Anthony JC, Khachaturian AS, Stone SV, Gustafson D, Tschanz JT, et al. (2004). Reduced risk of Alzheimer disease in users of antioxidant vitamin supplements: the Cache County Study. *Arch Neurol*, Vol.61, No.1, pp. 82-8

Zhao, W., Richardson, J.S., Mombourquette, M.J. & Weil, J.A. (1995). An in vitro EPR study of the free-radical scavenging actions of the lazaroid antioxidants U-74500A and U-78517F. *Free Radic. Biol. Med.*, Vol.19, pp.21– 30.

Zimmermann, A.K.; Loucks, F.A.; Schroeder, E.K.; Bouchard, R.J.; Tyler, K.L. & Linseman, D.A. (2007). Glutathione binding to the Bcl-2 homology-3 domain groove: a molecular basis for Bcl-2 antioxidant function at mitochondria. *J. Biol. Chem*, Vol.282, pp.29296-29304.

Part 3

Intracellular Signaling of Neurodegeneration

8

Neuropathological Disorders and Calcium Independent Forms of Phospholipase A_2 Activities in the Brain

Julie Allyson and Guy Massicotte
Université du Québec à Trois-Rivières
Trois-Rivières, Québec,
Canada

1. Introduction

Phospholipases A_2 (PLA_2s) constitute a large and diverse group of enzymes with broad biological functions, ranging from membrane synthesis and turnover to the generation of signaling molecules. So far, more than 20 isoforms of PLA_2 presenting diverse characteristics, including calcium requirement and subcellular localization, have been documented. Based on their nucleotide sequence and other properties, PLA_2 enzymes have been categorized into 15 groups (I-XV) – according to the classification of Dennis (Burke & Dennis, 2009a, 2009b). Released by cells, several groups of PLA_2s are relatively small proteins (~14 kDa) that require millimolar amounts of calcium for their optimal activation. These groups of enzymes have historically been called the secreted forms of PLA_2 (or $sPLA_2$). The remaining groups are larger proteins, localized in intracellular compartments, which are either dependent or not on calcium ions.

The first intracellular PLA_2 to be cloned was a 85-kD protein, classified as a group IV PLA_2 (Dennis, 1997; Leslie, 1997). This enzyme, now designated as cytosolic $PLA_2\alpha$ ($cPLA_2\alpha$), is known to be under the influence of extracellular signals likely to induce calcium mobilization and phosphorylation (Leslie, 1997). Another group of PLA_2 (group VI), which does not require calcium variations for its activity, has been cloned (Balboa et al., 1997; Ma et al., 1997; Tang et al., 1997). This PLA_2 isoform has been designated as calcium-independent PLA_2 ($iPLA_2$) (Balsinde & Dennis, 1997; Dennis, 1997) and, according to numerous lines of biochemical evidence, may account for most of the PLA_2 activity detected in resting cells. From a pharmacological perspective, $iPLA_2$ activity is markedly reduced by bromoenol lactone (BEL) suicide substrate, which is not an effective inhibitor of $sPLA_2$ or $cPLA_2$ enzymes at comparable concentrations (Balboa et al., 1997; Kudo & Murakami, 2002). Several interesting reviews have considered the functional and pathological implications of PLA_2 enzymes (Balsinde & Balboa, 2005; Bazan et al., 1993; Brown et al., 2003; Farooqui & Horrocks, 2004; Farooqui et al., 2004; Hooks & Cummings, 2008; Kolko et al., 2007; Kudo & Murakami, 2002; Leslie, 2004; Phillis & O'Regan, 2004; Sun et al., 2004; Sun et al., 2005). In this report, we will describe new and unique functional roles of $iPLA_2$ in the regulation of brain glutamate receptor functions, neuronal plasticity and neurodegenerative processes.

2. $iPLA_2$ isoforms and functions

Among PLA_2 enzymes, group IV ($cPLA_2$) and group VI ($iPLA_2$) families represent intracellular enzymes with a catalytic serine in their lipase consensus motif. Various studies, including gene targeting, have indicated that group IVA $cPLA_2$ (cPLA2α), which is regulated by calcium-dependent membrane translocation and mitogen-activated protein kinase (MAPK)-dependent phosphorylation, is central in stimulus-dependent eicosanoid biosynthesis (Bonventre et al., 1997; Uozumi et al., 1997). On the other hand, group VIA $iPLA_2$ (iPLA2β) and group VIB $iPLA_2$ ($iPLA_2\gamma$) isoforms mainly exhibit PLA_2 activity, whereas other $iPLA_2$ isoforms δ, ε, ξ and η display triglyceride lipase and transacylase activities (Table 1) in marked preference to PLA_2 activity (Jenkins et al., 2004; Quistad et al., 2003). Group VIA $iPLA_2\beta$, the most extensively studied $iPLA_2$ isoform, has been implicated in various cellular events, such as phospholipid remodelling (Balsinde et al., 1997; Balsinde & Dennis, 1997), eicosanoid formation (Tay & Melendez, 2004), cell proliferation (Herbert & Walker, 2006), apoptosis (Atsumi et al., 1998), and activation of store-operated channels and capacitative calcium influx (Smani et al., 2004). Disruption of the $iPLA_2\beta$ gene causes impaired sperm motility (Bao et al., 2004), mitigated insulin secretion (Bao, Bohrer et al., 2006; Bao, Song et al., 2006) and neuronal disorders presenting iron dyshomeostasis (Morgan et al., 2006).

Group	Source	Molecular Mass (kDa)	Feature	Alternate names
VIA-1	Human/Murine	84-85	8 ankyrin repeats	$iPLA_2$
VIA-2	Human/Murine	88-90	7 ankyrin repeats	$iPLA_2\beta$
VIB	Human/Murine	88-91	Membrane-bound	$iPLA_2\gamma$
VIC	Human/Murine	146	Integral membrane protein	$iPLA_2\delta$
VID	Human	53	Acylglycerol transacylase,triglycerol lipase	$iPLA_2\varepsilon$
VIE	Human	57	Acylglycerol transacylase,triglycerol lipase	$iPLA_2\zeta$
VIF	Human	28	Acylglycerol transacylase,triglycerol lipase	$iPLA_2\eta$

Table 1. Calcium-independent group VI phospholipase A_2 ($iPLA_2$) (Adapted from (Schaloske & Dennis, 2006))

Group VIB iPLA$_{2}\gamma$ is a membrane-bound iPLA$_2$ enzyme with unique features, such as utilization of distinct translation initiation sites producing different sizes of enzymes with distinct subcellular localizations (Kinsey,McHowat,Beckett et al., 2007; Mancuso et al., 2000; Mancuso et al., 2004; Murakami et al., 2005; Tanaka et al., 2000; J. Yang et al., 2003) and phospholipid selectivity in terms of sn-1/sn-2 positional specificity that differs among substrates (Yan et al., 2005) iPLA$_{2}\gamma$ has a mitochondrial localization signal in the N-terminal region and a peroxisomal localization signal near the C-terminus, and the 88-kDa full-length and 63-kDa translation products of iPLA$_{2}\gamma$ are preferentially distributed in mitochondria and peroxisomes, respectively (Kinsey,McHowat,Beckett et al., 2007; Mancuso et al., 2004; Murakami et al., 2005). In the brain, iPLA$_2$ represents predominant phospholipase activity in cells under resting conditions (Wolf et al., 1995; H. C. Yang et al., 1999). Reverse transcription-polymerase chain reaction experiments have revealed that rat brains constitutively express messenger RNAs for at least 3 calcium-independent PLA$_2$ isoforms, iPLA$_{2}\beta$, iPLA$_{2}\gamma$ and cPLA2γ (Kinsey et al., 2005; Tang et al., 1997; Underwood et al., 1998). These isoforms are characterized by differential sensitivity to PLA$_2$ inhibitors and, by isolating each enantiomer of the iPLA$_2$ inhibitor BEL, Jenkins et al. (Jenkins et al., 2002) established that the (S)-enantiomer of BEL selectively reduces iPLA$_{2}\beta$ activity, while its (R)-enantiomer blocks the iPLA$_{2}\gamma$ isoform more efficiently.

Although little is known about iPLA$_2$ functions in neurons, a growing body of evidence suggests their involvement in hippocampal long-term potentiation (LTP) of excitatory synaptic transmission (Fujita et al., 2001; Wolf et al., 1995). Hippocampal LTP, first described by Bliss and Lomo in 1973, is commonly regarded as a functional model of synaptic adaptation (i.e. plasticity) that likely participates in learning and memory (Bliss & Collingridge, 1993). PLA$_2$ activities are increased in membranes of slices prepared from the dentate gyrus after LTP induction in anaesthetized rats (Clements et al., 1991) and could be involved in hippocampal LTP expression by elevating the production of arachidonic acid (AA) that retrogradely increases transmitter release at glutamatergic synapses (Drapeau et al., 1990; J. H. Williams et al., 1989). Facilitation of transmitter release by PLA$_2$s during LTP is also reinforced by the fact that iPLA$_2$ activity plays an important role in membrane fusion processes required for exocytosis (Brown et al., 2003; Takuma & Ichida, 1997).

The notion that iPLA$_2$ activity may facilitate LTP expression by increasing glutamate release is complicated, however, by an abundant number of reports demonstrating that synaptic potentiation, at least in area CA1 of the hippocampus, is not dependent on changes in transmitter release, but is rather mediated by mechanisms involving the up-regulation of postsynaptic responses mediated by alpha-amino-3-hydroxy-5-methyl-4-isoxazole-propionic acid (AMPA) receptors at glutamatergic synapses (Hayashi et al., 2000). Several alterations have been reported at postsynaptic sites during LTP, including faster kinetics of receptor-associated ion channels (Ambros-Ingerson & Lynch, 1993; Ambros-Ingerson et al., 1993), redistribution of existing receptors within the postsynaptic density (Xie et al., 1997) and insertion of new receptors at synapses (Lu et al., 2001; Pickard et al., 2001). Consistent with these observations, we recently demonstrated that pretreatment of hippocampal slices with the iPLA$_2$ inhibitor BEL completely abolishes AMPA receptor translocation in synaptic membranes and expression of CA1 hippocampal LTP (Martel et al., 2006). Interestingly, both LTP and AMPA receptor translocation display enantio-selective impairment by the iPLA$_{2}\gamma$ blocker (R)-BEL but not by the iPLA$_{2}\beta$ inhibitor (S)-BEL, suggesting that iPLA$_{2}\gamma$ represents the crucial isoform governing hippocampal synaptic strengthening.

$iPLA_2\gamma$ mRNAs and proteins are enriched in the endoplasmic reticulum (ER)-Golgi apparatus in several cell types (Kinsey et al., 2005), where they may be essential for diverse intracellular trafficking pathways, such as retrograde movement from the Golgi complex to the ER, transport of material from the trans-Golgi network to the plasma membrane or recycling of membrane and receptors through endocytic pathways (Brown et al., 2003). In this matter, Pechoux et al. (Pechoux et al., 2005) reported that $iPLA_2$ inhibition slowed down the transport of caseins from the ER to the Golgi apparatus and from the trans-Golgi network to the plasma membrane, indicating that $iPLA_2$ could participate in membrane trafficking events leading to the secretion of milk proteins. Interestingly, translocation of AMPA receptors originating from the ER-Golgi complex to postsynaptic membranes might be critically involved in LTP (Broutman & Baudry, 2001). Thus, the $iPLA_2\gamma$ isoform may be well-suited to favour AMPA receptor translocation from intracellular pools to synaptic membranes during LTP.

Interestingly, impairment in synaptic plasticity by PLA_2 inhibition is correlated with loss of animal abilities to perform on memory tasks. For instance, intracerebral injection of wide-spectrum PLA_2 inhibitors into the chick intermediate medial hyperstriatum ventrale curbs the learning of a passive avoidance task (Holscher & Rose, 1994), while intraperitoneal injections in rats impede spatial learning tested in the Morris water maze (Holscher et al., 1995). Additionally, intracerebroventricular injection of specific $iPLA_2$ inhibitors 30 min before a learning session impairs spatial working memory in rodents (Fujita et al., 2000). Acquisition of 1-trial step-down inhibitory avoidance in rats correlates with $iPLA_2$ activity in the hippocampus, and bilateral injection of $iPLA_2$ inhibitors in region CA1 of the dorsal hippocampus prior to training hinders both short-term and long-term memory (Schaeffer & Gattaz, 2005). Hence, intact $iPLA_2$ activity seems important for proper acquisition of new memories. In a modified protocol developed to test memory retrieval, the same group recently showed that injection of the dual $cPLA_2$ and $iPLA_2$ inhibitor palmitoyl trifluoromethylketone in region CA1 of the rat dorsal hippocampus before performance testing impaired trained behavior in the step-down inhibitory avoidance task (Schaeffer & Gattaz, 2007). Importantly, memory retrieval was re-established after recovery of PLA_2 activity, indicating that these PLA_2s are indeed necessary for memory retrieval. However, identification of $iPLA_2$ isoforms in memory acquisition and retrieval remains to be addressed.

3. $iPLA_2$ and neuronal cell death mechanisms

Recently, evidence from non-neuronal cells has suggested that $iPLA_2$ enzymes may have diverse effects on cell death. First, constitutive $iPLA_2$ activity may contribute to cell death since $iPLA_2\beta$ overexpression amplifies thapsigargin-induced apoptosis in INS-1 insulinoma cells (Ramanadham et al., 2004) and accelerates U937 cell death after long-term exposure to hydrogen peroxide (Perez et al., 2004). $iPLA_2$ has been shown to play a pivotal role in oxidant damage of astrocytes (Xu et al., 2003), and its blockade by BEL dampens oligomeric amyloid-beta (Aβ1-42-induced mitochondrial membrane potential loss and reactive oxygen species production in these cells (Zhu et al., 2006). Moreover, $iPLA_2$ inhibition reduces the size of infarcts produced by global ischemia (S. D. Williams & Gottlieb, 2002). On the other hand, $iPLA_2$ activity has also been shown to protect against cell death, as inhibition of $iPLA_2$ accentuates oxidant-induced cell death in renal proximal tubule cells and astrocytes (Cummings et al., 2002; Peterson et al., 2007). Likewise, $iPLA_2$ activity may also have deleterious or beneficial effects on neurons. For instance, acute inhibition of $iPLA_2$ activity by racemic BEL has been found to be neuroprotective in organotypic hippocampal slices exposed to oxygen-glucose deprivation (Strokin et al., 2006). In contrast, immature cultures of primary cortical neurons exposed for several days to BEL show decreased neuritogenesis and cellular viability (Forlenza et al., 2007; Mendes et al., 2005). Moreover, $iPLA_2\beta$ knockout mice exhibit abnormal motor behaviors accompanied by the appearance of vacuoles and ubiquitin-positive axonal swelling (spheroids) in many brain regions (Malik et al., 2008; Shinzawa et al., 2008), suggesting that $iPLA_2\beta$ dysfunction leads to neuroaxonal dystrophy.

While the reported impact of $iPLA_2$ on cell viablility is mostly attributable to $iPLA_2\beta$, involvement of the $iPLA_2\gamma$ isoform is much less understood. A previous report demonstrated that $iPLA_2\gamma$ localized in mitochondria catalyzes AA liberation that mediates mitochondrial permeability transition, a key control point for apoptosis (Kinsey,McHowat,Patrick et al., 2007). On the other hand, $iPLA_2\gamma$ expression may exert cytoprotective effects during complement-mediated glomerular epithelial cell injury (Cohen et al., 2008). In addition, recent findings from our laboratory have revealed that constitutive $iPLA_2\gamma$ activity might represent an important neuroprotective system capable of limiting brain excitotoxic damage. We have shown that inhibition of $iPLA_2\gamma$ by the enantio-specific inhibitor (R)-BEL makes hippocampal slice cultures more vulnerable to AMPA-mediated excitotoxicity (Menard et al., 2007). Overactivation of N-methyl-D-aspartic acid (NMDA) or AMPA glutamatergic receptors, allowing the entry of high cation levels into cells, activates a number of enzymes, including ATPases, lipases, proteases and endonucleases that, in turn, deplete energy stores or damage cell membranes, cytoarchitecture or nucleus, respectively. Excitotoxicity has been reported to contribute to a variety of neuropathological disorders, including ischemic stroke, epilepsy, amyotrophic lateral sclerosis and Alzheimer's disease (AD) (Kwak & Weiss, 2006; Villmann & Becker, 2007).

Interestingly, the harmful effect of $iPLA_2\gamma$ inhibition on AMPA-mediated toxicity is associated with selective up-regulation of AMPA receptor GluR1 subunit (but not GluR2) phosphorylation with a subsequently increased level in synaptic membrane fractions (Menard et al., 2007; Menard et al., 2005; Villmann & Becker, 2007). In the hippocampus, AMPA receptors generally form heterodimers containing 2 copies of each of the GluR1 and GluR2 subunits. It is now well-recognized that GluR2 subunits render AMPA receptors impermeable to calcium. Consequently, its presence or absence plays a critical role in cellular calcium homeostasis and in determining susceptibility to excitotoxicity (Geiger et al., 1995; Sommer et al., 1991). Hence, the reduction of $iPLA_2\gamma$ activity, by promoting surface expression of the GluR1 subunit over the GluR2 subunit (which is reflected by a rise in the GluR1/GluR2 ratio in the membrane fraction), could exacerbate excitotoxic cell death through the formation of GluR2-lacking AMPA receptors that would allow adverse Ca2+ influx upon prolonged AMPA receptor activation. Consistent with this possibility, the greater cell death observed under $iPLA_2\gamma$ inhibition is prevented by GluR2-lacking AMPA receptor antagonists (Menard et al., 2007). How inhibition of $iPLA_2\gamma$ influences the expression of AMPA receptor subtypes in synaptic membranes remains an open question. As mentioned earlier, this may occur by the sorting of protein transport through intracellular secretory pathways (Pechoux et al., 2005). There are other circumstances in which GluR1 subunits are selectively up-regulated in hippocampal neurons, such as after activity deprivation elicited by prolonged blockade of AMPA receptors (Thiagarajan et al., 2005) or tumor necrosis factor-alpha receptor activation (Stellwagen et al., 2005). In the latter case, it has been proposed that up-regulation of GluR1 homomeric receptors could derive from a reserve pool of non-GluR2-containing AMPA receptors existing near the membrane.

4. $iPLA_2$ dysfunction and neuropathological disorders

Whereas $cPLA_2$ and $sPLA_2$ are commonly believed to be preferentially involved in AA release, emerging evidence indicates that $iPLA_2$ activity can contribute to docosahexaenoic acid (DHA) release from brain phospholipids (J. T. Green et al., 2008). To our knowledge, the first suggestion that brain $iPLA_2$ activity may be crucial for DHA release came from a study by Strokin et al. (Strokin et al., 2003) who showed that racemic BEL inhibited DHA release from astrocytes. Later, using siRNA silencing procedures, the same group demonstrated that DHA release from phospholipids of astrocytes was mainly dependent on $iPLA_{2}\gamma$ activity (Strokin et al., 2007). DHA is one of the most abundant omega-3 polyunsaturated fatty acids (PUFA) present in phospholipids of the mammalian brain (Glomset, 2006), where it is recognized to be important for the maintenance of neural membranes and brain function integrity (Youdim et al., 2000). Deficient dietary intake of DHA has been associated with lower performance of learning abilities in rodents (Catalan et al., 2002; Fedorova & Salem, 2006; Takeuchi et al., 2002). On the other hand, DHA dietary supplementation could decrease the risk of developing AD (Calon & Cole, 2007; Calon et al., 2005; Calon et al., 2004) or exert neuroprotective actions in a mouse model presenting numerous aspects of Parkinson's disease (Bousquet et al., 2008), while high-fat consumption combined with low omega-3 PUFA intake promotes AD-like neuropathology (Julien et al., 2008).

Both $iPLA_2$ activity and DHA levels have been reported to be decreased in the plasma of AD patients (Conquer et al., 2000; Gattaz et al., 2004). $iPLA_2$ activity is also lower in AD brains (Ross et al., 1999; Talbot et al., 2000). Whether or not decreased $iPLA_{2}\gamma$ activity, through its capacity to alter DHA release from brain astrocytes, is a factor that contributes to AD pathology remains to be established. Numerous neurobiological studies have demonstrated that DHA may be acting at different fundamental levels to counteract the cellular manifestations of AD. There are, for instance, strong indications that DHA release in the brain may diminish oxidative stress (Wu et al., 2004; Yavin et al., 2002) and glutamate-induced toxicity (Wang et al., 2003). In this line, DHA-induced reduction of excitotoxic damage in the hippocampus might, in fact, be dependent on internalization of AMPA receptors (Menard et al., 2009). The potential ability of DHA to reduce caspase activation (Calon et al., 2005; Calon et al., 2004), Aβ peptide accumulation and tau hyperphosphorylation (K. N. Green et al., 2007; Oksman et al., 2006) also strongly supports the notion that DHA deficiency, through $iPLA_2$ down-regulation, could represent a precursor event that likely initiates the cellular manifestations of AD pathology.

This has been the premise of our recent investigation on the influence of $iPLA_2$ inhibition on microtubule-associated protein tau phosphorylation. We determined whether $iPLA_2$ blockade could contribute to the development of tau hyperphosphorylation in cultured hippocampal slices from transgenic P301L mice expressing human tau. In this experimental model, treatment for up to 12 h with the specific $iPLA_{2}\gamma$ inhibitor (R)-BEL resulted in significantly increased tau phosphorylation at Thr231, Ser199/202 and Ser404 sites, and in total tau levels. High-resolution imaging studies have demonstrated that hyperphosphorylation is primarily localized in cell bodies and dendrites of hippocampal pyramidal neurons (Fig. 1).

These changes appear to be associated with up-regulation of P25, an activator of cyclin-dependent kinase 5, and phosphorylation/activation of MAPK. These data provide strong evidence that constitutive iPLA$_{2}\gamma$ activity is important in the regulation of tau hyperphosphorylation in hippocampal pyramidal neurons, raising the possibility that iPLA$_2$ dysfunctions might contribute to the development of tauopathies in AD. In this line, a putative biochemical model that accounts for the potential influence of iPLA$_{2}\gamma$ on Tau pathology is represented in Figure 2

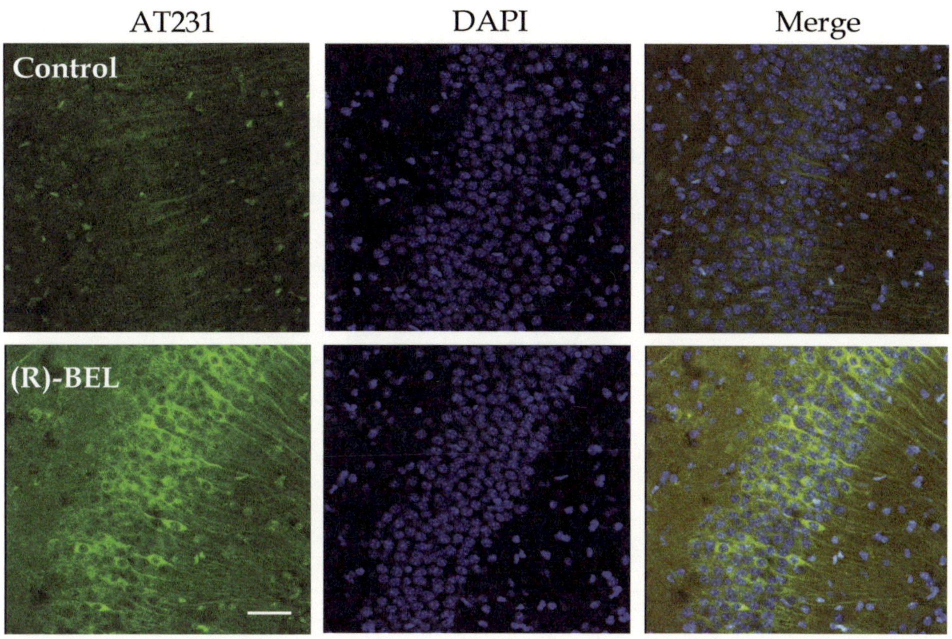

Fig. 1. Inhibition of iPLA$_{2}\gamma$ induces Tau phosphorylation in area CA1 of the hippocampus. Cultured hippocampal slices from P301L tau transgenic mice were pre-exposed to the iPLA$_{2}\gamma$ inhibitor R-BEL. Slices were then processed for confocal immunofluorescence microscopy with an antibody known to recognize the Thr-231 Tau epitope (AT231, in green). When compared to controls (upper panel), immunostaining revealed increased phosphorylation in the CA1 region of cultured hippocampal slices pre-exposed to 3 μM (R)-BEL for a period of 12 h (lower panel). DAPI (in blue) was included in the mounting medium to label nuclei. Scale bar = 25 μm

One of the central hypotheses underlying the pathophysiology of AD is the production of cytotoxic Aβ peptides that impairs neuronal activity and leads to a decline in memory and cognition (Palop et al., 2006). The exact mechanisms by which Aβ peptides contribute to AD pathogenesis remain uncertain. PLA$_2$ enzymes may be involved in this condition, as Aβ peptides accentuate cPLA$_{2}\alpha$ activity in neuronal cultures (Zhu et al., 2006) and primary cortical astrocytes (Sanchez-Mejia et al., 2008), while Aβ-induced learning and memory deficits in a transgenic mouse model of AD are prevented after genetic ablation of cPLA$_{2}\alpha$ activity in the brain (Sanchez-Mejia et al., 2008). Regarding the iPLA$_2$ system, it appears that its activity is essential for maintaining membrane phospholipid integrity by reducing peroxidative damage, especially injuries originating in the mitochondria. In this regard, $iPLA_2$ expression prevents the loss of mitochondrial membrane potential and attenuates the release of cytochrome c as well as apoptotic proteins, and ultimately diminishes apoptosis in INS-1 cells exposed to staurosporine (Seleznev et al., 2006). Furthermore, Kinsey et al. (Kinsey et al., 2008; Kinsey,McHowat,Patrick et al., 2007) reported that prominent PLA_2 activity in the mitochondria of rabbit renal proximal tubular cells comes from $iPLA_2\gamma$ and is of capital importance for the prevention and repair of basal lipid peroxidation and the maintenance of mitochondrial viability. Based on recent studies, it has been proposed that Aβ-induced neurotoxicity might derive from mitochondrial defects. Indeed, in vitro experiments have shown that Aβ peptides can be internalized by cells, imported into mitochondria and ultimately elicit mitochondrial dysfunctions (Hansson Petersen et al., 2008). Given its localization, it is thus tempting to propose that $iPLA_2\gamma$ might represent an important cellular component that prevents mitochondrial dysfunctions. Experiments are required to determine whether $iPLA_2\gamma$ overexpression activity might exert protective effects against Aβ peptide-induced mitochondrial dysfunctions.

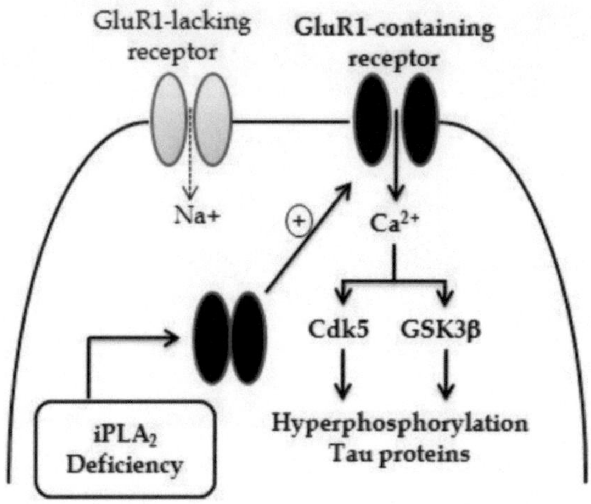

Fig. 2. A putative model illustrating the potential implication of $iPLA_2\gamma$ in Alzheimer's disease. In this simplified model, $iPLA_2$ dysfunction leads to delivery of new GluR1-containing receptors on neuronal membranes. These receptors are then inclined to induce calcium influx and, eventually, Tau phosphorylation by calcium-dependent protein kinases such as Cdk5 and GSK-3β

5. Conclusion

Besides AD, aberrant function of $iPLA_2$s has also been observed in several other neurological disorders. For instance, increased $iPLA_2$ activity might be an important factor that contributes to phospholipid abnormalities in schizophrenia or bipolar patients with a history of psychosis (Ross et al., 2006; Ross et al., 1999). However, the relationship between $iPLA_2$ up-regulation and cellular manifestations of schizophrenia requires further investigation. As mentioned earlier, because $iPLA_2\gamma$ regulates glutamate receptor subunit expression on cell membranes and functions, it will be interesting to examine whether the increase in $iPLA_2\gamma$ activity can lead to down-regulation of the AMPA receptor GluR1 subunit. This is of particular importance, since GluR1 down-regulation may evoke striatal hyperdopaminergia (Wiedholz et al., 2008), a well-established biological defect involved in schizophrenia-related behaviours. Interestingly, the relationship between $iPLA_2$s and the dopaminergic system is reinforced by the fact that $iPLA_2$ inhibition or knockdown in the rat striatum, motor cortex and thalamus results in the apparition of Parkinson-related behaviours (Lee et al., 2007), which are also known to depend on dopamine dysfunction. Thus, given the growing evidence relating the importance of $iPLA_2$s in physiological and pathological conditions, targeting $iPLA_2$ activity may represent a potentially new therapeutic strategy against several neurological disorders.

6. References

Ambros-Ingerson, J., & Lynch, G. (1993). Channel gating kinetics and synaptic efficacy: a hypothesis for expression of long-term potentiation. *Proc Natl Acad Sci U S A,* Vol. 90, No. 16, pp.7903-7907.

Ambros-Ingerson, J., Xiao, P., Larson, J., & Lynch, G. (1993). Waveform analysis suggests that LTP alters the kinetics of synaptic receptor channels. *Brain Res,* Vol. 620, No. 2, pp.237-244.

Atsumi, G., Tajima, M., Hadano, A., Nakatani, Y., Murakami, M., & Kudo, I. (1998). Fas-induced arachidonic acid release is mediated by Ca2+-independent phospholipase A2 but not cytosolic phospholipase A2, which undergoes proteolytic inactivation. *J Biol Chem,* Vol. 273, No. 22, pp.13870-13877.

Balboa, M. A., Balsinde, J., Jones, S. S., & Dennis, E. A. (1997). Identity between the Ca2+-independent phospholipase A2 enzymes from P388D1 macrophages and Chinese hamster ovary cells. *J Biol Chem,* Vol. 272, No. 13, pp.8576-8580.

Balsinde, J., & Balboa, M. A. (2005). Cellular regulation and proposed biological functions of group VIA calcium-independent phospholipase A2 in activated cells. *Cell Signal,* Vol. 17, No. 9, pp.1052-1062.

Balsinde, J., Balboa, M. A., & Dennis, E. A. (1997). Antisense inhibition of group VI Ca2+-independent phospholipase A2 blocks phospholipid fatty acid remodeling in murine P388D1 macrophages. *J Biol Chem,* Vol. 272, No. 46, pp.29317-29321.

Balsinde, J., & Dennis, E. A. (1997). Function and inhibition of intracellular calcium-independent phospholipase A2. *J Biol Chem,* Vol. 272, No. 26, pp.16069-16072.

Bao, S., Bohrer, A., Ramanadham, S., Jin, W., Zhang, S., & Turk, J. (2006). Effects of stable suppression of Group VIA phospholipase A2 expression on phospholipid content and composition, insulin secretion, and proliferation of INS-1 insulinoma cells. *J Biol Chem,* Vol. 281, No. 1, pp.187-198.

Bao, S., Miller, D. J., Ma, Z., Wohltmann, M., Eng, G., Ramanadham, S., et al. (2004). Male mice that do not express group VIA phospholipase A2 produce spermatozoa with impaired motility and have greatly reduced fertility. *J Biol Chem,* Vol. 279, No. 37, pp.38194-38200.

Bao, S., Song, H., Wohltmann, M., Ramanadham, S., Jin, W., Bohrer, A., et al. (2006). Insulin secretory responses and phospholipid composition of pancreatic islets from mice that do not express Group VIA phospholipase A2 and effects of metabolic stress on glucose homeostasis. *J Biol Chem,* Vol. 281, No. 30, pp.20958-20973.

Bazan, N. G., Allan, G., & Rodriguez de Turco, E. B. (1993). Role of phospholipase A2 and membrane-derived lipid second messengers in membrane function and transcriptional activation of genes: implications in cerebral ischemia and neuronal excitability. *Prog Brain Res,* Vol. 96, pp.247-257.

Bliss, T. V., & Collingridge, G. L. (1993). A synaptic model of memory: long-term potentiation in the hippocampus. *Nature,*Vol. 361, No. 6407, pp.31-39.

Bonventre, J. V., Huang, Z., Taheri, M. R., O'Leary, E., Li, E., Moskowitz, M. A., et al. (1997). Reduced fertility and postischaemic brain injury in mice deficient in cytosolic phospholipase A2. *Nature,*Vol. 390, No. 6660, pp.622-625.

Bousquet, M., Saint-Pierre, M., Julien, C., Salem, N., Jr., Cicchetti, F., & Calon, F. (2008). Beneficial effects of dietary omega-3 polyunsaturated fatty acid on toxin-induced neuronal degeneration in an animal model of Parkinson's disease. *FASEB J,*Vol. 22, No. 4, pp.1213-1225.

Broutman, G., & Baudry, M. (2001). Involvement of the secretory pathway for AMPA receptors in NMDA-induced potentiation in hippocampus. *J Neurosci,*Vol. 21, No. 1, pp.27-34.

Brown, W. J., Chambers, K., & Doody, A. (2003). Phospholipase A2 (PLA2) enzymes in membrane trafficking: mediators of membrane shape and function. *Traffic,*Vol. 4, No. 4, pp.214-221.

Burke, J. E., & Dennis, E. A. (2009a). Phospholipase A2 biochemistry. *Cardiovasc Drugs Ther,*Vol. 23, No. 1, pp.49-59.

Burke, J. E., & Dennis, E. A. (2009b). Phospholipase A2 structure/function, mechanism, and signaling. *J Lipid Res,*Vol. 50 Suppl, pp.S237-242.

Calon, F., & Cole, G. (2007). Neuroprotective action of omega-3 polyunsaturated fatty acids against neurodegenerative diseases: evidence from animal studies. *Prostaglandins Leukot Essent Fatty Acids,*Vol. 77, No. 5-6, pp.287-293.

Calon, F., Lim, G. P., Morihara, T., Yang, F., Ubeda, O., Salem, N., Jr., et al. (2005). Dietary n-3 polyunsaturated fatty acid depletion activates caspases and decreases NMDA receptors in the brain of a transgenic mouse model of Alzheimer's disease. *Eur J Neurosci,*Vol. 22, No. 3, pp.617-626.

Calon, F., Lim, G. P., Yang, F., Morihara, T., Teter, B., Ubeda, O., et al. (2004). Docosahexaenoic acid protects from dendritic pathology in an Alzheimer's disease mouse model. *Neuron,*Vol. 43, No. 5, pp.633-645.

Catalan, J., Moriguchi, T., Slotnick, B., Murthy, M., Greiner, R. S., & Salem, N., Jr. (2002). Cognitive deficits in docosahexaenoic acid-deficient rats. *Behav Neurosci,*Vol. 116, No. 6, pp.1022-1031.

Clements, M. P., Bliss, T. V., & Lynch, M. A. (1991). Increase in arachidonic acid concentration in a postsynaptic membrane fraction following the induction of long-term potentiation in the dentate gyrus. *Neuroscience,*Vol. 45, No. 2, pp.379-389.

Cohen, D., Papillon, J., Aoudjit, L., Li, H., Cybulsky, A. V., & Takano, T. (2008). Role of calcium-independent phospholipase A2 in complement-mediated glomerular epithelial cell injury. *Am J Physiol Renal Physiol,*Vol. 294, No. 3, pp.F469-479.

Conquer, J. A., Tierney, M. C., Zecevic, J., Bettger, W. J., & Fisher, R. H. (2000). Fatty acid analysis of blood plasma of patients with Alzheimer's disease, other types of dementia, and cognitive impairment. *Lipids,*Vol. 35, No. 12, pp.1305-1312.

Cummings, B. S., McHowat, J., & Schnellmann, R. G. (2002). Role of an endoplasmic reticulum Ca(2+)-independent phospholipase A(2) in oxidant-induced renal cell death. *Am J Physiol Renal Physiol,*Vol. 283, No. 3, pp.F492-498.

Dennis, E. A. (1997). The growing phospholipase A2 superfamily of signal transduction enzymes. *Trends Biochem Sci,*Vol. 22, No. 1, pp.1-2.

Drapeau, C., Pellerin, L., Wolfe, L. S., & Avoli, M. (1990). Long-term changes of synaptic transmission induced by arachidonic acid in the CA1 subfield of the rat hippocampus. *Neurosci Lett,*Vol. 115, No. 2-3, pp.286-292.

Farooqui, A. A., & Horrocks, L. A. (2004). Brain phospholipases A2: a perspective on the history. *Prostaglandins Leukot Essent Fatty Acids,*Vol. 71, No. 3, pp.161-169.

Farooqui, A. A., Ong, W. Y., & Horrocks, L. A. (2004). Biochemical aspects of neurodegeneration in human brain: involvement of neural membrane phospholipids and phospholipases A2. *Neurochem Res,*Vol. 29, No. 11, pp.1961-1977.

Fedorova, I., & Salem, N., Jr. (2006). Omega-3 fatty acids and rodent behavior. *Prostaglandins Leukot Essent Fatty Acids,*Vol. 75, No. 4-5, pp.271-289.

Forlenza, O. V., Mendes, C. T., Marie, S. K., & Gattaz, W. F. (2007). Inhibition of phospholipase A2 reduces neurite outgrowth and neuronal viability. *Prostaglandins Leukot Essent Fatty Acids,*Vol. 76, No. 1, pp.47-55.

Fujita, S., Ikegaya, Y., Nishikawa, M., Nishiyama, N., & Matsuki, N. (2001). Docosahexaenoic acid improves long-term potentiation attenuated by phospholipase A(2) inhibitor in rat hippocampal slices. *Br J Pharmacol,*Vol. 132, No. 7, pp.1417-1422.

Fujita, S., Ikegaya, Y., Nishiyama, N., & Matsuki, N. (2000). Ca2+-independent phospholipase A2 inhibitor impairs spatial memory of mice. *Jpn J Pharmacol,*Vol. 83, No. 3, pp.277-278.

Gattaz, W. F., Forlenza, O. V., Talib, L. L., Barbosa, N. R., & Bottino, C. M. (2004). Platelet phospholipase A(2) activity in Alzheimer's disease and mild cognitive impairment. *J Neural Transm,*Vol. 111, No. 5, pp.591-601.

Geiger, J. R., Melcher, T., Koh, D. S., Sakmann, B., Seeburg, P. H., Jonas, P., et al. (1995). Relative abundance of subunit mRNAs determines gating and Ca2+ permeability of AMPA receptors in principal neurons and interneurons in rat CNS. *Neuron,*Vol. 15, No. 1, pp.193-204.

Glomset, J. A. (2006). Role of docosahexaenoic acid in neuronal plasma membranes. *Sci STKE,*Vol. 2006, No. 321, pp.pe6.

Green, J. T., Orr, S. K., & Bazinet, R. P. (2008). The emerging role of group VI calcium-independent phospholipase A2 in releasing docosahexaenoic acid from brain phospholipids. *J Lipid Res,*Vol. 49, No. 5, pp.939-944.

Green, K. N., Martinez-Coria, H., Khashwji, H., Hall, E. B., Yurko-Mauro, K. A., Ellis, L., et al. (2007). Dietary docosahexaenoic acid and docosapentaenoic acid ameliorate amyloid-beta and tau pathology via a mechanism involving presenilin 1 levels. *J Neurosci,*Vol. 27, No. 16, pp.4385-4395.

Hansson Petersen, C. A., Alikhani, N., Behbahani, H., Wiehager, B., Pavlov, P. F., Alafuzoff, I., et al. (2008). The amyloid beta-peptide is imported into mitochondria via the TOM import machinery and localized to mitochondrial cristae. *Proc Natl Acad Sci U S A,*Vol. 105, No. 35, pp.13145-13150.

Hayashi, Y., Shi, S. H., Esteban, J. A., Piccini, A., Poncer, J. C., & Malinow, R. (2000). Driving AMPA receptors into synapses by LTP and CaMKII: requirement for GluR1 and PDZ domain interaction. *Science,*Vol. 287, No. 5461, pp.2262-2267.

Herbert, S. P., & Walker, J. H. (2006). Group VIA calcium-independent phospholipase A2 mediates endothelial cell S phase progression. *J Biol Chem,*Vol. 281, No. 47, pp.35709-35716.

Holscher, C., Canevari, L., & Richter-Levin, G. (1995). Inhibitors of PLA2 and NO synthase cooperate in producing amnesia of a spatial task. *Neuroreport,*Vol. 6, No. 5, pp.730-732.

Holscher, C., & Rose, S. P. (1994). Inhibitors of phospholipase A2 produce amnesia for a passive avoidance task in the chick. *Behav Neural Biol,*Vol. 61, No. 3, pp.225-232.

Hooks, S. B., & Cummings, B. S. (2008). Role of Ca2+-independent phospholipase A2 in cell growth and signaling. *Biochem Pharmacol,*Vol. 76, No. 9, pp.1059-1067.

Jenkins, C. M., Han, X., Mancuso, D. J., & Gross, R. W. (2002). Identification of calcium-independent phospholipase A2 (iPLA2) beta, and not iPLA2gamma, as the mediator of arginine vasopressin-induced arachidonic acid release in A-10 smooth muscle cells. Enantioselective mechanism-based discrimination of mammalian iPLA2s. *J Biol Chem,*Vol. 277, No. 36, pp.32807-32814.

Jenkins, C. M., Mancuso, D. J., Yan, W., Sims, H. F., Gibson, B., & Gross, R. W. (2004). Identification, cloning, expression, and purification of three novel human calcium-independent phospholipase A2 family members possessing triacylglycerol lipase and acylglycerol transacylase activities. *J Biol Chem,*Vol. 279, No. 47, pp.48968-48975.

Julien, C., Tremblay, C., Phivilay, A., Berthiaume, L., Emond, V., Julien, P., et al. (2008). High-fat diet aggravates amyloid-beta and tau pathologies in the 3xTg-AD mouse model. *Neurobiol Aging,*Vol. 31, No. 9, pp.1516-1531.

Kinsey, G. R., Blum, J. L., Covington, M. D., Cummings, B. S., McHowat, J., & Schnellmann, R. G. (2008). Decreased iPLA2gamma expression induces lipid peroxidation and cell death and sensitizes cells to oxidant-induced apoptosis. *J Lipid Res,*Vol. 49, No. 7, pp.1477-1487.

Kinsey, G. R., Cummings, B. S., Beckett, C. S., Saavedra, G., Zhang, W., McHowat, J., et al. (2005). Identification and distribution of endoplasmic reticulum iPLA2. *Biochem Biophys Res Commun,*Vol. 327, No. 1, pp.287-293.

Kinsey, G. R., McHowat, J., Beckett, C. S., & Schnellmann, R. G. (2007). Identification of calcium-independent phospholipase A2gamma in mitochondria and its role in mitochondrial oxidative stress. *Am J Physiol Renal Physiol,*Vol. 292, No. 2, pp.F853-860.

Kinsey, G. R., McHowat, J., Patrick, K. S., & Schnellmann, R. G. (2007). Role of Ca2+-independent phospholipase A2gamma in Ca2+-induced mitochondrial permeability transition. *J Pharmacol Exp Ther,*Vol. 321, No. 2, pp.707-715.

Kolko, M., Prause, J. U., Bazan, N. G., & Heegaard, S. (2007). Human secretory phospholipase A(2), group IB in normal eyes and in eye diseases. *Acta Ophthalmol Scand,*Vol. 85, No. 3, pp.317-323.

Kudo, I., & Murakami, M. (2002). Phospholipase A2 enzymes. *Prostaglandins Other Lipid Mediat,*Vol. 68-69, pp.3-58.

Kwak, S., & Weiss, J. H. (2006). Calcium-permeable AMPA channels in neurodegenerative disease and ischemia. *Curr Opin Neurobiol,*Vol. 16, No. 3, pp.281-287.

Lee, L. Y., Ong, W. Y., Farooqui, A. A., & Burgunder, J. M. (2007). Role of calcium-independent phospholipase A2 in cortex striatum thalamus cortex circuitry-enzyme inhibition causes vacuous chewing movements in rats. *Psychopharmacology (Berl),*Vol. 195, No. 3, pp.387-395.

Leslie, C. C. (1997). Properties and regulation of cytosolic phospholipase A2. *J Biol Chem,*Vol. 272, No. 27, pp.16709-16712.

Leslie, C. C. (2004). Regulation of arachidonic acid availability for eicosanoid production. *Biochem Cell Biol,*Vol. 82, No. 1, pp.1-17.

Lu, W., Man, H., Ju, W., Trimble, W. S., MacDonald, J. F., & Wang, Y. T. (2001). Activation of synaptic NMDA receptors induces membrane insertion of new AMPA receptors and LTP in cultured hippocampal neurons. *Neuron,*Vol. 29, No. 1, pp.243-254.

Ma, Z., Ramanadham, S., Kempe, K., Chi, X. S., Ladenson, J., & Turk, J. (1997). Pancreatic islets express a Ca2+-independent phospholipase A2 enzyme that contains a repeated structural motif homologous to the integral membrane protein binding domain of ankyrin. *J Biol Chem,*Vol. 272, No. 17, pp.11118-11127.

Malik, I., Turk, J., Mancuso, D. J., Montier, L., Wohltmann, M., Wozniak, D. F., et al. (2008). Disrupted membrane homeostasis and accumulation of ubiquitinated proteins in a mouse model of infantile neuroaxonal dystrophy caused by PLA2G6 mutations. *Am J Pathol,*Vol. 172, No. 2, pp.406-416.

Mancuso, D. J., Jenkins, C. M., & Gross, R. W. (2000). The genomic organization, complete mRNA sequence, cloning, and expression of a novel human intracellular membrane-associated calcium-independent phospholipase A(2). *J Biol Chem,*Vol. 275, No. 14, pp.9937-9945.

Mancuso, D. J., Jenkins, C. M., Sims, H. F., Cohen, J. M., Yang, J., & Gross, R. W. (2004). Complex transcriptional and translational regulation of iPLAgamma resulting in multiple gene products containing dual competing sites for mitochondrial or peroxisomal localization. *Eur J Biochem,*Vol. 271, No. 23-24, pp.4709-4724.

Martel, M. A., Patenaude, C., Menard, C., Alaux, S., Cummings, B. S., & Massicotte, G. (2006). A novel role for calcium-independent phospholipase A in alpha-amino-3-hydroxy-5-methylisoxazole-propionate receptor regulation during long-term potentiation. *Eur J Neurosci,*Vol. 23, No. 2, pp.505-513.

Menard, C., Chartier, E., Patenaude, C., Robinson, P., Cyr, M., Baudry, M., et al. (2007). Calcium-independent phospholipase A(2) influences AMPA-mediated toxicity of hippocampal slices by regulating the GluR1 subunit in synaptic membranes. *Hippocampus,*Vol. 17, No. 11, pp.1109-1120.

Menard, C., Patenaude, C., Gagne, A. M., & Massicotte, G. (2009). AMPA receptor-mediated cell death is reduced by docosahexaenoic acid but not by eicosapentaenoic acid in area CA1 of hippocampal slice cultures. *J Neurosci Res,*Vol. 87, No. 4, pp.876-886.

Menard, C., Patenaude, C., & Massicotte, G. (2005). Phosphorylation of AMPA receptor subunits is differentially regulated by phospholipase A2 inhibitors. *Neurosci Lett,*Vol. 389, No. 1, pp.51-56.

Mendes, C. T., Gattaz, W. F., Schaeffer, E. L., & Forlenza, O. V. (2005). Modulation of phospholipase A2 activity in primary cultures of rat cortical neurons. *J Neural Transm,*Vol. 112, No. 10, pp.1297-1308.

Morgan, N. V., Westaway, S. K., Morton, J. E., Gregory, A., Gissen, P., Sonek, S., et al. (2006). PLA2G6, encoding a phospholipase A2, is mutated in neurodegenerative disorders with high brain iron. *Nat Genet,*Vol. 38, No. 7, pp.752-754.

Murakami, M., Masuda, S., Ueda-Semmyo, K., Yoda, E., Kuwata, H., Takanezawa, Y., et al. (2005). Group VIB Ca2+-independent phospholipase A2gamma promotes cellular membrane hydrolysis and prostaglandin production in a manner distinct from other intracellular phospholipases A2. *J Biol Chem,*Vol. 280, No. 14, pp.14028-14041.

Oksman, M., Iivonen, H., Hogyes, E., Amtul, Z., Penke, B., Leenders, I., et al. (2006). Impact of different saturated fatty acid, polyunsaturated fatty acid and cholesterol containing diets on beta-amyloid accumulation in APP/PS1 transgenic mice. *Neurobiol Dis,* Vol. 23, No. 3, pp.563-572.

Palop, J. J., Chin, J., & Mucke, L. (2006). A network dysfunction perspective on neurodegenerative diseases. *Nature,*Vol. 443, No. 7113, pp.768-773.

Pechoux, C., Boisgard, R., Chanat, E., & Lavialle, F. (2005). Ca(2+)-independent phospholipase A2 participates in the vesicular transport of milk proteins. *Biochim Biophys Acta,* Vol. 1743, No. 3, pp.317-329.

Perez, R., Melero, R., Balboa, M. A., & Balsinde, J. (2004). Role of group VIA calcium-independent phospholipase A2 in arachidonic acid release, phospholipid fatty acid incorporation, and apoptosis in U937 cells responding to hydrogen peroxide. *J Biol Chem,*Vol. 279, No. 39, pp.40385-40391.

Peterson, B., Knotts, T., & Cummings, B. S. (2007). Involvement of Ca2+-independent phospholipase A2 isoforms in oxidant-induced neural cell death. *Neurotoxicology,* Vol. 28, No. 1, pp.150-160.

Phillis, J. W., & O'Regan, M. H. (2004). A potentially critical role of phospholipases in central nervous system ischemic, traumatic, and neurodegenerative disorders. *Brain Res Brain Res Rev,*Vol. 44, No. 1, pp.13-47.

Pickard, L., Noel, J., Duckworth, J. K., Fitzjohn, S. M., Henley, J. M., Collingridge, G. L., et al. (2001). Transient synaptic activation of NMDA receptors leads to the insertion of native AMPA receptors at hippocampal neuronal plasma membranes. *Neuropharmacology,*Vol. 41, No. 6, pp.700-713.

Quistad, G. B., Barlow, C., Winrow, C. J., Sparks, S. E., & Casida, J. E. (2003). Evidence that mouse brain neuropathy target esterase is a lysophospholipase. *Proc Natl Acad Sci U S A,*Vol. 100, No. 13, pp.7983-7987.

Ramanadham, S., Hsu, F. F., Zhang, S., Jin, C., Bohrer, A., Song, H., et al. (2004). Apoptosis of insulin-secreting cells induced by endoplasmic reticulum stress is amplified by overexpression of group VIA calcium-independent phospholipase A2 (iPLA2 beta) and suppressed by inhibition of iPLA2 beta. *Biochemistry,*Vol. 43, No. 4, pp.918-930.

Ross, B. M., Hughes, B., Kish, S. J., & Warsh, J. J. (2006). Serum calcium-independent phospholipase A2 activity in bipolar affective disorder. *Bipolar Disord,*Vol. 8, No. 3, pp.265-270.

Ross, B. M., Turenne, S., Moszczynska, A., Warsh, J. J., & Kish, S. J. (1999). Differential alteration of phospholipase A2 activities in brain of patients with schizophrenia. *Brain Res,*Vol. 821, No. 2, pp.407-413.

Sanchez-Mejia, R. O., Newman, J. W., Toh, S., Yu, G. Q., Zhou, Y., Halabisky, B., et al. (2008). Phospholipase A2 reduction ameliorates cognitive deficits in a mouse model of Alzheimer's disease. *Nat Neurosci,*Vol. 11, No. 11, pp.1311-1318.

Schaeffer, E. L., & Gattaz, W. F. (2005). Inhibition of calcium-independent phospholipase A2 activity in rat hippocampus impairs acquisition of short- and long-term memory. *Psychopharmacology (Berl),*Vol. 181, No. 2, pp.392-400.

Schaeffer, E. L., & Gattaz, W. F. (2007). Requirement of hippocampal phospholipase A2 activity for long-term memory retrieval in rats. *J Neural Transm,*Vol. 114, No. 3, pp.379-385.

Schaloske, R. H., & Dennis, E. A. (2006). The phospholipase A2 superfamily and its group numbering system. *Biochim Biophys Acta,*Vol. 1761, No. 11, pp.1246-1259.

Seleznev, K., Zhao, C., Zhang, X. H., Song, K., & Ma, Z. A. (2006). Calcium-independent phospholipase A2 localizes in and protects mitochondria during apoptotic induction by staurosporine. *J Biol Chem,*Vol. 281, No. 31, pp.22275-22288.

Shinzawa, K., Sumi, H., Ikawa, M., Matsuoka, Y., Okabe, M., Sakoda, S., et al. (2008). Neuroaxonal dystrophy caused by group VIA phospholipase A2 deficiency in mice: a model of human neurodegenerative disease. *J Neurosci,*Vol. 28, No. 9, pp.2212-2220.

Smani, T., Zakharov, S. I., Csutora, P., Leno, E., Trepakova, E. S., & Bolotina, V. M. (2004). A novel mechanism for the store-operated calcium influx pathway. *Nat Cell Biol,*Vol. 6, No. 2, pp.113-120.

Sommer, B., Kohler, M., Sprengel, R., & Seeburg, P. H. (1991). RNA editing in brain controls a determinant of ion flow in glutamate-gated channels. *Cell,* Vol. 67, No. 1, pp.11-19.

Stellwagen, D., Beattie, E. C., Seo, J. Y., & Malenka, R. C. (2005). Differential regulation of AMPA receptor and GABA receptor trafficking by tumor necrosis factor-alpha. *J Neurosci,* Vol. 25, No. 12, pp.3219-3228.

Strokin, M., Chechneva, O., Reymann, K. G., & Reiser, G. (2006). Neuroprotection of rat hippocampal slices exposed to oxygen-glucose deprivation by enrichment with docosahexaenoic acid and by inhibition of hydrolysis of docosahexaenoic acid-containing phospholipids by calcium independent phospholipase A2. *Neuroscience,* Vol. 140, No. 2, pp.547-553.

Strokin, M., Sergeeva, M., & Reiser, G. (2003). Docosahexaenoic acid and arachidonic acid release in rat brain astrocytes is mediated by two separate isoforms of phospholipase A2 and is differently regulated by cyclic AMP and Ca2+. *Br J Pharmacol,* Vol. 139, No. 5, pp.1014-1022.

Strokin, M., Sergeeva, M., & Reiser, G. (2007). Prostaglandin synthesis in rat brain astrocytes is under the control of the n-3 docosahexaenoic acid, released by group VIB calcium-independent phospholipase A2. *J Neurochem,* Vol. 102, No. 6, pp.1771-1782.

Sun, G. Y., Xu, J., Jensen, M. D., & Simonyi, A. (2004). Phospholipase A2 in the central nervous system: implications for neurodegenerative diseases. *J Lipid Res,* Vol. 45, No. 2, pp.205-213.

Sun, G. Y., Xu, J., Jensen, M. D., Yu, S., Wood, W. G., Gonzalez, F. A., et al. (2005). Phospholipase A2 in astrocytes: responses to oxidative stress, inflammation, and G protein-coupled receptor agonists. *Mol Neurobiol,* Vol. 31, No. 1-3, pp.27-41.

Takeuchi, T., Fukumoto, Y., & Harada, E. (2002). Influence of a dietary n-3 fatty acid deficiency on the cerebral catecholamine contents, EEG and learning ability in rat. *Behav Brain Res,* Vol. 131, No. 1-2, pp.193-203.

Takuma, T., & Ichida, T. (1997). Role of Ca2+-independent phospholipase A2 in exocytosis of amylase from parotid acinar cells. *J Biochem,* Vol. 121, No. 6, pp.1018-1024.

Talbot, K., Young, R. A., Jolly-Tornetta, C., Lee, V. M., Trojanowski, J. Q., & Wolf, B. A. (2000). A frontal variant of Alzheimer's disease exhibits decreased calcium-independent phospholipase A2 activity in the prefrontal cortex. *Neurochem Int,* Vol. 37, No. 1, pp.17-31.

Tanaka, H., Takeya, R., & Sumimoto, H. (2000). A novel intracellular membrane-bound calcium-independent phospholipase A(2). *Biochem Biophys Res Commun,* Vol. 272, No. 2, pp.320-326.

Tang, J., Kriz, R. W., Wolfman, N., Shaffer, M., Seehra, J., & Jones, S. S. (1997). A novel cytosolic calcium-independent phospholipase A2 contains eight ankyrin motifs. *J Biol Chem,* Vol. 272, No. 13, pp.8567-8575.

Tay, H. K., & Melendez, A. J. (2004). Fcgamma RI-triggered generation of arachidonic acid and eicosanoids requires iPLA2 but not cPLA2 in human monocytic cells. *J Biol Chem,* Vol. 279, No. 21, pp.22505-22513.

Thiagarajan, T. C., Lindskog, M., & Tsien, R. W. (2005). Adaptation to synaptic inactivity in hippocampal neurons. *Neuron,* Vol. 47, No. 5, pp.725-737.

Underwood, K. W., Song, C., Kriz, R. W., Chang, X. J., Knopf, J. L., & Lin, L. L. (1998). A novel calcium-independent phospholipase A2, cPLA2-gamma, that is prenylated and contains homology to cPLA2. *J Biol Chem,* Vol. 273, No. 34, pp.21926-21932.

Uozumi, N., Kume, K., Nagase, T., Nakatani, N., Ishii, S., Tashiro, F., et al. (1997). Role of cytosolic phospholipase A2 in allergic response and parturition. *Nature,*Vol. 390, No. 6660, pp.618-622.

Villmann, C., & Becker, C. M. (2007). On the hypes and falls in neuroprotection: targeting the NMDA receptor. *Neuroscientist,*Vol. 13, No. 6, pp.594-615.

Wang, X., Zhao, X., Mao, Z. Y., Wang, X. M., & Liu, Z. L. (2003). Neuroprotective effect of docosahexaenoic acid on glutamate-induced cytotoxicity in rat hippocampal cultures. *Neuroreport,*Vol. 14, No. 18, pp.2457-2461.

Wiedholz, L. M., Owens, W. A., Horton, R. E., Feyder, M., Karlsson, R. M., Hefner, K., et al. (2008). Mice lacking the AMPA GluR1 receptor exhibit striatal hyperdopaminergia and 'schizophrenia-related' behaviors. *Mol Psychiatry,*Vol. 13, No. 6, pp.631-640.

Williams, J. H., Errington, M. L., Lynch, M. A., & Bliss, T. V. (1989). Arachidonic acid induces a long-term activity-dependent enhancement of synaptic transmission in the hippocampus. *Nature,*Vol. 341, No. 6244, pp.739-742.

Williams, S. D., & Gottlieb, R. A. (2002). Inhibition of mitochondrial calcium-independent phospholipase A2 (iPLA2) attenuates mitochondrial phospholipid loss and is cardioprotective. *Biochem J,*Vol. 362, No. Pt 1, pp.23-32.

Wolf, M. J., Izumi, Y., Zorumski, C. F., & Gross, R. W. (1995). Long-term potentiation requires activation of calcium-independent phospholipase A2. *FEBS Lett,*Vol. 377, No. 3, pp.358-362.

Wu, A., Ying, Z., & Gomez-Pinilla, F. (2004). Dietary omega-3 fatty acids normalize BDNF levels, reduce oxidative damage, and counteract learning disability after traumatic brain injury in rats. *J Neurotrauma,*Vol. 21, No. 10, pp.1457-1467.

Xie, X., Liaw, J. S., Baudry, M., & Berger, T. W. (1997). Novel expression mechanism for synaptic potentiation: alignment of presynaptic release site and postsynaptic receptor. *Proc Natl Acad Sci U S A,*Vol. 94, No. 13, pp.6983-6988.

Xu, J., Yu, S., Sun, A. Y., & Sun, G. Y. (2003). Oxidant-mediated AA release from astrocytes involves cPLA(2) and iPLA(2). *Free Radic Biol Med,*Vol. 34, No. 12, pp.1531-1543.

Yan, W., Jenkins, C. M., Han, X., Mancuso, D. J., Sims, H. F., Yang, K., et al. (2005). The highly selective production of 2-arachidonoyl lysophosphatidylcholine catalyzed by purified calcium-independent phospholipase A2gamma: identification of a novel enzymatic mediator for the generation of a key branch point intermediate in eicosanoid signaling. *J Biol Chem,*Vol. 280, No. 29, pp.26669-26679.

Yang, H. C., Mosior, M., Ni, B., & Dennis, E. A. (1999). Regional distribution, ontogeny, purification, and characterization of the Ca2+-independent phospholipase A2 from rat brain. *J Neurochem,*Vol. 73, No. 3, pp.1278-1287.

Yang, J., Han, X., & Gross, R. W. (2003). Identification of hepatic peroxisomal phospholipase A(2) and characterization of arachidonic acid-containing choline glycerophospholipids in hepatic peroxisomes. *FEBS Lett,*Vol. 546, No. 2-3, pp.247-250.

Yavin, E., Brand, A., & Green, P. (2002). Docosahexaenoic acid abundance in the brain: a biodevice to combat oxidative stress. *Nutr Neurosci,*Vol. 5, No. 3, pp.149-157.

Youdim, K. A., Martin, A., & Joseph, J. A. (2000). Essential fatty acids and the brain: possible health implications. *Int J Dev Neurosci,*Vol. 18, No. 4-5, pp.383-399.

Zhu, D., Lai, Y., Shelat, P. B., Hu, C., Sun, G. Y., & Lee, J. C. (2006). Phospholipases A2 mediate amyloid-beta peptide-induced mitochondrial dysfunction. *J Neurosci,*Vol. 26, No. 43, pp.11111-11119.

9

ASK1 and Its Role in Neurodegenerative Diseases

Emmanuel Sturchler, Daniel Feurstein,
Patricia McDonald and Derek Duckett
Department of Molecular Therapeutics and Translational Research Institute Scripps Florida Jupiter, FL USA

1. Introduction

The apoptosis signal-regulating kinase 1 (ASK1) is a ubiquitously expressed serine/threonine protein kinase and one of more than 20 members that make up the triple MAP kinase (MAP3K) family of enzymes. Over the past decade, genetic studies have revealed that ASK1 plays a pivitol role in the cellular response to a wide variety of environmental and biological stressors including; reactive oxygen species (ROS) such as hydrogen peroxide (H_2O_2), endoplasmic reticulum (ER) stress caused by protein aggregation, influx of calcium ions, and receptor-mediated signals transduced via lipopolysaccharides (LPS), Fas ligand, cytokines (TNFα) and certain G protein-coupled receptor (GPCR) agonists [1-5]. In addition, exogenous expression of ASK1 in cells has shown that ASK1 signaling engages the intrinsic apoptosis pathway promoting cytochrome *c* release from mitochondria and subsequent activation of caspase 3 and 9 [1, 6, 7]. Conversely, ASK1 deficient cells are resistant to cell death induced by oxidative and ER stress, indicating that ASK1 acts as the lynch pin in certain forms of stress-induced cell death [8].

Once activated, ASK1 relays cellular stress signals via the classical three tierd mitogen activated protein kinase (MAPK) signaling cascade, whereby a MAP3K phosphorylates and activates a MAP2K, that in turn phosphorylates and activates a MAPK [9] (Figure 1). More specifically, the ASK1 signaling axis activates the p38 and the c-jun NH2-terminal kinases (JNK) family of MAPKs, via activation of MKK3/MKK6 and MKK4/MKK7 respectively [1, 2, 4]. In addition to its role in the cellular stress response, ASK1 also regulates physiological processes including neuronal differentiation, synaptic plasticity and the innate immune response [10-13]. Thus, ASK1 acts as an important regulator of several important biological processess and not surprisingly, ASK1 activation is under tight regulatory control.

Regulation of ASK1 activity is accomplished via a number of mechanisms including; protein-protein interactions as well as both spatial and temporal control. Firstly, more than 30 ASK1 interacting partners have been shown to regulate ASK1 activity (either positively or negatively) by posttranslational modifications and/or by inducing conformational changes through protein-protein interactions. Secondly, ASK1 signaling complexes are located in both the cytoplasm and mitochondria [14], with nuclear translocation observed upon stress induction indicating that ASK1 localization might also dictate the biological outcome [15,16] and thirdly, duration of ASK1 signaling can influence the nature of the cellular response. In this context, defects in the fine tuning of ASK1 activity can contribute to a number of pathological conditions including inflammatory, cardiac and several neurodegenerative diseases. In this chapter, we will discuss in detail the molecular mechanisms that regulate ASK1 activity, and focus on the contribution of ASK1 to neurodegenerative diseases such as Alzheimer's Disease, Parkinson's Disease, Polyglutamine (polyQ) Diseases, amyotrophic lateral sclerosis and stroke, together with the potential of ASK1 as a therapeutic target for the treatment of such disorders.

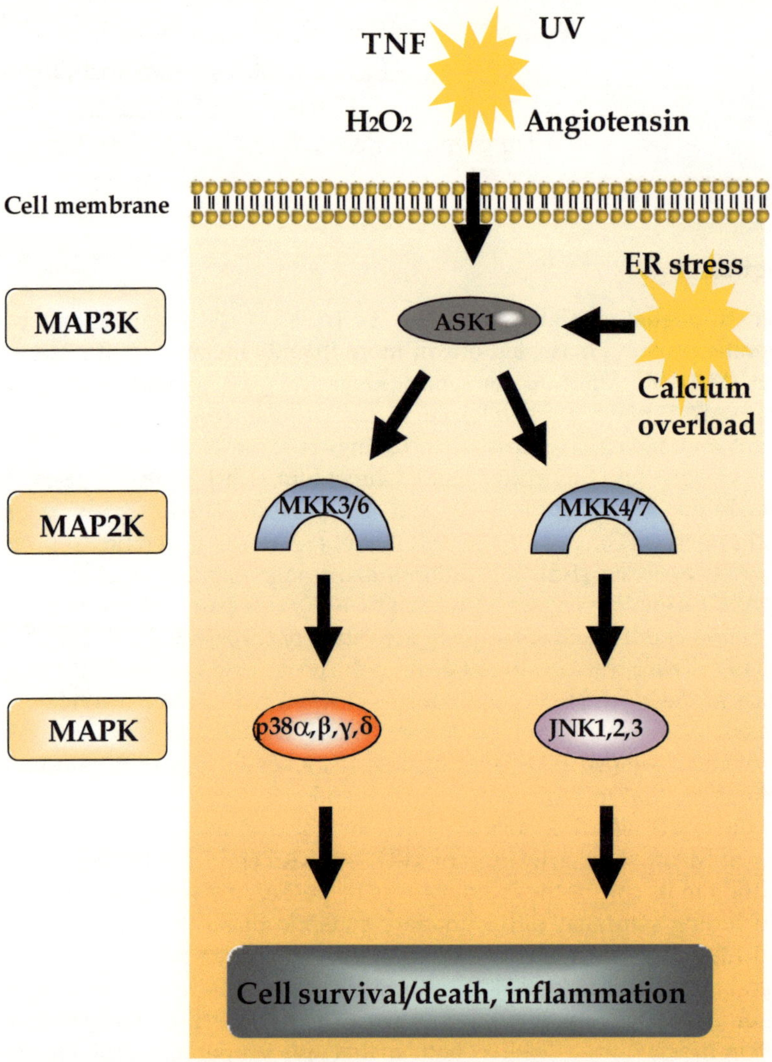

Fig. 1. ASK1, along with at least 20 other kinases belongs to the MAP3K family of enzymes. MAP3K selectively activate MAP2Ks with in turn activate members of the MAPK family. There are 7 MAP2K and 11 MAPK family members with the global MAPK family constituting 8% of the kinome. Specifically, ASK1 responds to multiple extracellular and intracellular stimuli by selectively phosphorylating MKK3/6 and/or MKK4/7 leading to the specific activation of the p38 and JNK MAPK pathways

2. Regulation of ASK1 activity

Based on sequence homology, three human ASK1 related genes have been identified, namely ASK1 (MAP3K5), ASK2 (MAP3K6) and ASK3 (MAP3K15). In this review we will focus specifically on the biology of ASK1, commenting only on ASK2 and 3 where appropriate. ASK1 is a 170 kDa protein composed of an inhibitiory N-terminal domain, an internal kinase domain and a C-terminal regulatory domain. Although the primary stuctures of the N- and C regulatory domains within the ASK family exhibit a fair degree of divergence, those within the kinase domains are highly consevd. High resolution crystal structure studies revealed that the ASK1 catalytic domain structure displays a typical protein kinase fold, comprised of five β sheets and helix αC constituting the small lobe and a larger mainly α helical C-terminal lobe. The hinge region connecting the two domains lines the catalytic ATP binding site and although catalytically active, the recombinant enzyme adopts a non-active conformation in the crystal state [17].

It is well established that both the subcellular localization as well as the magnitude and duration of MAPK activation are important for determining cellular fate. Thus, specific mechanisms may enable ASK1 modules to be rapidly activated or inactivated in a spatial and temporal manner. Increasing evidence indicates that depending on the stimulus and the cellular context, ASK1 activity is tightly regulated by multiple and distinct molecular events including phosphorylation/dephosphorylation of key residues, protein-protein interactions, and ubiquitination, resulting in ASK1 degradation and feedback regulation. Defects in these mechanisms may lead to aberrant ASK1 activity and to certain pathologies in humans.

3. Modulation of ASK1 activity by postranslational modification

In resting cells, ASK1 forms homo-oligomers through protein interactions via the C-terminal coiled-coiled domain (CCC). Cell-based and biochemical studies have demonstrated that ASK1 is associated with a number of interacting proteins which can lead to the formation of high molecular weight complexes (1000-3000 kDa), designated the ASK1 signalosome [18, 19]. To date, over 30 proteins have been shown to interact with ASK1 and regulate its activity. While the presice nature of the ASK1 signalosome remains to be fully characterised, it is postulated to be highly dynamic, serving as a foundation for the assembly of specific signaling modules and the subsets of regulatory proteins that it recruits depends upon the context of the initial stress.

Through genetic screening for ASK1-binding proteins, the redox protein Thioredoxin (Trx1) was one of the first ASK1 interacting proteins identified and has been shown to play a key role in the regulation of ASK1 in response to oxidative stress induced by H_2O_2 or tumor necrosis factor-α (TNFα) (Figure 2) [20, 21]. The thiol reductase activity of Trx1 is provided by cysteines 32 (Cys32) and 35 (Cys35) which forms a redox cataylitic CXPC motif [22]. Several studies demonstrated that tight association of a reduced form of Trx1 with the N-terminus of ASK1 suppresses ASK1 kinase activity by inhibiting N-terminal interactions between ASK1 monomers. The interaction has been shown to involve the catalytic cysteines Cys32 and Cys35 of Trx1, as mutation of either is sufficient to inhibit the dissociation of Trx1 from ASK1 [21]. Moreover, antioxidants such as catalase and N-acetylycysteine (NAC) block the release of Trx1 from ASK1 after challenge with H_2O_2, preventing ASK1 activation and associated cell death [23, 24]. These studies led to a model whereby upon H_2O_2 stimulation, Trx-1 is oxidized on Cys32 and Cys35 promoting formation of an intramolecular disulfide bond beetween these two cysteines. This allows dissociation of Trx1 from ASK1 promoting multimerization and activation of ASK1 [20, 23].

Studies conducted by Nadeau *et al.*, revealed an alternative mechanism for the function of Trx1 in the regulation of ASK1 in response to H_2O_2. These studies demonstrated that H_2O_2 induces ASK1 oxidation leading to the formation of interchain disulfide bond-linked ASK1 multimers [25, 26]. These authors demonstrated that changing all oxidation sensitive cysteine residues responsible for disulfide bond-linked multimers, prevented H_2O_2-induced ASK1 proapototic activity. Specifically, the cysteine residue at position 250 (Cys250) in ASK1 was identified as an essential residue for JNK activation in response to H_2O_2-induced stress. Recently, redox sensitive molecules such as the Parkinson's associated protein DJ-1 (a.k.a PARK7) and Peroxiredoxin-2 have also been shown to attenuate ASK1 activity in response to toxic stress in dopaminergic neurons [27-29]. Interestingly, mutation analyses demonstrated, that the ER stress-inducing agent thapsigargin, while inducing ASK1 activation (as determined by Thr838 phosphorylation) was observed to be independent of Cys250 [25]. In attempting to address the role of Cys250 and the role of Trx1 in regulating

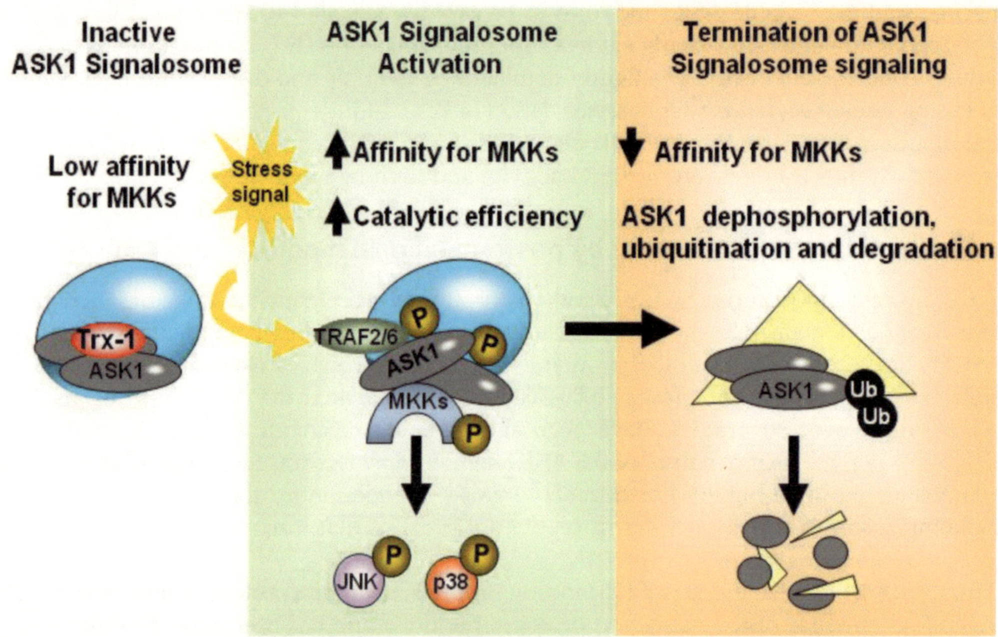

Fig. 2. ASK1-MKKs-JNK/p38 signaling cascade. Under basal conditions, ASK1 forms a high molecular mass complex with multiple interacting proteins including thioredoxin (Trx). In response to oxidative stress, ER stress, or calcium overload, firstly Trx is oxidized and released from the signalosome, secondly the TNF receptor associated factors 2 and 6 (TRAF2/6) are recruited to the complex leading to ASK1 autophosphorylation/transphosphorylation and activation. Subsequently, the affinity of the signalosome for its substrates, (MKKs) is increased, favoring ASK1-MKK6/4 interaction and MKK6/4 phosphoryation which in turn activate JNK/p38. Depending upon the cell type and initial stressor, a complex ASK1 regulatory mechanism is invoked, balancing the processes of phosphorylation/dephosphorylation together with ubiquitination/deubiquitination which fine tunes the specificity and duration of the ASK1 signaling cascade and ultimately the cellular response

ASK1 activity, it was demonstrated that mutation of ASK1 Cys250 to alanine (Cys250A) blocks the binding of Trx1. In this instance, ASK1 is still able to form disulfide bond-linked multimers but it is not constitutively phosphorylated on Thr838, nor can it activate downstream MAPK pathway members. These results suggest that simple dissociation of Trx1 from ASK1, while a trigger is not sufficient to activate ASK1. Further studies are required to define the regulatory role that Cys250 plays in the activation of ASK1 in response to H_2O_2 signaling.

Additional studies have demonstrated that in the absence of Trx1, tumor necrosis factor-α receptor-associated factors (TRAF) 2 and 6 are recruited to the ASK1 signalosome [14, 19, 30]. Recruitment of TRAF2 and 6 induces ASK1 phosphorylation and activation and stabilizes a higher molecular weight ASK1 signalosome complex. Consistent with this, H_2O_2-induced activation of ASK1 was strongly inhibited in mouse embyonic fibroblats (MEF's) deficient in TRAF 2 and 6 [19]. In addition, the residue Thr838 (Thr845 in mouse) located in the activation loop of the kinase is trans/auto-phosphorylated [18] and the affinity of ASK1 for its substrate MKK6, was observed to be significantly increased [31].

ASK1 is phosphorylated at multiple sites and to date, seven phosphorylation sites have been identified *in vitro*. As mentioned above phosphorylation of Thr838 located in the kinase activation loop is required for ASK1 kinase activity. In addition to ASK1 autophosphorylation, positive regulators of ASK1 activity including the family member ASK2 [32], and the murine protein serine/threonine kinase 38 (MPK38), a member of the AMP-activated protein kinase-related serine/threonine kinase family [33], were found to complex with ASK1 and to stimulate its activity by phosphorylating the Thr838 residue in response to H_2O_2 or TNF treatment. Conversely, several mechanisms negatively regulate ASK1 activity by modulating the phosphorylation status of this critical residue (Figure 3). For example, the protein phosphatase 5 (PP5), a member of the serine/threonine protein phosphatase family is reported to be recruited into the ASK1 signalosome and to dephosphorylate Thr838 subsequent to H_2O_2 treatment [34]. By dephosphorylating this critical residue, PP5 was shown to inhibit H_2O_2-induced ASK1 catalytic activity as well as ASK1-mediated apoptosis. Dephosphorylation of Thr838 inactivates ASK1 in a negative feedback manner and thereby modulates the activation of JNK/p38 and apoptosis. Such a negative feedback system most likely interplays with other cellular signal transduction pathways and is critical for determining cell fate (survival or cell death) in response to cellular stressors. Interestingly, overexpression of PP5 was shown to prevent amyloid-β-induced MAPK activation and neurotoxicity [35].

The calcium and intergrin binding protein 1 (CIB1) was also found to inhibit autophosphorylation of ASK1 at Thr838, by directly interacting with ASK1. This interaction was observed to compete with and inhibit TRAF2 recruitment to the ASK1 complex [36], repressing ASK1 activation in response to both tunicomycin, an ER stressor and 6-hydroxydopamine (6-OHDA) in dopaminergic cells. Furthermore, the block to ASK1 activation occured in a Ca^{2+}-dependent manner indicating that CIB1 functions as a Ca^{2+}-sensitive negative regulator of ASK1 activity. Thus, in an aging brain where calcium homeostasis is dysregulated [37, 38], the function of this calcium sensitive ASK1 repressor may be altered, leading to abnormal ASK1 activity and to the development of age-related neurodegenerative disorders.

ASK1 activity is further regulated by additional phosphorylation/dephosphorylation events that occur at serine-83 (Ser83), serine-967 (Ser967), serine-1034 (Ser1034), and tyrosine-718 (Tyr718). The N-terminal domain of ASK1, surrounding the Ser83 residue was found to contain a consensus Akt phorphorylation site and biochemical and cell-based studies confirmed this site as a substrate for Akt [39]. In addition, Hsp90 was found to form a complex with Akt and ASK1 in unstimulated cells, and to stabilize the Akt-ASK1 interaction under oxidative stress conditions in order to suppress apoptosis [40]. Importantly, Akt-induced inhibition of ASK1 was observed to promote cell survival and to mediate selenite-induced neuroprotection after cerebral ischemia in rat hippocampus [41]. In a study conducted by Nakagami *et al.*, activation of Akt was also observed to inhibit the toxic action of amyloid-β and to protect neurons from apoptosis [42]. These authors hypothesized that the suppression of cell death was mediated at least in part, by the ability of Akt to repress ASK1 activity. More recently, the proto-oncogene serine/threonine kinase, PIM1 was also shown to interact with and to phosphorylate ASK1 on Ser83 [43]. PIM1 phosphorylation of ASK1 decreased ASK1 activity and attenuated H_2O_2-induced ASK1 mediated activation of JNK/p38 and caspase-3. Thus, phosphorylation of ASK1 on Ser83 by Akt or PIM1 maintains ASK1 in an inactive state and suppresses ASK1-mediated p38/JNK downstream signaling.

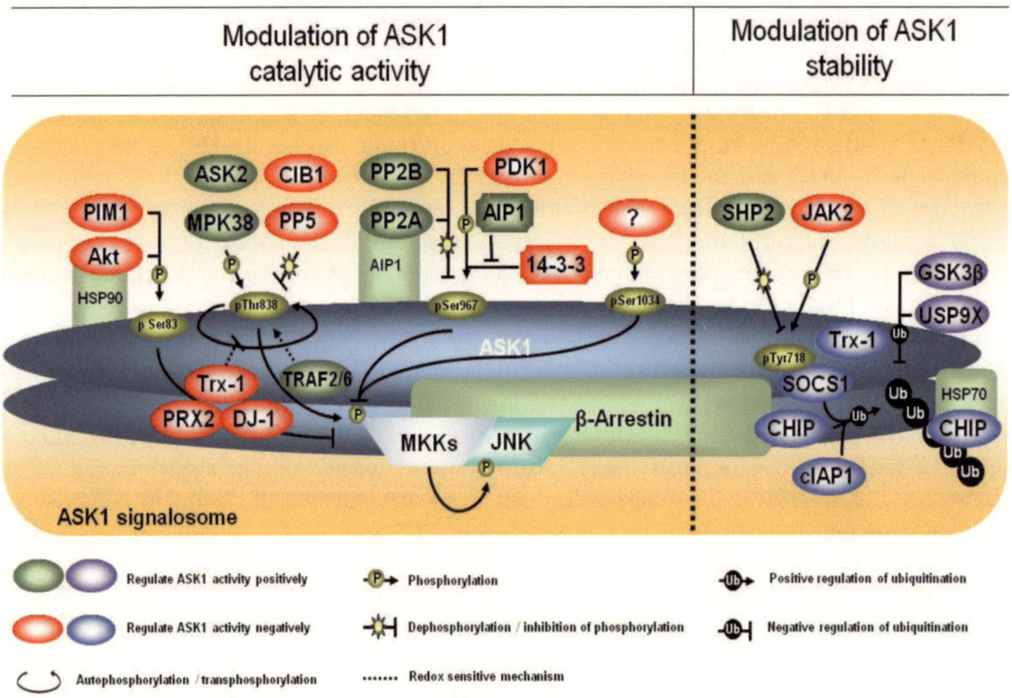

Fig. 3. Schematic representation of the multiple mechanisms regulating the catalytic activity and the stablility of ASK1 signalosome. ASK1 catalytic activity is modulated by the phosphorylation/dephosphorylation of critical residues as well as by the interaction with redox sensitive molecules. In addition, ASK1 signaling can be regulated by proteins that modulate ubiquitination of the complex and thus its stability. Green and purple represent the proteins involved in mechanisms that enhance ASK1 activity whereas red and blue represent proteins that inhibit ASK1 signaling. Together, it's the complex regulation of these mechanisms that are thought to modulate the specificity and strength of the ASK1-MKKs-JNK/p38 signaling cascade

A study conducted by Zhang *et al.*, revealed that the association of ASK1 with 14-3-3 protein suppresses ASK1-mediated apoptosis [44]. These authors demonstrated that phosphorylation of Ser967, a residue located C-terminal to the ASK1 kinase domain, is critical for ASK1/14-3-3 complex formation. Interestingly, the 14-3-3 binding motif in ASK1 is conserved among its homologues from human, mouse and Drosophila, suggesting the evolutionary importance of this interaction. Importantly, exogenous expression of $ASK1^{S967A}$, a 14-3-3 defective mutant, dramatically enhanced cell death, suggesting that 14-3-3 association inhibits the death promoting activity of ASK1. More recently, Seong *et al.*, demonstrated that Ser967 was phosphorylated by the 3-phosphoinositide-dependent protein kinase 1 (PDK1), a member of the protein kinase A,G, and C subfamily of protein kinases [45] and that binding of PDK1 to ASK1 was mediated through the pleckstrin homology domain of PDK1 and the C-terminal regulatory domain of ASK1. This interaction was shown to suppress H_2O_2-induced ASK1-JNK-p38 signaling as well as ASK1-mediated apoptosis. In addition, ASK1 was also observed to phosphorylate and inhibit PDK1 acitivity, suggesting a novel mechanism whereby ASK1 and PDK1 negatively regulate their respective kinase activity in a reciprocal manner [45].

Oxidative stress such as H_2O_2, was found to increase ASK1 catalytic activity by inducing dephosphorylation of ASK1 at Ser967 leading to ASK1/14-3-3 complex dissociation [46]. Two phosphatases that dephosphorylate ASK1 at Ser967 have been identified so far; Calcineurin B (protein phosphatase 2B) and protein phosphatse 2A (PP2A). Calcineurin B was found to directly interact with the ASK1 C-terminus and to dephosphorylate ASK1 at Ser967 leading to the disassociation of ASK1 from 14-3-3 proteins, ASK1 activation and enhanced cardiomyocyte apoptosis [47]. A study conducted in vascular endothelial cells demonstrated that in resting cells PP2A forms a complex with the ASK1-interacting protein (AIP1), a ras GTPase-activating protein [48]. Upon TNFα treatment the AIP1/PP2A complex was found to interact with and dephophorylate ASK1 at Ser967, leading to the dissociation of its inhibitor 14-3-3 and ASK1 activation [49]. Furthermore, Aβ was found to induce ASK1 Ser967 dephosphorylation and its dissociation from the 14-3-3 protein leading to p38 activation, and induction of the pro-apoptopic BCl-2 family member, Bax [50]. Selective inhibition of PP2A prevented the activation of this signaling cascade linking ASK1 Ser967 phosphorylation status to Aβ-induced toxicity.

Similar to phosphorylation at Ser967, phosphorylation at Ser1034, a residue contained with in the C-terminal regulatory domain of ASK1 was also found to negatively regulate its kinase and proapoptotic activity [51]. While distinct from the Akt and 14-3-3 mechanisms, candidate kinases/phosphatases implicated in the modulation of Ser1034 phosphorylation status remain to be identified.

4. Regulation of ASK1 protein levels

As outlined above, ASK1 cellular activity is tightly controlled in both a spatial and temporal fashion by distinct and multiple mechanisms (Figure 3). In addition to phosphorylation, other posttranslational modifications such as ubiquitination have been observed to play an important role in regulating ASK1 activity. Ubiquitination, is a reversible posttranslational modification that is reciprocally regulated by E3 ubiquitin ligases and deubiquitinating enzymes (DUBs). A study conducted by Liu *et al.*, demonstrated that the association of Trx with ASK1 suppresses ASK1 kinase activity not only by inhibiting N-terminal interactions between ASK1 molecules, but also by controling

ASK1 protein levels through ubiquitination and degradation via the 26S proteosome [23]. This work provided the first evidence that ASK1 protein expression is regulated by ubiquitination. Recently, our laboratory demonstrated that the duration of the ASK1 signal in response to oxidative stress is regulated by mechanisms modulating the degradation of the ASK1 signalosome [31]. LC-MS/MS analysis of the ASK1 signalosome, purified from cells treated with H_2O_2, revealed the presence of ubiquitinated ASK1 together with several proteins associated with the process of protein degradation such as the 26S proteasome regulatory subunit, ubiquitin-like modifier-activating enzyme1 and ubiquitin specific protease 9 X-linked (USP9X). USP9X belongs to the USP subfamiliy of deubiquitinating enzymes and is thought to regulate multiple cellular functions. In an earlier study conducted by Nagai *et al.*, a ubiquitin-like sequence in ASK1 responsible for USP9X recognition was identified [52]. These authors demonstrated that in response to oxidative stress, ubiquitination of ASK1 C-termini mediates the proteosomal degredation of ASK1. In addition, it was demonstrated that in complex with ASK1, USP9X cleaves ubiquitin from the C-terminus of stress induced ASK1, preventing degradation and stabilizing the activated form of ASK1. In keeping with this observation, knockdown of USP9X mediated by siRNA in HeLa cells, reduced H_2O_2 induced JNK and p38 activation equivalent to that observed in ASK1 deficient cells. H_2O_2-induced ASK1 activity is therefore regulated by a complex mechanism involving a balance between phosphorylation/dephosphorylation and ubiquitination levels, whereby ubiquitin dependent regulation of ASK1 is closely coupled to its activity. In this regard these authors postulated that USP9X may be a key regulator that fine-tunes the ASK1-dependent signaling cascade. Recently, Zhang *et al.* characterized region specific protein level changes in the brains of mice treated with the neurotoxin MPTP [53]. In comparison to normal brain, USP9X was significantly upregulated within the striatum, cerebellum and cortex of the MPTP treated mice, raising the possibility of a role for USP9X in neurodegeneration.

Several additional reports have emerged describing the ubiquitin dependent regulation of ASK1. It is well established that activation of the TNF receptor 2 (TNFR2) leads to activation of ASK1 and duration of TNFR2 mediated ASK1 signaling is proposed to be controled by ubiquitin-dependent proteosomal degradation of ASK1 [54]. This mechanism was shown to involve the ubiquitin protein ligase activity of the cellular inhibitor of apoptosis protein 1 (cIAP1) and genetic knockdown experiments confirmed that cIAP1 was critical for limiting TNFR2 mediated p38 and JNK activation. Moreover, in a model of glaucoma, a neurodegenerative disease leading to impaired visual function, Kisiswa *et al.* observed an age dependent down-regulation of cIAP1 accompanied by accumulation of TRAF2 in the retinal ganglion cell layer [55]. Interestingly, dysregulated ASK1 activity was recently reported to be involved in glaucoma, indicating that interrupting ASK1 dependent pathways may be beneficial in the treatment of this pathology [56]. In addition to identifying USP9X in H_2O_2 induced ASK1 signalosome complexes, we also confirmed the presence of Hsp70 in these complexes. Previous studies demonstrate that Hsp70 mediates ASK1 degradation by recruiting the chaperone and ubiquitin ligase CHIP (C-terminus of Hsp70-interacting protein) [57]. Hsp70 together with CHIP have been implicated in protecting cells against cellular stress that cause neurodegenerative diseases, including Alzheimer's Disease (AD), Parkinson's Disease (PD), Huntington Disease (HD), and Amyotrophic Lateral Sclerosis (ALS). The suppressor of cytokine signaling 1 (SOCS1), another protein regulating proteosomal degradation, was also reported to interact with ASK1 and to mediate its degradation [58]. Phosphorylation of ASK1 Tyr718 residue by JAK2 was demonstrated to be critical for complex formation between ASK1 and SOCS1. In unstimulated cells this residue is phophorylated, allowing SOCS1 to interact with ASK1 and repress its activity by decreasing its stability. Conversely, stimulation with TNF induced SHP2-mediated dephosphorylation of Tyr718 and activation of ASK1 signaling leading to cell death. More recently, the glycogen synthase kinase-3 (GSK-3β) was found to mediate TLR4-induced ASK1 activation by increasing ASK1 stability [59].

In addition to posttranslational modifications, ASK1 protein levels may also be transcriptionally regulated via upregulation of *ASK1* gene expression. Studies have demonstrated that the E2F family of transcription factors (E2 promoter-binding factors) regulate the expression of ASK1 [60]. Suzuki *et al.*, recently found that onset of spinal and bulbar muscular atrophy (SBMA), a neurodegenerative disorder caused by a polyglutamine repeat (polyQ) expansion within the human androgen receptor correlates with aberrant E2F activation [61]. Thus, multiple posttranslational modifications and other regulatory events work in concert to govern the activity of ASK1 under both physiological and pathological conditions. The aberrant activation of ASK1 observed in neurodegenerative diseases may be triggered by multiple stimuli (e.g. oxidative stress, ER stress) by acting directly on ASK1 molecules or by impairing the activity of other proteins implicated in regulating its activity.

5. ASK1 in Alzheimer's Disease

Alzheimer's Disease (AD), the most common form of dementia, was first described by Alois Alzheimer 100 years ago. It is a neurodegenerative disorder characterized clinically by the progressive loss of memory and cognitive impairment. AD is pathologically characterized by the accumulation of cerebral neuritic plaques of amyloid-β (Aβ), neurofibrillary tangle (NFT) formation as well as by neuronal cell death. Accumulation of misfolded proteins together with increased oxidative stress and mitochondrial dysfunction are mechanisms that correlate with the pathogenesis of the disease [62, 63]. Although age is the greatest risk factor for AD, the molecular mechanisms underlying the cause of the disease remain mainly elusive. As ASK1 is activated by ROS and ER-stress (UPR), several studies have implicated ASK1 in cell death processes associated with AD. Cell-based studies including, studies employing primary hybrid neuron cells (F11, hybrid cells of rat embryonic day 13 primary cultured neurons and a mouse neuroblastoma) demonstrated that ASK1 can form a complex with the amyloid precursor protein (APP) via JIP-1b (JNK-interacting protein), phospho-MKK6 and JNK1 [65-67] resulting in caspase dependent neuronal cell death [65]. In addition, the resulting neurotoxicity was significantly blocked by exogenous expression of a dominant negative mutant form of ASK1 as well as by the JNK inhibitor SP600125 [65] strongly suggesting an ASK1/JNK-mediated death pathway in AD.

The ASK1/APP complex formation was also confirmed by three-dimensional reconstruction of confocal microscopic Z-stacks obtained from fixed brains of APP transgenic mice that revealed an up-regulation of ASK1 expression in these mice compared to non-transgenic controls [66]. Beside ROS-induced ASK1 activation, Aβ, a toxic cleavage product of APP, was also demonstrated to activate ASK1 and subsequently JNK [68]. Whereas primary neuronal cultures derived from E14.5 $ASK^{+/+}$ mice demonstrated an 80% reduction in cell viability after exposure to $A\beta_{25-35}$, the survival in $ASK^{-/-}$ derived neurons treated with $A\beta_{25-35}$ was significantly elevated (only 30% reduction in viability). Furthermore, postmortem analysis of AD patient brains compared with age-matched controls revealed strong expression of the downstream ASK1 substrate MKK6 [69]. The activated phospho-MKK6 also co-immunoprecipitated with the paired helical filament Tau from human AD hippocampal supernatants [67] and overlapped with active p38. Both are found to be exclusively localized in classic pathological AD structures like NFT and senile plaques [69]. These data strongly suggest that ASK1 could play a significant role in the pathogenesis of AD by mediating ROS and/or Aβ induced neuronal cell death via the MKK6/JNK/p38 pathway. In addition, Aβ was not only shown to cause neuron-specific toxicity, but also demonstrated to cause vascular degeneration in cerebral amyloid angiopathy; Hsu and co-workers employed primary murine cerebral endothelial cells (CEC) to investigate the mode of cell death mediated by Aβ in ASK1 transfected CECs [50]. Aβ exposure was observed to result in an induction of the ASK1-MKK3/6-p38-p53 signaling machinery and increased levels of the pro-apoptotic protein Bax resulting in CEC programmed cell death. ASK1 activity is also known to be modulated by oxidized thioredoxin-1 (TRX1) and glutaredoxin-1 (GRX1). Postmortem brain samples of AD patients revealed that whereas TRX1 was decreased in neurons (frontal cortex and hippocampal CA1 regions) GRX1 expression was increased [70]. In addition, the same authors demonstrated that in SH-SY5Y cells, $A\beta_{1\text{-}41}$ exposure resulted in TRX1/GRX1 oxidation with subsequent induction of apoptosis. Current studies therefore suggest that ER-stress and ROS-mediated ASK1 activation represents an important signal transduction mechanism in AD.

6. ASK1 in Parkinson Disease

Parkinson's Disease (PD) is the second most common neurodegenerative disease after AD. The main pathology of PD is characterized by the severe loss of dopaminergic neurons from the substantia nigra pars compacta (SNpc) that project into the striatum. PD is also characterized by the misfolding of α-synuclein which generates protein aggregates called Lewy bodies [71]. Clinical signs of PD, which include rest tremor, rigidity and bradykinesia become evident when approximately 80% of striatal dopamine and 50% of nigral neurons are lost [72]. Like AD, age is the greatest known risk factor for PD. While the mechanism underlying the 'area-specific' neuronal loss in PD remains unclear, both oxidative and ER-stress are strongly implicated as contributing factors of the disease state [73-76].

The neurotoxin, 1-methyl-4-phenyl-1,2,3,6-tetrahydropyridine (MPTP) causes the selective loss of dopaminergic neurons in SNpc in mice in a manner similar to that seen in PD and is often used in mouse models to study the molecular mechanisms in PD pathogenesis. Activation of JNK and p38 appear to be critical in mediating MPTP induced toxicity, as dopaminergic neurons in JNK3 knockout mice were significantly protected from the toxic effects of MPTP [77, 78]. The activation of JNK and p38 in dopaminergic neurons is thought to be mediated by ASK1 [79]. Karunakaran and co-workers demonstrated that administration of the neurotoxin MPTP, induced ASK1 activation and the subsequent activation of its downstream targets MKK4 and JNK [80]. This pathway triggered the nucleus to cytoplasmic translocalization of the death-associated protein Daxx, specifically in neurons located in the SNpc. Co-administration of MPTP with α-lipoic acid, a thiol antioxidant inhibited the activation of ASK1 and subsequent activation of its downstream targets [80]. Recently, peroxiredoxin2 (PRX2), an antioxidant enzyme, was demonstrated to protect against 6-OHDA induced neurotoxicity both *in vitro* and *in vivo* [27]. The proposed mechanism of inhibition was through blockade of ASK1 activation and its downstream JNK/p38 signaling pathway. Infusion of a lentiviral vector expressing a short hairpin RNA (shRNA) to specifically knock down ASK1 protein expression in the left SNpc of C57BL/6 mice was evaluated. Inhibition of ASK1 was observed to significantly attenuate the 6-OHDA induced ASK1/JNK signaling axis. Moreover, knockdown of ASK1 significantly protected against 6-OHDA induced death of dopaminergic neurons, improved motor function and significantly elevated dopamine levels in the striatum. Interestingly, immunological analysis of postmortem PD brain sections clearly indicate that active-ASK1 is frequently observed in SNpc neurons and co-localized in 33% of the cases with Lewy bodies and more than 60% of phospho-ASK1 neurons also revealed abnormal α-synuclein staining [27]. Taken together, the data demonstrate that redox sensitive molecules (e.g. PRX2) are able to modulate apoptotic pathways by influencing ASK1 activity and suggest that targeting either PRX2 or ASK1 may be a promising approach for neuroprotective intervention in PD.

7. ASK1 in Huntington's Disease

The expansion of CAG trinucleotide repeat units which encode for uninterrupted glutamine residues or (polyQ) is the underlying cause of at least nine inherited human neurodegenerative disorders including Huntington's Disease (HD), Spinobulbar Muscular Atrophy (SBMA) and several forms of spinocereballar ataxia (SCA) [81, 82]. HD is clinically characterized by abnormal involuntary movements, including chorea and dystonia, and cognitive impairment through a selective loss of neurons mainly in the basal ganglia and cerebral cortex [83]. HD is caused by a mutation in the *huntingtin* gene (abnormal CAG repeats in the open reading frame) which encodes a large protein (350 kDa) with an expanded polyglutamine (polyQ) tract. Interestingly, the number of polyglutamine repeats is correlated with the severity of symptoms and once expanded over a repeat of 40, HD occurs [84]. It has been demonstrated that the expanded polyQ repeats form intracellular cytoplasmic and/or nuclear aggregates with subsequent neurotoxic effects *in vitro*, in transgenic animals (overexpressing polyQ proteins) and in postmortem brains of polyQ disease patients. The neurotoxic insult is mediated by dysfunction of the ubiquitin proteosome function resulting in ER stress [85, 86].

As described above, the accumulation of misfolded proteins and induction of ER stress is a process that is known to activate ASK1. Thus, it was hypothesized that ASK1 could play a significant role in HD by modifying huntingtin [87], acting as a signal transducer at the protein level as well as a cell death modulator at the post-translational level [88]. Indeed, by comparison to wild type cells, neuronal cell viability derived from ASK1 knockout mice was significantly protected against cell death mediated by expression of polyQ79 (i.e. 79 glutamine repeats) [8]. In addition, neurons derived from ASK1 knockout mice, were also observed to be defective in proteasome inhibitor and ER stress-induced JNK activation. Recently, it was shown that inhibition of ASK1 through administration of ASK1 antibodies using a micro-osmotic pump reduces ER stress and toxicity in a HD mouse model. In addition, nuclear translocation of huntington fragments was observed in cells harboring active ASK1 enzyme, whereas inactivated ASK1-bound huntingtin prevented its nuclear translocation and improved motor dysfunction in mice [89]. Similarly, ASK1 protein levels are also increased in the striatum following injection of 3-nitropropionic acid (3-NP), a mitochondrial toxin producing age-dependent oxidative stress and a model of Huntington's Disease [90], whereas reduction of ASK1 expression using siRNA was accompanied by a reduction in cell death. Therefore, regulating the activity of ASK1 by small molecule inhibitors and/or antibodies could also reveal promising treatment strategies for HD.

8. ASK1 in Amyotrophic Lateral Sclerosis

Amyotrophic Lateral Sclerosis (ALS) is a late onset neurodegenerative disorder, characterized by a selective loss of motor neurons in the spinal cord, brain stem and cerebral cortex [89]. Although the precise mechanism(s) for the pathogenesis of ALS remains unclear, studies highlight oxidative stress, excitotoxicity, protein aggregation and ER-stress as culprits in motor neuron demise. About 10% of ALS cases are familial (FALS) and about 1-2% are caused by mutations in the Cu/Zn-superoxide dismutase (SOD1) gene. SOD1$^{-/-}$ mice show no ALS phenotypes, indicating that the gain of function mutations in SOD1 (and over 120 have been identified in FALS) is critical for the death of motor neurons and FALS.
At the cellular level mutant SOD1 was suggested to play several roles in the pathogenesis of ALS, such as triggering abnormal protein interactions and activating caspases [92] [93]. Studies in transgenic mice expressing the ALS-linked SOD1 mutants showed an increase in the number of motor neurons with activated ASK1 and p38, strongly suggesting that ASK1-p38 pathway may be involved in neuronal cell death in FALS [94, 95]. Furthermore, several groups have demonstrated both *in vitro* and *in vivo* that the activation of ASK1 and/or its downstream pathways are associated with a selective motor neuron loss induced by the mutant SOD1 [96, 97]. Taken together these studies suggest a functional link between ER-stress and ASK1/p38 signaling axis in FALS. In a recent study by Nishitoh *et al.*, a specific interaction of SOD-1 and Derlin-1, a protein of the ER-associated degradation (ERAD) complex was observed to trigger ER-stress through dysfunction of ERAD [98]. The resulting ERAD dysfunction promoted ASK1 activation and subsequent apoptosis. These authors demonstrated that motor neuron death could be significantly reduced by the forced dissociation of mutant SOD1 from Derlin-1. Additional *in vivo* experiments revealed that deletion of ASK1 reduced the motor neuron loss and prolonged the lifespan of mutant SOD1 transgenic mice. These results suggest that Derlin-1/SOD-1 interaction promotes ER-stress, ASK1/p38 activation resulting in motor neuron cell death, a mechanism that is a key component of the disease progression of familial ALS [98].

9. ASK1 in ischemic brain injury

Ischemic brain injury is an acute or chronic disorder induced by insufficient blood flow into the brain. Hypoxic, or in the case of no oxygen supply, anoxic conditions trigger the induction of complex and overlapping signaling pathways, leading ultimately to neuronal cell death. Experimental models have demonstrated the involvement of pathways involving excitotoxicity, ionic imbalance, oxidative and nitrosactive stress resulting in neuronal cell death [99]. The activation of JNK was demonstrated in a murine model of transient focal ischemia to be a crucial signaling component mediating neuronal cell death [100] and strong evidence indicating a potential role for ASK1 in the pathogenesis of ischemic brain injury has emerged [101]. Using a cerebral ischemia rat model as well as in an *in vitro* kinase assay, ASK1 exhibited increased autophosphorylation and activity at various time points after the induction of cerebral ischemia. Furthermore, ASK1 autophosphorylation and activity were inhibited by the pre-administration of the antioxidant N-acetylcystein. Thus, activation of ASK1 may play a significant role in the apoptotic pathway following cerebral ischemia.
The heat shock protein-27 (Hsp27) was observed to be upregulated in cells surviving ischemic insults [102] and in ischemic preconditioning models [103], suggesting that Hsp-27 is associated with pro-survival cascades. Recently, studies overexpressing human Hsp-27 by viral mediated transfer and in Hsp27 transgenic mice demonstrated that Hsp-27 promoted

long-term neuroprotection against cerebral ischemia, as measured by infarct volume and sensory motor function. In addition, improvement in postischemic neurobehavioral recovery was also observed up to three weeks following cerebral ischemia [104]. At the molecular level, Hsp-27 was demonstrated to physically interact with ASK1 resulting in inhibition of ASK1 activity. Subsequent genetic knockdown of ASK1 or inhibition of the ASK1/MKK4 cascade also effectively abolished neuronal ischemia. Hsp-27 mediated inhibition of the pro-apoptotic ASK1 pathway may be a promising novel neuroprotective strategy for stroke.

10. Conclusion

Aberrant regulation of ASK1 activity is observed in a variety of neurodegenerative stress associated diseases and genetic knockout studies have delivered a strong case for ASK1 as a candidate therapeutic target in the treatment of such disorders. While ASK1 inhibitors have been claimed in the patent literature, no small molecule ASK1 inhibitors have obtained sufficient optimization characteristics for candidate selection and approval for first time in human studies. As such, there is little data available in the peer-reviewed literature concerning these inhibitors. In addition to their potential as future therapeutics, there is little doubt that small molecule inhibitors targeting ASK1 would be highly useful assets to facilitate understanding of the complex biology of ASK1. To rely on a molecular probe to make firm mechanistic conclusions about ASK1's role in cellular signaling, the selectivity of the final compound must be devoid of off-target activity. Recent characterization of the structure of the ASK1 kinase domain may facilitate development of ASK1-specific inhibitors [17]. Interestingly, Bunkoczi *et al.* observed that apart from its closely related isoform (ASK2), the nearest phylogenic neighbor to ASK1 shares sequence identity of only 50% within the kinase domain. In this regard, ASK1 may form a chemically diverse catalytic domain, which may allow a high level of kinase selectivity even with an inhibitor with an ATP competitive mode of action. Our laboratory has recently developed a biochemical assay using the full length ASK1 signalosome complex and full length substrate to identify inhibitors that are not only ATP competitive, but also substrate competitive and non-competitive with respect to ATP or substrate [31]. Since several ASK1 interacting proteins have been shown to modulate the activity of ASK1 within the signalosome complex, identification of cell permeable peptide inhibitors or development of ATP-noncompetative small molecule inhibitors that alter conformation or block ASK1 regultory protein interactions could serve as highly specific probes for ASK1. Regardless of the approach taken, careful analysis of the first generation of ASK1 inhibitors will be needed to define both the benefits and potential liabilities of mechanistically inhibiting ASK1 in cellular and animal systems.

11. References

[1] Ichijo, H., et al., Induction of apoptosis by ASK1, a mammalian MAPKKK that activates SAPK/JNK and p38 signaling pathways. *Science*, 1997. 275(5296): p. 90-4.

[2] Chen, Z., et al., ASK1 mediates apoptotic cell death induced by genotoxic stress. *Oncogene*, 1999. 18(1): p. 173-80.

[3] Matsukawa, J., et al., The ASK1-MAP kinase cascades in mammalian stress response. *J Biochem*, 2004. 136(3): p. 261-5.

[4] McDonald, P.H., et al., Beta-arrestin 2: a receptor-regulated MAPK scaffold for the activation of JNK3. *Science*, 2000. 290(5496): p. 1574-7.

[5] Matsuzawa, A., et al., Physiological roles of ASK1-mediated signal transduction in oxidative stress- and endoplasmic reticulum stress-induced apoptosis: advanced findings from ASK1 knockout mice. *Antioxid Redox Signal*, 2002. 4(3): p. 415-25.
[6] Hatai, T., et al., Execution of apoptosis signal-regulating kinase 1 (ASK1)-induced apoptosis by the mitochondria-dependent caspase activation. *J Biol Chem*, 2000. 275(34): p. 26576-81.
[7] Hao, W., et al., Induction of apoptosis by the Ste20-like kinase SLK, a germinal center kinase that activates apoptosis signal-regulating kinase and p38. *J Biol Chem*, 2006. 281(6): p. 3075-84.
[8] Nishitoh, H., et al., ASK1 is essential for endoplasmic reticulum stress-induced neuronal cell death triggered by expanded polyglutamine repeats. *Genes Dev*, 2002. 16(11): p. 1345-55.
[9] Schaeffer, H.J. and M.J. Weber, Mitogen-activated protein kinases: specific messages from ubiquitous messengers. *Mol Cell Biol*, 1999. 19(4): p. 2435-44.
[10] Faigle, R., et al., ASK1 inhibits astroglial development via p38 mitogen-activated protein kinase and promotes neuronal differentiation in adult hippocampus-derived progenitor cells. *Mol Cell Biol*, 2004. 24(1): p. 280-93.
[11] Takeda, K., et al., Apoptosis signal-regulating kinase 1 (ASK1) induces neuronal differentiation and survival of PC12 cells. *J Biol Chem*, 2000. 275(13): p. 9805-13.
[12] Matsuzawa, A., et al., ROS-dependent activation of the TRAF6-ASK1-p38 pathway is selectively required for TLR4-mediated innate immunity. *Nat Immunol*, 2005. 6(6): p. 587-92.
[13] Sayama, K., et al., Apoptosis signal-regulating kinase 1 (ASK1) is an intracellular inducer of keratinocyte differentiation. *J Biol Chem*, 2001. 276(2): p. 999-1004.
[14] Zhang, R., et al., Thioredoxin-2 inhibits mitochondria-located ASK1-mediated apoptosis in a JNK-independent manner. *Circ Res*, 2004. 94(11): p. 1483-91.
[15] Hwang, I.S., Y.S. Jung, and E. Kim, Interaction of ALG-2 with ASK1 influences ASK1 localization and subsequent JNK activation. FEBS Lett, 2002. 529(2-3): p. 183-7.
[16] Sturchler, E., et al., Identification of a nuclear localization signal within ASK1 and its role in stress-induced ASK1 nucleocytoplasmic transport. FEBS Lett. submitted.
[17] Bunkoczi, G., et al., Structural and functional characterization of the human protein kinase ASK1. *Structure*, 2007. 15(10): p. 1215-26.
[18] Tobiume, K., M. Saitoh, and H. Ichijo, Activation of apoptosis signal-regulating kinase 1 by the stress-induced activating phosphorylation of pre-formed oligomer. *J Cell Physiol*, 2002. 191(1): p. 95-104.
[19] Noguchi, T., et al., Recruitment of tumor necrosis factor receptor-associated factor family proteins to apoptosis signal-regulating kinase 1 signalosome is essential for oxidative stress-induced cell death. *J Biol Chem*, 2005. 280(44): p. 37033-40.
[20] Saitoh, M., et al., Mammalian thioredoxin is a direct inhibitor of apoptosis signal-regulating kinase (ASK) 1. *Embo J*, 1998. 17(9): p. 2596-606.
[21] Gotoh, Y. and J.A. Cooper, Reactive oxygen species- and dimerization-induced activation of apoptosis signal-regulating kinase 1 in tumor necrosis factor-alpha signal transduction. *J Biol Chem*, 1998. 273(28): p. 17477-82.
[22] Holmgren, A., Thioredoxin structure and mechanism: conformational changes on oxidation of the active-site sulfhydryls to a disulfide. *Structure*, 1995. 3(3): p. 239-43.
[23] Liu, Y. and W. Min, Thioredoxin promotes ASK1 ubiquitination and degradation to inhibit ASK1-mediated apoptosis in a redox activity-independent manner. *Circ Res*, 2002. 90(12): p. 1259-66.

[24] Song, J.J. and Y.J. Lee, Differential role of glutaredoxin and thioredoxin in metabolic oxidative stress-induced activation of apoptosis signal-regulating kinase 1. *Biochem J*, 2003. 373(Pt 3): p. 845-53.
[25] Nadeau, P.J., et al., Disulfide Bond-mediated multimerization of Ask1 and its reduction by thioredoxin-1 regulate H(2)O(2)-induced c-Jun NH(2)-terminal kinase activation and apoptosis. *Mol Biol Cell*, 2007. 18(10): p. 3903-13.
[26] Nadeau, P.J., S.J. Charette, and J. Landry, REDOX reaction at ASK1-Cys250 is essential for activation of JNK and induction of apoptosis. *Mol Biol Cell*, 2009. 20(16): p. 3628-37.
[27] Hu, X., et al., Peroxiredoxin-2 protects against 6-hydroxydopamine-induced dopaminergic neurodegeneration via attenuation of the apoptosis signal-regulating kinase (ASK1) signaling cascade. *J Neurosci*, 2011. 31(1): p. 247-61.
[28] Waak, J., et al., Oxidizable residues mediating protein stability and cytoprotective interaction of DJ-1 with apoptosis signal-regulating kinase 1. *J Biol Chem*, 2009. 284(21): p. 14245-57.
[29] Hu, X., et al., Peroxiredoxin-2 protects against 6-hydroxydopamine-induced dopaminergic neurodegeneration via attenuation of the apoptosis signal-regulating kinase (ASK1) signaling cascade. *J Neurosci*. 31(1): p. 247-61.
[30] Nishitoh, H., et al., ASK1 is essential for JNK/SAPK activation by TRAF2. *Mol Cell*, 1998. 2(3): p. 389-95.
[31] Sturchler, E., et al., Mechanism of oxidative stress-induced ASK1-catalyzed MKK6 phosphorylation. *Biochemistry*, 2010. 49(19): p. 4094-102.
[32] Takeda, K., et al., Apoptosis signal-regulating kinase (ASK) 2 functions as a mitogen-activated protein kinase kinase kinase in a heteromeric complex with ASK1. *J Biol Chem*, 2007. 282(10): p. 7522-31.
[33] Jung, H., H.A. Seong, and H. Ha, Murine protein serine/threonine kinase 38 activates apoptosis signal-regulating kinase 1 via Thr 838 phosphorylation. *J Biol Chem*, 2008. 283(50): p. 34541-53.
[34] Morita, K., et al., Negative feedback regulation of ASK1 by protein phosphatase 5 (PP5) in response to oxidative stress. *Embo J*, 2001. 20(21): p. 6028-36.
[35] Sanchez-Ortiz, E., et al., Protein phosphatase 5 protects neurons against amyloid-beta toxicity. *J Neurochem*, 2009. 111(2): p. 391-402.
[36] Yoon, K.W., et al., CIB1 functions as a Ca(2+)-sensitive modulator of stress-induced signaling by targeting ASK1. *Proc Natl Acad Sci U S A*, 2009. 106(41): p. 17389-94.
[37] Peterson, C., et al., Changes in calcium homeostasis during aging and Alzheimer's disease. *Ann N Y Acad Sci*, 1989. 568: p. 262-70.
[38] Gleichmann, M. and M.P. Mattson, Neuronal calcium homeostasis and dysregulation. *Antioxid Redox Signal*. 14(7): p. 1261-73.
[39] Kim, A.H., et al., Akt phosphorylates and negatively regulates apoptosis signal-regulating kinase 1. *Mol Cell Biol*, 2001. 21(3): p. 893-901.
[40] Zhang, R., et al., Hsp90-Akt phosphorylates ASK1 and inhibits ASK1-mediated apoptosis. *Oncogene*, 2005. 24(24): p. 3954-63.
[41] Wang, Q., et al., Neuroprotection of selenite against ischemic brain injury through negatively regulating early activation of ASK1/JNK cascade via activation of PI3K/AKT pathway. *Acta Pharmacol Sin*, 2007. 28(1): p. 19-27.
[42] Nakagami, Y., Inhibitors beta-amyloid-induced toxicity by modulating the Akt signaling pathway. *Drug News Perspect*, 2004. 17(10): p. 655-60.
[43] Gu, J.J., et al., PIM1 phosphorylates and negatively regulates ASK1-mediated apoptosis. *Oncogene*, 2009. 28(48): p. 4261-71.

[44] Zhang, L., J. Chen, and H. Fu, Suppression of apoptosis signal-regulating kinase 1-induced cell death by 14-3-3 proteins. *Proc Natl Acad Sci U S A*, 1999. 96(15): p. 8511-5.
[45] Seong, H.A., et al., Reciprocal negative regulation of PDK1 and ASK1 signaling by direct interaction and phosphorylation. *J Biol Chem*, 2010. 285(4): p. 2397-414.
[46] Goldman, E.H., L. Chen, and H. Fu, Activation of apoptosis signal-regulating kinase 1 by reactive oxygen species through dephosphorylation at serine 967 and 14-3-3 dissociation. *J Biol Chem*, 2004. 279(11): p. 10442-9.
[47] Liu, Q., et al., Direct interaction and reciprocal regulation between ASK1 and calcineurin-NFAT control cardiomyocyte death and growth. *Mol Cell Biol*, 2006. 26(10): p. 3785-97.
[48] Min, W., et al., AIP1 recruits phosphatase PP2A to ASK1 in tumor necrosis factor-induced ASK1-JNK activation. *Circ Res*, 2008. 102(7): p. 840-8.
[49] Zhang, R., et al., AIP1 mediates TNF-alpha-induced ASK1 activation by facilitating dissociation of ASK1 from its inhibitor 14-3-3. *J Clin Invest*, 2003. 111(12): p. 1933-43.
[50] Hsu, M.J., et al., Apoptosis signal-regulating kinase 1 in amyloid beta peptide-induced cerebral endothelial cell apoptosis. *J Neurosci*, 2007. 27(21): p. 5719-29.
[51] Fujii, K., et al., Negative control of apoptosis signal-regulating kinase 1 through phosphorylation of Ser-1034. *Oncogene*, 2004. 23(29): p. 5099-104.
[52] Nagai, H., et al., Ubiquitin-like sequence in ASK1 plays critical roles in the recognition and stabilization by USP9X and oxidative stress-induced cell death. *Mol Cell*, 2009. 36(5): p. 805-18.
[53] Zhang, X., et al., Region-specific protein abundance changes in the brain of MPTP-induced Parkinson's disease mouse model. *J Proteome Res*. 9(3): p. 1496-509.
[54] Zhao, Y., et al., Tumor necrosis factor receptor 2 signaling induces selective c-IAP1-dependent ASK1 ubiquitination and terminates mitogen-activated protein kinase signaling. *J Biol Chem*, 2007. 282(11): p. 7777-82.
[55] Kisiswa, L., et al., Cellular inhibitor of apoptosis (cIAP1) is down-regulated during retinal ganglion cell (RGC) maturation. *Exp Eye Res*. 91(5): p. 739-47.
[56] Harada, C., et al., ASK1 deficiency attenuates neural cell death in GLAST-deficient mice, a model of normal tension glaucoma. *Cell Death Differ*. 17(11): p. 1751-9.
[57] Hwang, J.R., C. Zhang, and C. Patterson, C-terminus of heat shock protein 70-interacting protein facilitates degradation of apoptosis signal-regulating kinase 1 and inhibits apoptosis signal-regulating kinase 1-dependent apoptosis. *Cell Stress Chaperones*, 2005. 10(2): p. 147-56.
[58] Yu, L., et al., JAK2 and SHP2 reciprocally regulate tyrosine phosphorylation and stability of proapoptotic protein ASK1. *J Biol Chem*, 2009. 284(20): p. 13481-8.
[59] Noh, K.T., et al., GSK-3beta-induced ASK1 stabilization is crucial in LPS-induced endotoxin shock. *Exp Cell Res*. 317(12): p. 1663-8.
[60] Kherrouche, Z., et al., ASK-1 (apoptosis signal-regulating kinase 1) is a direct E2F target gene. *Biochem J*, 2006. 396(3): p. 547-56.
[61] Suzuki, E., et al., Aberrant E2F activation by polyglutamine expansion of androgen receptor in SBMA neurotoxicity. *Proc Natl Acad Sci U S A*, 2009. 106(10): p. 3818-22.
[62] Smith, M.A., et al., Early AGEing and Alzheimer's. *Nature*, 1995. 374(6520): p. 316.
[63] Behl, C., et al., Amyloid beta peptide induces necrosis rather than apoptosis. *Brain Res*, 1994. 645(1-2): p. 253-64.
[64] Hashimoto, Y., et al., The cytoplasmic domain of Alzheimer's amyloid-beta protein precursor causes sustained apoptosis signal-regulating kinase 1/c-Jun NH2-terminal kinase-mediated neurotoxic signal via dimerization. *J Pharmacol Exp Ther*, 2003. 306(3): p. 889-902.

[65] Galvan, V., et al., Interaction of ASK1 and the beta-amyloid precursor protein in a stress-signaling complex. *Neurobiol Dis*, 2007. 28(1): p. 65-75.

[66] Peel, A.L., et al., Tau phosphorylation in Alzheimer's disease: potential involvement of an APP-MAP kinase complex. *Neuromolecular Med*, 2004. 5(3): p. 205-18.

[67] Kadowaki, H., et al., Amyloid beta induces neuronal cell death through ROS-mediated ASK1 activation. *Cell Death Differ*, 2005. 12(1): p. 19-24.

[68] Zhu, X., et al., Activation of MKK6, an upstream activator of p38, in Alzheimer's disease. *J Neurochem*, 2001. 79(2): p. 311-8.

[69] Akterin, S., et al., Involvement of glutaredoxin-1 and thioredoxin-1 in beta-amyloid toxicity and Alzheimer's disease. *Cell Death Differ*, 2006. 13(9): p. 1454-65.

[70] Samii, A., J.G. Nutt, and B.R. Ransom, Parkinson's disease. *Lancet*, 2004. 363(9423): p. 1783-93.

[71] Fearnley, J.M. and A.J. Lees, Ageing and Parkinson's disease: substantia nigra regional selectivity. *Brain*, 1991. 114 (Pt 5): p. 2283-301.

[72] Tsang, A.H. and K.K. Chung, Oxidative and nitrosative stress in Parkinson's disease. *Biochim Biophys Acta*, 2009. 1792(7): p. 643-50.

[73] Przedborski, S., Pathogenesis of nigral cell death in Parkinson's disease. *Parkinsonism Relat Disord*, 2005. 11 Suppl 1: p. S3-7.

[74] Przedborski, S. and H. Ischiropoulos, Reactive oxygen and nitrogen species: weapons of neuronal destruction in models of Parkinson's disease. *Antioxid Redox Signal*, 2005. 7(5-6): p. 685-93.

[75] Farrer, M.J., Genetics of Parkinson disease: paradigm shifts and future prospects. *Nat Rev Genet*, 2006. 7(4): p. 306-18.

[76] Hunot, S., et al., JNK-mediated induction of cyclooxygenase 2 is required for neurodegeneration in a mouse model of Parkinson's disease. *Proc Natl Acad Sci U S A*, 2004. 101(2): p. 665-70.

[77] Choi, W.S., et al., Phosphorylation of p38 MAPK induced by oxidative stress is linked to activation of both caspase-8- and -9-mediated apoptotic pathways in dopaminergic neurons. *J Biol Chem*, 2004. 279(19): p. 20451-60.

[78] Ouyang, M. and X. Shen, Critical role of ASK1 in the 6-hydroxydopamine-induced apoptosis in human neuroblastoma SH-SY5Y cells. *J Neurochem*, 2006. 97(1): p. 234-44.

[79] Karunakaran, S., et al., Activation of apoptosis signal regulating kinase 1 (ASK1) and translocation of death-associated protein, Daxx, in substantia nigra pars compacta in a mouse model of Parkinson's disease: protection by alpha-lipoic acid. *FASEB J*, 2007. 21(9): p. 2226-36.

[80] Kakizuka, A., Protein precipitation: a common etiology in neurodegenerative disorders? *Trends Genet*, 1998. 14(10): p. 396-402.

[81] Paulson, H.L., N.M. Bonini, and K.A. Roth, Polyglutamine disease and neuronal cell death. *Proc Natl Acad Sci U S A*, 2000. 97(24): p. 12957-8.

[82] Sawa, A., Mechanisms for neuronal cell death and dysfunction in Huntington's disease: pathological cross-talk between the nucleus and the mitochondria? *J Mol Med* (Berl), 2001. 79(7): p. 375-81.

[83] Sawa, A., T. Tomoda, and B.I. Bae, Mechanisms of neuronal cell death in Huntington's disease. *Cytogenet Genome Res*, 2003. 100(1-4): p. 287-95.

[84] Bence, N.F., R.M. Sampat, and R.R. Kopito, Impairment of the ubiquitin-proteasome system by protein aggregation. *Science*, 2001. 292(5521): p. 1552-5.

[85] Warrick, J.M., et al., Suppression of polyglutamine-mediated neurodegeneration in Drosophila by the molecular chaperone HSP70. *Nat Genet*, 1999. 23(4): p. 425-8.

[86] Arning, L., et al., ASK1 and MAP2K6 as modifiers of age at onset in Huntington's disease. *J Mol Med* (Berl), 2008. 86(4): p. 485-90.

[87] Sekine, Y., K. Takeda, and H. Ichijo, The ASK1-MAP kinase signaling in ER stress and neurodegenerative diseases. *Curr Mol Med*, 2006. 6(1): p. 87-97.

[88] Cho, K.J., et al., Inhibition of apoptosis signal-regulating kinase 1 reduces endoplasmic reticulum stress and nuclear huntingtin fragments in a mouse model of Huntington disease. *Neuroscience*, 2009. 163(4): p. 1128-34.

[89] Minn, Y., et al., Induction of apoptosis signal-regulating kinase 1 and oxidative stress mediate age-dependent vulnerability to 3-nitropropionic acid in the mouse striatum. *Neurosci Lett*, 2008. 430(2): p. 142-6.

[90] Cleveland, D.W. and J.D. Rothstein, From Charcot to Lou Gehrig: deciphering selective motor neuron death in ALS. *Nat Rev Neurosci*, 2001. 2(11): p. 806-19.

[91] Kunst, C.B., et al., Mutations in SOD1 associated with amyotrophic lateral sclerosis cause novel protein interactions. *Nat Genet*, 1997. 15(1): p. 91-4.

[92] Li, M., et al., Functional role of caspase-1 and caspase-3 in an ALS transgenic mouse model. *Science*, 2000. 288(5464): p. 335-9.

[93] Wengenack, T.M., et al., Activation of programmed cell death markers in ventral horn motor neurons during early presymptomatic stages of amyotrophic lateral sclerosis in a transgenic mouse model. *Brain Res*, 2004. 1027(1-2): p. 73-86.

[94] Holasek, S.S., et al., Activation of the stress-activated MAP kinase, p38, but not JNK in cortical motor neurons during early presymptomatic stages of amyotrophic lateral sclerosis in transgenic mice. *Brain Res*, 2005. 1045(1-2): p. 185-98.

[95] Raoul, C., et al., Motoneuron death triggered by a specific pathway downstream of Fas. potentiation by ALS-linked SOD1 mutations. *Neuron*, 2002. 35(6): p. 1067-83.

[96] Veglianese, P., et al., Activation of the p38MAPK cascade is associated with upregulation of TNF alpha receptors in the spinal motor neurons of mouse models of familial ALS. *Mol Cell Neurosci*, 2006. 31(2): p. 218-31.

[97] Nishitoh, H. and H. Ichijo, [Molecular mechanisms of ALS-linked mutant SOD1-induced motor neuron death] . Tanpakushitsu Kakusan Koso, 2009. 54(3): p. 237-44.

[98] Lo, E.H., T. Dalkara, and M.A. Moskowitz, Mechanisms, challenges and opportunities in stroke. *Nat Rev Neurosci*, 2003. 4(5): p. 399-415.

[99] Gao, Y.H., et al., [The protective effect of cholic acid on an in vitro injury model of ischemia-reperfusion in cerebral microvascular endothelial cells] . *Zhongguo Zhong Yao Za Zhi*, 2005. 30(12): p. 930-2.

[100] Zhang, Q. and G. Zhang, Activation and autophosphorylation of apoptosis signal-regulating kinase 1 (ASK1) following cerebral ischemia in rat hippocampus. *Neurosci Lett*, 2002. 329(2): p. 232-6.

[101] Kato, H., et al., Immunohistochemical localization of the low molecular weight stress protein HSP27 following focal cerebral ischemia in the rat. *Brain Res*, 1995. 679(1): p. 1-7.

[102] Currie, R.W., et al., Benign focal ischemic preconditioning induces neuronal Hsp70 and prolonged astrogliosis with expression of Hsp27. *Brain Res*, 2000. 863(1-2): p. 169-81.

[103] Stetler, R.A., et al., Hsp27 protects against ischemic brain injury via attenuation of a novel stress-response cascade upstream of mitochondrial cell death signaling. *J Neurosci*, 2008. 28(49): p. 13038-55.

10

Role of Connexin Hemichannels in Neurodegeneration

Juan A. Orellana[1,2], Christian Giaume[3] and Juan C. Sáez[1,4]
[1]*Departamento de Fisiología; Facultad de Ciencias Biológicas*
[2]*Departamento de Neurología; Facultad de Medicina*
Pontificia Universidad Católica de Chile, Santiago,
[3]*CIRB; UMR CNRS 7241/ INSERM U1050, Collège de France, Paris*
[4]*Instituto milenio, Centro Interdiciplinario de Neurociencias de Valparaiso, Valparaiso,*
[1,2,4]*Chile*
[3]*France*

1. Introduction

Progressive loss of neuronal structure and function occur in several neurodegenerative diseases. Cellular responses to brain injury depend on properties of the cells (e.g., hormonal nutritional status) and insult (e.g., duration, intensity, and quality), whereas, tissue responses depend on interactions between their constituent cells, including chemical and electrical transmission as well as paracrine and autocrine signaling. In vertebrate cells, autocrine and paracrine communication occur in part via release of chemical signals through connexin hemichannels (Sáez et al. 2010), the precursors of gap junction channels that are formed by two hemichannels provided by one of each apposed cells (Fig. 1). Each hemichannel is composed of six protein subunits termed connexins, which are highly conserved proteins encoded by 21 genes in human and 20 in mouse with orthologs in other vertebrate species (Cruciani and Mikalsen 2005). Connexins are abundantly expressed in cells of the central nervous system (CNS) (Orellana et al. 2009) (Fig. 2), and they are named after their predicted molecular mass expressed in kDa, so that connexin43 (Cx43) has a molecular mass of ~43 kDa.

For a long time the main function attributed to connexin hemichannels was the formation of gap junction channels. Nevertheless, in the last decade, the presence of functional connexin hemichannels in nonjunctional membranes has been demonstrated by several experimental approaches (Sáez et al. 2010). These channels allow cellular release of relevant quantities of autocrine/paracrine signaling molecules (e.g., ATP, glutamate, NAD^+ and PGE_2) to the extracellular milieu (Bruzzone et al. 2001; Cherian et al. 2005; Stout et al. 2002), as well as uptake of small molecules (e.g., glucose) (Retamal et al. 2007a). Recently, another gene family encoding a set of three membrane proteins, named pannexins (Panxs 1-3), has been identified (Bruzzone et al. 2003). Up to now, only Panx3 has been shown to form gap junctions in osteoblasts (Ishikawa et al. 2011) and further studies will be required to identify pannexin gap junctions in other cell types. Connexins and pannexins present similar membrane topology, with four α-helical transmembrane domains connected by two extracellular loops, where both N- and C-termini are intracellular. However, there is only 16% overall identity when their full-length amino acid sequences are compared.

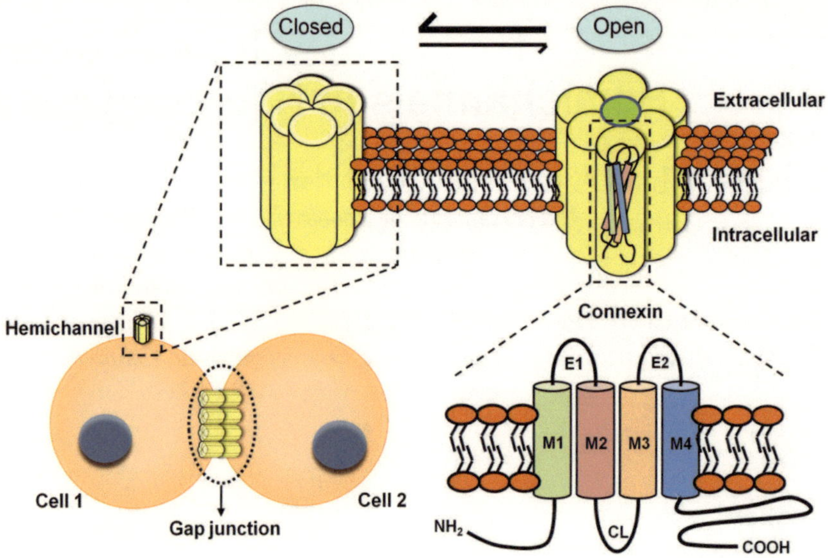

Fig. 1. Diagram illustrating basic structures of connexins and undocked hemichannels present at the cell surface. The membrane topology of a connexin consists of 4 membrane-spanning domains (M1-M4), 2 extracellular loops (E1 and E2) and 1 cytoplasmic loop (CL). The amino ($-NH_2$) and carboxy (-COOH) terminal tail are intracellular. A hemichannel is formed by six connexins that oligomerize laterally leaving a central pore. In cultured cells under resting conditions hemichannels remain preferentially closed, but they can be activated by diverse physiological and pathological conditions, offering a diffusional transmembrane route between the intra and extracellular milieu. [Modified from Orellana et al. 2011a]

A main role in cellular proliferation and tissue remodelling has been attributed to hemichannels (Burra and Jiang 2009; Schalper et al. 2008), while in the CNS they have been proposed to mediate ischemic tolerance (Lin et al. 2008; Schock et al. 2008) and establish adhesive interactions (Cotrina et al. 2008). To date, most studies suggest that under normal brain conditions hemichannels release physiological molecules relevant for intercellular signalling, including propagation of intercellular Ca^{2+} waves (Orellana et al. 2011a). However, an increasing body of evidence has situated the hemichannels as potential regulators of the beginning and maintenance of homeostatic imbalances present in diverse brain diseases (Orellana et al. 2009). Pioneering findings by Contreras and co-workers (Contreras et al. 2002) showed that astroglial death induced by ischemia-like conditions is accelerated by the opening of Cx43 hemichannels. In this sense, a constant increase of $[Ca^{2+}]_i$ mediated by augmented Ca^{2+} entry through hemichannels, which are permeable to Ca^{2+} (Schalper et al. 2010), and deficient or insufficient Ca^{2+} handling by injured cells could lead to cell death.
Here, we review and discuss the current evidence about the role of hemichannels in three major neurodegenerative diseases, namely, bacterial meningitis, stroke and Alzheimer's disease.

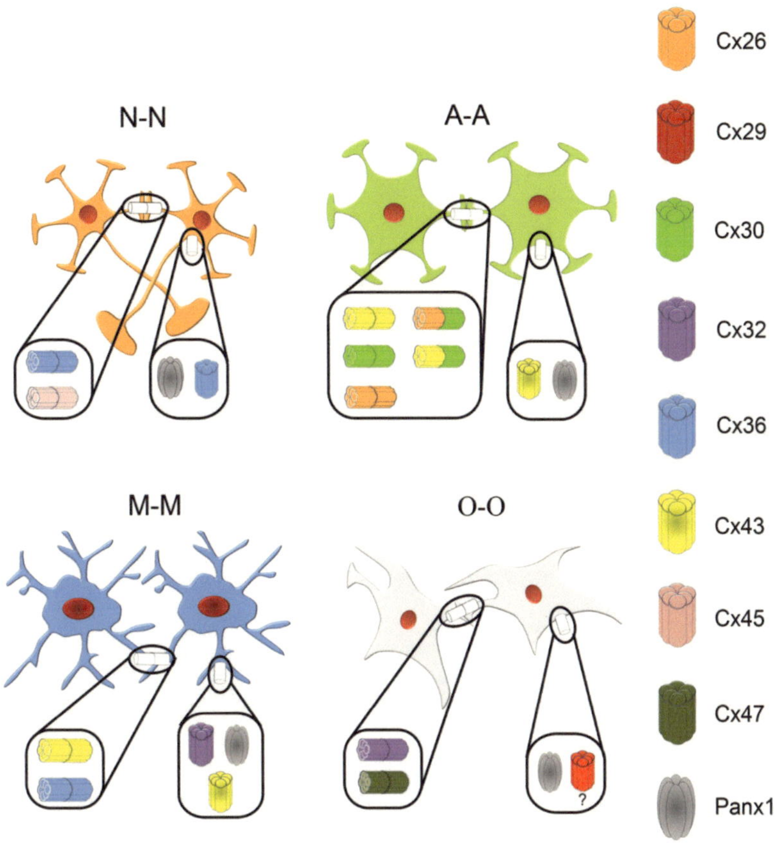

Fig. 2. Cellular distribution of pannexin and connexin hemichannels and connexin gap junctions in brain cells. This figure includes only those cases in which the available information has been obtained *in vivo* and/or *in vitro* with more than one experimental approach. Homocellular connexin gap junction channels and connexin and pannexin hemichannels are indicated within the encircled regions. Neuron (N), astrocyte (A), microglia (M) and oligodendrocyte (O). [Modified from Orellana et al. 2009]

2. What is known about hemichannels in neurological disorders?

2.1 Bacterial meningitis

Despite the advances in the understanding of infectious diseases, including bacterial meningitis, pathogen-host interactions and the widespread use of chemotherapeutic agents, infections are still an important cause of mortality, morbidity and social burden worldwide. Bacterial meningitis promotes inflammation of the pia, arachnoid, and subarachnoid space. Inflammation may also affect the brain parenchyma leading to encephalitis. Bacteria present in the bloodstream induce an innate immune response which produces systemic release of cytokines, mainly TNF-α (Dietzman et al. 1974; Ring et al. 1998). Then, bacteria colonize and cross the inflamed blood-brain barrier (BBB) and components of their wall, such as lipopolysaccharide (LPS) (Bannerman et al. 1998), peptidoglycan (PGN) (Bannerman et al. 1998), or streptococcal hemolysin/cytolysin (Doran et al. 2003), induce BBB activation and permeabilization (Freyer et al. 1999) (Fig. 3). BBB activation is characterized by numerous

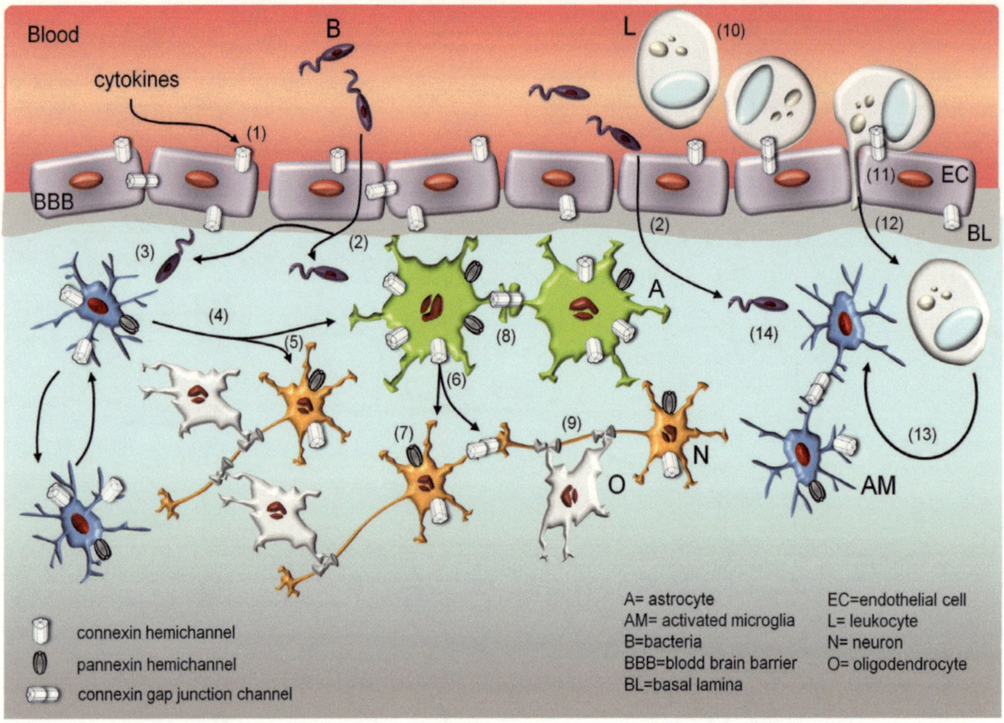

Fig. 3. Connexin based channels in brain cells during bacterial meningitis. During bacterial infection blood levels of cytokine (e.g., TNF-α and IL-1β) are elevated. Both, TNF-α and IL-1β enhance the hemichannel activity (1) of brain endothelial cells. Furthermore, these cytokines induce BBB discontinuity favoring bacterial extravasation (2). Once in the interstitium, bacteria and their extracellular wall components such as LPS and PGN are recognized by microglia (3), which are activated and release cytokines that further activate them (reciprocal arrows). ATP released via hemichannels from microglia (4) promotes microglial migration from less affected regions. Activated microglia can also release glutamate through hemichannels and oxygen and nitrogen derived free radicals that are neurotoxic (5). The enhanced hemichannel activity of activated astrocytes induces neuronal damage through the release of neurotoxic and/or inflammatory compounds such glutamate and PGE_2 (6). These compounds may also increase the activity of neuronal connexin/pannexin hemichannels (7) causing electrochemical imbalance and Ca^{2+} overload in neurons. In contrast to increased opening of hemichannels, astroglial gap junction communication is reduced (8), impairing glutamate and K^+ spatial buffering that enhances neuronal susceptibility to insults. Bacterial meningitis can also induce demyelination (9), possibly via microglial cytokine release. Severe inflammation induces recruitment of leukocytes (10) to the infected loci. Gap junction communication between leukocytes and endothelial cells (11) may contribute to strength heterocellular adhesion and allow transfer of signals that regulate leukocyte diapedesis across the endothelium (12). Activated microglia may perform antigen cross-presentation interaction with infiltrating leukocytes in which gap junctions between them may play an important role (13). Direct microglial interaction with LPS or PGN induces gap junction communication between microglia, which can coordinate microglial function (14). [Modified from Orellana et al. 2009]

changes including cytokine production, overexpression of cell adhesion molecules and NO synthesis (Freyer et al. 1999). Recently, hemichannels have been implicated in the pathogenesis of bacterial meningitis. Using a model of bacterial brain abscess, Karpuk and co-workers (Karpuk et al. 2011) showed that a transient hemichannel activity is induced in astrocytes within close proximity to the abscess border, which dissipates with increasing distance from the inflammatory site. Moreover, this transient hemichannel opening was blocked with the Cx43 mimetic peptide Gap26, carbenoxolone, the Panx1 mimetic peptide ^{10}panx1, and probenecid (Karpuk et al. 2011), indicating the involvement of both Cx43 and Panx1 hemichannels in this response. In addition, astroglial gap junction coupling was significantly reduced in areas immediately surrounding the abscess margins, while regions far from abscess presented normal coupling (Karpuk et al. 2011). These data are consistent with previous studies showing opposite regulation of gap junction channels versus hemichannels in astrocytes subjected to pro-inflammatory conditions (Froger et al. 2010; Froger et al. 2009; Orellana et al. 2011b; Orellana et al. 2010; Retamal et al. 2007a).

Pioneering findings by Retamal and co-workers (Retamal et al. 2007a) showed that TNF-α and IL-1β released from LPS-treated microglia induce an increase and decrease in astroglial hemichannel and gap junction channel activity, respectively (Retamal et al. 2007a).

The consequence of this opposite regulation on the homeostasis of the infected and uninfected brain parenchyma and how they may influence CNS function remain to be elucidated. A possible consequence of increased astroglial hemichannel opening could be an enhanced glucose uptake, which might explain the observed changes in the metabolic status of astrocytes under inflammatory conditions (Rtamal et al. 2007a). Moreover, hemichannel-mediated astroglial release of neurotoxic and/or inflammatory compounds such as glutamate and ATP could promote paracrine neuronal damage (Iglesias et al. 2009; Jiang et al. 2011; Kang et al. 2008; Orellana et al. 2011b; Orellana et al. 2011c; Ye et al. 2003).

Since the BBB critically regulates the passage of molecules into the CNS, the possibility of defective hemichannels in cells of the BBB during bacterial meningitis may be relevant. In this regard, TNF-α blocks the ATP release induced by photoliberation of $InsP_3$ or zero $[Ca^{2+}]_o$, but increases the basal ATP release and hemichannel-mediated dye uptake in brain cortical endothelium derived cell lines, RBE4 and GP8 (Vandamme et al. 2004). Since the increase in basal ATP release induced by TNF-α is not affected by the mimetic peptide Gap26, a prominent blocker of $InsP_3$- and zero Ca^{2+}-triggered connexin-dependent ATP release (Braet et al. 2003), it was concluded that the $InsP_3$- and zero Ca^{2+}-induced ATP release would involve a mechanism distinct from the one involved in the TNF-α induced elevation of basal ATP release (Vandamme et al. 2004). However, the authors did not rule out the involvement of other type of hemichannels (connexin/pannexins), including hemichannels formed by Cx40, which is highly expressed in brain endothelial cells (Nagasawa et al. 2006). Thus, the rise in basal activity induced by TNF-α could be related to Cx40 and/or pannexin hemichannels. At least in peripheral endothelial cells, the ATP release induced by brief exposure to PGN depends exclusively on Cx43 hemichannels (Robertson et al. 2010).

Enhanced endothelial hemichannel activity could elevate the ATP release, which would recruit microglia to the injury site (Davalos et al. 2005). In agreement with a role of hemichannels in ATP release during inflammatory conditions triggered by bacterial infections, Shigella infection of epithelial cells promote ATP release through Cx26 hemichannels, resulting in the activation of purinergic receptors on neighboring cells and bacterial dissemination (Tran Van Nhieu et al. 2003). In the same way, normal calcium signaling between astrocytes could be affected under pro-inflammatory conditions, eliciting one of the two calcium waves reported (Orellana et al. 2011a) (Fig. 4). In one of them, Ca^{2+} waves propagate by diffusion of cytoplasmic inositol (1,4,5)-trisphosphate (IP_3) through gap junctions between astrocytes, after phospholipase C (PLC) activation (Fig. 4). Evidence for this mechanism includes: (i) the waves are dependent on gap junctional communication; (ii) the waves are not blocked by extracellular apyrase, which is an ATPase; (iii) are not blocked by purine-receptor antagonists such as suramin; and (iv) do not jump a gap between cells (Orellana et al. 2011a). Other possible mechanism for astroglial Ca^{2+} waves is through the ATP released by Cx43 and/or Panx1 hemichannels after ATP-mediated P2 receptor activation (Fig. 4). Evidence for this mechanism include: (i) the waves require Cx43 and/or Panx1 expression (ii) hemichannel blockers prevent the waves; (iii) ATP is released by the

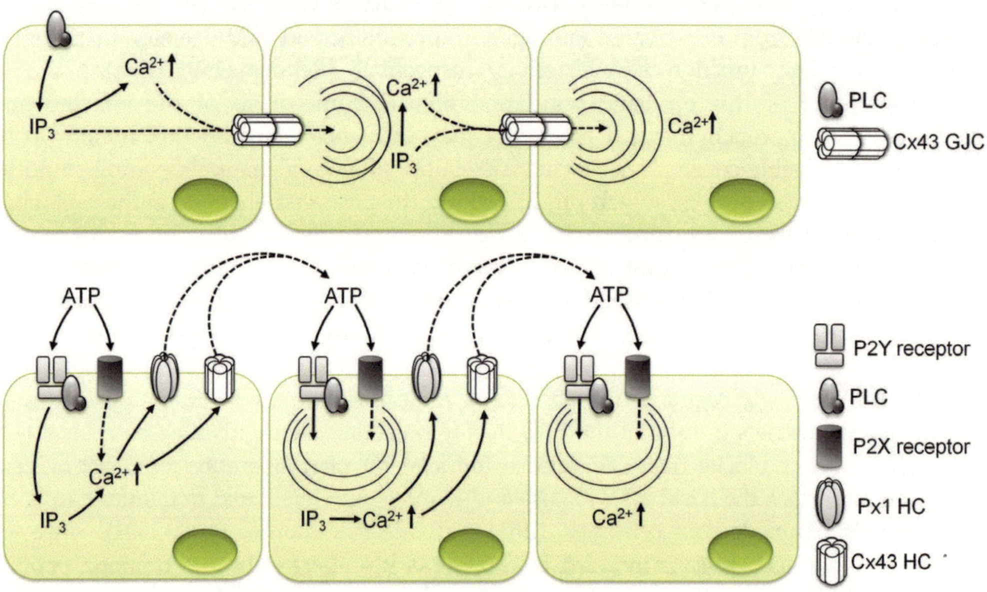

Fig. 4. Two models for conduction of Ca^{2+} waves in astrocytes. (Top panel) Upstream receptor stimulation leads to activation of phospholipase C (PLC) and formation of cytoplasmic inositol (1,4,5)-trisphosphate (IP_3), which promote the release of Ca^{2+} stored in the endoplasmic reticulum. Both IP_3 and Ca^{2+} diffuse to neighboring cells through gap junction channels generating waves of rises in intracellular Ca^{2+} concentration $[Ca^{2+}]_i$. (Bottom panel) ATP released from vesicles and/or ion channels diffuses through the extracellular space and activates membrane purinergic (P2) receptors. Stimulation of metabotropic P2Y receptors leads to activation of phospholipase C (PLC) and formation of IP_3. Whereas, activation of ionotropic P2X receptors leads to Ca^{2+} influx. The increase in free $[Ca^{2+}]_i$ induced by IP_3 and P2X receptor opening could promote ATP release through Cx43 and Px1 hemichannels, extending the Ca^{2+} wave to neighboring cells. [Modified from Orellana et al. 2011a]

initiator cell, and the Ca^{2+} waves extend as far as the ATP diffuses; (iv) the waves are blocked by extracellular apyrase; (v) are blocked by suramin (P2 receptor blocker); and (vi) jump cell-free gaps and are deflected by flow of medium (Orellana et al. 2011a). Probably, *in vivo* these two mechanisms coexist and are subjected to regulation by neuro- and gliotransmitters, playing a key role in the functional synchronization of neurovascular coupling.

As mentioned before, in the brain parenchyma, bacteria may undergo lysis and thus, they release pro-inflammatory and toxic factors such as PGN and LPS (Stuertz et al. 1998; Stuertz et al. 1999), while microglia interact directly with intact bacteria (Kim 2003). Bacterial derived pro-inflammatory factors such as LPS induce neurodegeneration (Qin et al. 2007). PGN and LPS stimulate microglial Toll-like receptors (TLRs), induce translocation of nuclear factor (NF) κB (Schwandner et al. 1999), and activation of MAPK signaling and transcription of genes encoding inflammatory cytokines (Laflamme and Rivest 2001; Nau and Bruck 2002). Moreover, PGN increases microglial Cx43 mRNA and protein expression, which correlates with development of gap junction communication *in vitro* (Garg et al. 2005). Similarly, treatment with LPS plus IFN-γ increases Cx43 expression in rat microglia and induces gap junction communication (Eugenín et al. 2001). In addition, brain stab wounds induce recruitment of Cx43 immunoreactive microglia to the injured foci, suggesting that Cx43 is important for coordinating microglial responses (Eugenín et al. 2001). However, up to now, the functional state of hemichannels in microglia has been not examined in model of bacterial brain infection.

Bacterial meningitis also causes axonal damage and demyelination (Nau et al. 2004). These effects may be related to microglial cytokine release, which could promote opening of oligodendrocyte hemichannels, possibly composed of Panx1, Cx32 or Cx29 [Cx29 does not form gap junctions and faces the periaxonal space (Li et al. 2002)] and, thus, promoting ion gradient imbalance and Ca^{2+} overload.

Adhesion between leukocytes and endothelial cells could result in part from leuko-endothelial gap junction formation (Veliz et al. 2008). In fact, treatment with diverse gap junction channel blockers reduces leukocyte adhesion to venular endothelium *in vivo* (Veliz et al. 2008) as well as transmigration across a BBB model (Eugenín et al. 2003). Gap junctions between lymphoma and endothelial cells have also been demonstrated, and α-GA attenuates the transmigration of lymphoma cells across an endothelial barrier (Haddad et al. 2008). However, it is important to keep in mind that most gap junction blockers will also block hemichannels and that connexin knockout animals will also have impaired transmembrane diffusional transport mediated by hemichannels. Indeed, the autocrine release of ATP through Cx37 hemichannels in monocyte/macrophages limits their adhesion to the endothelial wall and recruitment to the subendothelial compartment (Wong et al. 2006). Recent findings also suggest that connexin and pannexin hemichannels participate in acute and chronic inflammatory responses mediated by macrophagic cells. In fact, LPS or TNF-α promote microglial release of neurotoxic glutamate concentrations via Cx32 hemichannels (Takeuchi et al. 2006). Panx1 hemichannel opening occur in primary macrophages, macrophage cell lines and microglia exposed to pro-inflammatory conditions (Orellana et al. 2011c; Pelegrin and Surprenant 2006; Pelegrin and Surprenant 2007). In addition, caspase-1/inflammasome-mediated release of members of the IL-1 family including IL-1β from mouse peritoneal macrophages requires hemichannel activation through $P2X_7$ purinergic receptors (Pelegrin and Surprenant 2006).

2.2 Stroke

Stroke is a major cause of death in industrialized countries and results from a transient or permanent reduction in cerebral blood flow produced, in most cases, by cerebral artery occlusion by an embolus or local thrombosis, i.e., focal ischemia (Dirnagl et al. 1999). Severe and/or prolonged reduction in cerebral blood flow leads to deprivation of oxygen and glucose as well as build-up of potentially toxic substances. During stroke, decreased cellular oxygen levels, loss of oxidative phosphorylation and reduced ATP synthesis are the initial steps leading to cell death (Dirnagl et al. 1999). The ATP depletion may induce a rapid decrease in ATPase activity, leading to imbalanced electrochemical gradients across the plasma membrane. Notably, increased pannexin and/or connexin hemichannel activity occur in cortical astrocytes (Contreras et al. 2002; Orellana et al. 2011b; Orellana et al. 2010; Retamal et al. 2006), olygodendrocytes (Domercq et al. 2010) and hippocampal neurons (Lin et al. 2008; Schock et al. 2008; Thompson et al. 2006) subjected to ischemic like conditions. The enhanced hemichannel activity induced by ischemic like conditions accelerates cell death, at least in cultured rat astrocytes (Contreras et al. 2002; Orellana et al. 2010) (Fig. 5). Possibly, sustained hemichannel opening contribute to increased $[Ca^{2+}]_i$, which in turn may favour even more the connexin hemichannel activity (De Vuyst et al. 2007; Schalper et al. 2008), inducing Ca^{2+} and Na^+ intracellular overload (Fig. 5). The ionic (or electrolyte) imbalance leads to an osmotic imbalance that results in cell swelling and plasma membrane phospholipase A_2, with the subsequent generation of arachidonic acid and activation of

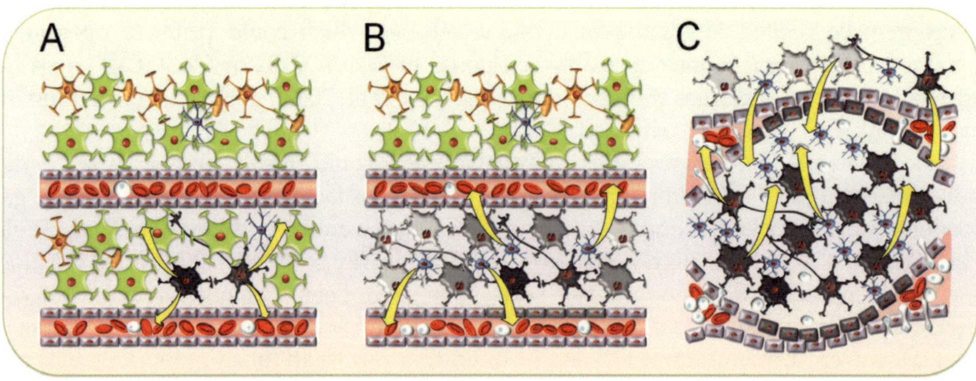

Fig. 5. Three mechanisms of death amplification. (A) Initially, a brain injury produced by ischemia, infection or necrosis affecting astrocytes (green), neurons (orange) or resting microglia (blue), could start a wave of death propagated (yellow arrows) and amplified through diffusible toxins and molecules (e.g., Ca^{2+}, NO, superoxide ion, peroxinitrite, glutamate, and NAD^+) present in high concentration in injured cells (depicted in the figure as dark colored cells). These molecules could be transferred through connexin gap junctions and connexin and pannexin hemichannels from injured cells (less and more affected cells in gray and black, respectively) to healthier cells. (B) Later, a second wave of death (yellow arrows) may be mediated by microglial cells overactivated by ATP and cytokines released by injured cells. (C) Still later inflammation-induced edema that reduces tissue perfusion could worsen the inflammatory response, recruiting leucocytes and increasing the extent of the lesion. [Modified from Orellana et al. 2009]

breakdown as observed in astrocytes exposed to ischemic conditions (Kimelberg 2005) (Fig. 5). Calcium overload induced in part by hemichannel opening may also activate cyclooxygenase/lipoxygenase pathways leading to increased free radicals, lipid peroxidation and further plasma membrane damage. It is noteworthy that arachidonic acid and decrease in the intracellular redox potential also activates Cx43 hemichannels, which may exacerbate cell damage (De Vuyst et al. 2009; Retamal et al. 2007b).

The first *in vivo* evidence for the involvement of connexin-based channels in the spread of death signals came from experiments in which octanol, a non-selective gap junction and hemichannel blocker, reduced the infarct size after focal cerebral ischemia (Rawanduzy et al. 1997). However, these observations disagree with the findings obtained in heterozygous Cx43 knockout mice or mouse astrocytes lacking Cx43 expression, in which focal ischemia causes larger lesions (Nakase et al. 2003; Nakase et al. 2004; Siushansian et al. 2001). In a rat model of transient global ischemia, pretreatment with compounds that block both hemichannels and gap junction channels (i.e. CBX, α-GA and endothelin) reduces the number of apoptotic neurons as compared to the contralateral hippocampus treated with saline (Perez Velazquez et al. 2006). In addition, hemichannels present in surrounding cells or in the stromal component of diverse organs may also participate in the ischemic responses. For example, the CA1 region of Cx32- deficient mice show increased sensitivity to global ischemia (Oguro et al. 2001). Since Cx32 forms hemichannels in activated microglia (Takeuchi et al. 2006), it is possible that Cx32 knockout animals may show attenuated microglial release of regulatory paracrine signals. When acute diseases like stroke have the presence of other pro-inflammatory components (e.g. high glucose produced by diabetes mellitus), brain damage and cognitive functions in patients is worse (Pasquier et al. 2006). Indeed, it has long been known that hyperglycemia worsens the outcome of acute brain ischemia by increasing the extent of tissue injury in animals and humans (Kagansky et al. 2001). Recently, we showed in astrocytes that high levels of extracellular glucose increase hemichannel activity and decrease gap junction permeability induced by hypoxia (Orellana et al. 2010). These changes are transient after 3 hours of hypoxia in high glucose. However, they are more prominent after 6 hours of hypoxia and last for over 3 hours followed by death of numerous astrocytes (Orellana et al. 2010). Because high glucose worsens the effect on ischemia-induced cell damage in endothelial cells, neurons, and microglia (Kagansky et al. 2001; Lin et al. 1998a; Tsuruta et al. ; Wang et al. 2001), it would be of interest to study if elevated hemichannel activity plays a relevant role as in astrocytes. Importantly, we also demonstrated that microglia treated with amyloid β peptide (Aβ) potentiate the increase in astroglial hemichannel activity and reduction in gap junctional communication induced by hypoxia in high glucose, suggesting that these changes are a common denominator of inflamed or activated astrocytes (Orellana et al. 2011b) (Fig. 6).

In addition, the extracellular media of activated astrocytes was neurotoxic due to its glutamate and ATP content that activate neuronal Panx1 hemichannels via NMDA/P2X receptors leading to neuronal death (Orellana et al. 2011b). Therefore, in a more integrated system (e.g., brain or brain slices) neurons could be efficiently protected from ischemia and neurotoxicity by blocking NMDA and P2X receptors as already proposed (Dirnagl et al. 1999), but also by targeting either glial or neuronal hemichannels composed by Cx43 and Panx1, respectively.

Hemichannels may also be involved in tissue response to stroke through their participation in a phenomenon known as ischemic preconditioning, in which a sublethal ischemic insult induces resistance to a subsequent more severe insult (Gidday 2006). It was recently shown

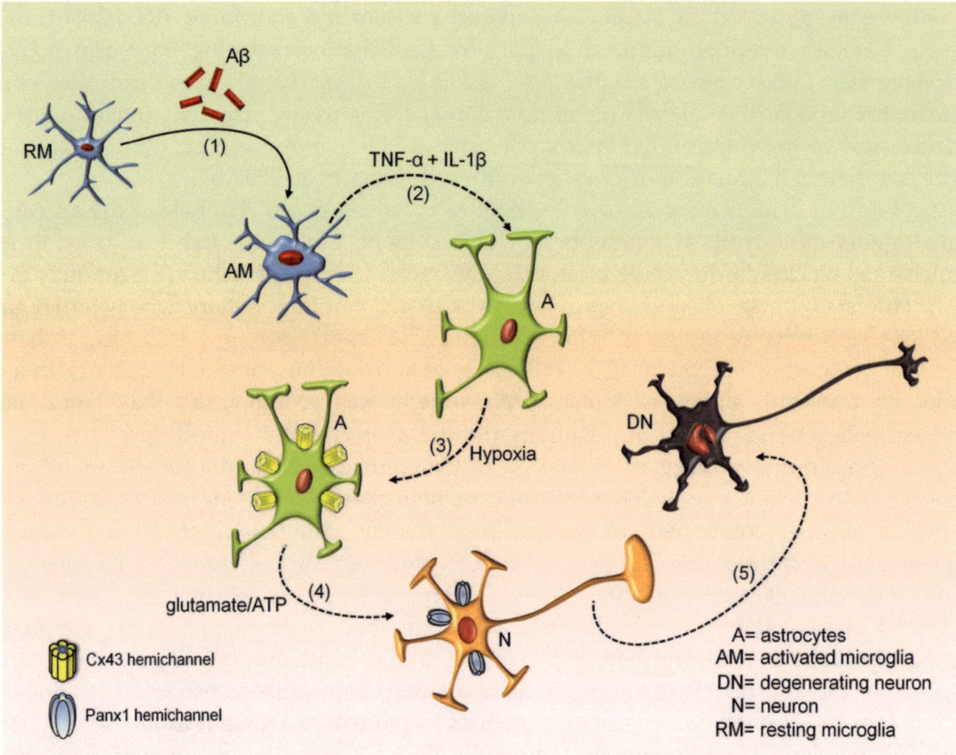

Fig. 6. Involvement of extracellular signals released by inflamed glial cells in neuronal death. Activated microglia (by for example Aβ) release pro-inflammatory cytokines (e.g., TNF-α /IL-1β), which increase astroglial hemichannel activity when another pro-inflammatory agent is involved (e.g., hypoxia). Then, astrocytes release glutamate and ATP via Cx43 hemichannels, which can activate more microglia and could promote activation of neuronal NMDA and P2X receptors and further opening of Panx1 hemichannels in neurons. ATP released as a result of Panx1 hemichannel opening could contribute to the progression of neuronal death by a vicious cycle since it will activate more P2X receptors leading to more Ca^{2+} entry and activation of intracellular neurotoxic cascades. Moreover, dead neurons can activate more microglia and thus, can either restart or potentiate the toxic circuit. [Modified from Orellana et al. 2011b]

that preconditioning reduces degradation of Cx43 in astrocytes, leading to a marked increase in the amount of surface Cx43 hemichannels (Lin et al. 2008). In agreement with the possible involvement of hemichannels in preconditioning responses, Cx43 null mice are insensitive to hypoxic preconditioning whereas wild-type littermates mice exhibit a prominent reduction in infarct volume after induction of preconditioning through occlusion of the middle cerebral artery (Lin et al. 2008). The mechanism of neuroprotection in this model involves the release of ATP through Cx43 hemichannels to the extracellular milieu, where it becomes hydrolyzed to adenosine, a potent neuroprotective molecule. The involvement of Cx36 hemichannels in the preconditioning response of cultured cerebellar granule neurons has been also recently demonstrated (Schock et al. 2008). The possible involvement of pannexin based hemichannels in brain preconditioning responses remains unknown. Final demonstration of the relative importance of enhanced hemichannel activity on cell viability during ischemia *in vivo* will require new approaches including better controlled experimental models and molecules that selectively block connexin- or pannexin-based hemichannels.

2.3 Alzheimer's Disease

Alzheimer's Disease (AD) is an age-related neurodegenerative disease that results in memory loss, behaviour and personality changes, among other symptoms. This disorder is characterized by the accumulation of the Aβ into amyloid plaques in the extracellular brain parenchyma, formation of tangles inside neurons as a result of abnormal phosphorylation of the microtubule associated protein tau, dendritic atrophy, and changes in neurotransmission in specific brain regions (Parihar and Hemnani 2004). Aβ is generated by proteolytic cleavage of the amyloid precursor protein (APP), which plays a role in neuronal adhesion, synaptogenesis, and axonal growth (Parihar and Hemnani 2004). High concentrations of Aβ are toxic to several neuronal types (Loo et al. 1993; Parihar and Hemnani 2004; Pike et al. 1995). The mechanisms underlying Aβ-neurotoxicity are complex but involve activation of NMDA receptors, sustained elevations of $[Ca^{2+}]_i$, and oxidative stress (Ekinci et al. 2000; Forloni et al. 1993), which are effects common to those induced by ischemia-reperfusion but on a different time scale.

In addition to the above, the cerebral cortex of individuals with AD present activated microglia and astroglia closely associated with amyloid plaques (Kalaria 1999; Wisniewski and Wegiel 1991). Notably, increased Cx43 immunoreactivity is detected in about 80% of Aβ plaques in postmortem human samples from AD patients (Nagy et al. 1996). Accordingly, a recent study performed in a murine model of AD showed that the immunoreactivity for Cxs 30 and 43 is increased at the proximity of most Aβ plaques (Mei et al. 2010). Imbalance in brain homeostasis may explain the increase expression of Cxs 30 and 43 close to amyloid plaques as compensatory mechanism to ensure normal brain function (Mei et al. 2010)(Nagy et al. 1996). Alternatively, increased astroglial gap junctions may serve as a pathway for the propagation of neuronal damage, transferring death signals generated in the microenvironment of amyloid plaques to distant neurons, as death signals can propagate from C6 glioma cells injured with calcium ionophore (Lin et al. 1998b). In agreement with this interpretation, inhibition of gap junctions with octanol abolishes the ability of Aβ to enhance the velocity and extent of propagation of astroglial calcium waves (Haughey and Mattson 2003). However, octanol also blocks $P2X_7$ receptors expressed by spinal astrocytes that also show calcium waves (Suadicani et al. 2006). In support of P2 receptor mediation of the Aβ-induced increase of calcium wave velocity in cortical astrocytes is the fact that suramin, a P2Y and P2X receptors blocker, reduces this response (Haughey and Mattson 2003).

Recently, it was shown that the treatment with the neurotoxic fragment of Aβ, 25-35 ($Aβ_{25-35}$) increases hemichannel opening in microglia, astrocytes and neurons monitored by single-channel recordings and by time-lapse ethidium uptake (Orellana et al. 2011c). The hemichannel forming proteins responsible of this activity were Cx43 and Panx1 in the case of microglia, Cx43 in the case of astrocytes and Panx1 and possibly Cx36 in neurons (Orellana et al. 2011c). Moreover, $Aβ_{25-35}$ increased the surface level of Cx43 in microglia and astrocytes and for the first time it was detected an increase in surface Panx1 in $Aβ_{25-35}$-treated microglia (Orellana et al. 2011c). Panx1 was also detected in astrocytes, but not at their surface, either in the absence or presence of $A\beta_{25-35}$, which is in disagreement with a recent study in which astroglial Panx1 hemichannels were activated by extracellular ATP (Iglesias et al. 2009). Importantly, conditioned media harvested either from $A\beta_{25-35}$-treated microglia or astrocytes, increased neuronal ethidium uptake and mortality, an effect prevented by inhibitors of P2X/NMDA receptors and Panx1 hemichannels, indicating that ATP and glutamate contribute to these changes (Orellana et al. 2011c). The contribution of these two molecules in neurotoxicity is well known (Lipton and Rosenberg 1994) and the involvement of hemichannels in glutamate and ATP release has also been documented

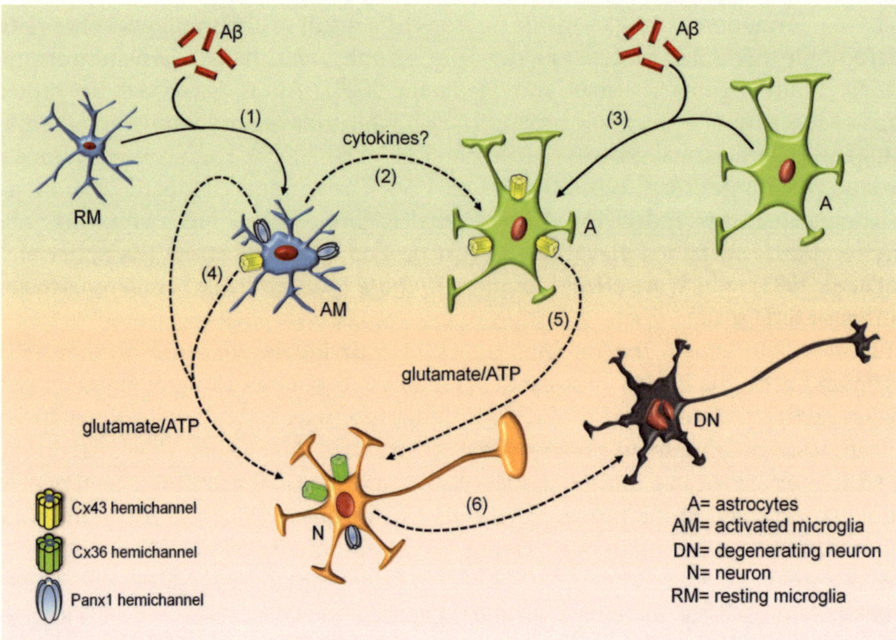

Fig. 7. Model of Aβ-induced cascade resulting in glial and neuronal hemichannel activation that leads to neuronal death. Microglia exposed to the amyloid β (Aβ) peptide become first activated (1), enhancing the opening of Cx43 and Panx1 hemichannels. Under these conditions, they release pro-inflammatory cytokines (2) that contribute to the Aβ-induced Cx43 hemichannel opening in astrocytes (3). Activated microglia might release glutamate and ATP through hemichannels (4), while astrocytes could release the same molecules through Cx43 hemichannels (5). This gliotransmission activates neuronal purinergic and NMDA receptors, resulting in an elevation of the intracellular free Ca^{2+} concentration that might trigger massive Cx36 and Panx1 hemichannel opening and further neuronal death (6). [Modified from Orellana et al. 2011c]

(Iglesias et al. 2009; Jiang et al.; Kang et al. 2008; Orellana et al. 2011b; Orellana et al. 2011c; Takeuchi et al. 2006; Ye et al. 2003). Moreover, these two molecules were shown to induce neuronal death via activation of Panx1 hemichannels in neurons (Orellana et al. 2011b). Their effect on neuronal death may proceed according to at least two mechanisms: 1) through the stimulation of NMDA and/or P2X receptors or 2) through Cx36 and Panx1 hemichannels themselves that could evoke large Ca^{2+} influxes resulting in neuronal death (Orellana et al. 2009) (Fig. 7).

Moreover, these two mechanisms could also be linked since transient activation of NMDA receptors induced a nonselective cationic current that develops slowly and mediates Ca^{2+} influx directly linked to neuronal death. Interestingly, this secondary current was reported recently to be mediated by neuronal Panx1 hemichannels (Thompson et al. 2008). Moreover, activation of Panx1 hemichannels might be triggered by protein-protein interaction with activated P2 receptors (Iglesias et al. 2008). Alternatively, Panx1 hemichannels could be activated by the rise in $[Ca^{2+}]_i$ caused by opening of NMDA and P2X receptors (Locovei et al. 2006). In this mechanism, neuronal ATP released as a result of Panx1 hemichannel opening is also likely to contribute in the progression of neuronal death by a vicious cycle since it will activate more ionotropic P2 receptors enhancing the Ca^{2+} entry and activation of intracellular neurotoxic cascades (Fig. 7). Studies in AD models will help to confirm or reject the above interpretations.

3. Conclusions

In the last decade, connexin hemichannels have been implicated in paracrine and autocrine cellular communication in several normal and pathologic conditions (Sáez et al. 2010). Currently, most of the available data regarding hemichannel involvement in brain pathologic events are from cultured cells and animal models of diseases. However, the current knowledge of human brain disease processes and the documented presence of hemichannels forming proteins in most studied human CNS tissues allows to speculate about the involvement of hemichannels in neurodegenerative processes. The role of glial cells in mediating nervous tissue inflammation has been recognized previously as leading to neuronal death; these cells can be bad neighbours for neurons (Block et al. 2007). Dysfunction of astroglial and microglial hemichannels, as well as gap junction channels, are likely mechanisms commonly elicited in all brain diseases associated with inflammatory responses. Therefore, normalization of connexin- and pannexin-based channel dysfunctions should confer tissue protection, improve quality of life, and extend survival of patients suffering acute or chronic brain inflammatory responses. Thus, it is proposed that chronic or acute processes of neurodegeneration might be prevented by blocking glial and neuronal hemichannels. Prevention might also be accomplished by reducing the effects of soluble factors (i.e., glutamate, ATP, prostaglandins, and cytokines) accumulated in the microenvironment of the inflamed CNS.

4. Acknowledgment

This work was partially supported by the CONICYT 24080055 (to JAO); CONICYT 79090028 (to JAO); CRPCEN (to CG); INSERM (to CG); FONDECYT 1070591 (to JCS); FONDEF DO7I1086 (to JCS); ANILLO ACT-71 (to JCS) and ECOS/CONICYT C10S01 (to CG and JCS) grants.

5. References

Bannerman DD, Fitzpatrick MJ, Anderson DY, Bhattacharjee AK, Novitsky TJ, Hasday JD, Cross AS, Goldblum SE. 1998. Endotoxin-neutralizing protein protects against endotoxin-induced endothelial barrier dysfunction. Infect Immun 66(4):1400-7.

Block ML, Zecca L, Hong JS. 2007. Microglia-mediated neurotoxicity: uncovering the molecular mechanisms. Nat Rev Neurosci 8(1):57-69.

Braet K, Vandamme W, Martin PE, Evans WH, Leybaert L. 2003. Photoliberating inositol-1,4,5-trisphosphate triggers ATP release that is blocked by the connexin mimetic peptide gap 26. Cell Calcium 33(1):37-48.

Bruzzone R, Hormuzdi SG, Barbe MT, Herb A, Monyer H. 2003. Pannexins, a family of gap junction proteins expressed in brain. Proc Natl Acad Sci U S A 100(23):13644-9.

Bruzzone S, Guida L, Zocchi E, Franco L, De Flora A. 2001. Connexin 43 hemi channels mediate Ca2+-regulated transmembrane NAD+ fluxes in intact cells. FASEB J 15(1):10-12.

Burra S, Jiang JX. 2009. Connexin 43 hemichannel opening associated with Prostaglandin E(2) release is adaptively regulated by mechanical stimulation. Commun Integr Biol 2(3):239-40.

Contreras JE, Sánchez HA, Eugenín EA, Speidel D, Theis M, Willecke K, Bukauskas FF, Bennett MV, Sáez JC. 2002. Metabolic inhibition induces opening of unapposed connexin 43 gap junction hemichannels and reduces gap junctional communication in cortical astrocytes in culture. Proc Natl Acad Sci U S A 99(1):495-500.

Cotrina ML, Lin JH, Nedergaard M. 2008. Adhesive properties of connexin hemichannels. Glia 56(16):1791-8.

Cruciani V, Mikalsen SO. 2005. The connexin gene family in mammals. Biol Chem 386(4):325-32.

Cherian PP, Siller-Jackson AJ, Gu S, Wang X, Bonewald LF, Sprague E, Jiang JX. 2005. Mechanical strain opens connexin 43 hemichannels in osteocytes: a novel mechanism for the release of prostaglandin. Mol Biol Cell 16(7):3100-6.

Davalos D, Grutzendler J, Yang G, Kim JV, Zuo Y, Jung S, Littman DR, Dustin ML, Gan WB. 2005. ATP mediates rapid microglial response to local brain injury in vivo. Nat Neurosci 8(6):752-8.

De Vuyst E, Decrock E, De Bock M, Yamasaki H, Naus CC, Evans WH, Leybaert L. 2007. Connexin hemichannels and gap junction channels are differentially influenced by lipopolysaccharide and basic fibroblast growth factor. Mol Biol Cell 18(1):34-46.

De Vuyst E, Wang N, Decrock E, De Bock M, Vinken M, Van Moorhem M, Lai C, Culot M, Rogiers V, Cecchelli R and others. 2009. Ca(2+) regulation of connexin 43 hemichannels in C6 glioma and glial cells. Cell Calcium 46(3):176-87.

Dietzman DE, Fischer GW, Schoenknecht FD. 1974. Neonatal Escherichia coli septicemia--bacterial counts in blood. J Pediatr 85(1):128-30.

Dirnagl U, Iadecola C, Moskowitz MA. 1999. Pathobiology of ischaemic stroke: an integrated view. Trends Neurosci 22(9):391-7.

Domercq M, Perez-Samartin A, Aparicio D, Alberdi E, Pampliega O, Matute C. 2010. P2X7 receptors mediate ischemic damage to oligodendrocytes. Glia 58(6):730-40.

Doran KS, Liu GY, Nizet V. 2003. Group B streptococcal beta-hemolysin/cytolysin activates neutrophil signaling pathways in brain endothelium and contributes to development of meningitis. J Clin Invest 112(5):736-44.

Ekinci FJ, Linsley MD, Shea TB. 2000. Beta-amyloid-induced calcium influx induces apoptosis in culture by oxidative stress rather than tau phosphorylation. Brain Res Mol Brain Res 76(2):389-95.

Eugenín EA, Branes MC, Berman JW, Sáez JC. 2003. TNF-alpha plus IFN-gamma induce connexin43 expression and formation of gap junctions between human monocytes/macrophages that enhance physiological responses. J Immunol 170(3):1320-8.

Eugenín EA, Eckardt D, Theis M, Willecke K, Bennett MV, Sáez JC. 2001. Microglia at brain stab wounds express connexin 43 and in vitro form functional gap junctions after treatment with interferon-gamma and tumor necrosis factor-alpha. Proc Natl Acad Sci U S A 98(7):4190-5.

Forloni G, Chiesa R, Smiroldo S, Verga L, Salmona M, Tagliavini F, Angeretti N. 1993. Apoptosis mediated neurotoxicity induced by chronic application of beta amyloid fragment 25-35. Neuroreport 4(5):523-6.

Freyer D, Manz R, Ziegenhorn A, Weih M, Angstwurm K, Docke WD, Meisel A, Schumann RR, Schonfelder G, Dirnagl U and others. 1999. Cerebral endothelial cells release TNF-alpha after stimulation with cell walls of Streptococcus pneumoniae and regulate inducible nitric oxide synthase and ICAM-1 expression via autocrine loops. J Immunol 163(8):4308-14.

Froger N, Orellana JA, Calvo CF, Amigou E, Kozoriz MG, Naus CC, Saez JC, Giaume C. 2010. Inhibition of cytokine-induced connexin43 hemichannel activity in astrocytes is neuroprotective. Mol Cell Neurosci 45(1):37-46.

Froger N, Orellana JA, Cohen-Salmon M, Ezan P, Amigou E, Saez JC, Giaume C. 2009. Cannabinoids prevent the opposite regulation of astroglial connexin43 hemichannels and gap junction channels induced by pro-inflammatory treatments. J Neurochem 111(6):1383-97.

Garg S, Md Syed M, Kielian T. 2005. Staphylococcus aureus-derived peptidoglycan induces Cx43 expression and functional gap junction intercellular communication in microglia. J Neurochem 95(2):475-83.

Gidday JM. 2006. Cerebral preconditioning and ischaemic tolerance. Nat Rev Neurosci 7(6):437-48.

Haddad L, El Hajj H, Abou-Merhi R, Kfoury Y, Mahieux R, El-Sabban M, Bazarbachi A. 2008. KSHV-transformed primary effusion lymphoma cells induce a VEGF-dependent angiogenesis and establish functional gap junctions with endothelial cells. Leukemia 22(4):826-34.

Haughey NJ, Mattson MP. 2003. Alzheimer's amyloid beta-peptide enhances ATP/gap junction-mediated calcium-wave propagation in astrocytes. Neuromolecular Med 3(3):173-80.

Iglesias R, Dahl G, Qiu F, Spray DC, Scemes E. 2009. Pannexin 1: the molecular substrate of astrocyte "hemichannels". J Neurosci 29(21):7092-7.

Iglesias R, Locovei S, Roque A, Alberto AP, Dahl G, Spray DC, Scemes E. 2008. P2X7 receptor-Pannexin1 complex: pharmacology and signaling. Am J Physiol Cell Physiol 295(3):C752-60.

Ishikawa M, Iwamoto T, Nakamura T, Doyle A, Fukumoto S, Yamada Y. 2011. Pannexin 3 functions as an ER Ca2+ channel, hemichannel, and gap junction to promote osteoblast differentiation. J Cell Biol 193(7):1257-74.

Jiang S, Yuan H, Duan L, Cao R, Gao B, Xiong YF, Rao ZR. 2011. Glutamate release through connexin 43 by cultured astrocytes in a stimulated hypertonicity model. Brain Res 1392:8-15.

Kagansky N, Levy S, Knobler H. 2001. The role of hyperglycemia in acute stroke. Arch Neurol 58(8):1209-12.

Kalaria RN. 1999. Microglia and Alzheimer's disease. Curr Opin Hematol 6(1):15-24.

Kang J, Kang N, Lovatt D, Torres A, Zhao Z, Lin J, Nedergaard M. 2008. Connexin 43 hemichannels are permeable to ATP. J Neurosci 28(18):4702-11.

Karpuk N, Burkovetskaya M, Fritz T, Angle A, Kielian T. 2011. Neuroinflammation leads to region-dependent alterations in astrocyte gap junction communication and hemichannel activity. J Neurosci 31(2):414-25.

Kim KS. 2003. Pathogenesis of bacterial meningitis: from bacteraemia to neuronal injury. Nat Rev Neurosci 4(5):376-85.

Kimelberg HK. 2005. Astrocytic swelling in cerebral ischemia as a possible cause of injury and target for therapy. Glia 50(4):389-97.

Laflamme N, Rivest S. 2001. Toll-like receptor 4: the missing link of the cerebral innate immune response triggered by circulating gram-negative bacterial cell wall components. FASEB J 15(1):155-163.

Li X, Lynn BD, Olson C, Meier C, Davidson KG, Yasumura T, Rash JE, Nagy JI. 2002. Connexin29 expression, immunocytochemistry and freeze-fracture replica immunogold labelling (FRIL) in sciatic nerve. Eur J Neurosci 16(5):795-806.

Lin B, Ginsberg MD, Busto R. 1998a. Hyperglycemic exacerbation of neuronal damage following forebrain ischemia: microglial, astrocytic and endothelial alterations. Acta Neuropathol 96(6):610-20.

Lin JH, Lou N, Kang N, Takano T, Hu F, Han X, Xu Q, Lovatt D, Torres A, Willecke K and others. 2008. A central role of connexin 43 in hypoxic preconditioning. J Neurosci 28(3):681-95.

Lin JH, Weigel H, Cotrina ML, Liu S, Bueno E, Hansen AJ, Hansen TW, Goldman S, Nedergaard M. 1998b. Gap-junction-mediated propagation and amplification of cell injury. Nat Neurosci 1(6):494-500.

Lipton SA, Rosenberg PA. 1994. Excitatory amino acids as a final common pathway for neurologic disorders. N Engl J Med 330(9):613-22.

Locovei S, Wang J, Dahl G. 2006. Activation of pannexin 1 channels by ATP through P2Y receptors and by cytoplasmic calcium. FEBS Lett 580(1):239-44.

Loo DT, Copani A, Pike CJ, Whittemore ER, Walencewicz AJ, Cotman CW. 1993. Apoptosis is induced by beta-amyloid in cultured central nervous system neurons. Proc Natl Acad Sci U S A 90(17):7951-5.

Mei X, Ezan P, Giaume C, Koulakoff A. 2010. Astroglial connexin immunoreactivity is specifically altered at beta-amyloid plaques in beta-amyloid precursor protein/presenilin1 mice. Neuroscience 171(1):92-105.

Nagasawa K, Chiba H, Fujita H, Kojima T, Saito T, Endo T, Sawada N. 2006. Possible involvement of gap junctions in the barrier function of tight junctions of brain and lung endothelial cells. J Cell Physiol 208(1):123-32.

Nagy JI, Li W, Hertzberg EL, Marotta CA. 1996. Elevated connexin43 immunoreactivity at sites of amyloid plaques in Alzheimer's disease. Brain Res 717(1-2):173-8.

Nakase T, Fushiki S, Sohl G, Theis M, Willecke K, Naus CC. 2003. Neuroprotective role of astrocytic gap junctions in ischemic stroke. Cell Commun Adhes 10(4-6):413-7.

Nakase T, Sohl G, Theis M, Willecke K, Naus CC. 2004. Increased apoptosis and inflammation after focal brain ischemia in mice lacking connexin43 in astrocytes. Am J Pathol 164(6):2067-75.

Nau R, Bruck W. 2002. Neuronal injury in bacterial meningitis: mechanisms and implications for therapy. Trends Neurosci 25(1):38-45.

Nau R, Gerber J, Bunkowski S, Bruck W. 2004. Axonal injury, a neglected cause of CNS damage in bacterial meningitis. Neurology 62(3):509-11.

Oguro K, Jover T, Tanaka H, Lin Y, Kojima T, Oguro N, Grooms SY, Bennett MV, Zukin RS. 2001. Global ischemia-induced increases in the gap junctional proteins connexin 32 (Cx32) and Cx36 in hippocampus and enhanced vulnerability of Cx32 knock-out mice. J Neurosci 21(19):7534-42.

Orellana JA, Figueroa XF, Sanchez HA, Contreras-Duarte S, Velarde V, Sáez JC. 2011a. Hemichannels in the neurovascular unit and white matter under normal and inflamed conditions. CNS Neurol Disord Drug Targets 10(3):404-14.

Orellana JA, Froger N, Ezan P, Jiang JX, Bennett MV, Naus CC, Giaume C, Sáez JC. 2011b. ATP and glutamate released via astroglial connexin 43 hemichannels mediate neuronal death through activation of pannexin 1 hemichannels. J Neurochem. In press.

Orellana JA, Shoji KF, Abudara V, Ezan P, Amigou E, Saez PJ, Jiang JX, Naus CC, Sáez JC, Giaume C. 2011c. Amyloid beta-induced death in neurons involves glial and neuronal hemichannels. J Neurosci 31(13):4962-77.

Orellana JA, Hernandez DE, Ezan P, Velarde V, Bennett MV, Giaume C, Sáez JC. 2010. Hypoxia in high glucose followed by reoxygenation in normal glucose reduces the viability of cortical astrocytes through increased permeability of connexin 43 hemichannels. Glia 58(3):329-43.

Orellana JA, Sáez PJ, Shoji KF, Schalper KA, Palacios-Prado N, Velarde V, Giaume C, Bennett MV, Sáez JC. 2009. Modulation of brain hemichannels and gap junction channels by pro-inflammatory agents and their possible role in neurodegeneration. Antioxid Redox Signal 11(2):369-99.

Parihar MS, Hemnani T. 2004. Alzheimer's disease pathogenesis and therapeutic interventions. J Clin Neurosci 11(5):456-67.

Pasquier F, Boulogne A, Leys D, Fontaine P. 2006. Diabetes mellitus and dementia. Diabetes Metab 32(5 Pt 1):403-14.

Pelegrin P, Surprenant A. 2006. Pannexin-1 mediates large pore formation and interleukin-1beta release by the ATP-gated P2X7 receptor. EMBO J 25(21):5071-82.

Pelegrin P, Surprenant A. 2007. Pannexin-1 couples to maitotoxin- and nigericin-induced interleukin-1beta release through a dye uptake-independent pathway. J Biol Chem 282(4):2386-94.

Perez Velazquez JL, Kokarovtseva L, Sarbaziha R, Jeyapalan Z, Leshchenko Y. 2006. Role of gap junctional coupling in astrocytic networks in the determination of global ischaemia-induced oxidative stress and hippocampal damage. Eur J Neurosci 23(1):1-10.

Pike CJ, Walencewicz-Wasserman AJ, Kosmoski J, Cribbs DH, Glabe CG, Cotman CW. 1995. Structure-activity analyses of beta-amyloid peptides: contributions of the beta 25-35 region to aggregation and neurotoxicity. J Neurochem 64(1):253-65.

Qin L, Wu X, Block ML, Liu Y, Breese GR, Hong JS, Knapp DJ, Crews FT. 2007. Systemic LPS causes chronic neuroinflammation and progressive neurodegeneration. Glia 55(5):453-62.

Rawanduzy A, Hansen A, Hansen TW, Nedergaard M. 1997. Effective reduction of infarct volume by gap junction blockade in a rodent model of stroke. J Neurosurg 87(6):916-20.

Retamal MA, Cortes CJ, Reuss L, Bennett MV, Sáez JC. 2006. S-nitrosylation and permeation through connexin 43 hemichannels in astrocytes: induction by oxidant stress and reversal by reducing agents. Proc Natl Acad Sci U S A 103(12):4475-80.

Retamal MA, Froger N, Palacios-Prado N, Ezan P, Saez PJ, Sáez JC, Giaume C. 2007a. Cx43 hemichannels and gap junction channels in astrocytes are regulated oppositely by proinflammatory cytokines released from activated microglia. J Neurosci 27(50):13781-92.

Retamal MA, Schalper KA, Shoji KF, Bennett MV, Sáez JC. 2007b. Opening of connexin 43 hemichannels is increased by lowering intracellular redox potential. Proc Natl Acad Sci U S A 104(20):8322-7.

Ring A, Weiser JN, Tuomanen EI. 1998. Pneumococcal trafficking across the blood-brain barrier. Molecular analysis of a novel bidirectional pathway. J Clin Invest 102(2):347-60.

Robertson J, Lang S, Lambert PA, Martin PE. Peptidoglycan derived from Staphylococcus epidermidis induces Connexin43 hemichannel activity with consequences on the innate immune response in endothelial cells. Biochem J 432(1):133-43.

Sáez JC, Schalper KA, Retamal MA, Orellana JA, Shoji KF, Bennett MV. Cell membrane permeabilization via connexin hemichannels in living and dying cells. Exp Cell Res 316(15):2377-89.

Schalper KA, Palacios-Prado, N., Retamal, M.A., Shoji, K.F., Martínez, A.D., Sáez, J.C. 2008. Connexin hemichannels composition determines the FGF-1-induced membrane permeability and free $[Ca^{2+}]_i$ responses. Mol Biol Cell . 19: 3501-13.

Schalper KA, Sanchez HA, Lee SC, Altenberg GA, Nathanson MH, Sáez JC. Connexin 43 hemichannels mediate the Ca2+ influx induced by extracellular alkalinization. Am J Physiol Cell Physiol 299(6):C1504-15.

Schock SC, Leblanc D, Hakim AM, Thompson CS. 2008. ATP release by way of connexin 36 hemichannels mediates ischemic tolerance in vitro. Biochem Biophys Res Commun 368(1):138-44.

Schwandner R, Dziarski R, Wesche H, Rothe M, Kirschning CJ. 1999. Peptidoglycan- and lipoteichoic acid-induced cell activation is mediated by toll-like receptor 2. J Biol Chem 274(25):17406-9.

Siushansian R, Bechberger JF, Cechetto DF, Hachinski VC, Naus CC. 2001. Connexin43 null mutation increases infarct size after stroke. J Comp Neurol 440(4):387-94.

Stout CE, Costantin JL, Naus CC, Charles AC. 2002. Intercellular calcium signaling in astrocytes via ATP release through connexin hemichannels. J Biol Chem 277(12):10482-8.

Stuertz K, Schmidt H, Eiffert H, Schwartz P, Mader M, Nau R. 1998. Differential release of lipoteichoic and teichoic acids from Streptococcus pneumoniae as a result of exposure to beta-lactam antibiotics, rifamycins, trovafloxacin, and quinupristin-dalfopristin. Antimicrob Agents Chemother 42(2):277-81.

Stuertz K, Schmidt H, Trostdorf F, Eiffert H, Mader M, Nau R. 1999. Lower lipoteichoic and teichoic acid CSF concentrations during treatment of pneumococcal meningitis with non-bacteriolytic antibiotics than with ceftriaxone. Scand J Infect Dis 31(4):367-70.

Suadicani SO, Brosnan CF, Scemes E. 2006. P2X7 receptors mediate ATP release and amplification of astrocytic intercellular Ca2+ signaling. J Neurosci 26(5):1378-85.

Takeuchi H, Jin S, Wang J, Zhang G, Kawanokuchi J, Kuno R, Sonobe Y, Mizuno T, Suzumura A. 2006. Tumor necrosis factor-alpha induces neurotoxicity via glutamate release from hemichannels of activated microglia in an autocrine manner. J Biol Chem 281(30):21362-8.

Thompson RJ, Jackson MF, Olah ME, Rungta RL, Hines DJ, Beazely MA, MacDonald JF, MacVicar BA. 2008. Activation of pannexin-1 hemichannels augments aberrant bursting in the hippocampus. Science 322(5907):1555-9.

Thompson RJ, Zhou N, MacVicar BA. 2006. Ischemia opens neuronal gap junction hemichannels. Science 312(5775):924-7.

Tran Van Nhieu G, Clair C, Bruzzone R, Mesnil M, Sansonetti P, Combettes L. 2003. Connexin-dependent inter-cellular communication increases invasion and dissemination of Shigella in epithelial cells. Nat Cell Biol 5(8):720-6.

Tsuruta R, Fujita M, Ono T, Koda Y, Koga Y, Yamamoto T, Nanba M, Shitara M, Kasaoka S, Maruyama I and others. Hyperglycemia enhances excessive superoxide anion radical generation, oxidative stress, early inflammation, and endothelial injury in forebrain ischemia/reperfusion rats. Brain Res 1309:155-63.

Vandamme W, Braet K, Cabooter L, Leybaert L. 2004. Tumour necrosis factor alpha inhibits purinergic calcium signalling in blood-brain barrier endothelial cells. J Neurochem 88(2):411-21.

Veliz LP, Gonzalez FG, Duling BR, Saez JC, Boric MP. 2008. Functional role of gap junctions in cytokine-induced leukocyte adhesion to endothelium in vivo. Am J Physiol Heart Circ Physiol 295(3):H1056-H1066.

Wang JY, Yang JM, Tao PL, Yang SN. 2001. Synergistic apoptosis induced by bacterial endotoxin lipopolysaccharide and high glucose in rat microglia. Neurosci Lett 304(3):177-80.

Wisniewski HM, Wegiel J. 1991. Spatial relationships between astrocytes and classical plaque components. Neurobiol Aging 12(5):593-600.

Wong CW, Christen T, Roth I, Chadjichristos CE, Derouette JP, Foglia BF, Chanson M, Goodenough DA, Kwak BR. 2006. Connexin37 protects against atherosclerosis by regulating monocyte adhesion. Nat Med 12(8):950-4.

Ye ZC, Wyeth MS, Baltan-Tekkok S, Ransom BR. 2003. Functional hemichannels in astrocytes: a novel mechanism of glutamate release. J Neurosci 23(9):3588-96.

Part 4

Roles of Glial Cells in Neurodegeneration

11

Role of Astrocytes in Neurodegenerative Diseases

George E. Barreto[1], Janneth Gonzalez[1],
Francisco Capani[2] and Ludis Morales[1]
[1]*Departamento de Nutrición y Bioquímica, Facultad de Ciencias,*
Pontificia Universidad Javeriana, Bogotá D.C.,
[2]*Instituto de Investigaciones Cardiológicas, Prof. Dr. Alberto Taquini,*
CONICET-UBA Buenos Aires,
[1]*Colombia*
[2]*Argentina*

1. Introduction

The past several decades have given rise to many important discoveries and novel insights into the role of astrocytes in normal brain function and disease, firmly establishing concepts that describe the dynamic and reciprocal signaling networks between astrocytes, neurons and other cell types.

Brain aging, overt any neurodegenerative state, leads to inflammation, oxidative stress and cell death. Neurons are more susceptible to injury than astrocytes, as they have fewer antioxidant mechanisms and are therefore prone to excitotoxicity (Swanson *et al.,* 2004). Both normally and with aging, astrocytes support neurons by providing antioxidant protection, substrates for neuronal metabolism via neurovascular coupling, and glutamate clearance. Although astrocytes are generally more resilient than neurons, severe damage also results in astrocyte dysfunction, leading to increased neuronal death (Nedergaard & Dirnagl, 2005). Therefore, many recent efforts have focused on the astrocyte-neuron interaction and how astrocyte function can be improved to enhance neuronal support and survival (Swanson *et al.,* 2004). A growing body of data demonstrates that astrocytes play a multifaceted and complex role in the response to neuropathologies, including neurodegenerative, as they have potential to both enhance neuronal survival and regeneration and contribute to further injury (Sofroniew, 2000, 2009; Sofroniew & Vinters, 2010). Because of the diverse nature and complex biology of these cells, and the limited number of studies to date, their role in neurodegeneration deserves further study.

It is likely that diminished astrocytes function throughout the neurodegenerative process is a prominent determinant of both neuronal survival as well as survival of the entire organism (Shibata & Kobayashi, 2008). In this chapter we provide a brief overview of the pathophysiological events underlying brain aging, and in neurodegenerative diseases, and discusses how these events affect astrocytes response to these chronic neuropathologies, such as Alzheimer's AD and Parkinson´s PD diseases, Amyotrophic Lateral Syndrome (ALS), and Multiple Sclerosis (MS).

2. Astrocytes function in the brain

Astrocytes are the most common cell type in mammalian brain. Glial fibrillary acidic protein (GFAP) and vimentin (Vim) constitute intermediate filaments (known also as nanofilaments) as part of the cytoskeleton in astrocytes. Reactive gliosis is a response of astrocytes to a variety of brain insults that is characterized by hypertrophy of the cell bodies and processes, altered gene expression, increase in the expression of GFAP, Vim and the calcium binding protein S100β (Ridet *et al.*, 1997), and proliferation that may likely occur in some neurodegenerative diseases (Sofroniew, 2009; Sofroniew & Vinters, 2010). In contrast, because reactive astrocytes are ubiquitous in aged central nervous system (CNS) tissue, they are often regarded as uniformly harmful, provoking inflammation, releasing cytotoxins and chemokines that serve no purpose but to inhibit axonal regeneration and increase damage. The wide range of activities that astrocytes can exhibit *in vitro* contributes to uncertainty over whether these cells exert beneficial or detrimental effects after CNS degeneration. For example, potential protective effects could be provided by glutamate uptake and neurotrophin release, while potential detrimental effects might be caused by the release of inflammatory cytokines and cytotoxic radicals. Little information has been available on the roles played by reactive astrocytes in the response to experimental models of neurodegenerative diseases *in vivo*. For instance, aged astrocytes exhibit an elevated content of GFAP and of S100β (Barreto *et al.*, 2009; Nichols, 1999). Use of oligonucleotide arrays has yielded the first profile of gene expression from the aging brain of mice and evidence that aging seems to be associated with an inflammatory response and oxidative stress both in neocortex, hippocampus and in cerebellum (Lee *et al.*, 2000; Zeier *et al.*, 2011), with parallels to human neurodegenerative disorders. GFAP is also one of the genes that undergoes a twofold increase in expression. Thus, the GFAP increases of the aged astrocytes may be the result of a response to the inflammatory and oxidative state of the aging brain. Indeed, better comprehension of the features that distinguish a normal, "healthy" old brain from a brain that is at an early stage of a neurodegenerative disease is a key aspect in developing treatments.

It is interesting to note that one of the characteristics of astrocytes in the aging brain - the number of astrocytes - is increased by ~20% (Peinado *et al.*, 1998; Pilegaard & Ladefoged, 1996; Rozovsky *et al.*, 1998; Salminen *et al.*, 2011). This response has been compared with reactive gliosis in response to injured or damaged neurons during aging. However, an alternative explanation is that increased number of astrocytes in the aging brain is required to provide the same level of neuroprotection that is present in the brain of a young animal.

One hallmark of the cellular response to brain aging, and in neurodegenerative states, is a rapid, dramatic increase in damaging free radicals, including nitric oxide (NO), superoxide, and peroxynitrite (Shibata & Kobayashi, 2008). On the other hand, astrocytes produce the beneficial antioxidants glutathione, superoxide dismutases (SODs 1, 2 and 3), and ascorbate (Figure 1, Anderson & Swanson, 2000; Dringen, 2000; Dringen *et al.*, 2000; Lindenau *et al.*, 2000; Sims *et al.*, 2004). Interestingly, neurons cocultured with astrocyte exhibit higher levels of glutathione compared with neurons cultured alone (Giordano *et al.*, 2009), suggesting that astrocytes provide additional antioxidant defense to neurons (Slemmer *et al.*, 2008). Similarly, astrocytes upregulate HO-1 (heme-oxygenase 1, Figure 2), a 32 kDa stress protein that degrades heme to biliverdin, free iron and carbon monoxide. Although the upregulation of this enzyme has been previously reported to confer neuroprotection following various brain insults (Beschorner *et al.*, 2000; Chen *et al.*, 2000; Espada *et al.*, 2010;

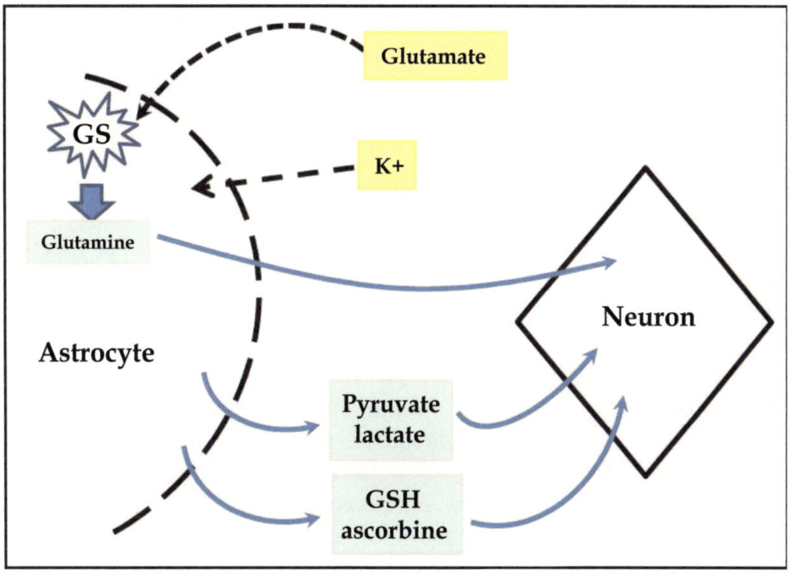

Fig. 1. Mechanisms of astrocyte support of neurons in the normal brain. Antioxidant defence includes release of glutathione and ascorbate. Regulation of extracellular levels of ions and neurotransmitters, especially K^+ and glutamate, strongly influence neuronal excitability. Elevated extracellular K^+ triggers astrocyte glycolysis and enhances lactate and pyruvate release which support neuronal metabolism. Sodium dependent glutamate uptake by astrocytes activates the Na^+/K^+ ATPase, stimulating glycolytic activity and production of lactate. Astrocytes and neurons are also coupled by the glutamate-glutamine cycle. Astrocytes take up glutamate, convert it to glutamine, release glutamine to the extracellular space where it is taken up by neurons and used to synthesize glutamate to replenishment the neurotransmitter pool. Any deregulation of these mechanisms, as a common situation in some neurodegenerative diseases, will likely influence neuronal survival

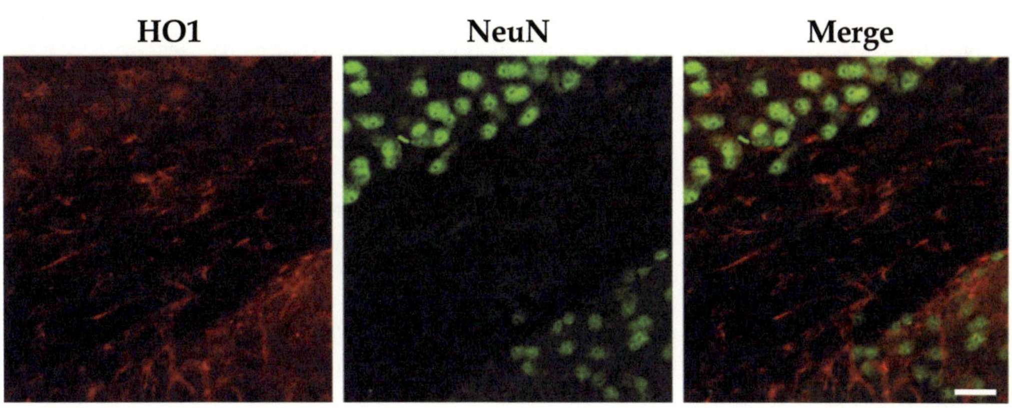

Fig. 2. Astrocytic HO-1 expression in corpus callosum. Immunostaining for HO-1 and NeuN (neuronal marker) was carried out in free floating brain sections of 3 months-old naïve male mice. Morphologically, HO-1 is expressed in shaped-like astrocytes, and does not seem to be expressed by neurons. Scale bar, 50 μm

Imuta *et al.*, 2007; Ku *et al.*, 2006; Le *et al.*, 1999; Takeda *et al.*, 2000), its overproduction in astrocytes may contribute to iron overload and mitochondrial insufficiency, characteristic of some neurodegenerative disorders (Fernandez-Checa *et al.*, 2010; Serviddio *et al.*, 2011). HO-1 is expressed by approximately 86% (Schipper *et al.*, 1995) and 77.1% (Schipper *et al.*, 1998) of GFAP-positive astrocytes in AD and PD, respectively, suggesting a possible role in the pathogenesis of these neurodegenerative diseases.

Control of energy metabolism is also controlled by astrocytes in the CNS. When astrocytes take up extracellular glutamate as a result of neuronal activity, the Na^+/ K^+-ATPase and AMPA signaling trigger astrocyte uptake of glucose from the blood, as astrocytic endfeet contact capillaries (Caesar *et al.*, 2008; Magistretti, 2006). The glucose is then made into lactate, a substrate for neuronal energy, to further "fuel" active neurons (Magistretti & Pellerin, 1999; Figure 1). As mentioned above, astrocytes produce glutathione. In addition to its antioxidant properties, glutathione is the enzyme needed for the conversion of methylglyoxal, a toxic by-product of metabolism, into D-lactate by glyoxalase 1 (Cliffe & Waley, 1961). Although the role of astrocyte metabolism is relatively well-established in normal tissues, the role of astrocyte metabolism maintenance with aging and in neurodegenerative diseases is less clear (Bartnik-Olson *et al.*, 2010; Bentzer *et al.*, 2000; Floyd & Lyeth, 2007).

Astrocytes are also key players in the production and regulation of neurotransmitters, antioxidant production, potassium uptake, energy metabolism and neurovascular coupling in the CNS. Notably, astrocytes make glutamine, the precursor for the neurotransmitters glutamate and GABA, from glucose (Zou *et al.*, 2010). In addition to providing the precursors for neurotransmitters, one important role of astrocytes in the normal brain is to take up glutamate using the glutamate transporters GLAST and GLT-1 (Anderson & Swanson, 2000; Romera *et al.*, 2004; Schousboe & Waagepetersen, 2006), as excess glutamate leads to cell death via excitotoxicity (Tilleux & Hermans, 2007).

Astrocytes regulate neuronal activation by extracellular potassium uptake, and proper maintenance of ion gradients, such as potassium, as an important mechanism for regulating cell volume in both normal and pathological conditions (Jayakumar & Norenberg, 2010; Lambert & Oberwinkler, 2005; Lang *et al.*, 1998; Obara *et al.*, 2008). Indeed, astrocytes upregulate glucose transporters in order to provide energy to dying neuronal cells (Floyd & Lyeth, 2007; Scafidi *et al.*, 2009; Yi & Hazell, 2006,) suggesting that astrocytes are necessary for improvement in chronic neurodegenerative diseases energy metabolism. In summary, astrocytes are important producers of antioxidants in the normal CNS, and astrocytic production of these molecules after brain injury may enhance neuronal survival and protect astrocyte function.

Astrocytes are critical in the development and/or maintenance of blood-brain barrier characteristics (Gordon *et al.*, 2007; Koehler *et al.*, 2009). Astrocytes are arranged in non-overlapping spatial domains (Bushong *et al.*, 2002; Halassa *et al.*, 2007), but coupled to each other in a syncytial network (Haydon & Carmignoto, 2006). Since one astrocyte maintains contacts with approximately 160,000 synapses (Bushong *et al.*, 2002), this cell population is well positioned to integrate neuronal activity and link neuronal activity to the vascular network (Ransom *et al.*, 2003).

Astrocytes terminal processes are also known as "endfeet" cover 99% of the abluminal vascular surface of capillaries, intracerebral arterioles, and venules (Simard *et al.*, 2003). The extent of contact between endfeet and penetrating and pial arterioles remains unclear. Pial arterioles and arteries lying free in the subarachnoid space are not covered (Jones, 1970).

Nevertheless, much of the pial circulation is in contact with the glia-limitans, a de-facto extension of astrocytic processes (Kontos *et al.,* 1971; Xu *et al.,* 2004). This domain organization has been proposed as being the key linking element of the neuronal-(astrocyte)-vascular unit (Volterra & Meldolesi, 2005). For example, working with neocortical slices, Zonta et al. (Zonta *et al.*, 2003) demonstrated that electrical stimulation of neuronal processes raises intracellular Ca^{2+} levels in astrocytic endfeet and leads to a slowly developing dilatation of local intracerebral arterioles. Additionally, electrical stimulation of individual astrocytes had the same effect. Since this initial report, several investigators observed a vascular response in conjunction with an elevation of intracellular Ca^{2+} levels in astrocytic endfeet. However, these studies reported inconsistent vascular responses ranging from vasorelaxation to vasodilatation or the combination of both (Gordon *et al.,* 2007; Iadecola & Nedergaard, 2007). Mediators implicated in this mechanism are vasoactive metabolites of the cyclooxygenase or cytochrome P450 ω-hydroxylase pathways. All of these studies were performed in brain slices in which the vessels are lacking in intraluminal pressure. This might account for disparate results. In vivo analysis with two-photon laser scanning microscopy revealed that increases of astrocytic Ca^{2+} by photolysis of caged Ca^{2+} evoked a vasodilatation of cortical arterioles (Takano *et al.,* 2006). This interaction between the vessel and the endfeet appeared to be mediated by metabolites of the COX-1 pathway, because inhibitors of nitric oxide synthetase (NOS), COX-2, p450 epoxygenases, and adenosine receptor antagonists had no effect. These and other studies strongly implicate a role for astrocytes in cerebral blood flow regulation during neuronal activation (Haydon & Carmignoto, 2006).

It is important to point that some, if not all, of these astrocytic functions may likely be altered or reduced in neurodegenerative states (Rossi & Volterra, 2009). The role of astrocytes in various neurodegenerative diseases will briefly be discussed more thoroughly below, specifically looking at their involvement during the pathologic processes of Alzheimer´s and Parkinson diseases, Amyotrophic Lateral Syndrome (ALS) and Multiple Sclerosis.

3. Astrocytes dysfunction in neurodegenerative diseases

Neurodegenerative diseases represent a heterogeneous group of disorders affecting the nervous system. In most instances, they affect adults, their causes are unknown, and progression is relentless. Some are genetic, but most are sporadic. They involve all parts of the nervous system, although the cerebral cortex and the basal ganglia are the most frequent loci of pathology. The historical classification of neurodegenerative diseases, based on clinical and pathological characteristics, is imperfect. New classifications are rather based on molecular determinants. Contrary to common belief, it is now recognized that neurodegenerative disorders are multisystemic, even if specific neuronal pathways are more affected than others. The death of astrocytes and specific types of neurons in neurodegenerative diseases is provoked, not by a single pathogenic factor, but rather by a cascade of multiple deleterious molecular and cellular events as described earlier.

3.1 Oxidative stress and neurodegeneration

Mitochondria are central neuronal organelles that play a vital role in neuronal life and death. Both mitochondrial dysfunction and proper function are essential components in neurodegeneration. Further elucidation of the mechanisms of interaction between mitochondria and neuronal death will allow better description of the pathogenesis of neurodegenerative diseases and provide potential targets for therapeutic intervention.

One of the hallmarks of various neurodegenerative and neuroinflammatory disorders is oxidative stress-induced CNS damage. Similarly, the natural aging process per se is associated with increased oxidative stress (Figure 3). Such oxidative stress can damage lipids, proteins and nucleic acids of cells and power-house mitochondria causing cell death in assorted cell types including astrocytes and neurons. However, astrocytes having high levels of anti-oxidant enzymes (glutathione peroxidase, catalase, glutathione reductase, and superoxide dismutase) and antioxidants (glutathione and ascorbic acid) try to absorb reactive oxygen species (O2 =, O2 −, and OH.) and reactive nitrogen species (NO, ONOO−), maintain redox homeostasis and defend the insulted CNS (Chen & Swanson, 2003; Dringen & Hirrlinger, 2003; Wilson, 1997). In addition, astrocytes also scavenge detrimental

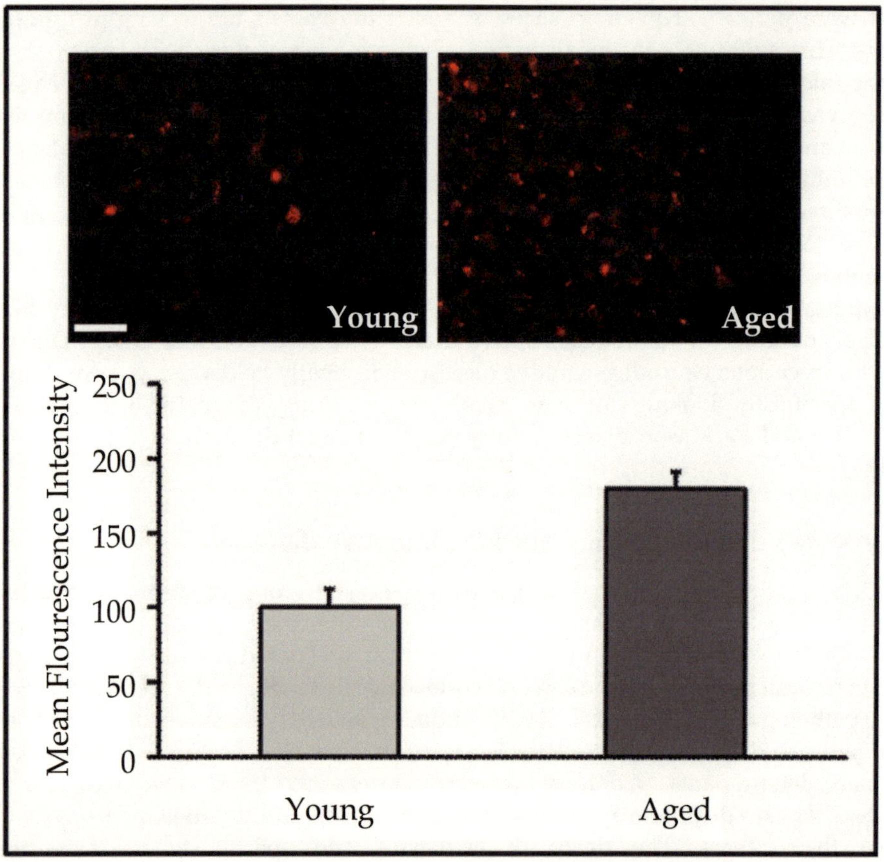

Fig. 3. Increased oxidative stress production in the normal aged brain. 3- or 18-months naïve old male mice were sacrificed and 40 µm brain sections were stained for 4-Hydroxynonenal (4-HNE), a marker of lipid peroxidation. Mean Fluorescence intensity assessed by ImageJ program showed that aged animals, overt any pathological condition, had an increased expression of 4-HNE in cortical layers II-III, compared to young mice. 3 sections/animal for 4 animals were analyzed in each condition. Data are represented as Means ± SEM. Scale bar, 100 µm

molecules such as glutamate, produced during synaptic transmission through neurons (Hertz & Zielke, 2004). This is, perhaps, the most common astrocytic dysfunction that likely occurs in some neurodegenerative states.

Astrocytes react to various neurodegenerative insults rapidly, leading to vigorous astrogliosis. This reactive gliosis is associated with alteration in morphology and structure of activated astrocytes along with its functional characteristics (Eddleston & Mucke, 1993). The astrocytic processes construct a bushy network surrounding the injury site, thus secluding the affected part from the rest of the CNS area. Subsequently, astrogliosis has been implicated in the pathogenesis of a variety of chronic neurodegenerative diseases, including Alzheimer's disease (AD), Parkinson's disease, Amyotrophic Lateral Syndrome (ALS), acute traumatic brain injury, stroke, and neuroinflammatory brain diseases (Axelsson *et al.*, 2011; Ciesielska *et al.*, 2009; Garcia-Matas *et al.*, 2010; Heales *et al.*, 2004; Li *et al.*, 2011; Simpson *et al.*, 2010; Sofroniew, 2000).

3.2 Alzheimer´s disease

AD is characterized clinically by cognitive loss in two or more domains, including memory, language, calculations, orientation and judgment; the loss must be of sufficient severity to cause social or occupational disability. These clinical features are the result of neuronal death and dysfunction in the cerebral cortex, entorhinal area, hippocampus, ventral striatum and basal forebrain, eventually resulting in severe dementia. Pathologically, the two hallmark findings of the disorder are neurofibrillary tangles and amyloid plaques (Veerhuis, 2011).

Senile plaques, a pathologic hallmark of Alzheimer's disease, are associated with GFAP-positive activated astrocytes (Nagele *et al.*, 2004). It is reported that in various neuropathological states, the increased GFAP expression corresponds to the severity of astroglial activation (Axelsson *et al.*, 2011; Kashon *et al.*, 2004; Notturno *et al.*, 2009; Pelinka *et al.*, 2004; Simpson *et al.*, 2010; Toft-Hansen *et al.*, 2011).

Concerning astrocytes, recent findings suggest that they play a role in the clearance of the Aβ- peptide and thus in preventing plaque formation (Li *et al.*, 2011). Similarly, this peptide decreases glutamate uptake in cultured astrocytes, thus increasing oxidative stress and and activation of mitogen-activated protein kinase cascades (Agostinho *et al.*, 2010; Matos *et al.*, 2008). High levels of pro-inflammatory cytokines such as interleukin 1β, interleukin 6 and TNFα, mostly produced by reactive astrocytes, are detected in the brain of AD subjects, so the consequences of this phenomenon are unclear, also because pro-inflammatory cytokines have varied effects depending on the biological context (Veerhuis, 2011).

A previous study indicated that activated astrocytes were closely associated with amyloid plaques in the molecular layer of the cerebral cortex (Wisniewski & Wegiel, 1991). Astrocytes might be activated by human amyloid-β (Aβ) (DeWitt *et al.*, 1998), indicating a correlation between this protein and subsequent alterations in astrocyte function. Astrocytes also accumulate neuron-derived amyloid material resulting from local neurodegeneration. Once substantial accumulation of this debris occurs, the astrocytes themselves might undergo cell death, resulting in the formation of $GFAP^{+}$ amyloid plaques (Nagele *et al.*, 2004). *In vitro* analyses also indicate that treatment of astrocytes with Aβ results in an increase in calcium-wave signaling between these cells (Haughey & Mattson, 2003). In cells expressing the familial AD presenilin 1 (*PSEN1*) mutation, calcium oscillations in astrocytes were found to occur at lower ATP and glutamate concentrations than in wild-type astrocytes (Johnston *et al.*, 2006). These data support a model in which calcium signaling between astrocytes is altered by the disease process, which might, in ways that are not fully understood, contribute to dysfunction or death of neurons.

Either prooxidant agents or amyloid beta peptide did not cause deleterious effects in the astrocytes, but the combined treatment let to oxidative stress and apoptosis in vitro and inflammation and degenerative traits in vivo. Therefore, a reduced oxidative stress defense capacity in frail aged astrocytes may contribute to neuron death by failure of astrocyte support. To preserve astrocyte function and reduce oxidative stress in old age is a new goal against AD (Aliev *et al.*, 2009a; Aliev *et al.*, 2009b; Garcia-Matas *et al.*, 2010).

3.3 Parkinson´s disease

PD is the second most prevalent neurodegenerative disease, after AD. PD is estimated to affect about 1 million Americans, or about 1% of the population over 60 years of age. PD is caused by the disruption of dopaminergic neurotransmission in the basal ganglia. On pathological examination, the numbers of dopaminergic neurons in the substantia nigra are markedly reduced, and Lewy bodies (cytoplasmic inclusions) are present in the residual dopaminergic neurons (Nutt & Wooten, 2005). The focus has always been on the loss of these dopamanergic neurons and subsequent depletion of dopamine, but a role for non-neuronal cells in producing neuropathological or neuroprotective functions in PD is becoming increasingly recognized.

The studies that have been carried out to date appear to support a neuroprotective role for astrocytes in PD. From pathological examinations, an increase in the number of astrocytes as well as in GFAP expression is observed in PD, (Ciesielska *et al.*, 2009; Muramatsu *et al.*, 2003), as with other neurodegenerative disorders. The pathological evidence indirectly indicates that antioxidant pathways might contribute to this neuroprotective effect, because in control brains the density of glutathione-peroxidase-positive cells was higher in the vicinity of the dopaminergic cell groups known to be resistant to the pathological process of PD. The increase in glutathione-peroxidase-containing cells was inversely correlated with the severity of dopaminergic cell loss in the respective cell groups in patients with PD. The quantity of glutathione-peroxidase-containing cells, therefore, might be critical for a protective effect against oxidative stress (Damier *et al.*, 1993). Conversely, the presence of synuclein-positive astrocytes in pathological samples has been shown to correlate with nigral neuronal cell death (Wakabayashi *et al.*, 2000).

Nitric oxide production and glutathione depletion also appear as consistent features in human PD. The release of glutathione represents another pathway by which astrocytes might be neuroprotective in PD models. Glutathione production appears to be increased by exposure of astrocytes to nitric oxide, and the increase in glutathione release by astrocytes might increase its availability to neurons, thereby making them less susceptible to reactive nitrogen species. This pattern is consistent with the data in PD patients, in whom glutathione-containing cells are in regions with preserved dopaminergic neurons (Heales *et al.*, 2004).

Evidence regarding regulation of glutamate transporter expression and function in PD has been somewhat mixed, with downregulation of glutamate transporters being reported in some studies and upregulation being reported in others. The differences in these studies might be related to the methods by which the lesions were induced (Maragakis & Rothstein, 2004).

3.4 Amyotrophic Lateral Syndrome (ALS)

Amyotrophic Lateral Syndrome is an inexorably progressive motor neuron disease, in which both the upper motor neurons and the lower motor neurons degenerate leading to muscle atrophy. Patients eventually experience respiratory failure, usually within three to five years from diagnosis. However, the onset of ALS may be subtle and early symptoms are frequently overlooked.

Common to familial and sporadic ALS is the loss of the astrocyte glutamate transporter EAAT2. Studies of the EAAT2 transporter in tissue from individuals with sporadic ALS showed a marked loss of up to 95% of astroglial EAAT2 protein expression and activity in affected areas of the CNS (Bristol & Rothstein, 1996). A clue to a possible mechanism for EAAT2 reduction or dysfunction was provided by the finding of aberrant *EAAT2* RNA species, which has been implicated in multiple neurodegenerative diseases. The production of truncated EAAT2 protein results in reduced function, and the retention of normal EAAT2 protein within the cytoplasm (Lin *et al.*, 1998). The significance of these aberrant *EAAT2* RNA species continues to be debated, however, as they have also been found in some normal controls (Flowers *et al.*, 2001; Meyer *et al.*, 1999).

In both human tissue and transgenic models of ALS, there is abundant evidence that astroglial abnormalities and physiological dysfunction precede clinical disease. These changes include reactive astrocytosis that can be seen many months before motor neuron degeneration (G85R) (Bruijn *et al.*, 1997), and loss of glutamate transport and GLT1 protein expression before the onset of clinical disease or overt motor neuron degeneration (Howland *et al.*, 2002). Similarly, increased astrocytes activation and expression of immune/inflammatory markers are hallmark of this pathology (Chiu *et al.*, 2008; Chiu *et al.*, 2009). Is the reduction in GLT1 protein in astrocytes significant? Guo and colleagues addressed this question by overexpressing the EAAT2 protein in astrocytes in the mSOD1 mouse model, and demonstrated an increase in motor neuron survival and a delay in disease onset; similar outcomes are seen with drugs that increase GLT1 expression (Guo *et al.*, 2003). This evidence indicates that EAAT2 expressed in astrocytes - and probably also glutamate- influences the timing of disease onset and motor neuron survival (Guo *et al.*, 2003). Other changes associated with ALS include increased expression of various proteins in astrocytes, including inducible nitric oxide synthase (iNOS), the copper chaperone CCS, and metallothioneins. Pathologically, early cytosolic proteinaceous aggregates have been found in spinal cord astrocytes from the entire mSOD1 mouse lines examined to date (Patel & Maragakis, 2002).

3.5 Multiple Sclerosis

Multiple Sclerosis is a chronic inflammatory demyelinating disease of the central nervous system in which glial cells play a prominent role. In murine experimental autoimmune encephalomyelitis (EAE), an established animal model of multiple sclerosis, astrocyte hypertrophy coincided with manifestation of axonal damage (Wang *et al.*, 2005). Astrocytes in multiple sclerosis plaques produce IL-6 (Okuda *et al.*, 1998), lack β-2 adrenergic receptors, and potentially serve as antigen-presenting cells (Zeinstra *et al.*, 2000b), thus facilitating T-cell invasion and activation. Repeated exposure of these astrocytes to inflammatory cytokines triggers unregulated inflammatory responses and increased noradrenalin levels, leading to focal areas of myelin and axonal damage (De Keyser *et al.*, 1999; Zeinstra *et al.*, 2000a).

Concerning the immune system, class II MHC expressing astrocytes have been shown to process and present antigens and activate both naïve and memory T cells (Nikcevich *et al.*, 1997; Soos *et al.*, 1998). In contrast, other investigators have shown that class II MHC expressing astrocytes are not capable of stimulating T-cell proliferation and instead induce apoptosis or down-regulation of T cells (Matsumoto *et al.*, 1992; Weber *et al.*, 1994). Such a response may be beneficial for astrocyte suppression of CNS autoimmunity like in multiple sclerosis.

4. Conclusions

Astrocytes play a critical role in normal function of the mammalian nervous system. Astrocytes regulate K^+ buffering, glutamate clearance, brain antioxidant defense, close metabolic coupling with neurons, and modulation of neuronal excitability. In numerous pathological states, such as AD, PD, ALS and ME, astrocytes are involved in both exacerbation of damage and neuroprotective mechanisms. As discussed in this chapter, they support neurons in many ways, all of which are essential for repair and regeneration. Disturbances in astrocytic functions are implicated in neurodegenerative diseases pathogenesis, therefore, modulation of astrocyte functioning may prove to be an efficient therapeutic strategy in many chronic CNS disorders.

5. References

Agostinho, P.; Cunha, R.A. & Oliveira, C. (2010). Neuroinflammation, oxidative stress and the pathogenesis of Alzheimer's disease. *Curr Pharm Des* 16, 2766-2778.

Aliev, G.; Palacios, H.H.; Lipsitt, A.E.; Fischbach, K.; Lamb, B.T.; Obrenovich, M.E.; Morales, L.; Gasimov, E. & Bragin, V. (2009a). Nitric oxide as an initiator of brain lesions during the development of Alzheimer disease. *Neurotox Res* 16, 293-305.

Aliev, G.; Palacios, H.H.; Walrafen, B.; Lipsitt, A.E.; Obrenovich, M.E. & Morales, L. (2009b). Brain mitochondria as a primary target in the development of treatment strategies for Alzheimer disease. *Int J Biochem Cell Biol* 41, 1989-2004.

Anderson, C.M. & Swanson, R.A. (2000): Astrocyte glutamate transport: review of properties, regulation, and physiological functions. *Glia* 32, 1-14.

Axelsson, M.; Malmestrom, C.; Nilsson, S.; Haghighi, S.; Rosengren, L. & Lycke, J. (2011). Glial fibrillary acidic protein: a potential biomarker for progression in multiple sclerosis. *J Neurol* 258, 882-888.

Barreto, G.; Santos-Galindo, M.; Diz-Chaves, Y.; Pernia, O.; Carrero, P.; Azcoitia, I. & Garcia-Segura, L.M. (2009). Selective estrogen receptor modulators decrease reactive astrogliosis in the injured brain: effects of aging and prolonged depletion of ovarian hormones. *Endocrinology* 150, 5010-5015.

Bartnik-Olson, B.L.; Oyoyo, U.; Hovda, D.A. & Sutton, R.L. (2010). Astrocyte oxidative metabolism and metabolite trafficking after fluid percussion brain injury in adult rats. *J Neurotrauma* 27, 2191-2202.

Bentzer, P.; Davidsson, H. & Grande, P.O. (2000). Microdialysis-based long-term measurements of energy-related metabolites in the rat brain following a fluid percussion trauma. *J Neurotrauma* 17, 441-447.

Beschorner, R.; Adjodah, D.; Schwab, J.M.; Mittelbronn, M.; Pedal, I.; Mattern R.; Schluesener, H.J. & Meyermann, R. (2000). Long-term expression of heme oxygenase-1 (HO-1, HSP-32) following focal cerebral infarctions and traumatic brain injury in humans. *Acta Neuropathol* 100, 377-384.

Bristol, L.A. & Rothstein, J.D. (1996). Glutamate transporter gene expression in amyotrophic lateral sclerosis motor cortex. *Ann Neurol* 39, 676-679.

Bruijn, L.I.; Becher, M.W.; Lee, M.K.; Anderson, K.L.; Jenkins, N.A.; Copeland, N.G.; Sisodia, S.S.; Rothstein, J.D.; Borchelt, D.R.; Price, D.L. & Cleveland, D.W. (1997). ALS-linked SOD1 mutant G85R mediates damage to astrocytes and promotes rapidly progressive disease with SOD1-containing inclusions. *Neuron* 18, 327-338.

Bushong, E.A.; Martone, M.E.; Jones, Y.Z. & Ellisman, M.H. (2002). Protoplasmic astrocytes in CA1 stratum radiatum occupy separate anatomical domains. *J Neurosci* 22, 183-192.

Caesar, K.; Hashemi, P.; Douhou, A.; Bonvento, G.; Boutelle, M.G.; Walls, A.B. & Lauritzen, M. (2008). Glutamate receptor-dependent increments in lactate, glucose and oxygen metabolism evoked in rat cerebellum in vivo. *J Physiol* 586, 1337-1349.

Ciesielska, A.; Joniec, I.; Kurkowska-Jastrzebska, I.; Cudna, A.; Przybylkowski, A.; Czlonkowska, A. & Czlonkowski, A. (2009). The impact of age and gender on the striatal astrocytes activation in murine model of Parkinson's disease. *Inflamm Res* 58, 747-753.

Cliffe, E.E. & Waley, S.G. (1961). The mechanism of the glyoxalase I reaction, and the effect of ophthalmic acid as an inhibitor. *Biochem J* 79, 475-482.

Chen, K.; Gunter, K. & Maines, M.D. (2000). Neurons overexpressing heme oxygenase-1 resist oxidative stress-mediated cell death. *J Neurochem* 75, 304-313.

Chen, Y. & Swanson, R.A. (2003). Astrocytes and brain injury. *J Cereb Blood Flow Metab* 23, 137-149.

Chiu, I.M.; Chen, A.; Zheng, Y.; Kosaras, B.; Tsiftsoglou, S.A.; Vartanian, T.K.; Brown, R.H.Jr. & Carroll, M.C. (2008). T lymphocytes potentiate endogenous neuroprotective inflammation in a mouse model of ALS. *Proc Natl Acad Sci U S A* 105, 17913-17918.

Chiu, I.M.; Phatnani, H.; Kuligowski, M.; Tapia, J.C.; Carrasco, M.A.; Zhang, M.; Maniatis, T. & Carroll, M.C. (2009). Activation of innate and humoral immunity in the peripheral nervous system of ALS transgenic mice. *Proc Natl Acad Sci U S A* 106, 20960-20965.

Damier, P.; Hirsch, E.C.; Zhang, P.; Agid, Y. & Javoy-Agid, F. (1993). Glutathione peroxidase, glial cells and Parkinson's disease. *Neuroscience* 52, 1-6.

De Keyser, J.; Wilczak, N.; Leta, R. & Streetland, C. (1999). Astrocytes in multiple sclerosis lack beta-2 adrenergic receptors. *Neurology* 53, 1628-1633.

DeWitt, D.A.; Perry, G.; Cohen, M.; Doller, C. & Silver, J. (1998). Astrocytes regulate microglial phagocytosis of senile plaque cores of Alzheimer's disease. *Exp Neurol* 149, 329-340.

Dringen, R. (2000): Metabolism and functions of glutathione in brain. *Prog Neurobiol* 62, 649-671.

Dringen, R.; Gutterer, J.M. & Hirrlinger, J. (2000). Glutathione metabolism in brain metabolic interaction between astrocytes and neurons in the defense against reactive oxygen species. *Eur J Biochem* 267, 4912-4916.

Dringen, R. & Hirrlinger, J. (2003). Glutathione pathways in the brain. *Biol Chem* 384, 505-516.

Eddleston, M. & Mucke, L. (1993): Molecular profile of reactive astrocytes--Implications for their role in neurologic disease. *Neuroscience* 54, 15-36.

Espada, S.; Ortega, F.; Molina-Jijon, E.; Rojo, A.I.; Perez-Sen, R.; Pedraza-Chaverri, J.; Miras-Portugal, M.T. & Cuadrado, A. (2010). The purinergic P2Y(13) receptor activates the Nrf2/HO-1 axis and protects against oxidative stress-induced neuronal death. *Free Radic Biol Med* 49, 416-426.

Fernandez-Checa, J.C.; Fernandez, A.; Morales, A.; Mari, M.; Garcia-Ruiz, C. & Colell, A. (2010). Oxidative stress and altered mitochondrial function in neurodegenerative diseases: lessons from mouse models. *CNS Neurol Disord Drug Targets* 9, 439-454.

Flowers, J.M.; Powell, J.F.; Leigh, P.N.; Andersen, P. & Shaw, C.E. (2001). Intron 7 retention and exon 9 skipping EAAT2 mRNA variants are not associated with amyotrophic lateral sclerosis. *Ann Neurol* 49, 643-649.

Floyd, C.L. & Lyeth, B.G. (2007). Astroglia: important mediators of traumatic brain injury. *Prog Brain Res* 161, 61-79.

Garcia-Matas, S.; de Vera, N.; Aznar, A.O.; Marimon, J.M.; Adell, A.; Planas, A.M.; Cristofol, R. & Sanfeliu, C. (2010). In vitro and in vivo activation of astrocytes by amyloid-beta is potentiated by pro-oxidant agents. *J Alzheimers Dis* 20, 229-245.

Giordano, G.; Kavanagh, T.J. & Costa, L.G. (2009). Mouse cerebellar astrocytes protect cerebellar granule neurons against toxicity of the polybrominated diphenyl ether (PBDE) mixture DE-71. *Neurotoxicology* 30, 326-329.

Gordon, G.R.; Mulligan, S.J. & MacVicar, B.A. (2007). Astrocyte control of the cerebrovasculature. *Glia* 55, 1214-1221.

Guo, H.; Lai, L.; Butchbach, M.E.; Stockinger, M.P.; Shan, X.; Bishop, G.A. & Lin, C.L. (2003). Increased expression of the glial glutamate transporter EAAT2 modulates excitotoxicity and delays the onset but not the outcome of ALS in mice. *Hum Mol Genet* 12, 2519-2532.

Halassa, M.M.; Fellin, T.; Takano, H.; Dong, J.H. & Haydon, P.G. (2007). Synaptic islands defined by the territory of a single astrocyte. *J Neurosci* 27, 6473-6477.

Haughey, N.J. & Mattson, M.P. (2003). Alzheimer's amyloid beta-peptide enhances ATP/gap junction-mediated calcium-wave propagation in astrocytes. *Neuromolecular Med* 3, 173-180.

Haydon, P.G. & Carmignoto, G. (2006). Astrocyte control of synaptic transmission and neurovascular coupling. *Physiol Rev* 86, 1009-1031.

Heales, S.J.; Lam, A.A.; Duncan, A.J. & Land, J.M. (2004). Neurodegeneration or neuroprotection: the pivotal role of astrocytes. *Neurochem Res* 29, 513-519.

Hertz, L. & Zielke, H.R. (2004). Astrocytic control of glutamatergic activity: astrocytes as stars of the show. *Trends Neurosci* 27, 735-743.

Howland, D.S.; Liu, J.; She, Y.; Goad, B.; Maragakis, N.J.; Kim, B.; Erickson, J.; Kulik, J.; DeVito, L.; Psaltis, G.; DeGennaro, L.J.; Cleveland, D.W. & Rothstein, J.D. (2002). Focal loss of the glutamate transporter EAAT2 in a transgenic rat model of SOD1 mutant-mediated amyotrophic lateral sclerosis (ALS). *Proc Natl Acad Sci U S A* 99, 1604-1609.

Iadecola, C. & Nedergaard, M. (2007). Glial regulation of the cerebral microvasculature. *Nat Neurosci* 10, 1369-1376.

Imuta, N.; Hori, O.; Kitao, Y.; Tabata, Y.; Yoshimoto, T.; Matsuyama, T. & Ogawa, S. (2007). Hypoxia-mediated induction of heme oxygenase type I and carbon monoxide release from astrocytes protects nearby cerebral neurons from hypoxia-mediated apoptosis. *Antioxid Redox Signal* 9, 543-552.

Jayakumar, A.R. & Norenberg, M.D. (2010). The Na-K-Cl Co-transporter in astrocyte swelling. *Metab Brain Dis* 25, 31-38.

Johnston, J.M.; Burnett, P.; Thomas, A.P. & Tezapsidis, N. (2006): Calcium oscillations in type-1 astrocytes, the effect of a presenilin 1 (PS1) mutation. *Neurosci Lett* 395, 159-164.

Jones, E.G. (1970). On the mode of entry of blood vessels into the cerebral cortex. *J Anat* 106, 507-520.

Kashon, M.L.; Ross, G.W.; O'Callaghan, J.P.; Miller, D.B.; Petrovitch, H.; Burchfiel, C.M.; Sharp, D.S.; Markesbery, W.R.; Davis, D.G.; Hardman, J.; Nelson, J. & White, L.R. (2004). Associations of cortical astrogliosis with cognitive performance and dementia status. *J Alzheimers Dis* 6, 595-604; discussion 673-581.

Koehler, R.C.; Roman, R.J. & Harder, D.R. (2009). Astrocytes and the regulation of cerebral blood flow. *Trends Neurosci* 32, 160-169.

Kontos, H.A.; Raper, A.J. & Patterson, J.L. Jr. (1971). Mechanisms of action of CO 2 on pial precapillary vessels. *Eur Neurol* 6, 114-118.

Ku, B.M.; Joo, Y.; Mun, J.; Roh, G.S.; Kang, S.S.; Cho, G.J.; Choi, W.S. & Kim, H.J. (2006). Heme oxygenase protects hippocampal neurons from ethanol-induced neurotoxicity. *Neurosci Lett* 405, 168-171.

Lambert, S. & Oberwinkler, J. (2005). Characterization of a proton-activated, outwardly rectifying anion channel. *J Physiol* 567, 191-213.

Lang, F.; Busch, G.L.; Ritter, M.; Volkl, H.; Waldegger, S.; Gulbins, E. & Haussinger, D. (1998). Functional significance of cell volume regulatory mechanisms. *Physiol Rev* 78, 247-306.

Le, W.D.; Xie, W.J. & Appel, S.H. (1999). Protective role of heme oxygenase-1 in oxidative stress-induced neuronal injury. *J Neurosci Res* 56, 652-658.

Lee, C.K.; Weindruch, R. & Prolla, T.A. (2000). Gene-expression profile of the ageing brain in mice. *Nat Genet* 25, 294-297.

Li, C.; Zhao, R.; Gao, K.; Wei, Z.; Yin, M.Y.; Lau, L.T.; Chui, D. & Hoi Yu, A.C. (2011). Astrocytes: implications for neuroinflammatory pathogenesis of Alzheimer's disease. *Curr Alzheimer Res* 8, 67-80.

Lin, C.L.; Bristol, L.A.; Jin, L.; Dykes-Hoberg, M.; Crawford, T.; Clawson, L. & Rothstein, J.D. (1998). Aberrant RNA processing in a neurodegenerative disease: the cause for absent EAAT2, a glutamate transporter, in amyotrophic lateral sclerosis. *Neuron* 20, 589-602.

Lindenau, J.; Noack, H.; Possel, H.; Asayama, K. & Wolf, G. (2000). Cellular distribution of superoxide dismutases in the rat CNS. *Glia* 29, 25-34.

Magistretti, P.J. (2006). Neuron-glia metabolic coupling and plasticity. *J Exp Biol* 209, 2304-2311.

Magistretti, P.J. & Pellerin, L. (1999). Cellular mechanisms of brain energy metabolism and their relevance to functional brain imaging. *Philos Trans R Soc Lond B Biol Sci* 354, 1155-1163.

Maragakis, N.J. & Rothstein, J.D. (2004). Glutamate transporters: animal models to neurologic disease. *Neurobiol Dis* 15, 461-473.

Matos, M.; Augusto E.; Oliveira, C.R. & Agostinho, P. (2008). Amyloid-beta peptide decreases glutamate uptake in cultured astrocytes: involvement of oxidative stress and mitogen-activated protein kinase cascades. *Neuroscience* 156, 898-910.

Matsumoto, Y.; Ohmori, K. & Fujiwara, M. (1992). Immune regulation by brain cells in the central nervous system: microglia but not astrocytes present myelin basic protein to encephalitogenic T cells under in vivo-mimicking conditions. *Immunology* 76, 209-216.

Meyer, T.; Fromm, A.; Munch, C.; Schwalenstocker, B.; Fray, A.E.; Ince, P.G.; Stamm, S.; Gron, G.; Ludolph, A.C. & Shaw, P.J. (1999). The RNA of the glutamate transporter

EAAT2 is variably spliced in amyotrophic lateral sclerosis and normal individuals. *J Neurol Sci* 170, 45-50.

Muramatsu, Y.; Kurosaki, R.; Watanabe, H.; Michimata, M.; Matsubara, M.; Imai, Y. & Araki, T. (2003). Cerebral alterations in a MPTP-mouse model of Parkinson's disease--an immunocytochemical study. *J Neural Transm* 110, 1129-1144.

Nagele, R.G.; Wegiel, J.; Venkataraman, V.; Imaki, H. & Wang, K.C. (2004). Contribution of glial cells to the development of amyloid plaques in Alzheimer's disease. *Neurobiol Aging* 25, 663-674.

Nedergaard, M. & Dirnagl, U. (2005). Role of glial cells in cerebral ischemia. *Glia* 50, 281-286.

Nichols, N.R. (1999). Glial responses to steroids as markers of brain aging. *J Neurobiol* 40, 585-601.

Nikcevich, K.M.; Gordon, K.B.; Tan, L.; Hurst, S.D.; Kroepfl, J.F.; Gardinier, M.; Barrett, T.A. & Miller, S.D. (1997). IFN-gamma-activated primary murine astrocytes express B7 costimulatory molecules and prime naive antigen-specific T cells. *J Immunol* 158, 614-621.

Notturno, F.; Capasso, M.; DeLauretis, A.; Carpo, M. & Uncini, A. (2009). Glial fibrillary acidic protein as a marker of axonal damage in chronic neuropathies. *Muscle Nerve* 40, 50-54.

Nutt, J.G. & Wooten, G.F. (2005). Clinical practice. Diagnosis and initial management of Parkinson's disease. *N Engl J Med* 353, 1021-1027.

Obara, M.; Szeliga, M. & Albrecht, J. (2008). Regulation of pH in the mammalian central nervous system under normal and pathological conditions: facts and hypotheses. *Neurochem Int* 52, 905-919.

Okuda, Y.; Sakoda, S.; Bernard, C.C. & Yanagihara, T. (1998). The development of autoimmune encephalomyelitis provoked by myelin oligodendrocyte glycoprotein is associated with an upregulation of both proinflammatory and immunoregulatory cytokines in the central nervous system. *J Interferon Cytokine Res* 18, 415-421.

Patel, S.A. & Maragakis, N.J. (2002). Amyotrophic lateral sclerosis: pathogenesis, differential diagnoses, and potential interventions. *J Spinal Cord Med* 25, 262-273.

Peinado, M.A.; Quesada, A.; Pedrosa, J.A.; Torres, M.I.; Martinez, M.; Esteban, F.J.; Del Moral, M.L.; Hernandez, R.; Rodrigo, J. & Peinado, J.M. (1998). Quantitative and ultrastructural changes in glia and pericytes in the parietal cortex of the aging rat. *Microsc Res Tech* 43, 34-42.

Pelinka, L.E.; Kroepfl, A.; Leixnering, M.; Buchinger, W.; Raabe, A. & Redl, H. (2004). GFAP versus S100B in serum after traumatic brain injury: relationship to brain damage and outcome. *J Neurotrauma* 21, 1553-1561.

Pilegaard, K. & Ladefoged, O. (1996). Total number of astrocytes in the molecular layer of the dentate gyrus of rats at different ages. *Anal Quant Cytol Histol* 18, 279-285.

Ransom, B.; Behar, T. & Nedergaard, M. (2003). New roles for astrocytes (stars at last). *Trends Neurosci* 26, 520-522.

Ridet, J.L.; Malhotra, S.K.; Privat, A. & Gage, F.H. (1997). Reactive astrocytes: cellular and molecular cues to biological function. *Trends Neurosci* 20, 570-577.

Romera, C.; Hurtado, O.; Botella, S.H.; Lizasoain, I.; Cardenas, A.; Fernandez-Tome, P.; Leza, J.C.; Lorenzo, P. & Moro, M.A. (2004). In vitro ischemic tolerance involves upregulation of glutamate transport partly mediated by the TACE/ADAM17-tumor necrosis factor-alpha pathway. *J Neurosci* 24, 1350-1357.

Rossi, D. & Volterra, A. (2009). Astrocytic dysfunction: insights on the role in neurodegeneration. *Brain Res Bull* 80, 224-232.

Rozovsky, I.; Finch, C.E. & Morgan, T.E. (1998). Age-related activation of microglia and astrocytes: in vitro studies show persistent phenotypes of aging, increased proliferation, and resistance to down-regulation. *Neurobiol Aging* 19, 97-103.

Salminen, A.; Ojala, J.; Kaarniranta, K.; Haapasalo, A.; Hiltunen, M. & Soininen, H. (2011). Astrocytes in the aging brain express characteristics of senescence-associated secretory phenotype. *Eur J Neurosci* 34, 3-11.

Scafidi, S.; O'Brien, J.; Hopkins, I.; Robertson, C.; Fiskum, G. & McKenna, M. (2009). Delayed cerebral oxidative glucose metabolism after traumatic brain injury in young rats. *J Neurochem* 109 Suppl 1, 189-197.

Schipper, H.M.; Cisse, S. & Stopa, E.G. (1995). Expression of heme oxygenase-1 in the senescent and Alzheimer-diseased brain. *Ann Neurol* 37, 758-768.

Schipper, H.M.; Liberman, A. & Stopa, E.G. (1998). Neural heme oxygenase-1 expression in idiopathic Parkinson's disease. *Exp Neurol* 150, 60-68.

Schousboe, A. & Waagepetersen, H.S. (2006). Glial modulation of GABAergic and glutamat ergic neurotransmission. *Curr Top Med Chem* 6, 929-934.

Serviddio, G.; Romano, A.D.; Cassano, T.; Bellanti, F.; Altomare, E. & Vendemiale, G. (2011). Principles and Therapeutic Relevance for Targeting Mitochondria in Aging and Neurodegenerative Diseases. *Curr Pharm Des.*

Shibata, N. & Kobayashi, M. (2008). [The role for oxidative stress in neurodegenerative diseases]. *Brain Nerve* 60, 157-170.

Simard, M.; Arcuino, G.; Takano, T.; Liu, Q.S. & Nedergaard, M. (2003). Signaling at the gliovascular interface. *J Neurosci* 23, 9254-9262.

Simpson, J.E.; Ince, P.G.; Lace, G.; Forster, G.; Shaw, P.J.; Matthews, F.; Savva, G.; Brayne, C. & Wharton, S.B. (2010). Astrocyte phenotype in relation to Alzheimer-type pathology in the ageing brain. *Neurobiol Aging* 31, 578-590.

Sims NR, Nilsson M & Muyderman H. (2004). Mitochondrial glutathione: a modulator of brain cell death. *J Bioenerg Biomembr* 36, 329-333.

Slemmer, J.E.; Shacka, J.J.; Sweeney, M.I. & Weber, J.T. (2008). Antioxidants and free radical scavengers for the treatment of stroke, traumatic brain injury and aging. *Curr Med Chem* 15, 404-414.

Sofroniew, M.V. (2000). Astrocyte failure as a cause of CNS dysfunction. *Mol Psychiatry* 5, 230-232.

Sofroniew, M.V. (2009). Molecular dissection of reactive astrogliosis and glial scar formation. *Trends Neurosci* 32, 638-647.

Sofroniew, M.V. & Vinters, H.V. (2010). Astrocytes: biology and pathology. *Acta Neuropathol* 119, 7-35.

Soos, J.M.; Morrow, J.; Ashley, T.A.; Szente, B.E.; Bikoff, E.K. & Zamvil, S.S. (1998). Astrocytes express elements of the class II endocytic pathway and process central nervous system autoantigen for presentation to encephalitogenic T cells. *J Immunol* 161, 5959-5966.

Swanson, R.A.; Ying, W. & Kauppinen, T.M. (2004). Astrocyte influences on ischemic neuronal death. *Curr Mol Med* 4, 193-205.

Takano, T.; Tian, G.F.; Peng, W.; Lou, N.; Libionka, W.; Han, X. & Nedergaard, M. (2006). Astrocyte-mediated control of cerebral blood flow. *Nat Neurosci* 9, 260-267.

Takeda, A.; Perry, G.; Abraham, N.G.; Dwyer, B.E.; Kutty, R.K.; Laitinen, J.T.; Petersen, R.B. & Smith, M.A. (2000). Overexpression of heme oxygenase in neuronal cells, the possible interaction with Tau. *J Biol Chem* 275, 5395-5399.

Tilleux, S. & Hermans, E. (2007). Neuroinflammation and regulation of glial glutamate uptake in neurological disorders. *J Neurosci Res* 85, 2059-2070.

Toft-Hansen, H.; Fuchtbauer, L. & Owens, T. (2011). Inhibition of reactive astrocytosis in established experimental autoimmune encephalomyelitis favors infiltration by myeloid cells over T cells and enhances severity of disease. *Glia* 59, 166-176.

Veerhuis, R. (2011). Histological and direct evidence for the role of complement in the neuroinflammation of AD. *Curr Alzheimer Res* 8, 34-58.

Volterra, A. & Meldolesi, J. (2005). Astrocytes, from brain glue to communication elements: the revolution continues. *Nat Rev Neurosci* 6, 626-640.

Wakabayashi, K.; Hayashi, S.; Yoshimoto, M.; Kudo, H. & Takahashi, H. (2000). NACP/alpha-synuclein-positive filamentous inclusions in astrocytes and oligodendrocytes of Parkinson's disease brains. *Acta Neuropathol* 99, 14-20.

Wang, D.; Ayers, M.M.; Catmull, D.V.; Hazelwood, L.J.; Bernard, C.C. & Orian, J.M. (2005). Astrocyte-associated axonal damage in pre-onset stages of experimental autoimmune encephalomyelitis. *Glia* 51, 235-240.

Weber, F.; Meinl, E.; Aloisi, F.; Nevinny-Stickel, C.; Albert, E.; Wekerle, H. & Hohlfeld, R. (1994). Human astrocytes are only partially competent antigen presenting cells. Possible implications for lesion development in multiple sclerosis. *Brain* 117 (Pt 1), 59-69.

Wilson, J.X. (1997). Antioxidant defense of the brain: a role for astrocytes. *Can J Physiol Pharmacol* 75, 1149-1163.

Wisniewski, H.M. & Wegiel, J. (1991). Spatial relationships between astrocytes and classical plaque components. *Neurobiol Aging* 12, 593-600.

Xu, H.L.; Koenig, H.M.; Ye, S.; Feinstein, D.L. & Pelligrino, D.A. (2004). Influence of the glia limitans on pial arteriolar relaxation in the rat. *Am J Physiol Heart Circ Physiol* 287, H331-339.

Yi, J.H. & Hazell, A.S. (2006). Excitotoxic mechanisms and the role of astrocytic glutamate transporters in traumatic brain injury. *Neurochem Int* 48, 394-403.

Zeier, Z.; Madorsky, I.; Xu, Y.; Ogle, W.O.; Notterpek, L. & Foster, T.C. (2011). Gene expression in the hippocampus: regionally specific effects of aging and caloric restriction. *Mech Ageing Dev* 132, 8-19.

Zeinstra, E.; Wilczak, N. & De Keyser, J. (2000a). [3H]dihydroalprenolol binding to beta adrenergic receptors in multiple sclerosis brain. *Neurosci Lett* 289, 75-77.

Zeinstra, E.; Wilczak, N.; Streefland, C. & De Keyser, J. (2000b). Astrocytes in chronic active multiple sclerosis plaques express MHC class II molecules. *Neuroreport* 11, 89-91.

Zonta, M.; Angulo, M.C.; Gobbo, S.; Rosengarten, B.; Hossmann, K.A.; Pozzan, T. & Carmignoto, G. (2003). Neuron-to-astrocyte signaling is central to the dynamic control of brain microcirculation. *Nat Neurosci* 6, 43-50.

Zou, J.; Wang, Y.X.; Dou, F.F.; Lu, H.Z.; Ma, Z.W.; Lu, P.H. & Xu, X.M. (2010). Glutamine synthetase down-regulation reduces astrocyte protection against glutamate excitotoxicity to neurons. *Neurochem Int* 56, 577-584.

12

Alteration of Neuron-Glia Interactions in Neurodegeneration: Molecular Biomarkers and Therapeutic Strategy

Alla B. Salmina et al.*
Krasnoyarsk State Medical University named after Prof. V.F.Voino-Yasenetsky
Russia

1. Introduction

Accumulating evidence suggests that alterations of neuron-astroglia interactions are associated with development of neurodegenerative diseases (Barres, 2008; Ricci et al., 2009; Verkhratsky et al., 2010). Astrocytes contribute to a variety of functions of neurons, including synapse formation and plasticity, energetic and redox metabolism, and synaptic homeostasis of neurotransmitters and ions (Bolton & Eroglu, 2009; Nimmerjahn, 2009; Salmina, 2009; Verkhratsky, 2010; Wang & Bordey, 2008). It is well known that astrocytes play important role in supporting energy production in neurons. Astrocytes produce lactate which is actively taken up by active neurons. They utilize lactate as an alternative energy fuel. In turn, neuronal activation results in glutamate-stimulated glycolysis in astroglial cells. Thus, neuron-astrocyte metabolic coupling provides tight interactions between the activated neuronal cells consuming lactate and lactate-producing astrocytes. Remodeling of astrocytes is required for adequate synapse turnover in the brain, and astrocytes or the closely related radial glial cells possess all the attributes of a neural stem cells, thereby playing a key role in neurogenesis (Steindler & Laywell, 2003; Theodosis et al., 2006).

Functional relationship between neurons, glial cells, and vascular cells within so-called neurovascular unit is very important in the context of pathogenesis of neurodegenerative disorders. A major function of the neurovascular unit is to regulate the transport and diffusion properties of brain capillary endothelial cells that compose the brain-blood barrier. Astrocytes exhibit anatomic relationships with cerebral arterioles and neurons. In the brain parenchyma, the extensive ensheatment of cerebral arterioles by astrocytic end-feet far exceeds any direct neural contacts with those perfusion-regulating microvessels. That unique arrangement permits astrocytes to transduce signals arising from activated neurons and to transmit that information to the cerebral microcirculation. Alteration of these processes may play a particularly significant role in the pathogenesis of neurodegenerative diseases. The early and mid-term stages of neurodegenerative processes are associated with generalised atrophy of astroglia, whereas the later stages are characterized with an

* Marina M. Petrova, Tatyana E. Taranushenko, Semen V. Prokopenko, Natalia A. Malinovskaya, Olesya S. Okuneva, Alyona I. Inzhutova, Andrei V. Morgun, Alexander A. Fursov
Krasnoyarsk State Medical University named after Prof. V.F.Voino-Yasenetsky; Russia

astrogliosis and microglial activation linked to neuropathological lesions such as senile plaques (Rodriguez & Verkhratsky, 2010).

Acute neurodegeneration is encountered during and following stroke, transient cardiac arrest, brain trauma, insulin-induced hypoglycemia and status epilepticus. All these severe clinical conditions are characterized by neuronal calcium overload, aberrant cell signaling, generation of free radicals and elevation of cellular free fatty acids, conditions that favor activation of the mitochondrial permeability transition pore (mtPTP) (Friberg & Wieloch, 2002).

Pathological cascade leading to clinical manifestations of chronic neurodegeneration (i.e. Parkinson's disease, Alzheimer's disease, Hungtington's disease) includes progressive loss of functional synapses, irreversible damage and loss of neurons, neurotoxicity, and excessive activation of astroglial (reactive astrogliosis) and microglial (neuroinflammation) cells. Neurodegeneration is associated with axonal and synapse degeneration which is triggered by mechanical, metabolic, infectious, toxic, hereditary and inflammatory stimuli. Several signaling pathways are implicated in axonal and synapse degeneration, but identification of an integrative mechanism for these self-destructive processes has remained elusive. Also, neurodegenerative events are known to be associated with alterations in cell-cell interactions, gene expression, dynamics of neuronal networks, development of oxidative stress, accumulation of lipid and protein oxidation products, production of fatty acids metabolites with biological activity, mitochondrial dysfunction, impairment of multiple signaling pathways, activation of programmed cell death (Salmina, 2009).

In general, the link between the character of astroglial activation and neuronal damage or repair in neurodegeneration is well established (Theodosis et al., 2008). The current conception includes impairment of astroglia-assisted synapse formation and plasticity, synapse elimination, neurogenesis, function of neural circuits, and functioning of the blood-brain barrier; dysregulation of gliovascular control and cerebral blood flow, alterations of neuronal metabolism, astrocyte-dependent augmentation of oxidative stress due to impaired antioxidant activity, stimulation of neuroinflammatory response, potentiation of excitotoxic insult, mitochondrial and glycolytic failure, impairment of glial calcium homeostasis, pathology of neurovascular unit, reactive astrogliosis accompanied by scar formation and initiation of brain repair (Bambrick et al., 2004; Barres, 2008; Buffo et al., 2008; L'Episcopo et al., 2010; Ricci, et al., 2009; Sofroniew, 2009; Stevens, 2008; Verkhratsky, et al., 2010; Verkhratsky et al., 1998).

Recent achievements in deciphering cell and molecular mechanisms of acute and chronic neurodegeneration suggest new prospective biomarkers and therapeutic targets for modulation of neuron-glia interactions. In this chapter, we will focus on several aspects of metabolism of nicotinamide adenine dinucleotide (NAD^+) in neurons and astrocytes as a critical factor in neurodegeneration-associated cell damage.

2. Neuronal and glial NAD^+-generating and NAD^+-converting enzymes in neurodegeneration

Few decades ago, the actions of NAD^+ have been extended from being an oxidoreductase cofactor for single enzymatic activities to acting as substrate for a wide range of proteins. These include NAD^+-converting enzymes, and transcription factors that affect a large array of cellular functions. Through these effects, NAD^+ provides a direct link between the cellular redox status and the control of signaling and transcriptional events (Houtkooper et al., 2010). Cellular bioenergetic homeostasis requires production and delivery of energy-rich phosphoryls and NAD^+. In cytosol, NAD^+ and NADH mediate glycolysis acting as co-factors for rate-limiting glycolytic enzyme glyceraldehyde 3-phosphate dehydrogenase, participate in lactate-pyruvate conversions, and affect mitochondrial oxidative phosphorylation. Also, NAD^+ serves as a substrate for NAD^+-converting enzymes (ADP-ribosyltransferases, poly(ADP-ribosyl)polymerase and ADP-ribosyl cyclase).

Synthesis of NAD^+ *in vivo* and *de novo* is possible by means of 4 pathways: 1) from nicotinic acid (niacin); 2) from nicotinamide (vitamin PP); 3) from tryptophan; 4) from aspartate (in plants only). Recently, a biosynthesis pathway which uses nicotinamide riboside as a precursor has been described. For the synthesis of NAD^+ from L-tryptophan, the indole ring should undergo transformation into the pyridine ring, and finally quinolinate is formed. Quinolinic acid undergoes further transformations resulting in NAD^+ formation. Indoleamine 2,3-dioxygenase (expressed in various tissues) and tryptophan 2,3-dioxygenase (expressed in liver) catalyze the formation of N-formylkynurenine in the reaction representing the first rate-limiting step in this pathway. Indoleamine 2,3-dioxygenase is a unique enzyme in that it can utilize as the substrate, in place of oxygen, the superoxide anion radical, thus acting as a radical scavenger. The second rate-limiting step in this pathway is represented by the reaction catalyzing by quinolinate phosphoribosyltransferase responsible for the conversion of quinolinic acid and 5-phospho-α-D-ribose 1-diphosphate to nicotinate mononucleotide, pyrophosphate and CO_2 (Magni et al., 2004).

Enzymes responsible for producing neuroactive compounds in the kynurenine pathway are preferentially localized in astrocytes and microglia. Astrocytes are well equipped with enzymes for kynurenine metabolism, i.e indoleamine 2,3-dioxygenase is highly expressed in these cells (Suh et al., 2007), thus raising the possibility that generation of the neuroactive compounds may play significant role in neuron-glial cell interactions (Ying, 2006). Interestingly, tryptophan and kynurenine stimulate expression of nerve growth factor in astrocytes (Dong-Ruyl et al., 1998), while interferon-gamma hyperactivates indoleamine 2,3-dioxygenase resulting in elevated production of kynunerines (i.e. quinolinic and picolinic acids) and stimulation of iNOS in human aged brain and vascular cognitive impairment (Oxenkrug, 2007). In general, kynurenine pathway is up-regulated in Alzheimer's disease brain, i.e. in hippocampus, where indoleamine 2,3-dioxygenase and quinolinic acid immunoreactivity was detected in astrocytes, microglia and neurons, with highest expression in glial cells in the perimeter of senile plaques. Quinolinic acid immunoreactivity was also present in granular deposits within the neuronal soma of cortex, and looks to label neurofibrillary tangles (Guillemin et al., 2005). Dysfunction of quinolinate metabolism in the human brain has been postulated to be involved in the pathogenesis of Alzheimer's disease ("quinolinate hypothesis") (Fukuoka et al., 2002). At the same time, it was suggested that astrocytes alone are neuroprotective by minimizing quinolinic acid production and maximizing synthesis of kynurenic acid (due to absence of kynurenine hydroxylase), but in the presence of macrophages and/or microglia, astrocytes become indirectly neurotoxic by the production of high concentrations of kynurenine that can be secondary metabolized by neighboring cells to quinolinic acid (Guillemin et al., 2001).

Mononucleotide adenylyltransferase (NMNAT) is a central enzyme in NAD^+ biosynthesis, catalyzing the condensation of nicotinamide mononucleotide or nicotinic acid mononucleotide with the AMP moiety of ATP to form NAD^+. NMNAT-1 has nuclear localization, and was proposed to have functional relations with poly (ADP-ribosyl) polymerase (PARP) in prevention of NAD^+ depletion during PARP over-activation. NMNAT-2 isoform has cytoplasmic localization, and is very prone to oxidation due to presence of nine cysteines versus four cysteines present in NMNAT-1. NMNAT-3 presents in cytoplasm and mitochondria, has much lower enzymatic activity comparing with NMNAT-1 and NMNAT-2 (Raffaelli et al., 2002). Extracelullar nucleotides (*e.g.* NAD^+ and NMN) undergo extracellular degradation resulting in the formation of permeable precursors which are further converted to NAD^+ in mitochondria due to activity of NMNAT3 localized to the mitochondrial matrix (Nikiforov et al., 2011). Interestingly enough, in genomewide screen for late-onset Alzheimer's disease, SNP of the NMNAT-3 gene was found, thus suggesting involvement of NAD^+ synthesizing pathways in pathogenesis of this neurodegenerative disorder (Liu et al., 2007)].

Recently, a role for mitochondrial permeability transition, and mitochondrial dysfunction, in development of axonal degeneration has been proposed. Axonal degeneration has been shown to be regulated by proapoptotic proteins (i.e. caspases 3 and 6) and/or NAD^+-sensitive pathways (Schoenmann et al., 2010). Since these degenerative processes can cause permanent loss of function, they represent a focus for neuroprotective strategies (Barrientos et al., 2011). Functioning of NMNAT as a chaperone acting through a proteasome-mediated pathway was found (Zhai et al., 2008), thus suggesting novel aspects in regulation of NAD^+ homeostasis under the conditions of cellular stress. Overexpression of NMNAT in the mitochondrial matrix resulted in suppression of axonal degeneration seen in neurodenegeration (Sasaki & Milbrandt, 2010; Sasaki et al., 2009; Yahata et al., 2009). In amyloid-treated cells, NMNAT-sensitive program is uniquely involved in axonal, but not cell body, degeneration (Vohra et al., 2010). Axonal degeneration can be slowed by the addition of extracellular NAD^+ (Billington et al., 2008).

Nicotinamide N-methyltransferase (NNMT) methylates pyridines, in particular nicotinamide, to N-methyl nicotinamide which is further used for synthesis of NAD(P) and NAD(P)H. Increased activity of NNMT leads to cellular nicotinamide deficiency. It was demonstrated that elevated levels of NNMT result in reduced Complex I activity in idiopathic Parkinson's disease (IPD) in two ways: (1) reduction in the levels of nicotinamide available for nicotinamide adenine dinucleotide synthesis; and (2) increased methylation of compounds such as tetrahydroisoquinolines and β-carbolines, which are potent Complex I inhibitors. Expression of NNMT is increased in Parkinson's disease which may ultimately lead to neurodegeneration via a reduction in Complex I activity (Parsons et al., 2003). A.C.Williams has proposed that elevated activity of NNMT may be responsible for dopaminergic toxicity of N-methylated pyridines (i.e. MPP^+) and for depletion of NAD^+ in the cells (Williams et al., 2005).

Apart from the pathways of NAD^+ synthesis *de novo*, there are some reactions for the regeneration of NAD^+ from molecules formed during its functioning and catabolism (reduced pyridine nucleotides (NADH, ADP-ribose, nicotinamide, $NAAD^+$). It should be noted that re-synthesis of NAD^+ from ADP-ribose and nicotinamide requires as many as four molecules of ATP, therefore being energetically unfavorable (Di Lisa & Ziegler, 2001). Regeneration of NAD^+ from NADH may be achieved through the activity of following enzymes and processes: 1) specific NADH flavin dehydrogenase acting in the respiratory chain; 2) transhydrogenase of the outer mitochondrial membrane; 3) specific NADH oxidases; 4) malate-aspartate shuttle. Regeneration of NAD^+ is very important not only for the economic using of cellular pool of pyridine nucleotides, but also for their effective intracellular redistribution at the appropriate moment under physiological and pathological conditions. Murine glial cells have been shown to synthesize NAD^+ from quinolinic acid, however, the pathway for NAD^+ regeneration from nicotinic acid is a preferred route for NAD^+ biosynthesis (Grant & Kapoor, 1998).

Among all the NAD^+-converting enzymes, poly(ADP-ribosyl) polymerase (PARP) and ADP-ribosyl cyclase attract the main attention in terms of neurodegenerative disorders (Kauppinen & Swanson, 2007). Poly(ADP-ribosyl) polymerase functions as DNA damage sensor and signaling molecule binding to single- and double-stranded DNA breaks. Upon binding to damaged DNA PARP forms homodimers and catalyzes the cleavage of NAD^+ into ADP-ribose and nicotinamide. ADP-ribose is then used to synthesize the branched polymer attached to nuclear (or mitochondrial) acceptor proteins. Variety of acceptor proteins has been described (histones, DNA repair enzymes, topoisomerases, transcription factors, DNA-dependent protein kinase, lamin B, p53), but the most efficient acceptor appears to be the enzyme itself (Ziegler, 2000).

There is a growing number of evidences on involvement of PARP and PARP-mediated depletion of intracellular NAD^+ in the acute and chronic injury of cells (ischemia/reperfusion, endothelial dysfunction, genotoxicity, inflammation, traumatic injury) (Oliver et al., 1999). In respect to the CNS, NAD^+ depletion and mitochondrial permeability transition were shown to be sequential and necessary steps in PARP-1 overactivation-dependent cell death in astrocytes (Alano et al., 2004). Increased poly(ADP-ribosylation) of nuclear proteins was demonstrated in neurons in Alzheimer's disease (Love et al., 1999). Intra-mitochondrial PARP contributes to NAD^+ depletion and cell death induced by oxidative stress in neurons (Du et al., 2003). Increased poly ADP-ribosylation of nuclear proteins in Alzheimer's disease has been detected, and double immunolabelling for poly(ADP-ribose) and markers of neuronal, astrocytic and microglial differentiation showed many of the cells containing poly(ADP-ribose) to be neurons, while few of the cells were astrocytes, and no poly(ADP-ribose) accumulation was found in microglia (Kauppinen & Swanson, 2007; Love, et al., 1999). Moreover, it was shown that β-amyloid affected cholinergic receptor-mediated signal transduction to PARP, probably, through free radical evoked inhibition of inositol-3-phosphate formation in the hippocampal cells (Adamczyk et al., 2005). Glutamate neurotransmission involving NMDA receptors and neuronal nitric oxide synthase activity in part mediates neuronal DNA strand breaks and PARP activation. These events are especially important for neurons since astrocytes able to maintain higher levels of NAD^+ comparing with neurons (Pieper et al., 2000), and much higher concentrations of oxidants are required for killing astrocytes (Ying et al., 2002). It should be taken into the consideration that excessive PARP activation leads to impairment of glycolysis in affected cells, thereby impaired glycolytic flux is involved into PARP-mediated neuronal and astroglial cell death. Since astrocyte-produced lactate is a major endogenous energy substrate used by neurons in brain, NAD^+ depletion caused by excessive PARP activation in neurons would result in alteration of lactate-pyruvate conversion thus affecting the efficacy of oxidative metabolism in neurons and astrocyte-neuronal lactate shuttle mechanism. In addition, neurological metabolic coupling implies subcellular compartmentation of pyruvate and monocarboxylate recycling through the plasma membrane of both neurons and glial cells, subcellular compartmentation of pyruvate allows neurons and astrocytes to select between glucose and lactate as alternative substrates depending of the concentrations and the operation of a redox switch (Cerdan et al., 2006). Pyruvate compartmentation results in effective transcellular coupling between the cytosolic NAD^+/NADH redox states of neuronal and glial cells, therefore, impairment of this mechanism due to PARP hyperactivation in neurons could directly affect restoring the basal redox state in astrocytes.

Another class of enzymes utilizing NAD^+ is represented by the CD38 family (EC 3.2.2.5, EC 3.2.2.6). Two ligands of CD38 - the substrate ligand NAD^+ acting either extracellularly or intracellularly, and the non-substrate ligand CD31 expressed in endothelial cells - have important functions in brain cells under (patho)physiological conditions (Higashida et al., 2001a; Higashida et al., 2007; Salmina et al., 2010a; Salmina et al., 2006b). CD38 possesses the capability to catalyze different reactions, such as the hydrolysis of NAD^+ and cADPR to ADP-ribose, and the cyclization of NAD^+ and nicotinamine guanine dinucleotide (NGD^+) to cADPR and cGDPR, respectively. The physiological meaning of the latter reaction is still unclear, but biological activity of cADPR is well defined in many cell types (Deaglio et al., 2008; Malavasi et al., 2008a). ADP-ribosyl cyclase attributable to CD38 was detected in the central nervous system where its activity and expression showed developmental changes. ADP-ribosyl cyclase synthesizes Ca^{2+} mobilizing messengers by cyclizing NAD^+ to produce cyclic ADP-ribose (cADPR) acting through activation/modulation of ryanodine receptor channels involving FKBP12.6. In addition, cADPR was also shown to affect some potassium currents and thereby could be involved in synaptic activity. In murine brain, CD38 was found in both neurons and glial cells, showed predominant intracellular location, and was enriched in neuronal perikarya. In human brain, CD38 immunoreactivity was demonstrated in neurons, astrocytes, and microglial cells. In rat astrocytes, ADP-ribosyl cyclase has been reported to have both intracellular and extracellular actions. Co-culture of astrocytes with neurons resulted in significantly increased expression of astrocytic CD38 both on the plasma membrane and cytosol, and this effect was attributed to neuron-released glutamate action on astrocytes (Bruzzone et al., 2004). It is known that astrocytic response to neuronal activity can be most readily detected by observing changes in the intracellular Ca^{2+} concentrations mediated via calcium flux trough the plasma membrane calcium channels or calcium release from intracellular stores. Subtype-specific coupling with ADP-ribosyl cyclase of various neurotransmitter receptors confirms the involvement of this enzyme in signal transduction in neuronal and glial cells. The expression of CD38 is regulated by various substances (cytokines, retinoic acid), while enzymatic activity of ADP-ribosyl cyclase/CD38 is controlled by the structure of the catalytic center, the integrity of the sulfhydryl cysteine residues in this center, the intracellular levels of ATP and NADH, intracellular localization of the enzyme (plasma membrane, mitochondrial membrane, nuclear membrane, and cytosol), conformational plasticity, ligands (NAD^+, CD31), and capacity to form dimers in a membrane for effective transport of reaction product.

In the cells of the CNS, ADP-ribosyl cyclase is expressed in different cell compartments (the nucleus, cytosol, and mitochondria), including the plasma membrane; however, the mechanisms that control translocation of the enzyme molecules, role of intracellular localization in the realization of enzymatic activity, and the mechanisms of directed transport of the enzyme to different cell compartments are unclear (Higashida et al., 2001; Salmina et al., 2008). Proposal exists that CD38 is a regulator of cellular NAD^+ levels under physiological conditions, while PARP is the key factor determining intracellular NAD^+ levels when significant DNA damage occurs (Ying et al., 2005).

A key role of CD38 in regulation of NAD^+ homeostasis in cells has been suggested (Aksoy et al., 2006). Thereby, CD38 may contribute to regulation of activity of SIRT proteins or TRPM (transient receptor potential) channels. SIRT1 promotes survival and stress tolerance in brain cells. SIRT expressed in neuronal and astroglial cells requires NAD^+ as an essential cofactor for their deacetylase activity, thus providing direct link between the metabolic and transcriptional response (Cohen et al., 2009; Kwon & Ott, 2008), while TRPM2 channels are expressed predominantly in neurons and microglia and are activated by cyclic ADP-ribose or by NAD^+ (Togashi et al., 2006).

It is known that astrocytic response to neuronal activity can be most readily detected by observing changes in the intracellular Ca^{2+} concentrations mediated via calcium flux through the plasma membrane calcium channels or calcium release from intracellular stores. Products of enzymatic activity of CD38 - cyclic ADP-ribose (cADPR) and nicotinic acid adenine dinucleotide phosphate ($NAADP^+$) - work as potent Ca^{2+} mobilizing second messengers acting at ryanodine receptors (Higashida, et al., 2001a). Immunocytochemical studies revealed association of altered Ca^{2+} regulation in astrocytes (i.e. calcineurin up-regulation) with their activation in aging or Alzheimer's disease models (Norris et al., 2005). Functional ryanodine receptors are required for astrocyte migration that is important component of regenerative process in the brain (Matyash et al., 2002). Therefore, expression and functional activity of CD38 in astrocytes and/or neurons, and ectocellular action of cADPR and $NAADP^+$ on astrocytes resulting in Ca^{2+} signaling (Heidemann et al., 2005; Pawlikowska et al., 1996) would have physiological and pathophysiological meaning as a mechanism of Ca^{2+} signaling involved in neuron-astroglia cell interactions. Alterations in ryanodine receptor binding and function are very early events in the pathogenesis of Alzheimer's disease (Kelliher et al., 1999) while Aβ increases ryanodine receptors expression and function in cortical neurons (Supnet et al., 2006). Taking into account importance of neuronal calcium mishandling in the development of Alzheimer's disease (Verkhratsky, et al., 1998), one can suggest involvement of cADPR-associated signaling pathways in observed ryanodine receptor dysfunction.

Figure 1 summarizes data on NAD^+-generating and NAD^+-converting pathways in mammalian cells.

3. Astroglial CD38 and Cx43 in neuron-glia metabolic coupling

Glial cells can communicate with each other by means of Ca^{2+} waves, and any perturbation of astrocytic intracellular concentration can propagate to other adjacent astrocytes through gap junction formed by connexins (Cx). Astroglial calcium signaling can be linked to synaptic transduction between neurons and neuronal-astroglial metabolic coupling (Allegrini et al., 2009). Cx43-formed gap junctions extensively couple neurons with glia (Nagy et al., 2004), and astrocytes represent the largest gap junction-coupled cellular network within the brain (Nakase & Naus, 2004). In the adult brain, Cx43 levels vary according to the developmental stage and brain region: Cx43 is expressed from early in development and further its expression increases.Cx43 is believed to be mediator of intercellular communication and operator between processes originating from a single astrocyte. In astrocytes, connexons are activated at metabolic inhibition, pro-inflammatory microenvironment, brain injury. Cx43 contributes to paracrine pathways in astroglial cells by regulating Ca^{2+} waves and uptake and release of glutamate, ATP, glucose, and glutathione (Giaume et al., 2010).

Astroglial cells express connexin-based gap junction channels and hemichannels that allow passage of molecules between the cytoplasm and extracellular cells or between the cells

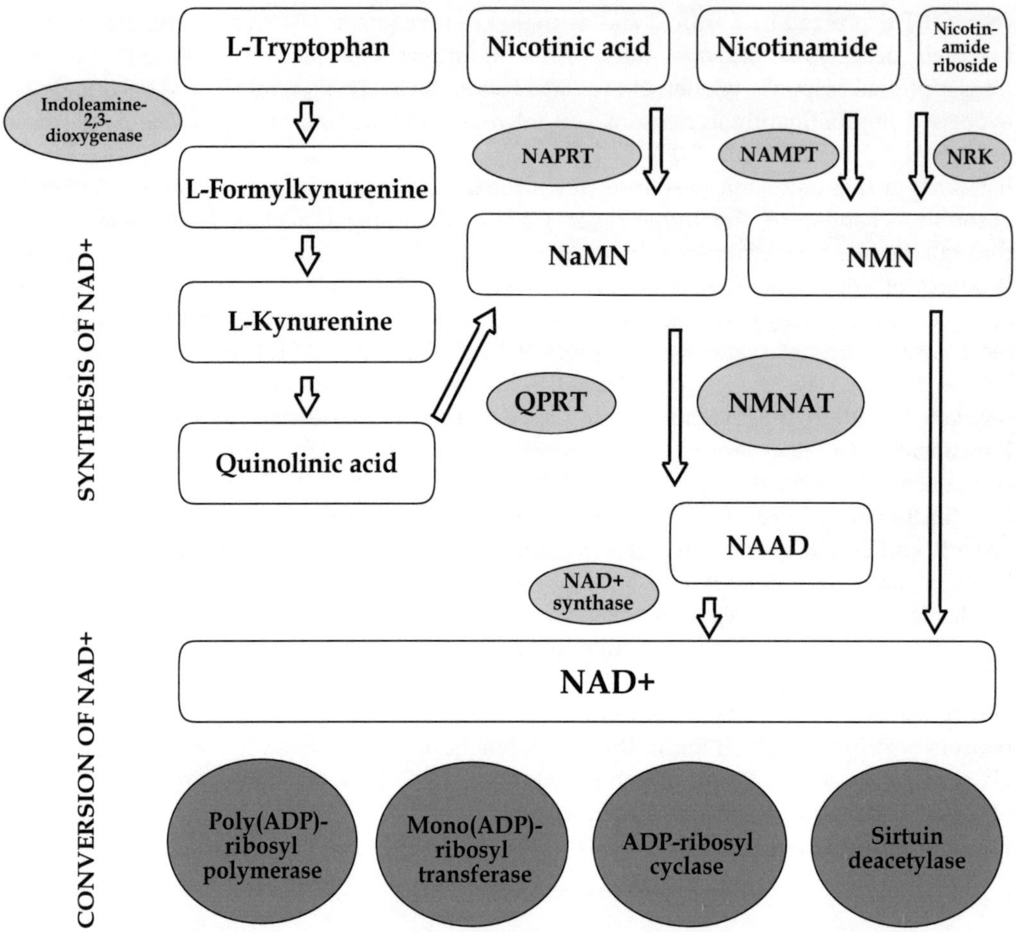

Fig. 1. Metabolism of NAD^+ in mammalian cells. Abbreviations used: NAPRT – nicotinic acid phosphoribosyltransferase, NAMPT – nicotinamide phosphoribosyltransferase, NRK – nicotinamide riboside kinase, NaMN – nicotinic acid mononucleotide, NMN – nicotinamide mononucleotide, QPRT – quinolinate phosphoribosyltransferase, NMNAT – nicotinamide mononucleotide adenylyltransferase, NAAD – nicotinic acid adenine dinucleotide, NAD^+ - nicotinamide dinucleotide

(Contreras et al., 2004). Synapse-glial interactions in the developing, adult and injured brain are very important for brain plasticity. Distinct phases of synapse development depend on assistance from glial cells (Pfrieger, 2010). Astrocytic hemichannels consisted of connexin 43 mediate release of glutamate and other amino acids (Ye et al., 2003). Gap junction channels allow the coordination of intrinsic or elicited metabolic and/or electrical responses of cells in a heterogenous population, and regulate poroliferative activity of astroglial cells. Astrocytes with a radial glia-like morphology in the subgranular zone of the dentate gyrus are considered as stem cells which give rise to neurons within different regions of the adult brain. Radial glia-like cells express GFAP, nestin, and Cx43. The latter contribute to controlling proliferation and differentiation of these cells since no other mechanisms (i.e. glutamatergic) have been detected in radial glia-like cells (Kunze, 2009).

Two primary hypotheses of gap junction coupling in the CNS are the following: (1) generalized coupling occurs between neurons and glia, with some connexins expressed in both neurons and glia, and (2) intercellular junctional coupling is restricted to specific coupling partners, with different connexins expressed in each cell type. The most important question is a role of connexon in mediating communication between different cell types in the brain (Rash et al., 2001). It is well-known that intercellular calcium signaling between different types of glial cells (astrocytes and oligodendocytes) is mediated by Cx43 (Parys et al., 2010). Several connexin proteins have been identified at gap junctions between neuronal and astroglial cells. Moreover, expression of Cx43 but at much lower levels comparing to astrocytes has been detected in oligodendrocytes, Schwann cells and neurons (Nagy, et al., 2004). However, astrocytes are still considered as connexin-dependent signaling cells (Saez, 2008). Expression of Cx43 is closely related to the role of astrocytes in coordinating the neuronal signals and local blood flow (neurovascular coupling).
In the CNS, expression and activity of Cx43 are modulated by cytokines, NO. Recently, novel protein interacting with Cx43 in astrocytes has been identified - brain-derived integrating factor-1 (BDIF-1) which is probably involved in regulating of astroglial activity (Ito et al., 2011). Pharmacological modulation of Cx43 can be achieved by various compounds (Dhein et al., 2002). T. Nakase et al. (Nakase & Naus, 2004) reported that the activation of astrocytes associated with an increase in the expression and activity of connexin 43 protects neurons from ischemia-induced damage. It should be noted that Cx43 can provide NAD^+ to the ectodomain of CD38. In fibroblasts, Cx43 hemichannels mediate release of NAD^+ to the extracellular medium, presumably allowing cytoplasmic NAD^+ to reach the active site of ADP-ribosyl cyclase/CD38 located at the extracellular part of plasma membrane (Franco et al., 2001). The same mechanism could work in astrocytes (Verderio et al., 2001) since glutamate-induced CD38 overexpression in astrocytes was observed in the model of neuronal-astroglial cell coupling. Functional cross-talk between Cx43 hemichannels and CD38 may be triggered by elevation of intracellular Ca^{2+} concentrations or by binding of a ligand to Cx43 or CD38. De Flora et al. (De Flora et al., 2004) suggested that extra phosphorylation of Cx43 induced by Ca^{2+} rise decreases the open-state probability of connexons, thereby downregulating NAD^+ transport across them and resulting in lower access of NAD^+ to the active site of CD38 and decreasing cADPR generation and limiting of Ca^{2+} levels inside the cell. Thus, autocrine and paracrine Ca^{2+} signaling is mediated by Cx43-CD38 system. Whether or not such system is operating in astrocytes in the context of neuronal-astroglial coupling remains to be elucidated. This mechanism is very important, because it helps to prevent NAD^+ loss from cells, depletion of intracellular NAD^+ due to elevated CD38 activity, and cADPR overproduction leading to calcium accumulation to toxic levels (Salmina et al., 2009a).
CD38 and Cx43 also may serve as transporters of nucleotides (NAD(H), cADPR, and $NAADP^+$) into the cell from the extracellular space (Billington, et al., 2008), thus contributing to maintaining NAD^+ homeostasis within the cell. NAD^+ itself can enter astrocytes via gap junction-mediated pathway (Ying, et al., 2005).
What are the possible roles for Cx43 hemichannes in neurodegenerative processes? Elevated expression of Cx43 in reactive astrocytes may reflect: 1) extensive buffering of neurotoxic substances by activated astroglial cells required for protecting the neurons from cell death (i.e. inhibition of gap junctions with octanol abolishes the ability of Aβ to enhance the velocity and extent of propagation of astroglial calcium waves (Orellana et al., 2009));

2) propagating Ca^{2+} waves between communicating astrocytes and/or individual processes of a single cell; 3) active proliferation and migration of Cx43-immunopositive progenitor cells to the site of neurodegeneration; 4) activation of autocrine and paracrine signaling in astrocytes and adjacent neurons; 5) action of stimuli (prooxidant and proinflammatory) able to increase Cx43 expression. In neurodegenerative diseases and ischemia, reactive astrocytes have increased levels of Cx43, and changes in Cx43 expression are dependent on the proximity of the reactive astrocytes to the focus of neurodegeneration. In the site of injury, reactive astrocytes can lose their non-overlapping domains (Giaume, et al., 2010).

Functional hemichannels that have a role in glutamate homeostasis may significantly contribute to astrocyte-mediated regulation of neuronal activity. It is interesting that in the Alzheimer's type of neurodegeneration, elevated expression of Cx43 has been detected at β-amyloid plaques due to reactive astrogliosis (Mei et al., 2010). It was suggested that in Alzheimer's disease, increased Cx43 expression might represent an attempt to maintain tissue homeostasis by augmented intercellular communication via gap junction formation between astrocytic processes that invest senile plaques. In addition, one can propose that elevated expression of Cx43 hemichannels could result in massive release of glutamate from astrocytes into the extracellular space resulting in excitotoxic injury of neurons. Connexin 43 regulates astrocytic migration and proliferation in response to injury. Reactive astrocytes display up-regulation of the gap junction protein Cx43, and astroglial cells with depleted expression of Cx43 show diminished ability to migrate and to proliferate in the wound area of the brain (Homkajorn et al., 2010). Drebrin as an actin binding protein whose level is greatly decreased in brains of Alzheimer's patients was found to be a binding partner of the Cx43 COOH-terminal domain in astrocytes. In experimental model, depletion of drebrin in cells results in impaired cell-cell coupling, internalization of gap junctions, and targeting of Cx43 to a degradative pathway (Butkevich et al., 2004)]. It was suggested that increased Cx43 expression in a close vicinity to amyloid plaques might represent aberrant induction of Cx43 expression stimulated by excessive degradative pathway. In support of this hypothesis, increased expression of Cx43 was found to be induced by β-amyloid precursor protein (Hallaq & Killick, 2006)], thus suggesting direct effect of amyloid deposites on the mechanism of glutamate release from astroglial cells and neuron-astrocyte communication.

Recently, changes in expression and activity of Cx43 have been registered in rotenone-induced model of Parkinson's disease: enhancement of Cx43 protein levels in cells treated with rotenone (mitochondrial complex I inhibitor) resulted in increased efficacy of gap junctional intercellular communication (Kawasaki et al., 2009). However, some authors registered inhibited expression of astrocytic Cx43 and gap junction permeability in astrocytes in rotenone models of Parkinson's disease. Moreover, rotenone-induced dysfunction of astrocytic Cx43 can be reversed by opening mitochondrial ATP-sensitive potassium channels (iptakalim and diazoxide) resulting in prevention of astrocyte apoptosis (Zhang et al., 2010). Thus, we believe that Cx43-CD38 functional coupling in astrocytes significantly contribute to controlling energy homeostasis in astroglial and neuronal cells.

Opening of the mitochondrial permeability transition pore is known to play a role in cell death. Its opening has been shown to cause activation of NAD^+ glycohydrolase located in the outer mitochondrial membrane following by NAD^+ hydrolysis in cardiomyocytes at postischemic reperfusion (Di Lisa et al., 2001). Since mitochondrial NAD^+ glycohydrolase has been identified as ADP-ribosyl cyclase (Ziegler et al., 1997), NAD^+ released from mitochondrial matrix could be transformed into cADPR which promoting Ca^{2+} release from intracellular stores. Thereby, amplification of initial rise in intracellular Ca^{2+} levels might be important in cell damage. It was reported that mitochondrial dysfucntion leads to postponed changes in CD38 expression (Mills et al., 1999). Thus, accumulating data suggest that ADP-ribosyl cyclase may affect mitochondrial functioning through various mechanisms.

Mitochondrial localization of Cx43 has been shown in cardiomyocytes, and the role for Cx43 as regulator of mitochondrial potassium uptake (Miro-Casas et al., 2009) or mitochondrial respiration (Boengler et al., 2008a) has been suggested. Stimulatory effect of Cx43 on mitochondrial KATP channels resulting in cytoprotectiion has been shown in cardiomyocytes (Rottlaender et al., 2010). It is intriguing to speculate that mitochondrial Cx43 contributes to regulation of respiration and potassium uptake in astroglial cells, thus providing adaptation of mitochondrial activity to altered microenvironment in activated astrocytes in the site of brain injury. It was proposed that Cx43 may directly regulate respiratory chain complex I activity and mitochondrial oxygen consumption: decrease in mitochondrial Cx43 levels reduced complex I activity (Boengler et al., 2008b).

Mitochondrial localization of CD38 is well documented. I. Balan et al. (Balan et al., 2010) detected NAD^+- glycohydrolase activity in isolated synaptosomes and also in intact brain mitochondria, confirming localization of CD38 also in outer mitochondrial membranes. Interestingly, the NAD^+- glycohydrolase activity appeared to be much higher in nonsynaptic mitochondria compared with mitochondria isolated from synaptosomes. Taken together, these data suggest that NAD^+ depletion can occur more rapidly in astrocytes following ischemic insult, compromising the ability of astrocytes to support neuronal functions. Interestingly, the NAD^+ catabolic activity is higher in brain regions that are vulnerable to ischemic insult, furthermore, the CD38 NAD^+ glycohydrolase activity is significantly increased in postischemic tissue, and the immunohistochemistry shows overexpression of this enzyme preferentially in neuroglial cells (Kristian et al., 2011; Salmina, et al., 2008; Salmina, et al., 2009a). Activation of CD38 can lead to rapid and almost complete tissue NAD^+ depletion (Balan, et al., 2010). A prolonged MPT results not only in dissipation of the mitochondrial electrochemical hydrogen ion gradient and swelling of mitochondria but also depletion of pyridine nucleotides from the matrix (Di Lisa & Ziegler, 2001), however, significant loss of matrix pyridine nucleotides can lead to inhibition of mitochondrial respiration but without irreversible damage to the respiratory complexes or mitochondrial membranes (Kristian, et al., 2011). It was proposed, that once the cellular CD38 enzymatic pool is saturated, cytosolic NAD^+ concentrations rise to a level that permits efflux into extracellular space where NAD^+ becomes to be the substrate for surface-expressed CD38 acting as autocrine or paracrine regulator of Ca^{2+} signaling.

Neurodegeneration is associated with altered energy metabolism in the brain; accumulation of glycolytic enzymes, such as enolase and glyceraldehyde 3-phosphate dehydrogenase, decrease in expression of voltage-dependent anion-selective channel protein-1 (VDAC-1), and decrease in expression of subunits of multiprotein enzyme complex NADH:ubiquinone oxidoreductase (complex I of the mitochondrial electron transport chain) have been registered in Alzheimer's disease (Butterfield et al., 2003)]. It is well known that astrocytes play important roles in supporting energy production in neurons. According to astrocyte-neuron lactate shuttle hypothesis, lactate is produced in an activity-dependent and glutamate-mediated manner by astrocytes and is then transferred to and used by active neurons (Pellerin et al., 1998). Neuronal activation results in uptake of glutamate by astrocytes leading to activation of glutamine synthetase and Na^+-K^+-ATPase, followed by activation of anaerobic glycolysis in astrocytes, and release of lactate supporting the activity-related energy required for neurons (Magistretti, 2000)]. In general, astrocytes metabolize glucose mainly to lactate and release it into the extracellular medium, while neurons appear to have a kinetic preference for oxidizing lactate imported from the external medium over pyruvate/lactate produced in neurons by glycolysis (Itoh et al., 2003). However, neurons die more intensively than astrocytes even though the apparent dysfunction takes place in astrocytes. Glycolysis is high in astrocytes, so they need a way to maintain the adequate levels of NAD^+. Probably, astrocytes can sustain themselves adequately with glycolytic metabolism, not significantly affected by mitochondrial dysfunction, thereby being more resistant to oxidative stress and NAD^+ depletion.

4. CD38 expression in acute and chronic neurodegeneration

Very few data are available on CD38 expression in neurodegeneration. In different experimental models of acute and chronic neurodegeneration in rats (focal brain ischemia, rotenone model of Parkinson's disease, and perinatal hypoxic-ischemic brain injury), we found elevated expression of CD38 in neurons and astroglial cells in the acute period of brain injury (Salmina, et al., 2008; Salmina, et al., 2009a; Salmina et al., 2006a).

In the model of perinatal hypoxic-ischemic brain damage, we found that changes in CD38 expression and ADP-ribosyl cyclase activity in neuronal and glial cells attribute to alterations in intracellular NAD^+ level as well as to susceptibility of the cells to the action of apoptogenic stimuli; acute period of perinatal hypoxic/ischemic brain injury is characterized by reactive astrogliosis and elevation of CD38 expression, changes in CD38 and Cx43 expression in astrocytes serving as markers of neuron-glial interactions in perinatal CNS injury; ADP-ribosyl cyclase activity in neurons in response to stimulation of NMDA is changed after perinatal hypoxic-ischemic brain injury. It has been demonstrated that, in the immature brain, the impairment of intracellular calcium homeostasis is the leading mechanism of perinatal damage to both neuronal and glial cells (Vannucci et al., 2001). Based on our data, we can conclude that the mechanisms of maintenance of intracellular calcium homeostasis, which are under the control of ADP-ribosyl cyclase and Cx43, play a special role in responses of neurons and glia to hypoxic–ischemic damage.

We demonstrated that most of the cells that expressed Cx43 were CD38-immunopositive in acute neurodegeneration. Interestingly, in the 10-day-old rats subjected to cerebral damage, the number of Cx43 and CD38 coexpressing cells was several times higher as compared to GFAP and CD38 coexpressing cells, whereas the fractions of cells that expressed both GFAP and CD38 were similar in the control and experimental groups. These data suggest that other types of Cx43-containing cells, such as microglia, substantially contributed to the total elevation in CD38 expression after perinatal brain damage. Taking into account the data on the functional coupling of CD38 ADP-ribosyl cyclase activity and connexin 43, we studied the effects of a connexin blocker, glycyrrhetinic acid (GRA), on ADP-ribosyl cyclase activity in astrocytes isolated from brain tissue of control and experimental animals. We found that a 30-minute incubation of astrocytes with 5μM GRA resulted in decrease in ADP-rybosyl cyclase activity in these cells (Salmina, et al., 2009a).

In the model of focal brain ischemia in adult animals, we confirmed that CD38 could be considered as a marker of neuron-glia interactions disturbances caused by acute ischemic injury, and that modulation of ADP-ribosyl cyclase/CD38 expression and activity in the brain significantly improved clinical manifestations of neurological dysfunction associated with ischemia-induced neurodegeneration (Salmina, et al., 2006a).

In patients with ischemic stroke, elevated expression of CD38 in peripheral blood leukocytes corresponds to formation of membrane-derived microparticles and progression of endothelial dysfunction due to CD38-CD31 interactions (Inzhutova et al., 2008; Salmina et al., 2010b). It is well known that astrocytes play important role in the formation, extent and configuration of the junctional complexes in the brain endothelium in a manner that astrocyte-induced enhanced tight junction communication is associated with the reduction of gap junctions. A major function of the neurovascular unit is to regulate the transport and diffusion properties of brain capillary endothelial cells that compose the brain-blood barrier (Banerjee & Bhat, 2007). Astrocytes exhibit anatomic relationships with cerebral arterioles and neurons. In the brain parenchyma, the extensive ensheatment of cerebral arterioles by astrocytic end-feet far exceeds any direct neural contacts with those perfusion-regulating microvessels. That unique arrangement permits astrocytes to transduce signals arising from activated neurons and to transmit that information to the cerebral microcirculation (Xu et al., 2008).

Coupling of NMDA receptors to ADP-ribosyl cyclase/CD38 in neuronal and glial cells, involvement of CD38 in neuronal-glial (Higashida et al., 2007a; Salmina, et al., 2009a) and leukocyte-endothelial interactions (Deaglio, et al., 2008; Inzhutova, et al., 2008; Malavasi et al., 2008) suggest new approach to treat endothelial dysfunction caused by various stimuli, i.e. by homocysteine (Boldyrev, 2010) in neurodegenerative processes.

As we mentioned above, in acute neurodegeneration, $CD38^+$-expressing cells were predominantly represented by $GFAP^+/Cx43^+$ cells of astroglial origin. We found that in neurons, elevated CD38 expression resulted in intracellular NAD^+ depletion and cell death, while in astrocytes high levels of CD38 expression relate to increased resistance to the action of apoptogenic stimuli, development of reactive gliosis, and changes in their glycolytic activity. Mitochondrial ADP-ribosyl cyclase activity was mainly induced by ischemic stimuli. Our data well fit the previous observations that intracellular NAD^+ levels regulate astroglial response to neuronal activation, NAD^+ released from astrocytes regulate apoptosis of neurons in postischemic period, and astrocytes are more resistant to hypoxia than neurons.

In the developing brain, direct correlation between the CD38 expression and apoptosis development in the given cell populations has been registered. We found stimulating effects of agonists of mGluRI, mGluRIII, suppressive effects of agonists of NMDAR on CD38 activity in premature injured brain cells. However, in the adult brain, reverse correlation between CD38 expression and apoptosis progression was observed. Under the pathophysiological conditions, development of cell death and ability of brain cells to maintain the levels of intracellular NAD^+ are determined by hypoxia/ischemia-induced disturbance in the dynamics of ADP-ribosyl cyclase activity in the brain cells. These data are in agreement with our report on the contribution of CD38 overexpression to development of plasma membrane blebbing in neuroblastoma x glioma NG108-15 hybrid cells (Egorova et al., 2000).

In the experimental model of Parkinson's disease, we found that loss of dopaminergic neurons via apoptosis was associated with elevation of expression and activity of ADP-ribosyl cyclase/CD38 in remaining tyrosine hydroxylase-immunopositive cells. Immunochemical studies with anti-CD38 antibodies indicated accumulation of CD38 antigen in the neurofibrillary tangles that occur in neuronal perikarya and proximal dendrites in Alzheimer's disease (Otsuka et al., 1994). Literature data suggest that in Alzheimer's disease, accumulation of CD38 antigen in the neurofibrillary tangles, an association of altered Ca^{2+} regulation in astrocytes, alterations in ryanodine receptors binding and functions are detectable.

Dramatic rise in CD38 messenger RNA levels in IL-1β-activated astrocytes was reported in HIV-associated neurodegeneration and dementia: in astrocytes, pre-treatment with the cADPR-specific antagonist 8-Br-cADPR and CD38 siRNA transfection returned elevated $[Ca^{2+}]_i$ to baseline, thus confirming a CD38-cADPR specific response. These data have broader implications in other inflammatory diseases involving astrocyte activation and CD38 dysregulation (Banerjee et al., 2008).

We suggest that possible causes of elevation of CD38 expression in brain cells are the following: 1) changes in NAD^+ bioavailability (release from mitochondria into cytosol, cell death, connexin Cx43 activation); 2) redistribution of the enzyme in the cells; 3) cytokine-dependent (IL, TNF) changes in expression of gene encoding for CD38 in the sites of brain injury of neurodegeneration; 4) action of neuro- and gliotransmitters. Since CD38 expression in astrocytes is stimulated by glutamate release from neurons, we can suggest that CD38 is a marker of altered neuron-astrocyte interactions under the conditions of excitotoxic insult. Also, since mitochondrial complex I dysfunction causes elevation of CD38 expression, we suggest that CD38 is a marker of mitochondrial dysfunction in the context of neuron-glia metabolic coupling. Activity of Cx43 prevents NAD^+ depletion in CD38-overexpressing astrocytes and provides enough NAD^+ for glycolysis, thus making astrocytes more resistant to the action of stimuli causing neurodegeneration.

Therefore, we propose that expression of CD38 in neuronal and glial cells: 1) is regulated under (patho)physiological conditions; 2) is associated with various signal transduction pathways (i.e. GluR in neurons and Cx43 in astrocytes) whose activity is important for molecular pathogenesis of neurodegeneration; 3) reflects - specifically or non-specifically - mitochondrial dysfunction; 4) could be considered as a target for pharmacological correction of neurodegeneration. Deciphering of CD38-associated molecules/events in neuronal and glial populations would give us new biomarkers for diagnostics of neurodegeneration, while pharmacological manipulation of ADP-ribosyl cyclase activity in brain cells would provide new therapeutic opportunities for the treatment of neurodegenerative disorders.

5. Modulation of NAD^+ metabolism in glial cells as therapeutic approach in neurodegeneration

Manipulating the neuron-glial cell interactions associated with changes in NAD^+ levels represent one of the promising approaches to treatment of Alzheimer's disease (Braidy et al., 2008; Henricksen & Federoff, 2004). Pharmacological manipulation may be targeted to the modulation of intracellular NAD^+ metabolism with substances affecting activity of NAD^+-synthesizing and NAD^+-converting enzymes, modulators of NAD^+-dependent enzymes (i.e. sirtuins, glycolytic enzymes), regulators of tryptophan kynurenine metabolism, substrates of NAD^+ synthetic pathways, ligands and regulators of CD38 expression and activity, modulators of NAD^+ and cyclic ADP-ribose transport across the membrane (i.e. Cx43).

Metabolism of NAD^+ could be efficiently regulated by inhibitors of mono(ADP-ribosyl) transferase and poly-ADP-ribosyl polymerase activities. Pharmacological interventions aimed at inhibiting PARP activity have been shown to be efficient in prevention of PARP-mediated death of neurons and astrocytes (Ying, et al., 2002). Several studies have suggested the therapeutic potential of sirtuins (NAD^+-dependent histone deacetylases consuming NAD^+) for Alzheimer's disease (Anekonda & Reddy, 2006). Inhibitors of kynurenine 3-hydroxylase can reduce the production of neurotoxic metabolites (Khan et al., 2007). It was reported that decreases in β-amyloid content in the brain can be achieved by governing cellular sirtuin activity (Qin et al., 2006). Improvement of cognitive functions was detected after treatment with oral stabilized NADH (Demarin et al., 2004), probably, due to ability of NADH to enter into astrocyets and block PARP-mediated astrocyte death (Zhu et al., 2005). However, efficacy of NADH to correction of cognitive dysfunction in dementia remains to be ambiguos (Rainer et al., 2000). Recently, CD38 was suggested as a new target for dementias including Alzheimer's disease (Chini et al., 2007). It is interesting enough that NAD^+ (and, probably, NADH) can be transported across the plasma membranes of astrocytes through connexin hemichannels (Verderio, et al., 2001) or purinergic receptors (Lu et al., 2007), thus suggesting new approach to manipulating its intracellular concentrations and metabolism.

Overexpression of NMNAT results in suppression of Wallerian degeneration in neurons, however, in Cd38-/- cells with higher levels of intracellular NAD^+ no difference in the axon degeneration patterns were registered. In general, increased NAD^+ synthesis is responsible for axonal protection (Yan et al., 2010). In vitro NNMT expression significantly decreased cell death which correlated with increased intracellular ATP content, ATP: ADP ratio, Complex I activity and a reduction in the degradation of the NDUFS3 subunit of Complex I. These effects were replicated by incubation of cells with 1-methylnicotinamide. In the context of pathogenesis of Parkinson's disease, it is important that both NNMT expression and 1-methylnicotinamide protected SH-SY5Y cells from the toxicity of the Complex I inhibitors MPP^+ and rotenone by reversing their effects upon ATP synthesis, ATP:ADP ratio, Complex I activity and the NDUFS3 subunit (Parsons et al., 2011). Overexpression of SIRT1 or its activation in neuronal and glial cells with resveratrol has been shown to protect the brain tissue from degeneration in Alzheimer's disease and Huntington's disease, and calorie restriction able to modulate SIRT activity is neuroprotective against Parkinson's disease and Alzheimer's disease (Outeiro et al., 2008). Modulation of TRPM channels which are abundantly expressed in the brain has neuroprotective activity in Parkinson's disease and Alzheimer's disease (Yamamoto et al., 2007). Protection of neurons from glutamate and β-amyloid toxicity was achieved by preloading neurons with creatine (Brewer & Wallimann, 2000) or by pyruvate (Massieu et al., 2001). The latter as well as another tricarboxilic acid cycle substrate - α-ketoglutarate - were also potent in preventing death of neurons and astrocytes caused by intracellular NAD^+ depletion (Ying, et al., 2002).

Experimental pharmacological intervention in the cADPR-signaling pathway are usually restricted to two targets, the cADPR-binding protein and the ADP-ribosyl cyclase (Guse, 2000). The agents used for such properties are: a) cADP-ribose and its analogues; b) modulators of ryanodine receptors activity such as caffeine, ryanodine, procaine, ruthenium red; c) ligands of FKBP. The usefulness of cADP-ribose as a pharmacological tool is limited by its rapid hydrolysis, therefore various cADPR analogues have been synthesized.

Among all inhibitors of NAD^+-consuming enzymes, nicotinamide attracts the biggest interest. Nicotinamide has several cellular functions in CNS and serves as an anxiolytic, increases brain choline concentrations and is endogenous ligand of benzodiazepine receptors (Maiese & Chong, 2003). Neuroprotective action of nicotinamide has been reported in neurons at oxidative stress even it may be attributed to changes in glycolysis, apoptotic machinery, MAP kinase activity etc. rather than inhibition of NAD^+

glycohydrolases. Age-dependent susceptibility of glial cells to the action of nicotinamide analogs has been reported (Krum, 1995). 6-aminonicotinamide as niacin antagonist produces neurotoxic activity by inducing inflammatory response of astroglial and microglial cells (Penkowa et al., 2003). But using of inhibitors of NAD^+ hydrolysis may have even unfavorable results: partial inhibition of poly-ADP-ribosylation with 5-iodo-6-amino-1,2-benzopyrone preserves NAD^+ and improves functional outcome after traumatic brain injury, whereas more complete inhibition impairs spatial memory acquisition independent of injury (Satchell et al., 2003). Therefore, cytoprotection with inhibitors of NAD^+-consuming enzymes might be concentration specific. We found that nicotinamide (500 mg/kg) reduced expression of CD38 in the brain cortex in the model of ischemia-induced acute neurodegeneration in adult rats in vivo and potentiate neurological dysfunction caused by ischemia, thereby further confirming ambiguity of nicotinamide action on neuronal and glial cells.

Retinoic acid (RA) is a potent inducer of CD38 in peripheral blood cells, and recently it was suggested that this compound can be used to 'rescue' cells exhibiting low CD38 synthesis and hence might be a novel therapeutic strategy in treatment of autism associated with impaired CD38 expression in neurosecretory cells (Ebstein et al., 2011). Cultured astrocytes express the key enzyme mRNAs of retinoic acid biosynthesis and actively produce retinoic acid acting at RA receptors (RAR). Synthesis of retinoic acid in astrocytes is provided by retinal dehydrogenase and alcohol dehydrogenase (Wagner et al., 2002). It was shown that blockage of retinoic acid signaling by the pan-RAR antagonist prevented glia-induced neuron formation by noncommitted stem cells, thus suggesting a role for retinoic acid in astroglia-induced neuronal differentiation (Kornyei et al., 2007). Retinoids control expression of wide spectrum of genes in neuronal and glial cells (Lane & Bailey, 2005).

We tested effect of all-trans retinoic acid in vivo (20 mg/kg with ethanol to suppress endogenous synthesis of retinoic acid) in rats with experimental model of perinatal ischemic-hypoxic acute neurodegeneration. We found that suppression of endogenous synthesis of retinoic acid with ethanol reduced expression of CD38 in the cortex, while retinoic acid itself partially restored the level of CD38 (Salmina et al., 2009b).

Retinoid and retinoid-associated signaling plays an essential role in normal neurodevelopment and appears to remain active in the adult CNS. Molecular factors involved in RA-mediated responses become up-regulated in the adult CNS as a consequence of injury or degeneration. Our data and recent findings of R. Ebstein et al. (Ebstein, et al., 2011) suggest that intervention that modulates RA-regulated CD38 may have therapeutic potential in CNS disorders. It is interesting that a prolonged regime of vitamin A deprivation in adult rats has been shown to cause a deposition of β-amyloid peptide in the forebrain, RA could regulate the expression of the tau protein, and in particular the level of phosphorylated forms of tau, as suggested by *in vitro* observations, vitamin A, as well as β-carotene and coenzyme Q10, have also been shown to dose-dependently inhibit the formation of α-synuclein fibrils *in vitro,* RA reduces the effect of β-amyloid, and thus inhibits the neurotoxic effect of activated microglia, by suppressing the production of these cytotoxic molecules (Malaspina & Michael Titus, 2008). Retinoid receptors are involved in the regulation of brain functions, and retinoic acid signaling defects may contribute to pathologies such as Parkinson's disease (Krezel et al., 1998). Whether or not these events are associated with NAD^+-converting activity of CD38 in neuronal and astroglial cells remains to be elucidated.

6. Concluding remarks and outstanding questions for further investigation

So far, several hypotheses have been suggested to explain pathogenesis of acute and chronic neurodegenration. Almost all of the proposed mechanisms include processes considered as gliopathy (Maragakis & Rothstein, 2006; Verkhratsky, 2010). Different molecules mark gliopathological changes, and CD38 expressed in astroglial cells should be considered as one of the markers of neuron-astrocyte metabolic coupling. Neuron-glia communication is responsible for establishment of vicious circles in the pathogenesis of neurodegeneration, therefore deciphering new molecular mechanisms of intercellular communication will provide us with new diagnostic and therapeutic strategies. To achieve this goal in the context of NAD^+-controlled neuronal-astroglial coupling, the following questions should be addressed:

1. Which glial- and neuronal-derived factors can affect NAD^+ metabolism in acute and chronic neurodegeneration? What is an integrative scheme for NAD^+ homeostatic mechanisms in neurons and astrocytes?
2. What is the role for CD38-Cx43 interactions in initiation and progression of mitochondrial dysfunction in neurodegeneration?
3. Which molecular mechanisms coupled to NAD^+ homeostasis in brain cells are involved in axonal degeneration and neuronal repair?
4. Which new biomarkers could be developed for early diagnostics of astroglial dysfunction in neurodegeneration? Which molecular targets in neurons and glial cells could be efficiently used for the appropriate treatment of neurodegeneration?

7. References

Adamczyk, A., Jesko, H. & Strosznajder, R.P. (2005) Alzheimer's disease related peptides affected cholinergic receptor mediated poly(ADP-ribose) polymerase activity in the hippocampus. *Folia Neuropathologica*. Vol. 43, No. 3, pp. 139-142

Aksoy, P., White, T.A., Thompson, M. & Chini, E.N. (2006) Regulation of intracellular levels of NAD: a novel role for CD38. *Biochemical and biophysical research communications*. Vol. 345, No. 4, pp. 1386-1392, ISSN 0006-291X

Alano, C.C., Ying, W. & Swanson, R.A. (2004) Poly(ADP-ribose) Polymerase-1-mediated Cell Death in Astrocytes Requires NAD^+ Depletion and Mitochondrial Permeability Transition. *J. Biol. Chem.* Vol. 279, No. 18, pp. 18895-18902

Allegrini, P., Fronzoni, L. & Pirino, D. (2009) The influence of the astrocyte field on neuronal dynamics and synchronization. *Journal of biological physics*. Vol. 35, No. 4, pp. 413-423, ISSN 0092-0606

Anekonda, T.S. & Reddy, P.H. (2006) Neuronal protection by sirtuins in Alzheimer's disease. *J Neurochem*. Vol. 96, pp. 305-313

Balan, I.S., Fiskum, G. & Kristian, T. (2010) Visualization and quantification of NAD (H) in brain sections by a novel histo-enzymatic nitrotetrazolium blue staining technique. *Brain Research*. Vol. 1316, pp. 112-119, ISSN 0006-8993

Bambrick, L., Kristian, T. & Fiskum, G. (2004) Astrocyte mitochondrial mechanisms of ischemic brain injury and neuroprotection. *Neurochemical research*. Vol. 29, No. 3, pp. 601-608, ISSN 0364-3190

Banerjee, S. & Bhat, M.A. Neuron-glial interactions in blood-brain barrier formation [Book Section] // Annual Review of Neuroscience, 2007: Vol. 30.

Banerjee, S., Walseth, T.F., Borgmann, K., Wu, L., Bidasee, K.R., Kannan, M.S. & Ghorpade, A. (2008) CD38/cyclic ADP-ribose regulates astrocyte calcium signaling: implications for neuroinflammation and HIV-1-associated dementia. *Journal of Neuroimmune Pharmacology*. Vol. 3, No. 3, pp. 154-164, ISSN 1557-1890

Barres, B.A. (2008) The mystery and magic of glia: a perspective on their roles in health and disease. *Neuron*. Vol. 60, No. 3, pp. 430-440, ISSN 0896-6273

Barrientos, S.A., Martinez, N.W., Yoo, S., Jara, J.S., Zamorano, S., Hetz, C., Twiss, J.L. & Alvarez, J. (2011) Axonal degeneration is mediated by the mitochondrial permeability transition pore. *The Journal of Neuroscience*. Vol. 31, No. 3, pp. 966-978, ISSN 0270-6474

Billington, R.A., Travelli, C., Ercolano, E., Galli, U., Roman, C.B., Grolla, A.A., Canonico, P.L., Condorelli, F. & Genazzani, A.A. (2008) Characterization of NAD Uptake in Mammalian Cells. *Journal of Biological Chemistry*. Vol. 283, No. 10, pp. 6367-6374

Boengler, K., Stahlhofen, S., Rohrbach, S., Ruiz-Meana, M., Garcia-Dorado, D., Heusch, G. & Shultz, R. (2008a) Connexin 43 regulates respiratory chain complex I activity and mitochondrial oxygen consumption. *European Hearty Journal*. Vol. 29 Suppl, pp. 797-798

Boengler, K., Stahlhofen, S., Ruiz-Meana, M., Miro-Casas, E., Garcia-Dorado, D., Heusch, G. & Schulz, R. (2008b) Orientation of Connexin 43 in the Inner Mitochondrial Membrane and its Role in Respiration. *Circulation*. Vol. 118, No. 18 Supplement, pp. S_354

Boldyrev, A. (2010) Molecular mechanisms of homocysteine toxicity and possible protection against hyperhomocysteinemia. *Recent Advances on Nutrition and the Prevention of Alzheimer's Disease*. pp. 127-143, ISSN 978-81-7895-470-7

Bolton, M.M.L. & Eroglu, C. (2009) Look who is weaving the neural web: glial control of synapse formation. *Current Opinion in Neurobiology*. Vol. 19, No. 5, pp. 491-497, ISSN 0959-4388

Braidy, N., Guillemin, G. & Grant, R. (2008) Promotion of cellular NAD($^+$) anabolism: therapeutic potential for oxidative stress in ageing and Alzheimer's disease. *Neurotox Res* Vol. 13, No. 3-4, pp. 173-184

Brewer, G.J. & Wallimann, T.W. (2000) Protective effect of the energy precursor creatine against toxicity of glutamate and b-amyloid in rat hippocampal neurons. *J Neurochem*. Vol. 74, pp. 1968-1978

Bruzzone, S., Verderio, C., Schenk, U., Fedele, E., Zocchi, E., Matteoli, M. & De Flora, A. (2004) Glutamate-mediated overexpression of CD38 in astrocytes cultured with neurones. *Journal of Neurochemistry*. Vol. 89, No. 1, pp. 264-272

Buffo, A., Rite, I., Tripathi, P., Lepier, A., Colak, D., Horn, A.P., Mori, T. & G tz, M. (2008) Origin and progeny of reactive gliosis: A source of multipotent cells in the injured brain. *Proceedings of the National Academy of Sciences*. Vol. 105, No. 9, pp. 3581-3586, ISSN 0027-8424

Butkevich, E., Hьlsmann, S., Wenzel, D., Shirao, T., Duden, R. & Majoul, I. (2004) Drebrin Is a Novel Connexin-43 Binding Partner that Links Gap Junctions to the Submembrane Cytoskeleton. *Current Biology*. Vol. 14, No. 8, pp. 650-658

Butterfield, D.A., Boyd-Kimball, D. & Castegna, A. (2003) Proteomics in Alzheimer's disease: insights into potential mechanisms of neurodegeneration. *Journal of Neurochemistry*. Vol. 86, No. 6, pp. 1313-1327

Cerdan, S., Rodrigues, T.B., Sierra, A., Benito, M., Fonseca, L.L., Fonseca, C.P. & GarcHa-MartHn, M.L. (2006) The redox switch/redox coupling hypothesis. *Neurochemistry International*. Vol. 48, No. 6-7, pp. 523-530

Chini, E.N., Barbosa, M.T.P. & Soares, S.M. (2007) CD38 as a target for obesity, metabolic syndrome related disorders, and dementia (including Alzheimer's disease). www.mayoclinictechnology.com/tc/therapeutics/2007-187-1462.html,

Cohen, D.E., Supinski, A.M., Bonkowski, M.S., Donmez, G. & Guarente, L.P. (2009) Neuronal SIRT1 regulates endocrine and behavioral responses to calorie restriction. *Genes & development*. Vol. 23, No. 24, pp. 2812-2817, ISSN 0890-9369

Contreras, J.E., Sanchez, H.A., Veliz, L.P., Bukauskas, F.F., Bennett, M.V.L. & Saez, J.C. (2004) Role of connexin-based gap junction channels and hemichannels in ischemia-induced cell death in nervous tissue. *Brain Research Reviews*. Vol. 47, No. 1-3, pp. 290-303

De Flora, A., Zocchi, E., Guida, L., Franco, L. & Bruzzone, S. (2004) Autocrine and Paracrine Calcium Signaling by the CD38/NAD^+/Cyclic ADP Ribose System. *Annals of the New York Academy of Sciences*. Vol. 1028, No. 1, pp. 176-191, ISSN 1749-6632

Deaglio, S., Aydin, S., Vaisitti, T., Bergui, L. & Malavasi, F. (2008) CD38 at the junction between prognostic marker and therapeutic target. *Trends in Molecular Medicine*. Vol. 14, No. 5, pp. 210-218, ISSN 1471-4914

Demarin, V., Podobnik, S.S., Storga-Tomic, D. & Kay, G. (2004) Treatment of Alzheimer's disease with stabilized oral nicotinamide adenine dinucleotide: a randomized, double-blind study. *Drugs Exp Clin Res*. Vol. 30, pp. 27-33,

Dhein, S., Polontchouk, L., Salameh, A. & Haefliger, J.A. (2002) Pharmacological modulation and differential regulation of the cardiac gap junction proteins connexin 43 and connexin 40. *Biology of the Cell*. Vol. 94, No. 7, pp. 409-422, ISSN 0248-4900

Di Lisa, F., Menab , R., Canton, M., Barile, M. & Bernardi, P. (2001) Opening of the mitochondrial permeability transition pore causes depletion of mitochondrial and cytosolic NAD^+ and is a causative event in the death of myocytes in postischemic reperfusion of the heart. *Journal of Biological Chemistry*. Vol. 276, No. 4, pp. 2571-2575, ISSN 0021-9258

Di Lisa, F. & Ziegler, M. (2001) Pathophysiological relevance of mitochondria in NAD^+ metabolism. *FEBS Letters*. Vol. 492, No. 1-2, pp. 4-8

Dong-Ruyl, L., Sawada, M. & Nakano, K. (1998) Tryptophan and its metabolite, kynurenine, stimulate expression of nerve growth factor in cultured mouse astroglial cells. *Neuroscience Letters*. Vol. 244, No. 1, pp. 17-20

Du, L., Zhang, X., Han, Y.Y., Burke, N.A., Kochanek, P.M., Watkins, S.C., Graham, S.H., Carcillo, J.A., Szabo, C. & Clark, R.S.B. (2003) Intra-mitochondrial Poly(ADP-ribosylation) Contributes to NAD^+ Depletion and Cell Death Induced by Oxidative Stress. *J. Biol. Chem*. Vol. 278, No. 20, pp. 18426-18433

Ebstein, R.P., Mankuta, D., Yirmiya, N. & Malavasi, F. (2011) Are retinoids potential therapeutic agents in disorders of social cognition including autism? *FEBS Letters*. pp. doi:10.1016/j.febslet.2011.05.004 ISSN 0014-5793

Egorova, A., Yokoyama, S., Fukami, H. & Higashida, H. (2000) Cell membrane blebbing is related to the CD38 redistribution in NG108-15 hybrid cells. *Neurophysiology*. Vol. 32, No. 3, pp. 240-241, ISSN 0090-2977

Franco, L., Zocchi, E., Usai, C., Guida, L., Bruzzone, S., Costa, A. & De Flora, A.G. (2001) Paracrine roles of NAD^+ and cyclic ADP-ribose in increasing intracellular calcium and enhancing cell proliferation of 3T3 fibroblasts. *J Biol Chem*. Vol. 276, pp. 21642-21648

Friberg, H. & Wieloch, T. (2002) Mitochondrial permeability transition in acute neurodegeneration. *Biochimie*. Vol. 84, No. 2-3, pp. 241-250, ISSN 0300-9084

Fukuoka, S.-I., Ishiguro, K., Yanagihara, K., Tanabe, A., Egashira, Y., Sanada, H. & Shibata, K. (2002) Identification and expression of a cDNA encoding human a-amino-b-carboxymuconate-e-semialdehyde decarboxylase (ACMSD). *J Biol Chem*. Vol. 277, No. 38, pp. 35162-35167

Giaume, C., Koulakoff, A., Roux, L., Holcman, D. & Rouach, N. (2010) Astroglial networks: a step further in neuroglial and gliovascular interactions. *Nature Reviews Neuroscience*. Vol. 11, No. 2, pp. 87-99, ISSN 1471-003X

Grant, R.S. & Kapoor, V. (1998) Murine Glial Cells Regenerate NAD, After Peroxide-Induced Depletion, Using Either Nicotinic Acid, Nicotinamide, or Quinolinic Acid as Substrates. *Journal of Neurochemistry*. Vol. 70, No. 4, pp. 1759-1763

Guillemin, G.J., Brew, B.J., Noonan, C.E., Takikawa, O. & Cullen, K.M. (2005) Indoleamine 2,3-dioxygenase and quinolinic acid immunoreactivity in Alzheimer's disease hippocampus. *Neuropath Appl Neurobiol*. Vol. 31, No. 4, pp. 395-404

Guillemin, G.J., Kerr, S.J., Smythe, G.A., Smith, M.A., Kapoor, V., Armati, P.J., Croitoru, J. & Brew, B.J. (2001) Kynurenine pathway metabolism in human astrocytes: a paradox for neuronal protection. *J Neurochem*. Vol. 78, No. 4, pp. 842-853

Guse, A.H. (2000) Cyclic ADP-ribose. *Journal of molecular medicine*. Vol. 78, No. 1, pp. 26-35, ISSN 0946-2716

Hallaq, R.Y. & Killick, R. (2006) P1-415: Connexin-43: A potential transduction target for amyloid intracellular domain? *Alzheimer's and Dementia*. Vol. 2, No. 3, Supplement 1, pp. S219-S219

Heidemann, A.C., Schipke, C.G. & Kettenmann, H. (2005) Extracellular Application of Nicotinic Acid Adenine Dinucleotide Phosphate Induces Ca^{2+} Signaling in Astrocytes in Situ. *J. Biol. Chem*. Vol. 280, No. 42, pp. 35630-35640

Henricksen, L.A. & Federoff, H.J. (2004) Redefining neuroprotective gene therapeutic strategies: Lessons learned from caloric restriction and NAD^+ metabolism. *Journal of Alzheimer's Disease*. Vol. 6, No. 6, pp. S43-S46

Higashida, H., Hashii, M., Yokoyama, S., Hoshi, N., Chen, X.L., Egorova, A., Noda, M. & Zhang, J.S. (2001) Cyclic ADP-ribose as a second messenger revisited from a new aspect of signal transduction from receptors to ADP-ribosyl cyclase. *Pharmacology & therapeutics*. Vol. 90, No. 2-3, pp. 283-296, ISSN 0163-7258

Higashida, H., Salmina, A.B., Olovyannikova, R.Y., Hashii, M., Yokoyama, S., Koizumi, K., Jin, D., Liu, H.X., Lopatina, O. & Amina, S. (2007) Cyclic ADP-ribose as a universal calcium signal molecule in the nervous system. *Neurochemistry international*. Vol. 51, No. 2-4, pp. 192-199, ISSN 0197-0186

Homkajorn, B., Sims, N. & Muyderman, H. (2010) Connexin 43 regulates astrocytic migration and proliferation in response to injury. *Neuroscience letters*. Vol. 486, No. 3, pp. 197-201, ISSN 0304-3940

Houtkooper, R.H., Cantó, C., Wanders, R.J. & Auwerx, J. (2010) The Secret Life of NAD+: An Old Metabolite Controlling New Metabolic Signaling Pathways. *Endocrine Reviews*. Vol. 31, No. 2, pp. 194-223

Inzhutova, A., Salmina, A., Petrova, M. & Larionov, A. (2008) Role of CD38 in cell-cell interactions under conditions of endothelial dysfunction. *Bulletin of Experimental Biology and Medicine*. Vol. 145, No. 6, pp. 703-706

Ito, T., Ueki, T., Furukawa, H. & Sato, K. (2011) The identification of novel protein, brain-derived integrating factor-1 (BDIF1), which interacts with astrocytic gap junctional protein. *Neuroscience Research*. Vol. 70, No. 3, pp. 330-333, ISSN 0168-0102

Itoh, Y., Esaki, T., Shimoji, K., Cook, M., Law, M.J., Kaufman, E. & Sokoloff, L. (2003) Dichloroacetate effects on glucose and lactate oxidation by neurons and astroglia in vitro and on glucose utilization by brain in vivo. *Proceedings of the National Academy of Sciences*. Vol. 100, No. 8, pp. 4879-4884

Kauppinen, T.M. & Swanson, R.A. (2007) The role of poly(ADP-ribose) polymerase-1 in CNS disease. *Neuroscience*. Vol. 145, No. 4, pp. 1267-1272

Kawasaki, A., Hayashi, T., Nakachi, K., Trosko, J., Sugihara, K., Kotake, Y. & Ohta, S. (2009) Modulation of connexin 43 in rotenone-induced model of Parkinson's disease. *Neuroscience*. Vol. 160, No. 1, pp. 61-68, ISSN 0306-4522

Kelliher, M., Fastbom, J., Cowburn, R.F., Bonkale, W., Ohm, T.G., Ravid, R., Sorrentino, V. & O'Neill, C. (1999) Alterations in the ryanodine receptor calcium release channel correlate with Alzheimer's disease neurofibrillary and b-amyloid pathologies. *Neuroscience*. Vol. 92, No. 2, pp. 499-513

Khan, J.A., Forouhar, F., Tao, X. & Tong, L. (2007) Nicotinamide adenine dinucleotide metabolism as an attractive target for drug discovery. *Expert Opinion on Therapeutic Targets*. Vol. 11, No. 5, pp. 695-705

Kornyei, Z., Gocza, E., R hl, R., Orsolits, B., V r s, E., Szab , B., V govits, B. & Madar sz, E. (2007) Astroglia-derived retinoic acid is a key factor in glia-induced neurogenesis. *The FASEB Journal*. Vol. 21, No. 10, pp. 2496-2509, ISSN 0892-6638

Krezel, W., Ghyselinck, N., Samad, T.A., Dupe, V., Kastner, P., Borrelli, E. & Chambon, P. (1998) Impaired locomotion and dopamine signaling in retinoid receptor mutant mice. *Science (New York, NY)*. Vol. 279, No. 5352, pp. 863-867, ISSN 0036-8075

Kristian, T., Balan, I., Schuh, R. & Onken, M. (2011) Mitochondrial dysfunction and nicotinamide dinucleotide catabolism as mechanisms of cell death and promising targets for neuroprotection. *Journal of Neuroscience Research*. Vol. in press, ISSN 1097-4547

Krum, J.M. (1995) Age-dependent susceptibility of CNS glial populations in situ to the antimetabolite 6-aminonicotinamide. *Molecular and chemical neuropathology*. Vol. 26, No. 2, pp. 79-94, ISSN 0734-600X

Kunze, A. (2009) Connexin expression by radial glia-like cells is required for neurogenesis in the adult dentate gyrus. *Proceedings of the National Academy of Sciences*. Vol. 106, No. 27, pp. 11336-11341, ISSN 0027-8424

Kwon, H.S. & Ott, M. (2008) The ups and downs of SIRT1. *Trends in biochemical sciences*. Vol. 33, No. 11, pp. 517-525, ISSN 0968-0004

L'Episcopo, F., Tirolo, C., Testa, N., Caniglia, S., Morale, M.C., Cossetti, C., D'Adamo, P., Zardini, E., Andreoni, L. & Ihekwaba, A.E.C. (2010) Reactive astrocytes and Wnt/[beta]-catenin signaling link nigrostriatal injury to repair in 1-methyl-4-

phenyl-1, 2, 3, 6-tetrahydropyridine model of Parkinson's disease. *Neurobiology of Disease*. Vol. 41, No. 2, pp. 508-527, ISSN 0969-9961

Lane, M.A. & Bailey, S.J. (2005) Role of retinoid signalling in the adult brain. *Progress in Neurobiology*. Vol. 75, No. 4, pp. 275-293, ISSN 0301-0082

Liu, F., Arias-Vasquez, A., Sleegers, K., Aulchenko, Y.S., Kayser, M., Sanchez-Juan, P., Feng, B.-J., Bertoli-Avella, A.M., Swieten, J.v., Axenovich, T.I., Heutink, P., Broeckhoven, C.v., Oostra, B.A. & Duijn, C.M.v. (2007) A genomewide screen for late-onset Alzheimer disease in a genetically isolated Dutch population. *Am J Hum Genet*. Vol. 81, No. 1, pp. 17-31

Love, S., Barber, R. & Wilcock, G.K. (1999) Increased poly(ADP-ribosyl)ation of nuclear proteins in Alzheimer's disease. *Brain*. Vol. 122, No. 2, pp. 247-253

Lu, H., Burns, D., Garnier, P., Wei, G., Zhu, K. & Ying, W. (2007) P2X7 receptors mediate NADH transport across the plasma membranes of astrocytes. *Biochemical and Biophysical Research Communications*. Vol. 362, No. 4, pp. 946-950

Magistretti, P.J. (2000) Cellular bases of functional brain imaging: insights from neuron-glia metabolic coupling. *Brain Res Rev*. Vol. 886, pp. 108-112

Magni, G., Amici, A., Emanuelli, M., Orsomando, G., Raffaelli, N. & Ruggieri, S. (2004) Enzymology of NAD^+ homeostasis in man. *Cell Mol Life Sci*. Vol. 61, pp. 19-34

Maiese, K. & Chong, Z.Z. (2003) Nicotinamide: necessary nutrient emerges as a novel cytoprotectant for the brain. *Trends in pharmacological sciences*. Vol. 24, No. 5, pp. 228-232, ISSN 0165-6147

Malaspina, A. & Michael Titus, A.T. (2008) Is the modulation of retinoid and retinoid associated signaling a future therapeutic strategy in neurological trauma and neurodegeneration? *Journal of neurochemistry*. Vol. 104, No. 3, pp. 584-595, ISSN 1471-4159

Malavasi, F., Deaglio, S., Funaro, A., Ferrero, E., Horenstein, A.L., Ortolan, E., Vaisitti, T. & Aydin, S. (2008) Evolution and function of the ADP ribosyl cyclase/CD38 gene family in physiology and pathology. *Physiological reviews*. Vol. 88, No. 3, pp. 841-886, ISSN 0031-9333

Maragakis, N.J. & Rothstein, J.D. (2006) Mechanisms of Disease: astrocytes in neurodegenerative disease. *Nat Clin Pract Neuro*. Vol. 2, No. 12, pp. 679-689, ISSN 1745-834X

Massieu, L., Del Rho, P. & Montiel, T. (2001) Neurotoxicity of glutamate uptake inhibition in vivo: correlation with succinate dehydrogenase activity and prevention by energy substrates. *Neuroscience*. Vol. 106, No. 4, pp. 669-677

Matyash, M., Matyash, V., Nolte, C., Sorrentino, V. & Kettenmann, H. (2002) Requirement of functional ryanodine receptor type 3 for astrocyte migration. *The FASEB Journal*. Vol. 16, No. 1, pp. 84-86, ISSN 0892-6638

Mei, X., Ezan, P., Giaume, C. & Koulakoff, A. (2010) Astroglial connexin immunoreactivity is specifically altered at [beta]-amyloid plaques in APP/PS1 mice. *Neuroscience*. Vol. 171, No. 1, pp. 92-105, ISSN 0306-4522

Mills, K., Woodgate, L., Gilkes, A., Walsh, V., Sweeney, M., Brown, G. & Burnett, A. (1999) Inhibition of Mitochondrial Function in HL60 Cells Is Associated with an Increased Apoptosis and Expression of CD14* 1. *Biochemical and biophysical research communications*. Vol. 263, No. 2, pp. 294-300, ISSN 0006-291X

Miro-Casas, E., Ruiz-Meana, M., Agullo, E., Stahlhofen, S., Rodr guez-Sinovas, A., Cabestrero, A., Jorge, I., Torre, I., Vazquez, J. & Boengler, K. (2009) Connexin43 in cardiomyocyte mitochondria contributes to mitochondrial potassium uptake. *Cardiovascular research*. Vol. 83, No. 4, pp. 747-756, ISSN 0008-6363

Nagy, J.I., Dudek, F.E. & Rash, J.E. (2004) Update on connexins and gap junctions in neurons and glia in the mammalian nervous system. *Brain Research Reviews*. Vol. 47, No. 1-3, pp. 191-215,

Nakase, T. & Naus, C.C. (2004) Gap junctions and neurological disorders of the central nervous system. *Biochim Biophys Acta*. Vol. 1662, No. 1-2, pp. 149-158

Nikiforov, A., Dölle, C., Niere, M. & Ziegler, M. (2011) Pathways and Subcellular Compartmentation of NAD Biosynthesis in Human Cells. *Journal of Biological Chemistry*. Vol. 286, No. 24, pp. 21767-21778

Nimmerjahn, A. (2009) Astrocytes going live: advances and challenges. *The Journal of physiology*. Vol. 587, No. 8, pp. 1639-1647, ISSN 1469-7793

Norris, C.M., Kadish, I., Blalock, E.M., Chen, K.-C., Thibault, V., Porter, N.M., Landfield, P.W. & Kraner, S.D. (2005) Calcineurin Triggers Reactive/Inflammatory Processes in Astrocytes and Is Upregulated in Aging and Alzheimer's Models. *J. Neurosci*. Vol. 25, No. 18, pp. 4649-4658

Oliver, F.J., Menissier-de Murcia, J. & de Murcia, G. (1999) Poly(ADP-Ribose) Polymerase in the Cellular Response to DNA Damage, Apoptosis, and Disease. *The American Journal of Human Genetics*. Vol. 64, No. 5, pp. 1282-1288

Orellana, J.A., S ez, P.J., Shoji, K.F., Schalper, K.A., Palacios–Prado, N., Velarde, V., Giaume, C., Bennett, M.V.L. & Saez, J.C. (2009) Modulation of brain hemichannels and gap junction channels by pro-inflammatory agents and their possible role in neurodegeneration. *Antioxidants & redox signaling*. Vol. 11, No. 2, pp. 369-399, ISSN 1523-0864

Otsuka, K., Mizuguchi, M., Aizawa, T., Haga, S., Sato, M., Inoya, H., Namba, Y., Hofbauer, J. & Marberger, M. (1994) Immunoreactivity in Alzheimer's neurofibrillary tangles. *Brain Pathol*. Vol. 4, pp. 558

Outeiro, T.F., Marques, O. & Kazantsev, A. (2008) Therapeutic role of sirtuins in neurodegenerative disease. *Biochimica et Biophysica Acta (BBA)-Molecular Basis of Disease*. Vol. 1782, No. 6, pp. 363-369, ISSN 0925-4439

Oxenkrug, G.F. (2007) Genetic and Hormonal Regulation of Tryptophan Kynurenine Metabolism: Implications for Vascular Cognitive Impairment, Major Depressive Disorder, and Aging. *Ann NY Acad Sci*. Vol. 1122, No. 1, pp. 35-49

Parsons, R.B., Aravindan, S., Kadampeswaran, A., Evans, E.A., Sandhu, K.K., Levy, E., Thomas, M.G., Austen, B.M. & Ramsden, D.B. (2011) The expression of nicotinamide N-methyltransferas increases ATP synthesis and protects SH-SY5Y neuroblastoma cells against the toxicity of complex I inhibitors. *Biochemical Journal*. Vol. 436, No. 1, pp. 145-155

Parsons, R.B., Smith, S.W., Waring, R.H., Williams, A.C. & Ramsden, D.B. (2003) High expression of nicotinamide N-methyltransferase in patients with idiopathic Parkinson's disease. *Neuroscience letters*. Vol. 342, No. 1-2, pp. 13-16, ISSN 0304-3940

Parys, B., C t , A., Gallo, V., De Koninck, P. & S k, A. (2010) Intercellular calcium signaling between astrocytes and oligodendrocytes via gap junctions in culture. *Neuroscience*. Vol. 167, No. 4, pp. 1032-1043, ISSN 0306-4522

Pawlikowska, L., Votrell, S.E., Harms, M.B., Li, Y. & Rosenberg, P.A. (1996) Extracellular synthesis of cADP-ribose from nicotinamide-adenine dinucleotide by rat cortical astrocytes in culture. *J Neurosci* Vol. 16, pp. 5372-5381

Pellerin, L., Pellegri, G., Bittar, P.G., Charnay, Y., Bouras, C., Martin, J.L., Stella, N. & Magistretti, P.J. (1998) Evidence supporting the existence of an activity-dependent astrocyte-neuron lactate shuttle. *Dev Neurosci*. Vol. 20, pp. 291-299

Penkowa, M., Camats, J., Hadberg, H., Quintana, A., Rojas, S., Giralt, M., Molinero, A., Campbell, I.L. & Hidalgo, J. (2003) Astrocyte targeted expression of interleukin 6 protects the central nervous system during neuroglial degeneration induced by 6 aminonicotinamide. *Journal of Neuroscience Research*. Vol. 73, No. 4, pp. 481-496, ISSN 1097-4547

Pfrieger, F.W. (2010) Role of glial cells in the formation and maintenance of synapses. *Brain research reviews*. Vol. 63, No. 1-2, pp. 39-46, ISSN 0165-0173

Pieper, A.A., Blackshaw, S., Clements, E.E., Brat, D.J., Krug, D.K., White, A.J., Pinto-Garcia, P., Favit, A., Conover, J.R., Snyder, S.H. & Verma, A. (2000) Poly(ADP-ribosyl)ation basally activated by DNA strand breaks reflects glutamate-nitric oxide neurotransmission. *Proceedings of the National Academy of Sciences*. Vol. 97, No. 4, pp. 1845-1850

Qin, W., Yang, T., Ho, L., Zhao, Z., Wang, J., Chen, L., Zhao, W., Thiyagarajan, M., MacGrogan, D., Rodgers, J.T., Puigserver, P., Sadoshima, J., Deng, H., Pedrini, S., Gandy, S., Sauve, A.A. & Pasinetti, G.M. (2006) Neuronal SIRT1 Activation as a Novel Mechanism Underlying the Prevention of Alzheimer Disease Amyloid Neuropathology by Calorie Restriction. *J. Biol. Chem.* Vol. 281, No. 31, pp. 21745-21754

Raffaelli, N., Sorci, L., Amici, A., Emanuelli, M., Mazzola, F. & Magni, G. (2002) Identification of a novel human nicotinamide mononucleotide adenylyltransferase. *Biochemical and Biophysical Research Communications*. Vol. 297, No. 4, pp. 835-840

Rainer, M., Kraxberger, E., Haushofer, M., Mucke, H.A.M. & Jellinger, K.A. (2000) No evidence for cognitive improvement from oral nicotinamide adenine dinucleotide (NADH) in dementia. *Journal of Neural Transmission*. Vol. 107, No. 12, pp. 1475-1481

Rash, J.E., Yasumura, T., Dudek, F.E. & Nagy, J.I. (2001) Cell-specific expression of connexins and evidence of restricted gap junctional coupling between glial cells and between neurons. *The Journal of Neuroscience*. Vol. 21, No. 6, pp. 1983-2000, ISSN 0270-6474

Ricci, G., Volpi, L., Pasquali, L., Petrozzi, L. & Siciliano, G. (2009) Astrocyte–neuron interactions in neurological disorders. *Journal of biological physics*. Vol. 35, No. 4, pp. 317-336, ISSN 0092-0606

Rodriguez, J.J. & Verkhratsky, A. (2010) Neuroglial Roots of Neurodegenerative Diseases? *Molecular neurobiology*. Vol. 43, No. 2, pp. 1-10, ISSN 0893-7648

Rottlaender, D., Boengler, K., Wolny, M., Michels, G., Endres-Becker, J., Motloch, L.J., Schwaiger, A., Buechert, A., Schulz, R. & Heusch, G. (2010) Connexin 43 acts as a cytoprotective mediator of signal transduction by stimulating mitochondrial KATP channels in mouse cardiomyocytes. *The Journal of clinical investigation*. Vol. 120, No. 5, pp. 1441-1453

Saez, J.C. (2008) Astrocytes as connexin-dependent signaling cells for local blood flow regulation. *American Journal of Physiology-Heart and Circulatory Physiology*. Vol. 294, No. 2, pp. H586, ISSN 0363-6135

Salmina, A., Lopatina, O., Ekimova, M., Mikhutkina, S. & Higashida, H. (2010a) CD38/Cyclic ADP ribose System: A New Player for Oxytocin Secretion and Regulation of Social Behaviour. *Journal of neuroendocrinology*. Vol. 22, No. 5, pp. 380-392, ISSN 1365-2826

Salmina, A., Malinovskaya, N., Okuneva, O., Taranushenko, T., Fursov, A., Mikhutkina, S., Morgun, A., Prokopenko, S. & Zykova, L. (2008) Perinatal Hypoxic and Ischemic Damage to the Central Nervous System Causes Changes in the Expression of Connexin 43 and CD38 and ADP-Ribosyl Cyclase Activity in Brain Cells. *Bulletin of experimental biology and medicine*. Vol. 146, No. 6, pp. 733-736, ISSN 0007-4888

Salmina, A., Okuneva, O., Malinovskaya, N., Zykova, L., Fursov, A., Morgun, A., Mikhutkina, S. & Taranushenko, T. (2009a) Changes in expression and activity of CD38 in astroglial cells after impairment of the neuron-glia relationship in the brain induced by perinatal hypoxia-ischemia. *Neurochemical Journal*. Vol. 3, No. 3, pp. 207-213, ISSN 1819-7124

Salmina, A.B. (2009) Neuron-glia interactions as therapeutic targets in neurodegeneration. *Journal of Alzheimer's Disease*. Vol. 16, No. 3, pp. 485-502, ISSN 1387-2877

Salmina, A.B., Fursov, A.A., Mikhutkina, S.V., Malinovskaya, N.A., Morgun, A.V., Zykova, L.D., Musaeva, O.F., Fursov, M.A., Laletin, D.I., Yudin, G.V., Trufanova, L.V. & Schnayder, N.A. (2006a) Progression of apoptosis and changes in ADP-ribosyl cyclase activity in ischemic brain injury. *Siberian Medical Review*. No. 4, pp. 22-27

Salmina, A.B., Inzhutova, A.I., Malinovskaya, N.A. & Petrova, M.M. (2010b) Endothelial dysfunction and repair in Alzheimer-type neurodegeneration: Neuronal and glial control. *Journal of Alzheimer's Disease*. Vol. 22, No. 1, pp. 17-36, ISSN 1387-2877

Salmina, A.B., Malinovaskaya, N.A., Okuneva, O.S., Zykova, L.D., Yudin, G.V., Laletin, D.I., Frolova, O.V., Fursov, A.A. & Fursova, A.A. (2009b) Modulation of CD38 expression in brain cells with retinoic acid. *Siberian Medical Review*. No. 1, pp. 22-26 (russ.)

Salmina, A.B., Olovyannikova, R.Y., Noda, M. & Higashida, H. (2006b) ADP-ribosyl cyclase as a therapeutic target for central nervous system diseases. *Curr Medic Chem*. Vol. 6, No. 3, pp. 193-210

Sasaki, Y. & Milbrandt, J. (2010) Axonal degeneration is blocked by nicotinamide mononucleotide adenylyltransferase (NMNAT) protein transduction into transected axons. *Journal of Biological Chemistry*. Vol. 285, No. 53, pp. 41211-41215, ISSN 0021-9258

Sasaki, Y., Vohra, B.P.S., Lund, F.E. & Milbrandt, J. (2009) Nicotinamide Mononucleotide Adenylyl Transferase-Mediated Axonal Protection Requires Enzymatic Activity But Not Increased Levels of Neuronal Nicotinamide Adenine Dinucleotide. *The Journal of Neuroscience*. Vol. 29, No. 17, pp. 5525-5535

Satchell, M.A., Zhang, X., Kochanek, P.M., Dixon, C.E., Jenkins, L.W., Melick, J., Szab , C. & Clark, R.S.B. (2003) A dual role for poly ADP ribosylation in spatial memory acquisition after traumatic brain injury in mice involving NAD^+ depletion and ribosylation of 14 3 3. *Journal of neurochemistry*. Vol. 85, No. 3, pp. 697-708, ISSN 1471-4159

Schoenmann, Z., Assa-Kunik, E., Tiomny, S., Minis, A., Haklai-Topper, L., Arama, E. & Yaron, A. (2010) Axonal Degeneration Is Regulated by the Apoptotic Machinery or a NAD^+-Sensitive Pathway in Insects and Mammals. *The Journal of Neuroscience*. Vol. 30, No. 18, pp. 6375-6386

Sofroniew, M.V. (2009) Molecular dissection of reactive astrogliosis and glial scar formation. *Trends in Neurosciences*. Vol. 32, No. 12, pp. 638-647, ISSN 0166-2236

Steindler, D.A. & Laywell, E.D. (2003) Astrocytes as stem cells: nomenclature, phenotype, and translation. *Glia*. Vol. 43, No. 1, pp. 62-69, ISSN 1098-1136

Stevens, B. (2008) Neuron-astrocyte signaling in the development and plasticity of neural circuits. *Neurosignals*. Vol. 16, No. 4, pp. 278–288

Suh, H.S., Zhao, M.L., Rivieccio, M., Choi, S., Connoly, E., Zhao, Y., Takikawa, O., Brosnan, C.F. & Lee, H.-G. (2007) Astrocyte indoleamine 2,3-dioxygenase is induced by the TLR3 ligand poly(I:C): mechanism of induction and role in antiviral response. *J Virol*. Vol. 81, No. 18, pp. 9838-9850

Supnet, C., Grant, J., Kong, H., Westaway, D. & Mayne, M. (2006) Amyloid-b-(1-42) Increases Ryanodine Receptor-3 Expression and Function in Neurons of TgCRND8 Mice. *J. Biol. Chem.* Vol. 281, No. 50, pp. 38440-38447

Theodosis, D.T., Poulain, D.A. & Oliet, S.H.R. (2008) Activity-dependent structural and functional plasticity of astrocyte-neuron interactions. *Physiological reviews*. Vol. 88, No. 3, pp. 983-1008, ISSN 0031-9333

Theodosis, D.T., Trailin, A. & Poulain, D.A. (2006) Remodeling of astrocytes, a prerequisite for synapse turnover in the adult brain? Insights from the oxytocin system of the hypothalamus. *American Journal of Physiology-Regulatory, Integrative and Comparative Physiology*. Vol. 290, No. 5, pp. R1175-R1182, ISSN 0363-6119

Togashi, K., Hara, Y., Tominaga, T., Higashi, T., Konishi, Y., Mori, Y. & Tominaga, M. (2006) TRPM2 activation by cyclic ADP-ribose at body temperature is involved in insulin secretion. *The EMBO journal*. Vol. 25, No. 9, pp. 1804-1815

Vannucci, R.C., Brucklacher, R.M. & Vannucci, S.J. (2001) Intracellular calcium accumulation during the evolution of hypoxic-ischemic brain damage in the immature rat. *Developmental Brain Research*. Vol. 126, No. 1, pp. 117-120, ISSN 0165-3806

Verderio, C., Bruzzone, S., Zocchi, E., Fedele, E., Schenk, U., Flora, A.D. & Matteoli, M. (2001) Evidence of a role for cyclic ADP-ribose in calcium signalling and neurotransmitter release in cultured astrocytes. *J Neurochem*. Vol. 78, pp. 646-657

Verkhratsky, A. (2010) Physiology of neuronal-glial networking. *Neurochemistry international*. Vol. 57, pp. 332-343, ISSN 0197-0186

Verkhratsky, A., Olabarria, M., Noristani, H.N., Yeh, C.Y. & Rodriguez, J.J. (2010) Astrocytes in Alzheimer's Disease. *Neurotherapeutics*. Vol. 7, No. 4, pp. 399-412, ISSN 1933-7213

Verkhratsky, A., Orkand, R.K. & Kettenmann, H. (1998) Glial calcium: homeostasis and signaling function. *Physiological reviews*. Vol. 78, No. 1, pp. 99-141, ISSN 0031-9333

Vohra, B.P.S., Sasaki, Y., Miller, B.R., Chang, J., DiAntonio, A. & Milbrandt, J. (2010) Amyloid precursor protein cleavage-dependent and-independent axonal degeneration programs share a common nicotinamide mononucleotide adenylyltransferase 1-sensitive pathway. *The Journal of Neuroscience*. Vol. 30, No. 41, pp. 13729-13738, ISSN 0270-6474

Wagner, E., Luo, T. & Dr ger, U.C. (2002) Retinoic acid synthesis in the postnatal mouse brain marks distinct developmental stages and functional systems. *Cerebral Cortex*. Vol. 12, No. 12, pp. 1244-1253, ISSN 1047-3211

Wang, D.D. & Bordey, A. (2008) The astrocyte odyssey. *Progress in Neurobiology*. Vol. 86, No. 4, pp. 342-367, ISSN 0301-0082

Williams, A., Cartwright, L. & Ramsden, D. (2005) Parkinson's disease: the first common neurological disease due to auto-intoxication? *Qjm*. Vol. 98, No. 3, pp. 215, ISSN 1460-2725

Xu, H.-L., Mao, L., Ye, S., Paisansathan, C., Vetri, F. & Pelligrino, D.A. (2008) Astrocytes are a key conduit for upstream signaling of vasodilation during cerebral cortical neuronal activation in vivo. *Am J Physiol Heart Circ Physiol*. Vol. 294, No. 2, pp. H622-632

Yahata, N., Yuasa, S. & Araki, T. (2009) Nicotinamide mononucleotide adenylyltransferase expression in mitochondrial matrix delays Wallerian degeneration. *The Journal of Neuroscience*. Vol. 29, No. 19, pp. 6276-6284, ISSN 0270-6474

Yamamoto, S., Wajima, T., Hara, Y., Nishida, M. & Mori, Y. (2007) Transient receptor potential channels in Alzheimer's disease. *Biochimica et Biophysica Acta (BBA)-Molecular Basis of Disease*. Vol. 1772, No. 8, pp. 958-967, ISSN 0925-4439

Yan, T., Feng, Y. & Zhai, Q. (2010) Axon degeneration: Mechanisms and implications of a distinct program from cell death. *Neurochemistry international*. Vol. 56, No. 4, pp. 529-534, ISSN 0197-0186

Ye, Z.-C., Wyeth, M.S., Baltan-Tekkok, S. & Ransom, B.R. (2003) Functional Hemichannels in Astrocytes: A Novel Mechanism of Glutamate Release. *J. Neurosci*. Vol. 23, No. 9, pp. 3588-3596

Ying, W. (2006) NAD^+ and NADH in cellular functions and cell death. *Front Biosci*. Vol. 11, pp. 3129-3148

Ying, W., Alano, C.C., Garnier, P. & Swanson, R.A. (2005) NAD^+ as a metabolic link netween DNA damage and cell death. *J Neurosci Res*. Vol. 79, pp. 216-223

Ying, W., Chen, Y., Alano, C.C. & Swanson, R.A. (2002) Tricarboxylic Acid Cycle Substrates Prevent PARP-Mediated Death of Neurons and Astrocytes. *J Cereb Blood Flow Metab*. Vol. 22, No. 7, pp. 774-779, ISSN 0271-678X

Zhai, R.G., Zhang, F., Hiesinger, P.R., Cao, Y., Haueter, C.M. & Bellen, H.J. (2008) NAD synthase NMNAT acts as a chaperone to protect against neurodegeneration. *Nature*. Vol. 452, No. 7189, pp. 887-891, ISSN 0028-0836

Zhang, S., Liang, R., Zhou, F., Huang, X., Ding, J.H. & Hu, G. (2010) Reversal of Rotenone-Induced Dysfunction of Astrocytic Connexin43 by Opening Mitochondrial ATP-Sensitive Potassium Channels. *Cellular and molecular neurobiology*. Vol. 31, No. 1, pp. 111-117, ISSN 0272-4340

Zhu, K., Swanson, R.A. & Ying, W.C. (2005) NADH can enter into astrocytes and block poly(ADP-ribose) polymerase-1-mediated astrocyte death. *Neuroreport*. Vol. 16, No. 11, pp. 1209-1212

Ziegler, M. (2000) New functions of a long-known molecule. Emerging roles of NAD in cellular signaling. *Eur J Biochem*. Vol. 267, pp. 1550-1564

Ziegler, M., Jorcke, D. & Schweiger, M. (1997) Identification of bovine liver mitochondrial NAD^+ glycohydrolase as ADP-ribosyl cyclase. *Biochemical Journal*. Vol. 326, No. Pt 2, pp. 401-405

13

Microglia, Calcification and Neurodegenerative Diseases

Jose M. Vidal-Taboada, Nicole Mahy and Manuel J. Rodríguez
Unitat de Bioquímica i Biologia Molecular, Facultat de Medicina, Institut d'Investigacions Biomèdiques August Pi i Sunyer (IDIBAPS), Universitat de Barcelona and Centro de Investigación Biomédica en Red sobre Enfermedades Neurodegenerativas (CIBERNED), Barcelona
Spain

1. Introduction

1.1 Neurodegeneration involve different cell types

Neurodegeneration is a complex process involving different cell types and neurotransmitters. A common characteristic of neurodegenerative disorders such as Alzheimer's disease (AD), Parkinson's disease (PD), multiple sclerosis, Huntington's disease (HD) and Amyotrophic Lateral Sclerosis (ALS) is the occurrence of a neuroinflammatory reaction in which cellular processes involving glial cells (mainly microglia and astrocytes) and T cells are activated in response to neuronal death. This inflammatory reaction has recently received attention as an unexpected potential target for the treatment of these diseases.

Microglial cells have a mesenchymal origin, invade the central nervous system (CNS) prenatally (Chan et al., 2007b) and are the resident macrophages in the CNS (Ransohoff & Perry, 2009). They comprise approximately 10-20% of adult glia and serve as the CNS innate immune system. In neurodegenerative diseases, microglia is activated by misfolded proteins. In the case of AD, amyloid-β (Aβ) peptides accumulate extracellularly and activate the microglia locally. In the case of PD, ALS and HD, the misfolded proteins accumulate intracellularly but are still associated with activation of the microglia (Perry et al., 2010). Reactive microglia in the substantia nigra and striatum of PD brains have been described, and increased levels of proinflammatory cytokines and inducible nitric oxide synthase have been detected in these brain regions, providing evidence of a local inflammatory reaction (Hirsch & Hunot, 2009). The injection of lipopolysaccharide (a potent microglia activator) into the substantia nigra produces microglial activation and the death of dopaminergic cells. These findings support the hypothesis that microglial activation and neuroinflammation contribute to PD pathogenesis (Herrera et al., 2000).

Astrocytes are ectodermal cells, and they are probably about ten times as numerous as neurons. Astroglial cells were initially believed to be passive support cells providing trophic support for surrounding neurons (Sofroniew & Vinters, 2010), maintaining extracellular ion homeostasis and capturing excess extracellular neurotransmitters such as glutamate, which is considered particularly important given its involvement in excitotoxicity. However, recent studies have implicated astrocytes in many complex CNS functions, such as physical structuring of the brain (they are the main cells involved in cholesterol synthesis), active control of synaptogenesis and plasticity (Graeber, 2010), regulation of blood flow and promotion of myelination (Halliday & Stevens, 2011). Astroglial activation is characterized by an increase in expression of intermediate filament glial fibrillary acidic protein (GFAP) and the gene aldehyde dehydrogenase 1 family member L1 (ALDH1L1). Astrocytes are not immune cells per se, but they can, under specific conditions, contribute to the immune response (Farina et al., 2007).

Several other cell types have been associated with neurodegeneration and neuroinflammation, such as T-cells, oligodendrocytes and ependymal and subependymal cells (Philips & Robberecht, 2011). Once infiltrated in the CNS, T-cell subpopulations modulate the neuroinflammatory reaction differently, depending on stage of disease progression (Beers et al., 2011, Philips & Robberecht, 2011). Oligodendrocyte cells are widely distributed in the adult nervous system and their precursors have been reported to differentiate into astrocytes and even neurons in specific conditions (Rivers et al., 2008); however, their role in neuroinflammation is still poorly understood, as is that of ependymal and subependymal (Chi et al., 2006).

In addition to the death of specific neuronal populations, there are many other parallels between different neurodegenerative disorders. These include alteration of a diversity of neurotransmitters and intracellular signals, in particular of glutamate and calcium, which play key roles in excitotoxicity. Thus, alterations in cellular and molecular steady states give rise to changes that cannot be counteracted by the tissue, and lead to chronic and progressive neurodegenerative processes from which a return to normality is impossible. As advances in research are made, more similarities between these neurodegenerative diseases have been found on many different levels, from molecular to tissular.

1.2 Inflammation and neurodegeneration

The term neuroinflammation describes endogenous CNS tissue response to injury. Classically known as reactive gliosis, neuroinflammation refers to the aggressive response of glia to activating stimuli, analogous to the response of activated immune cells in peripheral tissues. Neuroinflammation has been associated with chronic CNS diseases such as multiple sclerosis, which is an unequivocal example of an inflammatory CNS disease. Other neurodegenerative diseases such as AD, ALS, PD, and HD lack the prominent infiltrates of blood-derived mononuclear cells that characterize autoimmune diseases. However, many substances involved in the promotion of inflammatory processes are present in the CNS of patients with such neurodegenerative diseases (Block et al., 2007).

Microglia are transformed and activated by a range of signals, such as neuronal death, mechanical injury and toxins (Block et al., 2007, Streit et al., 2004), and once activated they form the first line of defense against infection or injury to the CNS (Schwartz et al., 2006). Activated microglia acquire an amoeboid phenotype morphology similar to macrophages expressing the same markers, such as MHCI, MHCII, Iba1 and GLUT5 (Halliday & Stevens, 2011), and secrete proinflammatory molecules such as tumor necrosis factor-alpha (TNF-α), interferon γ, and interleukin 1β; they also upregulate oxidant molecules such as nitric oxide (NO) and O_2, which can protect against pathogens. This proinflammatory reaction eliminates hazards and repairs any damage. Microglia also release anti-inflammatory and trophic factors such as insulin-like growth factor 1 (IGF-1), interleukin 4, and interleukin 10, contributing to the repair and limitation of the inflammatory process (Block et al., 2007, Stoll et al., 2002). The proinflammatory or anti-inflammatory responses of the microglia are influenced by surrounding astrocytes and inflammatory T-cell subsets, which can affect their phagocytic capacity and antigen-presenting cell properties.

All neurological disorders lead to activation of the microglia. Thus, microglial reaction represents the main mediator of the inflammatory process in neurodegenerative diseases, and microgliosis is directly related to the physiopathology of these. For example, microgliosis is associated with atypical and insoluble components caused by irregular protein folding and degradation pathways, altered subcellular localization, and the abnormal interactions with other cellular proteins found in AD, PD HD, Down syndrome and normal aging. Microgliosis is also associated with the formation of extracellular ionic precipitates, such as hydroxyapatites, which are frequently observed within the CNS areas involved in the disease (Rodriguez et al., 2009a, Saura et al., 1995), and is also present in encephalopathies caused by prions. This innate immune response is currently considered to be a potential pathogenic factor, since microglial reaction may engender neurodegenerative events, including amyloid-beta plaque formation, dystrophic neurite growth, and excessive tau phosphorylation.

1.3 Microglial reaction: Two sides of the same coin

In the healthy CNS, ramified resting microglia are active cells since they permanently scan their microenvironment (Wake et al., 2009). In response to any CNS injury or immunological stimuli, the microglia rapidly evolve from a surveillance state towards a more reactive one, through important phenotypical changes in response to activation signals released by the tissue (Schwartz et al., 2006). Microglia undergo a dramatic morphological transformation into amoeboid form and express an upregulated catalogue of molecules, such as CD14, major histocompatibility complex (MHC) molecules, chemokine receptors, CD11c, integrins, neurotrophins, and several other markers (Kettenmann et al., 2011). As such, reactive microglia can perform functions essential to neuron survival, such as phagocytosis to clear toxic and cellular debris, and innate immunity. Also involved in the release of trophic and anti-inflammatory factors, microglia facilitate repair through the guided migration of stem cells to the site of inflammation and injury.

In contrast, once microglia become overactivated they can produce detrimental effects through excessive production of a large array of cytotoxic factors, such as NO, TNF-α, reactive oxygen species, and pro-inflammatory cytokines (Lull & Block, 2010, Milligan & Watkins, 2009). Currently, the conditions that determine whether microglial reaction will be detrimental or beneficial to neuronal survival are poorly understood. However, it is becoming more widely accepted that although microglial activation is necessary and crucial for host defense and neuron survival, microglial overactivation leads to deleterious consequences.

Since every single microglial cell generates its own response to damage according to the nature and intensity of the signals released by the injured tissue, microglial cells do not constitute a homogenous cell population, but instead present a range of different phenotypes closely related to the evolution of the lesion process. In addition, some microglial cells become increasingly dysfunctional as they age, and may participate directly in the development of neurodegeneration (Block et al., 2007, Stoll et al., 2002). Microglia adopts a phenotype that mostly exacerbates tissue injury or promotes brain repair. Microglia can thus present two phenotypes, one of which is deleterious (also called M1 microglial phenotype) and the other benign (M2 microglial phenotype), depending on their intrinsic properties, interaction with the cellular microenvironment, and presence of pathogenic factors (Halliday & Stevens, 2011, Henkel et al., 2009). Therefore, controlling microglial cell activation and the acquisition of positive or negative phenotypes is of major therapeutic interest in all CNS disorders related to neuroinflammation.

1.4 Astrocyte-microglia interactions: Who's the bad guy after all?

The classical view of astroglia, as simply presenting non-excitable support to neurons, has changed radically in recent years. Astrocytes are now seen as elements that generate various local signals, including glutamate, to communicate with neurons and that influence the tissue outcome during neurodegeneration (Allaman et al., 2011). There is increasing evidence in support of this active role of astrocytes, suggesting that atypical astrocyte activation or astroglial dysfunction constitute maladaptive responses to brain injury that may feed the on-going pathologic process during neurodegeneration. For example, astrocyte dysfunction is a key factor in the pathogenesis of human neurological disorders (Seifert et al., 2006), and in the cognitive impairment of aged rats (Andrés et al., 2000). Furthermore, glutamate-induced chronic lesion in rat brain not only presents a lack of astrogliosis but also long term atrophy of astrocytes, suggesting a maladaptive response that may be a cause of the on-going pathologic process (Rodriguez et al., 2009a).

Moreover, astrocytes influence microglial behaviour (figure 1). For instance, astrocytes play a critical role in the activation of microglia under infectious conditions (Ovanesov et al., 2008). In addition, astroglial chemokines are involved in microglia/macrophage activation in multiple sclerosis with MCP-1/CCL2 and IP-10/CXCL10 directing reactive gliosis (Tanuma et al., 2006). Therefore, it is reasonable to assume that astrocytic activity can be influenced by microglial activation. Although a clear account of this dynamic relationship has yet to be proposed, the astrocyte-microglia interplay may determine the phenotype that microglial cells adopt during neurodegeneration.

Some findings have implicated astrocytes in chronic microgliosis, with a transition from an initial neuroprotective activity to a later cytotoxic one. TNF-α secretion is crucial for rapid autocrine microglial activation with both neuroprotective and cytotoxic effects, a process that is also fed by TNF-α released by reactive astrocytes (Suzumura et al., 2006). TNF-α actions leading to neuronal death or survival are dose dependent (Bernardino et al., 2008), since it can activate two specific receptors: TNFR1, with an intracellular death domain, and TNFR2, mainly involved in neuroprotection (Fontaine et al., 2002). Consequently, low concentrations of TNF-α would initially induce TNFR2-mediated neuroprotection, whereas a subsequent high concentration of TNF-α would be able to activate TNFR1 both in astrocytes and microglia and contribute to cell injury through the death domain of the receptor.

Astroglial S100β is another of the factors that control microglial activity. Astrocytes release S100β constitutively (Van Eldik & Wainwright, 2003) and increase this release upon stimulation by several factors, including TNF-α (Edwards & Robinson, 2006). Under normal conditions, released S100β acts as a neurotrophic factor, countering the stimulatory effect of neurotoxins on (Reali et al., 2005) and stimulating astrocyte glutamate uptake (Tramontina et al., 2006). Released S100β modifies astrocytic, neuronal and microglial activities, depending on the extracellular concentration of the former and the expression of the specific receptor for advanced glycation end-products (RAGE). At micromolar concentrations, S100β upregulates IL-1β and TNF-α expression in activated microglia via RAGE, with the requirement of concurrent activation of NF-κB and AP-1 transcription factors (Bianchi et al., 2010). Furthermore, factors that modulate microglial reactivity, such as Ca^{2+} concentration,

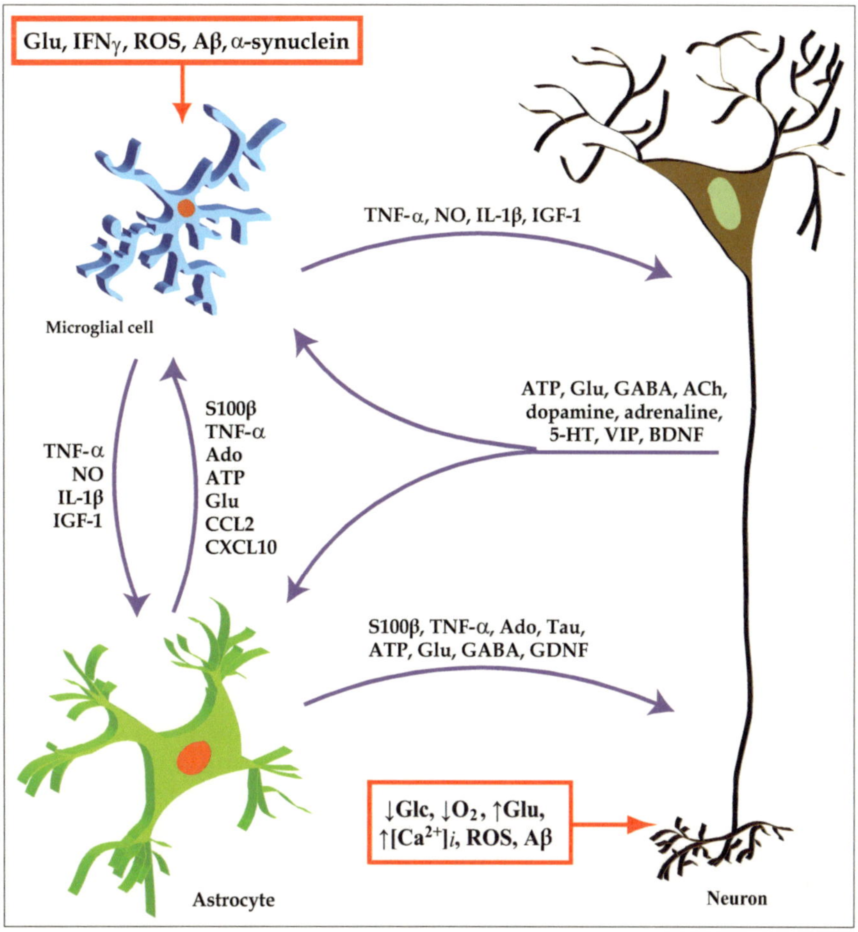

Fig. 1. Signalling systems in the microglia-astrocyte-neuron cross-talk. Astrocytes and microglia monitorize neuronal activity by sensing neurotransmitter release. In the same way, microglial cells have receptors to molecules released by astrocytes. Microglia integrate all these signals and release molecules that may modulate neuronal and astroglial activity. During neurodegeneration, changes in physiological parameters may trigger neuronal injury and/or microglial activation (molecules inside a red square) that modify those signal transduction systems. Aβ, amyloid beta; Ach, acetylcholine; Ado, adenosine; BDNF, Brain-derived neurotrophic factor; GABA, γ-aminobutyric acid; GDNF, Glial cell-derived neurotrophic factor; Glc, glucose; Glu, glutamate; 5-HT, serotonin; VIP, Vasoactive intestinal peptide; IFNγ, interferon gamma; ROS, reactive oxygen species; Tau, taurine

reactive oxygen species or TNF-α, also modify the RAGE response to S100β (Edwards & Robinson, 2006) in a microglia-astroglia cross-talk that integrates these signaling systems. In contrast, at high concentrations S100β binds the RAGE, which may mediate microglial activation during the course of brain damage (Bianchi et al., 2010). An increased release of S100β during neurodegeneration (Li et al., 2011) will enhance inflammatory cytokine production and potentiate the switch of microglia to chronic cytotoxic activity, feeding the neurotoxic process and leading to neurodegeneration.

Thus, CNS neurodegeneration involves chronic microgliosis with a putative transition from an initial neuroprotective activity to a later cytotoxic one, with S100β as a key modulator of microglial transition towards a cytotoxic response. This suggests a role for astrocytes in promoting the cytotoxic microglial phenotype through secretion of TNF-α, S100β and other signals (Donato et al., 2009, Suzumura et al., 2006). In this scenario, the interplay between trophic, neuroprotective, inflammatory and cytotoxic functions of both cell types during brain injury will determine the evolution of the neurodegenerative process. Precise control of these processes thus requires a dynamic view of their interactions so as to allow effective development of approaches to neuroprotection.

2. CNS calcification and neurodegeneration

2.1 Enduring effects of excessive synaptic glutamate

Glutamate accounts for most of the excitatory synaptic activity in the CNS and has been implicated in learning, memory, synaptic plasticity and neurotrophic activity processes. Glutamate receptors have been classified into three groups: two ionotropic groups -N-methyl-D-aspartate (NMDA) and α-amino-3-hydroxy-5-methyl-4-isoxazole propionic acid (AMPA)-kainate receptors-; and one group of metabotropic receptors, which are coupled to G proteins. Although non-NMDA receptors are not initially permeable to Ca^{2+}, glutamate release in the synaptic cleft increases post-synaptic and glial membrane permeability, leading to a transient increase in intracellular Ca^{2+} concentration ($[Ca^{2+}]_i$) (Obrenovitch et al., 2000).

Excessive activation of glutamate receptors can trigger neuronal death through a process characterized by chronic glutamate release and the consequent $[Ca^{2+}]_i$ dys-homeostasis in neurons and astrocytes (Arundine & Tymianski, 2004) and formation of $[Ca^{2+}]_i$ precipitates, the size and number of which depends on the CNS area involved and CNS maturation (Bernal et al., 2000b, Rodríguez et al., 2001). This process, defined as excitotoxicity, also involves cellular influxes of Na^+ and Cl^- and efflux of K^+, with ensuing cell swelling (Chen et al., 1998, Katayama et al., 1995). Because of the complexity and diversity of the processes taking place at the glutamatergic synapse, any disturbance at the pre-synaptic, post-synaptic, or astroglial level may trigger a chronic excitotoxic process. For example, ALS presents a loss of selectivity of ionotropic receptors (Obrenovitch et al., 2000) and deficiencies in glial re-uptake of glutamate (Liévens et al., 2000). These glutamate-related dysfunctions contribute to explaining phenomena such as the aging-associated hypoactivity of NMDA receptors observed in AD (Olney et al., 1997), and the specific AMPA-receptor increment detected in the hippocampus of aged, cognitive-impaired rats (Le Jeune et al., 1996).

One of the consequences of excitotoxic-induced neuronal loss is the alteration of other neurotransmitter systems and neuromodulators. For example, long-term ibotenic-induced lesion in the basal forebrain of rat leads to a loss of cholinergic afferences and to decreased extracellular noradrenaline, glutamate, and taurine (Boatell et al., 1995). This cortical reduction in glutamatergic transmission presents a temporal pattern which, together with the development of Ca^{2+} precipitates and a decrease in the cholinergic and noradrenergic functions (Saura et al., 1995), mimics the neurochemical modifications described in AD. Similarly, one year after acute lesion, the cortical and hippocampal decrease in brain-derived neurotrophic factor, fibroblastic growth factor and glucocorticoid receptor, and the increase in c-fos expression in the septal area were still significant (Boatell et al., 1992). Thus, excitotoxic lesions in basal forebrain can modify long-term cortical adaptative responses, and may modulate the expression of glutamate receptor. Some of these effects, such as the decrease in brain-derived neurotrophic factor and the increase in c-fos expression, also reflect the molecular alterations present in AD.

Given these toxic effects, adaptations that act to control glutamatergic neurotransmission and Ca^{2+} movements in the cell may be potentially protective. Over time, these defenses are developed to act at any time during an excitotoxic event, involve different cellular types such as neurons, astrocytes and microglia, and deal with the cellular and molecular mechanisms of glutamatergic neurotransmission. These mechanisms include defenses that: a) decrease neuronal excitability, b) decrease glutamate accumulation in the synapse, c) limit Ca^{2+} mobilization in the postsynaptic neuron and protect against calcium-dependent degenerative effects, and d) enhance neuronal energy (Rodriguez et al., 2009b, Sapolsky, 2001).

If the compensatory mechanisms are not sufficiently effective, the initial acute neuronal injury due to an increase in $[Ca^{2+}]_i$ leads, with time, to a chronic lesion. This secondary excitotoxicity appears in neurons after the massive entrance of Ca^{2+} and Na^+ through ionotropic glutamate receptors, an entrance that is supplemented by Ca^{2+} release from the endoplamic reticulum following activation of mGluRs. As a result, an excessive $[Ca^{2+}]_i$ increment occurs (Verkhratsky, 2007), which activates the mechanisms triggering neuronal death. Ca^{2+} extrusion and buffering are activated when $[Ca^{2+}]_i$ increases (Mattson & Chan, 2003), with high expenditure of energy through Ca^{2+}-ATPases. (Figure 4).

Calcium homeostasis disturbances are present in all neurodegenerative disorders (Mattson, 2006). Dysregulation of Ca^{2+} homeostasis alters the rapid and coherent activation of neurons, and is therefore ultimately responsible for many aspects of brain dysfunction and CNS diseases. For example, an increased rate of Ca^{2+}-mediated apoptosis may cause neuronal death in the penumbra of cerebral ischemia, or may underlie the etiology of chronic neurodegenerative disorders such as PD and AD. Calcium precipitation that coincides with microglial activation, amyloid deposits and other ion accumulations in AD may thus be a key element of the neurodegenerative process (Ramonet et al., 2006).

2.2 Neurodegeneration as a result of disturbances in calcium homeostasis

Regulation of intraneuronal Ca^{2+} movements is a key element to ensure adequate cellular response at all times and produce a physiological effect. Ca^{2+} participates in most cellular functions, including membrane excitability and secretion, energy production, synaptic transmission, gene regulation and plasticity, cell proliferation and cell death (Arundine & Tymianski, 2003). As a consequence, cell function requires tight control of Ca^{2+} homeostasis between extra- and intracellular compartments at all times, including the production of sufficient energy from glycolysis to maintain different gradient concentrations such as a 1/10,000 inside-outside cell concentration (Verkhratsky, 2005). Most calcium within cells is sequestered in the mitochondria and the endoplasmic reticulum. Intracellular free calcium concentrations fluctuate widely, from roughly 100 nM to over 1 μM, due to release from cellular stores or influx from extracellular fluid. These fluctuations are integral to the role of calcium, and unless compensated for by some other mechanism, any dysregulation will have severe cellular consequences, the effects of which will be propagated to the surrounding cells, namely, neurons and glial cells (Beck et al., 2004). For example, activation of glutamate receptors by excitatory signals leads to a massive increase in cytoplasm Ca^{2+} levels, which in turn activates a cascade of events to produce a neuronal response. A return

to basal activity requires a considerable expenditure of energy to bring Ca^{2+} back to initial levels. Any failure in these multiple, coordinated steps will alter neuronal signalling and interfere with neuronal network functions (Rodriguez et al., 2009b).
Reduction of $[Ca^{2+}]_i$ involves a high mitochondrial intake of Ca^{2+} that may lead to loss of the mitochondrial membrane potential and the production of reactive oxygen species, thereby decreasing cellular respiratory capacity and ATP formation from ADP and Pi (Chan et al., 2007a). As a result, there is an acceleration of anaerobic glycolysis with a net lactate production that contributes to tissue acidification and progression of damage. Disturbances in Ca^{2+} homeostasis in astrocytes reduce neuronal support, in particular through alteration of the glutamate/glutamine cycle and a reduction of glucose delivery to neurons (Pellerin et al., 2007, Ramonet et al., 2004) (Figure 4). Consequently, astrocyte dysfunction can lead to increased synaptic glutamate levels and glutamate receptor overactivation, combined with reduced neuronal energy, resulting in neuronal damage. Under these conditions of high Ca^{2+} and Pi and low ATP, formation of hydroxyapatite precipitates to reduce Ca^{2+} cytoplasm activity at low energy costs can occur in neurons and astrocytes (Rodriguez et al., 2000). This new step in calcium homeostasis temporarily helps the cell to resist excessive stimulatory signals and return to basal activity by dissolving paracrystal elements. However, in most cases, the hydroxyapatite crystals show progressive growth and participate in cell death and CNS damage.
Depending on the importance of the damage, microglial activation may take place, initially expressing neuroprotective signals to help avoid further neuronal death, but then changing progressively to an inflammatory phenotype (Graeber, 2010). Glycolysis, highly stimulated in microglia to ensure and maintain their activated stage, reduces neuronal glucose and oxygen availability. Consequently, microglial participation in neuronal death includes not only neuroinflammation, but also reduction in neuronal energy availability (Allaman et al., 2011). If, as asserted by Gyuri Buzsaki in Rhythms of the Brain (Buzsáki, 2006), "Brains are foretelling devices and their predictive powers emerge from the various rhythms they perpetually generate", any significant alteration of the neuronal rhythms caused by an abnormally high Ca^{2+} concentration in neurons or glia should alter the brain's ability to pause, adapt and learn, and can lead to disease. This is the case of neurodegenerative diseases, which exhibit diverse clinical and neuropathological phenotypes but share the common feature of progressively reduced cell function and survival within the nervous system, leading to neurological disability and often death. As such, several different CNS disorders can be induced following the same injury, due to the multi-directional interactions between the neurons, glial cells, extracellular matrix, endothelia and host immune cells that regulate tissue homeostasis and orchestrate neuroinflammation and degeneration. Furthermore, the characteristics of each neuronal population and network, the different gliopathic changes occurring between CNS areas, the various microglia phenotypes and the abundance and distribution of glutamate receptor subtypes and of Ca^{2+}-binding proteins, all participate directly in the properties of the neurodegenerative parameters (Graeber & Streit, 2010, Rodriguez et al., 2004, Rodriguez et al., 2009a) that will determine the dynamics and progression of the disease in the specific affected areas. For example, PD and AD are both regarded as diseases that are initiated by neuronal death to which the immune system responds, as evidenced by astroglial and microglial activation with pathogenic consequences (Agostinho et al., 2010, Halliday & Stevens, 2011). Similarly, multiple sclerosis is typically considered a neuroinflammatory disorder, but one in which neuronal injury plays an active role in

regulating neuroinflammation, as has been recently reported (Haider et al., 2011). In all of these diseases, dysregulation of Ca^{2+} homeostasis has been considered a pathophysiological factor linked to neuronal degeneration, and the formation of intracellular Ca^{2+} deposits with different characteristics as regards size and distribution - reflecting differential CNS area vulnerability - has frequently been reported (Hashimoto et al., 2003, Ramonet et al., 2006).

2.3 CNS calcification

In immature human CNS, Ca^{2+}-mediated excitotoxicity is associated with a calcification process that directly correlates with neuronal loss and the extent of injury. Revealed by Alizarin red staining and appearing in TEM and X-ray microanalyses of animal neurodegeneration models, small and large intracellular Ca^{2+} precipitates indicate the formation of a paracrystalline structure of hydroxyapatites localized within neurons and astrocytes (figure 2).

Glutamate analog microinjection in rat CNS leads to an intracellular Ca^{2+} precipitation similar to brain calcification in humans (Ramonet et al., 2006, 2002). As these Ca^{2+} deposits can be observed in several areas of rat brain after microinjection of different excitotoxins (Bernal et al., 2000b, Rodriguez et al., 2000, Saura et al., 1995), their formation does not depend on the glutamate receptor subtype initially stimulated. However, their size, number and distribution vary with both the activated receptor and the CNS area. For example, sensitivity to AMPA-induced calcification decreased from the globus pallidus, cerebral cortex, hippocampus, medial septum, to retina (Rodriguez et al., 2000). Moreover, in medial septum, the degeneration associated with microinjection of ibotenic and quisqualic acids was characterized by significant atrophy and no calcification (Mahy et al., 1996, Saura et al., 1995). In similar conditions, AMPA microinjection resulted in similar atrophy and Ca^{2+} deposits at the injection site (Rodriguez et al., 2009a).

Ca^{2+} deposits do not occur in all cells that degenerate in response to excitotoxins. For example, in the basal forebrain and medial septum, the calcification observed in GABAergic cells was not detected in cholinergic neurons. The former, together with astrocytes, seem to participate actively in the calcification process (Mahy et al., 1999). Differences in the neuronal phenotype of Ca^{2+} buffering and extrusion systems, specific energy needs, expression of the glutamate subtype receptor and different astroglial populations, should explain this variability. The ultrastructural study of tissue affected by excitotoxicity has also contributed to our understanding of calcification. Ca^{2+} deposits within hypertrophied astrocytes have been characterized in the basal forebrain and hippocampus which ranged from 0.5 to 10 μm in diameter and were formed by numerous, small, needle-shaped crystals associated with cellular organelles, such as microtubules, cisternae, vesicles or mitochondria, with no signs of neurodegeneration (figure 2). Larger inclusions were surrounded by reactive microglia, a finding that was also observed in tissue after specific localization by in vitro autoradiography (Bernal et al., 2000b, Petegnief et al., 1999). X-ray microanalysis has shown an electron-diffraction ring pattern characteristic of a crystalline structure similar to apatites (Kim, 1995), and a Ca/P ratio of 1.3±0.2 of cytoplasmic deposits (Figure 2). This ratio, lower than the theoretical apatite value of 1.67, is also typical of biological crystals, which do not present an ideal organization (Rodriguez et al., 2000). As biological hydroxyapatites, these deposits are similar to those observed in several human peripheral nervous system tissues (Kodaka et al., 1994).

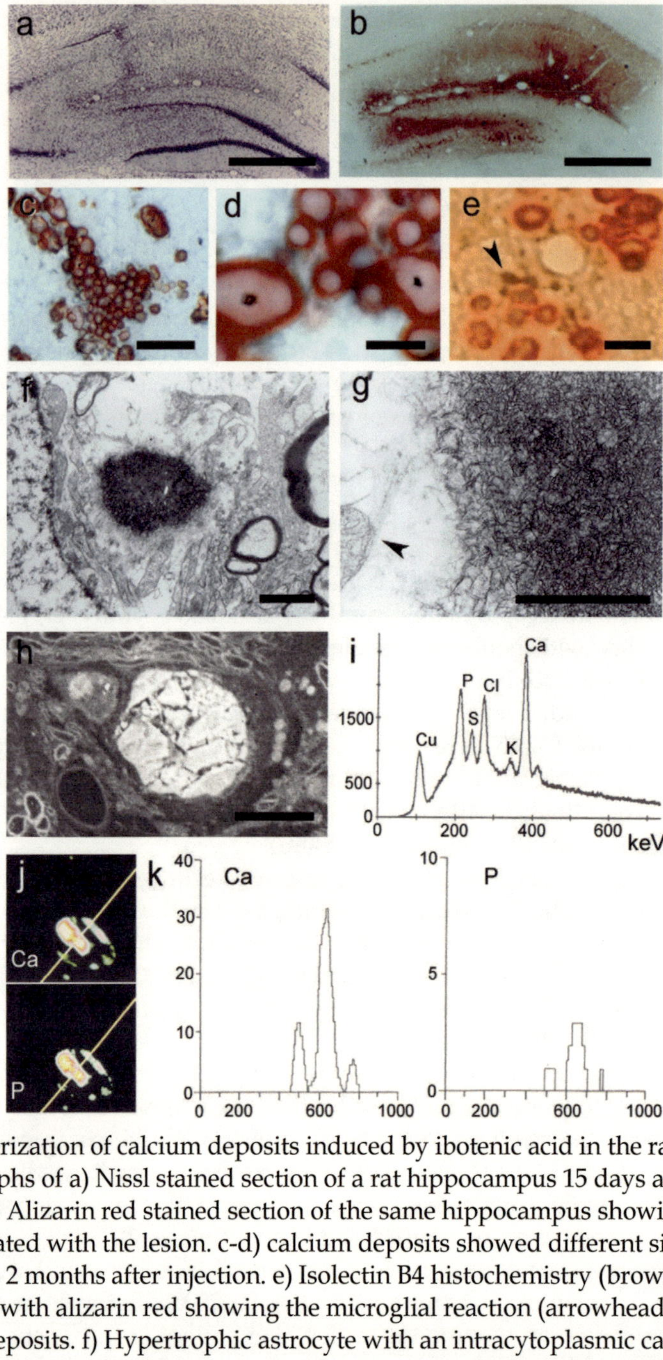

Fig. 2. Characterization of calcium deposits induced by ibotenic acid in the rat brain. Microphotographs of a) Nissl stained section of a rat hippocampus 15 days after the injection and b) Alizarin red stained section of the same hippocampus showing calcium deposits associated with the lesion. c-d) calcium deposits showed different sizes in the rat globus pallidus 2 months after injection. e) Isolectin B4 histochemistry (brown staining) counterstained with alizarin red showing the microglial reaction (arrowhead) associated with calcium deposits. f) Hypertrophic astrocyte with an intracytoplasmic calcium deposit by TEM. g) Detail of the ultrastructure of calcium deposit within an astrocyte. Note the normal appearance of the surrounding mitochondria (arrowhead). X-ray image h) and spectrum analysis i) of one calcium deposit in a non-osmificated sample with a calculated Ca/P ratio of 1.3. False colour X-ray image mapping j) and distribution plots k) of Ca and P of the same deposit. Bars; a-b, 1 mm; c, 100 μm; d-e, 20 μm; f, 0.6 μm, g, 0.2 μm; h, 10 μm

Experimental models of bone formation (i.e. hydroxyapatite formation in vitro) (Andre-Frei et al., 2000) have shown that rather than Ca^{2+}, a minimal amount of phosphorus, as inorganic phosphate, is crucial for crystal nucleation in a collagen matrix. Similarly, organic phosphate residues of the phosphoproteins also play a direct and significant role in the process of in vitro nucleation of apatite by bone collagen, whereas collagen itself does not promote the precipitation of Ca^{2+} or phosphate (Andre-Frei et al., 2000). Therefore, excitotoxicity-induced calcification in the rat brain depends on an increase in intracellular inorganic phosphate (i.e. ATP depletion) and, most importantly, on the degree of protein phosphorylation. Thus, the Ca^{2+}-binding-protein-dependent kinases and activity of the neurotrophic factor ultimately determine calcification.

In aqueous solutions, hydroxyapatite crystallization takes place in two sequential steps (Barat et al., 2011): in the first, crystal nucleation occurs spontaneously with subsequent growth to some nanometers, when phosphate and Ca^{2+} ions reach a certain concentration; in the second step, an accretion process of these nanocrystals on a proteinic net takes place until reaching a maximum size of 20 micrometers. While the first process facilitates re-solubilization of the crystal, the second produces a stable precipitate and requires a catalytic agent. These two mechanisms may help explain the size differences we found between several areas of the CNS. For example, the large insoluble Ca^{2+} precipitates (mean size 20 μm) found after AMPA microinjection in globus pallidus (Petegnief et al., 1999) fit well with the second step theory, whereas the small deposits (mean size lower than 3 μm) obtained in hippocampus after the same procedure (Rodriguez et al., 2004) may reflect the lack of a catalytic agent for accretion, or an equilibrium between crystal formation and solubilization. Furthermore, blockade of glial glutamate uptake in rat striatum (Liévens et al., 2000) produced a spherical lesion with a central necrotic core surrounded by a penumbra zone similar to that caused by focal ischemia. Three days after treatment, an astroglial reaction and small Ca^{2+} deposits (mean diameter < 1 μm) were observed in the penumbra area. Eleven days later, these deposits had disappeared, the penumbra zone had recovered from injury and the necrotic area was partially repaired (Liévens et al., 2000). In this scenario, compensatory mechanisms helped normalize Ca^{2+} homeostasis and avoid further neuronal death. The tissue recovered the ability to use extrusion mechanisms, and re-solubilization of Ca^{2+} precipitates took place.

When Ca^{2+} deposits are localized extracellularly due to cell death, a microglial reaction is activated for their phagocytic removal. This microglial reaction also participates in the neuronal death seen in chronic neurodegenerative processes, but is dissociated from astrogliosis. In some animal models of neurodegeneration, a recovery has been observed associated with the disappearance of Ca^{2+} deposits. In other excitotoxic rodent models, the on-going neurodegenerative process increased with time and the Ca^{2+} deposits remained present, associated with microglial reaction.

2.4 The calcification process and ageing

In the neonate mammalian brain, considered more resistant to hypoxia-ischemia than adult CNS, dysregulation of Ca^{2+} homeostasis together with lactate acidosis are considered the main factors causing neuronal death. As premature-neonates are more resistant to hypoxia-ischemia than term neonates, we studied the relationship between differences in human brain vulnerability to hypoxia-ischemia during the perinatal period and brain calcification in the basal ganglia, cerebral cortex, and hippocampus (Rodríguez et al., 2001). The number and size of the observed non-arteriosclerotic calcifications were area-specific and increased in term neonates (Figure 3). The basal ganglia presented the highest degree of calcification and the hippocampus the lowest, mainly in the CA1 subfield. In all cases, neuronal damage was associated with astroglial reaction and Ca^{2+} precipitates, with microglial reaction absent in the hippocampus. These data are consistent with those obtained following long-term excitotoxic lesions in adult rat brain and support the involvement of excitotoxic processes in hypoxia-ischemia damage.

A comparison between lifespan and degree of calcification (Figure 3) demonstrated that in all cases, highest calcification occurred within two months of hypoxia-ischemia, and that semi-calcification time was very short (less than 10 days). Independent of subjective measurements, this last parameter suggests that calcification depends on the degree of brain differentiation and initial cerebral injury, but not on the time-course of the lesion. Moreover, the mechanisms leading to Ca^{2+} precipitation seem to be similar for all brain areas. If this is true, neurons of each CNS structure degenerate through a common mechanism, which is linked to disturbances in Ca^{2+} homeostasis. As each area of the brain participates in specific physiological functions, the resultant pathology will depend on the specific neuronal death of the area affected.

Aging increases neuronal vulnerability to toxic compounds, including drugs that impair energy metabolism and induce secondary excitotoxic processes (Brouillet et al., 1993). However, a decreased susceptibility of aged rats to excitotoxins such as quinolinic or kainic acids has been reported (Kesslak et al., 1995). AMPA-induced Ca^{2+} deposits in rat hippocampus are age-dependent, since young rats (3 months old) present greater areas of calcification than middle-aged ones (15 months old) (Bernal et al., 2000a). In this study, glial reaction, γ-aminobutiric acid (GABA)-uptake activity and immunostaining of Ca^{2+} binding proteins showed the same response. Therefore, the vulnerability of hippocampal neurons to AMPA-induced neurodegeneration decreases with age between 3 and 15 months. Similar results have been found in other brain areas, such as the striatum and the nucleus basalis magnocellularis. This reduced vulnerability may be related to several factors: for example, age-associated variations in the relative abundance of glutamate receptors and pre-synaptic alterations of glutamate release may explain, at least in part, an increased resistance to excitotoxicity in the hippocampus (Mullany et al., 1996, Nicolle et al., 1996).

This effect is compatible with the increased vulnerability to excitotoxicity observed in the oldest animals (Brouillet et al., 1993), since some of the factors responsible for injury resistance may follow a biphasic pattern, with a progressive increase until reaching maturity followed by a subsequent decrease (Coleman et al., 1990). Many authors have also described biphasic variations in several parameters during aging, with an opposite tendency before and after middle age (Villa et al., 1994). We observed a biphasic variation in monoamine oxidase B (MAO-B) during aging in most human brain areas: up to the age of 50-60 years old, MAO-B levels remain constant, but start to increase thereafter (Saura et al., 1997). This finding may be due to the presence of MAO-B rich reactive astrocytes in response to neuronal degeneration. A similar increase in plaque-associated astrocytes has been found in patients with AD (Saura et al., 1994). As MAO-B activity is associated with reactive oxygen species production, astrocytes may contribute to the age-associated decline of neurological functions. The evidence that an increase in AMPA receptor correlates negatively with MAO-B in age-associated learning-impaired rats also suggests that a gliopathic reaction may be involved in neuronal dysfunction (Andrés et al., 2000).

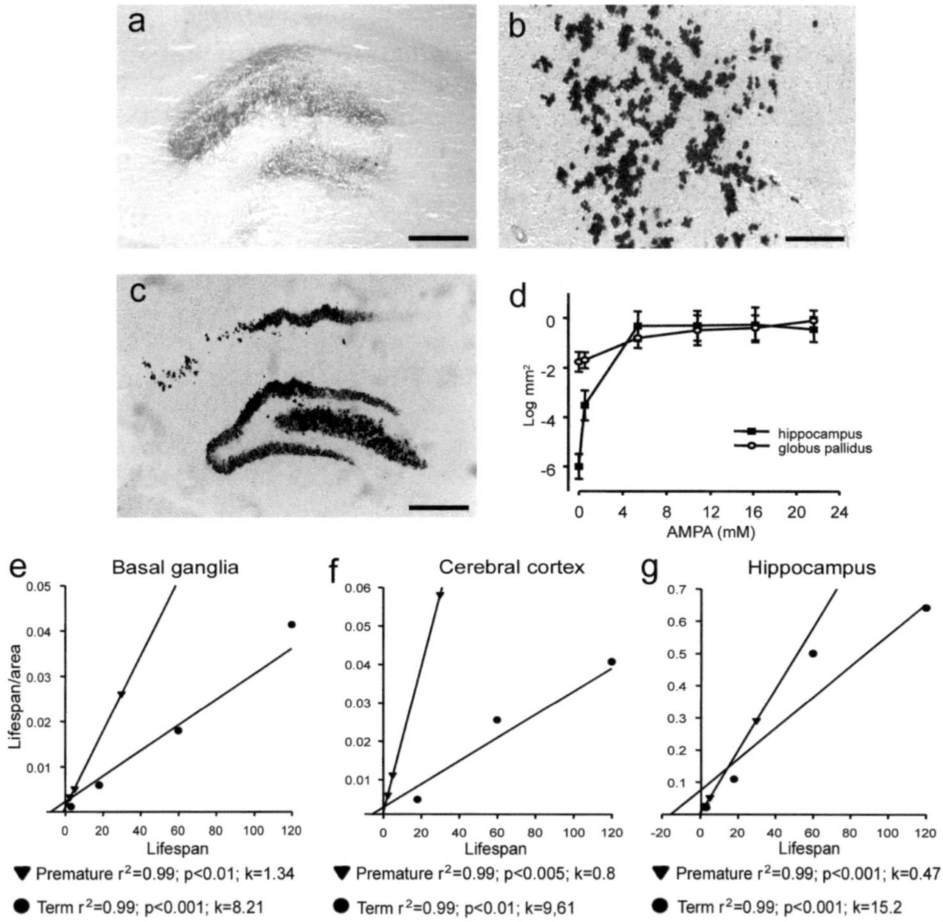

Fig. 3. Calcification depends on the brain area but also on the glutamate receptor involved. a) AMPA induces small calcium deposits in the rat hippocampus, affecting mainly the CA1 radiatum and lacunosum moleculare subfields. b) AMPA microinjection in the globus pallidus induces larger calcium deposits. c) NMDA microinjection in the hippocampus induces the formation of large calcium deposits located mainly in the pyramidal CA1 and granual dentate gyrus. d) The plots show comparison of the AMPA dose-response study in the hippocampus and the globus pallidus. e-f) Correlation plots of the hypoxia ischemia-induced calcification in the basal ganglia e), cerebral cortex f) and hippocampus g) of premature and term neonates. Calcification was calculated in a representative area (1 mm^2) and the lifespan corresponds to the time of injury in days. k, days to reach half of the maximal calcified area. Bars, 300 μm

Thus, the correlation between the calcification process, neuronal loss and the extent of CNS injury disappears with aging, but differences in CNS area vulnerability to calcification are maintained. The components that underlie the specific vulnerability of each brain area are thus already expressed in human neonates. The permanent area differences are associated with significant variations in the response to specific Ca^{2+} channel blockers such as nimodipine and TMB-8 (Bernal et al., 2009, Petegnief et al., 2004), and illustrate the functional diversity of each area and the difficulty encountered in ensuring the efficacy of such types of treatment. Similar results concerning differences between calcium precipitates and brain area susceptibility have been observed in congenital toxoplasmosis (Safadi et al., 2003, Surendrababu et al., 2006). Cerebral calcification has been described in 65% of these patients, with calcified foci distributed predominantly in the cortex in the form of tiny flecks, and as linear streaks in the basal ganglia.

The calcification process can thus be considered a new stage in cytoplasmic calcium homeostasis taking place in a diversity of CNS injuries to reduce calcium signalling at no energy cost. When located extracellularly due to cell-death, these precipitates activate a permanent microglial reaction aimed at their removal but which rapidly turns into chronic damage and aggravation of neurodegeneration.

2.5 Uncoupling of retaliatory systems and energy availability

The balance between retaliatory system actions and energy metabolism constitutes a fine equilibrium in physiological conditions, but it can be disrupted by glutamate-mediated neuronal injury to then participate in the evoked neurodegenerative process. For example, AMPA-microinjection in medial septum induces a progressive cholinergic and GABAergic loss associated with a long-term decline of the hippocampal functions and decreased glutamatergic activity (Rodriguez et al., 2005). Other effects of this lesion imply modifications of adenosine and taurine transmissions, glutamate recycling and glucose metabolism (Ramonet et al., 2004, Rodriguez et al., 2005). Over time, adenosine replaces GABA functions to avoid further excitotoxic damage when cholinergic and GABAergic processes are compromised.

Long-term septal lesion-induced neuronal loss in the hippocampus is apoptotic, with enhancement of neuronal glycolysis. Together with the cleavage of caspase 3, a glutamate-glutamine cycle displacement towards glutamine production reduces glutamate synthesis (Ramonet et al., 2004). In addition, synaptic glutamine is decreased, probably through expulsion to vessels, where it exerts a vasodilatory effect through NO synthesis inhibition (Mates et al., 2002). In this scenario, the reduction in glutamate signaling and increased neuronal energy metabolism both reflect a neurodegenerative process with deficient adaptation of the retaliatory systems and a chronic energy requirement to execute the apoptotic program.

This chronic energy requirement induces mitochondrial damage, in turn leading to acidosis in cells and the extracellular space (Hertz, 2008). Mitochondrial damage forces the cell to shift from an aerobic to an anaerobic metabolism, and as a result lactate is produced with the formation of two ATPs and the release of two protons. After trauma and ischemia, extracellular lactate increases dramatically and pH decreases. To ensure neuronal viability during and even after human hypoxia, glial glucose is only oxidized to lactate, which is rapidly transported into neurons for its complete oxidation (Sibson et al., 1998). In parallel, a Ca^{2+} influx causes rapid cytoplasmic acidification (Verkhratsky, 2007) through: a) activation of membrane Na^+/H^+ exchanger to restore the Na^+ gradient, and b) the Ca^{2+}-dependent displacement of protons bound to cytoplasmic anions (Arundine & Tymianski, 2004). Furthermore, H^+ also appears during some chemical reactions, such as phospholipid hydrolysis.

2.6 Functional relevance of the calcification process

The massive astroglial production of lactate to help compensate for the neuronal energy depletion caused by excitotoxicity is a key factor in brain calcification (Figure 4). pH reduction associated with increased lactate concentration facilitates solubility of Ca^{2+} and the formation of $H_2PO_4^-$, HPO_4^{2-} and PO_4^{3-} ions from inorganic phosphate (Rodriguez et al., 2000) and phosphorylated proteins. Because of the very high Ca^{2+} / $H_2PO_4^-$, HPO_4^{2-}, PO_4^{3-} affinity, apatite nucleation may occur, with the subsequent growth of crystalline formations together with neurodegeneration. In this case, calcification of each lesioned area will also depend on phosphate availability and the differential capacity of glial cells to release lactate during degeneration.

Wide variations have been described in the extent of calcification in pathological cases (Ramonet et al., 2002, Rodríguez et al., 2001) and animal species (Ramonet et al., 2006) However, the homogeneous morphology of these deposits suggests common synaptic processes (Ramonet et al., 2006) where variability depends on cellular type (astrocyte or neuron), glutamatergic activity, and energy availability (Figure 4). These factors modify Ca^{2+} homeostasis and may trigger cellular calcification through a common mechanism (Ramonet et al., 2006). Thus, hydroxyapatite formation, with the subsequent reduction of free Ca^{2+} ions, may take place as an alternative homeostatic step to reduce excitotoxicity (Ramonet et al., 2006, Rodriguez et al., 2000), and a number of findings lend support to this interpretation. For example, it has been observed that mitochondria close to Ca^{2+} deposits appear normal at electron microscopy level (Mahy et al., 1999, Rodriguez et al., 2000), despite

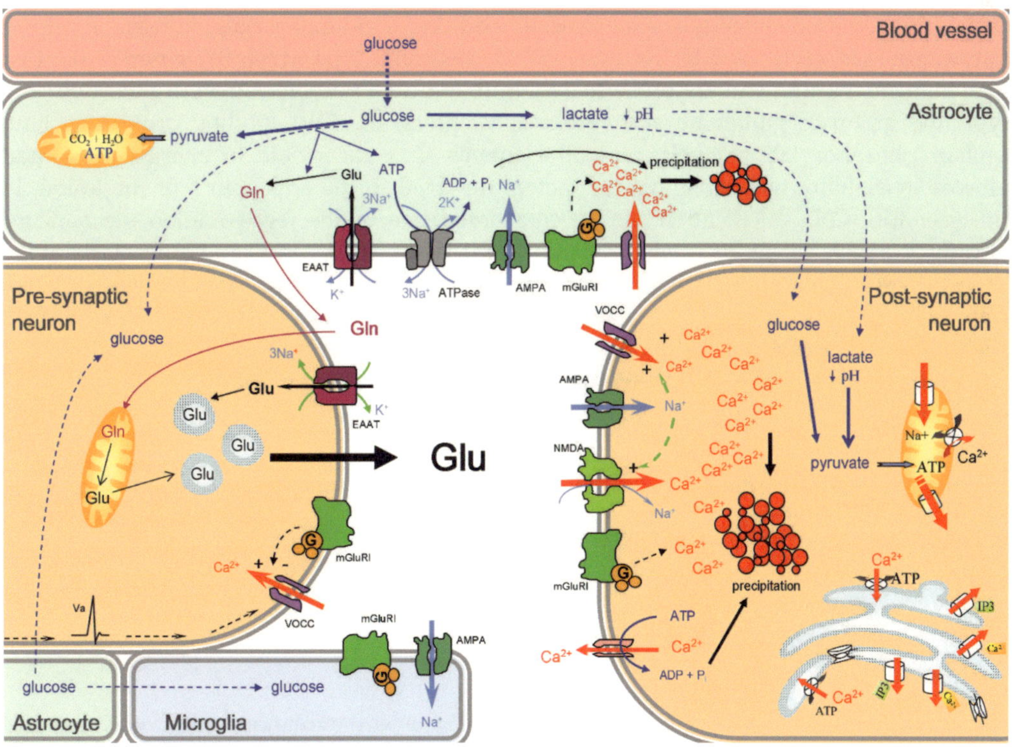

Fig. 4. Excitotoxicity modifies cell calcium homeostasis in the brain. Drawing of the excitotoxic process induced by glutamate, with the intercellular precipitation of calcium as part of the calcium homeostasis. The metabolic pathway of lactate with the communication between endothelial, astroglial, microglial and neuronal compartments is included in the diagram

the fact that mitochondrial dysfunction constitutes a primary event in NMDA-induced degeneration (Schinder et al., 1996). This hypothesis is also consistent with the finding that neurons undergoing prolonged stimulation of NMDA receptors can survive in the presence of $[Ca^{2+}]_i$ chelators. Very high levels of cytoplasmic Ca^{2+} are not necessarily neurotoxic, and an effective uptake of this element into mitochondria is required to trigger NMDA-receptor-stimulated neuronal death (Stout et al., 1998). Moreover, in rat globus pallidus, an AMPA-dose-response study has shown a dose-dependent increase in calcification, which was not accompanied by an increase in astrogliosis (Petegnief et al., 1999). In the hippocampus, AMPA induced a calcified area larger than the injured area. In this same structure, the selective adenosine-A2a-receptor antagonist 8-(3-chlorostyryl)-caffeine increased NMDA-induced neuronal loss while calcification was decreased (Robledo et al., 1999). All these data indicate that Ca^{2+} precipitation does not necessarily reflect neuronal death and that, as proposed for retinal excitotoxic damage (Chen et al., 1999), in addition to Ca^{2+} other factors such as Na^+ and Cl^- influx, cell swelling and acidosis induce excitotoxic neuronal damage.

3. Conclusions

Neurodegenerative disorders are characterized by the appearance of distinct neurodegenerative parameters that determine the induction of a chronic process with underlying glutamate-mediated excitotoxicity and Ca^{2+} dys-homeostasis. At tissue level, the pathogenesis of each disorder depends on the neuronal type involved, synaptic density, glial interactions, and vicinity of vascularization. For each neuron, astrocyte and microglial type, the group of glutamate and cytokine receptors, the Ca^{2+} binding protein content, protein phosphorylation levels, and all elements that participate in energy needs and glucose availability will constitute the factors involved in the appearance of the lesion. In this scenario, CNS calcification can be considered one of the few common mechanisms already available at an early age to help buffer disturbances in Ca^{2+} homeostasis at no energy cost. Over time, CNS maturation includes a massive increase in synaptic connections, the organization of inhibitory systems and greater cellular complexity. As it becomes more sophisticated, the CNS relies on a greater diversity of mechanisms to prevent CNS injury. This would explain why calcification is observed in neurodegenerative diseases, but does not correlate with CNS damage.

4. Acknowledgements

This research was supported by grants SAF2008-01902 and IPT-010000-2010-35 from the Ministerio de Ciencia e Innovación, and by grant 2009SGR1380 from the Generalitat de Catalunya, Spain.

5. References

Agostinho, P., Cunha, R.A. & Oliveira, C. (2010). Neuroinflammation, oxidative stress and the pathogenesis of Alzheimer's disease. *Curr Pharm Des*, Vol. 16, No. 25, pp. 2766-78, ISSN 1873-4286

Allaman, I., Belanger, M. & Magistretti, P.J. (2011). Astrocyte-neuron metabolic relationships: for better and for worse. *Trends Neurosci*, Vol. 34, No. 2, pp. 76-87, ISSN 1878-108X

Andre-Frei, V., Chevallay, B., Orly, I., Boundeulle, M., Huc, A. & Herbage, D. (2000). Acellular mineral deposition in collagen-based biomaterials incubated in cell culture media. *Calc Tissue Int*, Vol. 66, No. pp. 204-211, ISSN 1432-0827

Andrés, N., Rodríguez, M.J., Andrade, C., Rowe, W., Quirion, R. & Mahy, N. (2000). Increase in AMPA receptors in aged memory-impaired rats is not associated with increase in monoamine oxidase B levels. *Neuroscience*, Vol. 101, No. 4, pp. 807-810, ISSN 0306-4522

Arundine, M. & Tymianski, M. (2003). Molecular mechanisms of calcium-dependent neurodegeneration in excitotoxicity. *Cell Calcium*, Vol. 34, No. 4-5, pp. 325-337, ISSN 0143-4160

Arundine, M. & Tymianski, M. (2004). Molecular mechanisms of glutamate-dependent neurodegeneration in ischemia and traumatic brain injury. *Cell Mol Life Sci*, Vol. 61 No. 6, pp. 657-668, ISSN 1420-682X

Barat, R., Montoya, T., Seco, A. & Ferrer, J. (2011). Modelling biological and chemically induced precipitation of calcium phosphate in enhanced biological phosphorus removal systems. *Water Res*, Vol. 45, No. 12, pp. 3744-52, ISSN 1879-2448

Beck, A., Nieden, R.Z., Scheinder, H.P. & Deitmer, J.W. (2004). Calcium release from intracellular stores in rodent astrocytes and neurons in situ. *Cell Calcium*, Vol. 35 No. pp. 47-58, ISSN 0143-4160

Beers, D.R., Henkel, J.S., Zhao, W., Wang, J., Huang, A., Wen, S., Liao, B. & Appel, S.H. (2011). Endogenous regulatory T lymphocytes ameliorate amyotrophic lateral sclerosis in mice and correlate with disease progression in patients with amyotrophic lateral sclerosis. *Brain*, Vol. 134, No. Pt 5, pp. 1293-314, ISSN 1460-2156

Bernal, F., Andrés, N., Samuel, D., Kerkerian-Legoff, L. & Mahy, N. (2000a). Age-related resistance to α-amino-3-hydroxy-5-methyl-4-isoxazole propionic acid-induced hippocampal lesion. *Hippocampus*, Vol. 10, No. pp. 296-304, ISSN 1098-1063

Bernal, F., Petegnief, V., Rodriguez, M.J., Ursu, G., Pugliese, M. & Mahy, N. (2009). Nimodipine inhibits TMB-8 potentiation of AMPA-induced hippocampal neurodegeneration. *J Neurosci Res*, Vol. 87, No. 5, pp. 1240-1249, ISSN 0360-4012

Bernal, F., Saura, J., Ojuel, J. & Mahy, N. (2000b). Differential vulnerability of hippocampus, basal ganglia and prefrontal cortex to long-term NMDA excitotoxicity. *Exp Neurol*, Vol. 161, No. pp. 686-695, ISSN 0014-4886

Bernardino, L., Agasse, F., Silva, B., Ferreira, R., Grade, S. & Malva, J.O. (2008). Tumor necrosis factor-alpha modulates survival, proliferation, and neuronal differentiation in neonatal subventricular zone cell cultures. *Stem Cells*, Vol. 26, No. 9, pp. 2361-2371, ISSN 1066-5099

Bianchi, R., Giambanco, I. & Donato, R. (2010). S100B/RAGE-dependent activation of microglia via NF-kappaB and AP-1 Co-regulation of COX-2 expression by S100B, IL-1beta and TNF-alpha. *Neurobiol Aging*, Vol. 31, No. 4, pp. 665-77, ISSN 1558-1497

Block, M.L., Zecca, L. & Hong, J.S. (2007). Microglia-mediated neurotoxicity: uncovering the molecular mechanisms. *Nat Rev Neurosci*, Vol. 8, No. pp. 57-69, ISSN 1471-003X

Boatell, M.L., Bendahan, G. & Mahy, N. (1995). Time-related cortical amino acid changes after basal forebrain lesion: a microdialysis study. *J Neurochem*, Vol. 64, No. 1, pp. 285-291, ISSN 0022-3042

Boatell, M.L., Lindefors, N., Ballarín, M., Ernforns, P., Mahy, N. & Persson, H. (1992). Activation of basal forebrain cholinergic neurons differentially regulates brain-derived neurotrophic factor mRNA expression in different projection areas. *Neurosci Letters*, Vol. 136, No. pp. 203-208, ISSN 0304-3940

Brouillet, E., Jenkins, B.G., Hyman, B.T., Ferrante, R.J., Kowall, N.W., Srivastava, R., Roy, D.S., Rosen, B.R. & Beal, M.F. (1993). Age-dependent vulnerability of the striatum to the mitochondrial toxin 3-nitropropionic acid. *J Neurochem*, Vol. 60, No. pp. 356-359, ISSN 0022-3042

Buzsáki, G. (2006). *Rhyrhms of the brain* Oxford University Press, ISBN 0195301064, Oxford

Chan, S.L., Liu, D., Kyriazis, G.A., Bagsiyao, P., Ouyang, X. & Mattson, M.P. (2007a). Mitochondrial uncoupling protein-4 regulates calcium homeostasis and sensitivity to store-depletion-induced apoptosis in neural cells. *J Biol Chem*, Vol. 281, No. 49 pp. 3739-37403, ISSN 0021-9258

Chan, W.Y., Kohsaka, S. & Rezaie, P. (2007b). The origin and cell lineage of microglia: new concepts. *Brain Res Rev*, Vol. 53, No. 2, pp. 344-54, ISSN 0165-0173

Chen, Q., Moulder, K., Tenkova, T., Hardy, K., Olney, J.W. & Romano, C. (1999). Excitotoxic cell death dependent on inhibitory receptor activation. *Exp Neurol*, Vol. 160, No. pp. 215-225, ISSN 0014-4886

Chen, Q., Olney, J.W., Lukasiewicz, P.D., Almli, T. & Romano, C. (1998). Ca2+-independent excitotoxic neurodegeneration in isolated retina, an intact neural net: a role for Cl- and inhibitory transmitters. *Mol Pharmacol*, Vol. 53, No. 3, pp. 564-572, ISSN 0026-895X

Chi, L., Ke, Y., Luo, C., Li, B., Gozal, D., Kalyanaraman, B. & Liu, R. (2006). Motor neuron degeneration promotes neural progenitor cell proliferation, migration, and neurogenesis in the spinal cords of amyotrophic lateral sclerosis mice. *Stem Cells*, Vol. 24, No. 1, pp. 34-43, ISSN 1066-5099

Coleman, P., Finch, C. & Joseph, J. (1990). The need for multiple time points in aging studies. *Neurobiol Aging*, Vol. 11, No. pp. 1-2, ISSN 0197-4580

Donato, R., Sorci, G., Riuzzi, F., Arcuri, C., Bianchi, R., Brozzi, F., Tubaro, C. & Giambanco, I. (2009). S100B's double life: intracellular regulator and extracellular signal. *Biochim Biophys Acta*, Vol. 1793, No. 6, pp. 1008-1022, ISSN 0006-3002

Edwards, M.M. & Robinson, S.R. (2006). TNF alpha affects the expression of GFAP and S100B: implications for Alzheimer's disease. *J Neural Transm*, Vol. 113, No. 11, pp. 1709-15, ISSN 0300-9564

Farina, C., Aloisi, F. & Meinl, E. (2007). Astrocytes are active players in cerebral innate immunity. *Trends Immunol*, Vol. 28, No. 3, pp. 138-45, ISSN 1471-4906

Fontaine, V., Mohand-Said, S., Hanoteau, N., Fuchs, C., Pfizenmaier, K. & Eisel, U. (2002). Neurodegenerative and neuroprotective effects of tumor Necrosis factor (TNF) in retinal ischemia: opposite roles of TNF receptor 1 and TNF receptor 2. *J Neurosci*, Vol. 22, No. 7, pp. RC216, ISSN 1529-2401

Graeber, M.B. (2010). Changing face of microglia. *Science*, Vol. 330, No. 6005, pp. 783-8, ISSN 1095-9203

Graeber, M.B. & Streit, W.J. (2010). Microglia: biology and pathology. *Acta Neuropathol*, Vol. 119, No. 1, pp. 89-105, ISSN 1432-0533

Haider, L., Fischer, M.T., Frischer, J.M., Bauer, J., Hoftberger, R., Botond, G., Esterbauer, H., Binder, C.J., Witztum, J.L. & Lassmann, H. (2011). Oxidative damage in multiple sclerosis lesions. *Brain*, Vol. 134, No. Pt 7, pp. 1914-24, ISSN 1460-2156

Halliday, G.M. & Stevens, C.H. (2011). Glia: initiators and progressors of pathology in Parkinson's disease. *Mov Disord*, Vol. 26, No. 1, pp. 6-17, ISSN 1531-8257

Hashimoto, N., Takeuchi, T., Ishihara, R., Ukai, K., Kobayashi, H., Iwata, H., Iwai, K., Mizuno, Y., Yamaguchi, H. & Shibayama, H. (2003). Glial fibrillary tangles in diffuse neurofibrillary tangles with calcification. *Acta Neuropathol*, Vol. 106, No. 2, pp. 150-156, ISSN 0001-6322

Henkel, J.S., Beers, D.R., Zhao, W. & Appel, S.H. (2009). Microglia in ALS: the good, the bad, and the resting. *J Neuroimmune Pharmacol*, Vol. 4, No. 4, pp. 389-98, ISSN 1557-1904

Herrera, A.J., Castano, A., Venero, J.L., Cano, J. & Machado, A. (2000). The single intranigral injection of LPS as a new model for studying the selective effects of inflammatory reactions on dopaminergic system. *Neurobiol Dis*, Vol. 7, No. 4, pp. 429-47, ISSN 0969-9961

Hertz, L. (2008). Bioenergetics of cerebral ischemia: a cellular perspective. *Neuropharmacology*, Vol. 55, No. 3, pp. 289-309, ISSN 0028-3908

Hirsch, E.C. & Hunot, S. (2009). Neuroinflammation in Parkinson's disease: a target for neuroprotection? *Lancet Neurol*, Vol. 8, No. 4, pp. 382-97, ISSN 1474-4422

Katayama, Y., Maeda, T., Koshinaga, M., Kawamata, T. & Tsubokawa, T. (1995). Role of excitatory amino acid-mediated ionic fluxes in traumatic brain injury. *Brain Pathol*, Vol. 5, No. pp. 427-435, ISSN 1015-6305

Kesslak, J., Yuan, D., Neeper, S. & Cotman, C. (1995). Vulnerability of the hippocampus to kainate excitotoxicity in the aged, mature and young adult rat. *Neurosci Letters*, Vol. 188, No. pp. 117-120, ISSN 0304-3940

Kettenmann, H., Hanisch, U.K., Noda, M. & Verkhratsky, A. (2011). Physiology of microglia. *Physiol Rev*, Vol. 91, No. 2, pp. 461-553, ISSN 1522-1210

Kim, K.M. (1995). Apoptosis and calcification. *Scanning Microscopy*, Vol. 9, No. 4, pp. 1137-1178, ISSN 0891-7035

Kodaka, T., Mori, R., Debari, K. & Yamada, M. (1994). Scanning electron microscopy and electron probe microanalysis studies of human pineal concretions. *J Electron Microscopy*, Vol. 43, No. 5, pp. 307-317, ISSN 0022-0744

Le Jeune, H., Cçcyre, D., Rowe, W., Meaney, M.J. & Quirion, R. (1996). Ionotropic glutamate receptor subtypes in the aged memory-impaired and unimpaired Long-Evans rat. *Neuroscience*, Vol. 74, No. 2, pp. 349-363, ISSN 0306-4522

Li, C., Zhao, R., Gao, K., Wei, Z., Yin, M.Y., Lau, L.T., Chui, D. & Hoi Yu, A.C. (2011). Astrocytes: implications for neuroinflammatory pathogenesis of Alzheimer's disease. *Curr Alzheimer Res*, Vol. 8, No. 1, pp. 67-80, ISSN 1875-5828

Liévens, J.C., Bernal, F., Forni, C., Mahy, N. & Kerkerian-Legoff, L. (2000). Characterization of striatal lesions produced by glutamate uptake alteration: cell death, reactive gliosis and changes in GLT1 and GADD45 mRNA expression. *Glia*, Vol. 29, No. pp. 222-232, ISSN 1098-1136

Lull, M.E. & Block, M.L. (2010). Microglial activation and chronic neurodegeneration. *Neurotherapeutics*, Vol. 7, No. 4, pp. 354-65, ISSN 1878-7479

Mahy, N., Diaz, R., Andrés, N. & Fuxe, K. (1996). Ibotenic acid in the medial septum increases brain-derived neurotrophic factor mRNA levels in the dorsal rat hipocampal formation. *Neurosci Letters*, Vol. 213, No. pp. 169-172, ISSN 0304-3940

Mahy, N., Prats, A., Riveros, A., Andrés, N. & Bernal, F. (1999). Basal ganglia calcification induced by excitotoxicity: an experimental model characterised by electron microscopy and X-ray microanalysis. *Acta Neuropathol*, Vol. 98, No. 3, pp. 217-225, ISSN 0001-6322

Mates, J.M., Perez-Gomez, C., Nunez De Castro, I., Asenjo, M. & Marquez, J. (2002). Glutamine and its relationship with intracellular redox status, oxidative stress and cell proliferation/death. *Int J Biochem Cell Biol*, Vol. 34, No. 5, pp. 439-58, ISSN 1357-2725

Mattson, M.K. & Chan, S.L. (2003). Neuronal and glial calcium signalling in Alzheimer's disease. *Cell Calcium*, Vol. 34 No. pp. 385-397, ISSN 0143-4160

Mattson, M.P. (2006). Neuronal life-and-death signaling, apoptosis, and neurodegenerative disorders. *Antioxid Redox Signal.*, Vol. 8, No. 11-12, pp. 1997-2006, ISSN 1523-0864

Milligan, E.D. & Watkins, L.R. (2009). Pathological and protective roles of glia in chronic pain. *Nat Rev Neurosci*, Vol. 10, No. 1, pp. 23-36, ISSN 1471-0048

Mullany, P., Connolly, S. & Lynch, M.A. (1996). Ageing is associated with changes in glutamate release, protein tyrosine kinase and Ca 2+ /calmodulin-dependent protein kinase II in rat hippocampus. *Eur J Pharmacol*, Vol. 309, No. pp. 311-315, ISSN 0014-2999

Nicolle, M.M., Bizon, J.L. & Gallagher, M. (1996). In vitro autoradiography of ionotropic glutamate receptors in hippocampus and striatum of aged Long-Evans rats: relationship to spatial learning. *Neuroscience*, Vol. 74, No. 3, pp. 741-756, ISSN 0306-4522

Obrenovitch, T.P., Urenjak, J., Zilkha, E. & Jay, T.M. (2000). Excitotoxicity in neurological disorders--the glutamate paradox. *Int J Dev Neurosci*, Vol. 18, No. 2-3, pp. 281-287, ISSN 0736-5748

Olney, J.W., Wozniak, D.F. & Farber, N.B. (1997). Excitotoxic neurodegeneration in Alzheimer disease. *Arch Neurol*, Vol. 54, No. pp. 1234-1240, ISSN 0003-9942

Ovanesov, M.V., Ayhan, Y., Wolbert, C., Moldovan, K., Sauder, C. & Pletnikov, M.V. (2008). Astrocytes play a key role in activation of microglia by persistent Borna disease virus infection. *J Neuroinflammation*, Vol. 5, No. pp. 50, ISSN 1742-2094

Pellerin, L., Bouzier-Sore, A.K., Aubert, A., Serres, S., Merle, M., Costalat, R. & Magistretti, P.J. (2007). Activity-dependent regulation of energy metabolism by astrocytes: an update. *Glia*, Vol. 55, No. 12, pp. 1251-1262, ISSN 1098-1136

Perry, V.H., Nicoll, J.A. & Holmes, C. (2010). Microglia in neurodegenerative disease. *Nat Rev Neurol*, Vol. 6, No. 4, pp. 193-201, ISSN 1759-4766

Petegnief, V., Saura, J., Dewar, D., Cummins, D.J., Dragunow, M. & Mahy, N. (1999). Long-term effects of alpha-amino-3-hydroxy-5-methyl-4-isoxazole propionate and 6-nitro-7-sulphamoylbenzo(f)quinoxaline-2,3-dione in the rat basal ganglia: calcification, changes in glutamate receptors and glial reactions. *Neuroscience*, Vol. 94, No. 1, pp. 105-115, ISSN 0306-4522

Petegnief, V., Ursu, G., Bernal, F. & Mahy, N. (2004). Nimodipine and TMB-8 potentiate the AMPA-induced lesion in the basal ganglia. *Neurochem Int*, Vol. 44 No. pp. 287-291, ISSN 0197-0186

Philips, T. & Robberecht, W. (2011). Neuroinflammation in amyotrophic lateral sclerosis: role of glial activation in motor neuron disease. *Lancet Neurol*, Vol. 10, No. 3, pp. 253-63, ISSN 1474-4465

Ramonet, D., De Yebra, L., Fredriksson, K., Bernal, F., Ribalta, T. & Mahy, N. (2006). Similar calcification process in acute and chronic human brain pathologies. *J Neurosci Res*, Vol. 83 No. pp. 147-156, ISSN 0360-4012

Ramonet, D., Pugliese, M., Rodríguez, M.J., De Yebra, L., Andrade, C., Adroer, R., Ribalta, T., Mascort, J. & Mahy, N. (2002). Calcium precipitation in acute and chronic brain diseases. *J Physiol-Paris*, Vol. 96, No. pp. 307-312, ISSN 0928-4257

Ramonet, D., Rodríguez, M.J., Fredriksson, K., Bernal, F. & Mahy, N. (2004). In vivo neuroprotective adaptation of the glutamate/glutamine cycle to neuronal death. *Hippocampus*, Vol. 14, No. 5, pp. 586-594, ISSN 1098-1063

Ransohoff, R.M. & Perry, V.H. (2009). Microglial physiology: unique stimuli, specialized responses. *Annu Rev Immunol*, Vol. 27, No. pp. 119-45, ISSN 0732-0582

Reali, C., Scintu, F., Pillai, R., Donato, R., Michetti, F. & Sogos, V. (2005). S100b counteracts effects of the neurotoxicant trimethyltin on astrocytes and microglia. *J Neurosci Res*, Vol. 81, No. 5, pp. 677-86, ISSN 0360-4012

Rivers, L.E., Young, K.M., Rizzi, M., Jamen, F., Psachoulia, K., Wade, A., Kessaris, N. & Richardson, W.D. (2008). PDGFRA/NG2 glia generate myelinating oligodendrocytes and piriform projection neurons in adult mice. *Nat Neurosci*, Vol. 11, No. 12, pp. 1392-401, ISSN 1546-1726

Robledo, P., Ursu, G. & Mahy, N. (1999). Effects of adenosine and gamma-aminobutyric acid A receptor antagonists on N -methyl-D-aspartate induced neurotoxicity in the rat hippocampus. *Hippocampus*, Vol. 9, No. 5, pp. 527-533, ISSN 1098-1063

Rodriguez, M.J., Bernal, F., Andres, N., Malpesa, Y. & Mahy, N. (2000). Excitatory amino acids and neurodegeneration: a hypothetical role of calcium precipitation. *Int J Dev Neurosci*, Vol. 18, No. 2-3, pp. 299-307, ISSN 0736-5748

Rodriguez, M.J., Martinez-Sanchez, M., Bernal, F. & Mahy, N. (2004). Heterogeneity between hippocampal and septal astroglia as a contributing factor to differential in vivo AMPA excitotoxicity. *J Neurosci Res*, Vol. 77, No. 3, pp. 344-353, ISSN 0360-4012

Rodriguez, M.J., Prats, A., Malpesa, Y., Andres, N., Pugliese, M., Batlle, M. & Mahy, N. (2009a). Pattern of injury with a graded excitotoxic insult and ensuing chronic medial septal damage in the rat brain. *J Neurotrauma*, Vol. 26, No. 10, pp. 1823-34, ISSN 1557-9042

Rodriguez, M.J., Pugliese, M. & Mahy, N. (2009b). Drug abuse, brain calcification and glutamate-induced neurodegeneration. *Curr Drug Abuse Rev*, Vol. 2, No. 1, pp. 99-112, ISSN 1874-4745

Rodriguez, M.J., Robledo, P., Andrade, C. & Mahy, N. (2005). In vivo co-ordinated interactions between inhibitory systems to control glutamate-mediated hippocampal excitability. *J Neurochem*, Vol. 95, No. 3, pp. 651-661, ISSN 0022-3042

Rodríguez, M.J., Ursu, G., Bernal, F., Cusí, V. & Mahy, N. (2001). Perinatal human hypoxia-ischemia vulnerability correlates with brain calcification. *Neurobiol Dis*, Vol. 8, No. pp. 59-68, ISSN 0969-9961

Safadi, M.A., Berezin, E.N., Farhat, C.K. & Carvalho, E.S. (2003). Clinical presentation and follow up of children with congenital toxoplasmosis in Brazil. *Braz J Infect Dis*, Vol. 7, No. 5, pp. 325-31, ISSN 1413-8670

Sapolsky, R.M. (2001). Cellular defenses against excitotoxic insults. *J Neurochem*, Vol. 76, No. pp. 1601-1611, ISSN 0022-3042

Saura, J., Andrés, N., Andrade, C., Ojuel, J., Eriksson, K. & Mahy, N. (1997). Biphasic and region-specific MAO-B response to aging in normal human brain. *Neurobiol Aging*, Vol. 18, No. 5, pp. 497-507, ISSN 0197-4580

Saura, J., Boatell, M.L., Bendahan, G. & Mahy, N. (1995). Calcium deposit formation and glial reaction in rat brain after ibotenic acid-induced basal forebrain lesion. *Eur J Neurosci*, Vol. 7, No. 7, pp. 1569-1578, ISSN 0953-816X

Saura, J., Richards, J. & Mahy, N. (1994). Age-related changes of MAO in BL/C57 mouse tissues: A quantitative radioautographic study. *J Neural Transm*, Vol. 41, No. pp. 89-94, ISSN 1435-1463

Schinder, A.F., Olson, E.C., Spitzer, N.C. & Montal, M. (1996). Mitochondrial dysfunction is a primary event in glutamate neurotoxicity. *J Neurosci*, Vol. 16, No. 19, pp. 6125-6133, ISSN 0270-6474

Schwartz, M., Butovsky, O., Bråck, W. & Hanisch, U.K. (2006). Microglial phenotype: is the commitment reversible? *Trends Neurosci*, Vol. 29 No. 2, pp. 68-74, ISSN 0166-2236

Seifert, G., Schilling, K. & Steinhñuser, C. (2006). Astrocyte dysfunction in neurological disorders: a molecular perspective. *Nat Rev Neurosci.*, Vol. 7, No. pp. 194-206, ISSN 1471-003X

Sibson, N.R., Dhankhar, A., Mason, G.F., Rothman, D.L., Behar, K.L. & Shulman, R.G. (1998). Stoichiometric coupling of brain glucose metabolism and glutamatergic neuronal activity. *Proc Natl Acad Sci USA*, Vol. 95, No. pp. 316-321, ISSN 0027-8424

Sofroniew, M.V. & Vinters, H.V. (2010). Astrocytes: biology and pathology. *Acta Neuropathol*, Vol. 119, No. 1, pp. 7-35, ISSN 1432-0533

Stoll, G., Jander, S. & Schroeter, M. (2002). Detrimental and beneficial effects of injury-induced inflammation and cytokine expression in the nervous system. *Adv Exp Med Biol*, Vol. 513, No. pp. 87-113, ISSN 0065-2598

Stout, A.K., Raphael, H.M., Kanterewicz, B.I., Klann, E. & Reynolds, I.J. (1998). Glutamate-induced neuron death requires mitochondrial calcium uptake. *Nat Neurosci*, Vol. 1, No. 5, pp. 366-373, ISSN 1097-6256

Streit, W.J., Mark, R. & Griffin, S. (2004). Microglia and neuroinflammation: a pathological perspective. *J Neuroinflamation*, Vol. 1, No. pp. 14-17, ISSN 1742-2094

Surendrababu, N.R., Kuruvilla, K.A., Jana, A.K. & Cherian, R. (2006). Globe calcification in congenital toxoplasmosis. *Indian J Pediatr*, Vol. 73, No. 6, pp. 527-8, ISSN 0973-7693

Suzumura, A., Takeuchi, H., Zhang, G., Kuno, R. & Mizuno, T. (2006). Roles of glia-derived cytokines on neuronal degeneration and regeneration. *Ann N Y Acad Sci*, Vol. 1088, No. pp. 219-29, ISSN 0077-8923

Tanuma, N., Sakuma, H., Sasaki, A. & Matsumoto, Y. (2006). Chemokine expression by astrocytes plays a role in microglia/macrophage activation and subsequent neurodegeneration in secondary progressive multiple sclerosis. *Acta Neuropathol*, Vol. 112, No. 2, pp. 195-204, ISSN 0001-6322

Tramontina, F., Tramontina, A.C., Souza, D.F., Leite, M.C., Gottfried, C., Souza, D.O., Wofchuk, S.T. & Goncalves, C.A. (2006). Glutamate uptake is stimulated by extracellular S100B in hippocampal astrocytes. *Cell Mol Neurobiol*, Vol. 26, No. 1, pp. 81-6, ISSN 0272-4340

Van Eldik, L.J. & Wainwright, M.S. (2003). The Janus face of glial-derived S100B: beneficial and detrimental functions in the brain. *Restor Neurol Neurosci*, Vol. 21, No. 3-4, pp. 97-108, ISSN 0922-6028

Verkhratsky, A.J. (2007). Calcium and cell death. *Subcell Biochem.*, Vol. 45, No. pp. 465-480, ISSN 0096-8757

Verkhratsky, A.J. (2005). Physiology and pathophysiology of the calcium store in the endoplasmic reticulum of neurons. *Physiol Rev*, Vol. 85 No. pp. 201-279, ISSN 0031-9333

Villa, A., Podini, P., Panzeri, M.C., Racchetti, G. & Meldolesi, J. (1994). Cytosolic Ca^{2+} binding proteins during rat brain ageing: loss of calbindin and calretinin in the hippocampus, with no change in the cerebellum. *Eur J Neurosci*, Vol. 6, No. pp. 1491-1499, ISSN 0953-816X

Wake, H., Moorhouse, A.J., Jinno, S., Kohsaka, S. & Nabekura, J. (2009). Resting microglia directly monitor the functional state of synapses in vivo and determine the fate of ischemic terminals. *J Neurosci*, Vol. 29, No. 13, pp. 3974-80, ISSN 1529-2401

14

Analysis of the Impact of CD200 on Neurodegenerative Diseases

Anne-Marie Miller[1], Brian F. Deighan[1], Eric Downer[1], Anthony Lyons[1]
Petra Henrich-Noack[1], Yvonne Nolan[2] and Marina A. Lynch[1]
[1]Trinity College Institute of Neuroscience, Trinity College Dublin
[2]University College, Cork,
Ireland

1. Introduction

Neuroinflammation, accompanied by neuronal loss and dysfunction, is a characteristic of neurodegenerative disorders like Alzheimer's disease (AD) and Parkinson's disease (PD). It is well documented that inappropriate activation of glia is the primary cause of neuroinflammation (Masocha, 2009), but their role in the pathogenesis of neurodegenerative diseases is not known. However it is certainly the case that dying neurons act to stimulate glia since they release alarmins which activate pathogen recognition receptors (PRR) and therefore the possibility exists that activation of glia especially microglia, may be a consequence, rather than a cause, of neurodegenerative processes which characterize diseases like AD and PD. Understanding microglial function remains a major goal since it is widely believed that modulating glial function will provide a possible strategy for limiting the progression of neurodegenerative diseases. Consequently it is imperative to increase our understanding of the factors which control microglial function and the mechanisms by which expression of these factors are controlled.

2. Microglia adopt different activation states

Secreted factors including neurotrophins and growth factors like transforming growth factor (TGF)-β, as well as anti-inflammatory cytokines, impact on microglial activation and help to maintain these cells in a relatively quiescent state. Similarly, the interaction of microglia with other cells affects their activation state. However the recognition that macrophages, the peripheral cells which are derived from the same myeloid precursors as microglia, adopt different activation states has led to the acknowledgement that microglia can also adopt different activation states (Gordon, 2003). As the primary immune cells in the brain, microglia express PRR and therefore pathogen-associated molecular patterns (PAMPs) or damage-associated molecular patterns (DAMPs) interact with these receptors and trigger the innate immune response (Blasko et al., 2004, Koenigsknecht and Landreth, 2004). Microglia, like macrophages, are activated by the secreted proinflammatory cytokine, interferon-γ (IFNγ) inducing classical activation, and by the anti-inflammatory cytokines interleukin (IL)-4 and IL-13 to induce the alternative activation state (Gordon, 2003). Humoral activation of microglia, involving the complement system has also been described

(Griffiths et al., 2010). In addition to the modulatory effect of secreted factors like pro- and anti-inflammatory cytokines and factors like TGFβ, a deactivation/suppression state of microglia has been described, and this state is controlled by neuroimmunoregulatory proteins (NIRegs).

2.1 Neuroimmunoregulatory proteins modulate microglial activation

NIRegs act on specific receptors expressed on microglia and ensure that cell activation is checked. These NIRegs include CD200, CD22, CD47, semaphorin and fractalkine which interact with CD200R, CD45, SIRPα, plexin B1 or CD72, and fractalkine receptor respectively. In most of these cases, expression of the receptors is relatively restricted to cells of the myeloid lineage, whereas expression of the ligands is more widespread.

CD47 is a membrane glycoprotein and a member of the immunoglobulin superfamily. It is expressed on neurons and endothelial cells and its expression on macrophages has also been reported (Reinhold et al., 1995). CD47 is a 'don't eat me' signal and circulating cells lacking CD47 are rapidly cleared. Activation of SIRPα by CD47 leads to activation of an inhibitory signal as a consequence of the interaction between tyrosine phosphatases SHP-1 and SHP2 with cytoplasmic tyrosine-linked inhibition motifs (Hatherley et al., 2009). SIRPα, and another receptor for CD47, thrombospondin, are expressed on microglia, although SIRPα is also expressed on neurons (Brown and Frazier, 2001; Lamy et al., 2007).

CD45 is expressed on microglia, albeit at low levels when cells are unstimulated, contrasting with the higher expression on macrophages. It is a transmembrane protein tyrosine phosphatase which has been identified as a negative regulator of microglial activation (Tan et al., 2000). It has been known for 20 years that CD22 is a ligand for CD45 (Stamenkovic et al., 1991), but the fact that CD22 is expressed on neurons, and also released from neurons, has been established only relatively recently (Mott et al., 2004). These authors identified a role for CD22 in modulating tumour necrosis factor (TNF)-α release from microglia.

Fractalkine (also known as CX_3CL1) is the only member of the CX_3C subfamily of chemokines (Bazan et al., 1997). In the brain, it is expressed mainly on neurons (Harrison et al., 1998, Maciejewski-Lenoir et al., 1999), whereas its receptor is expressed chiefly on microglial cells (Harrison et al., 1998). However this expression pattern is probably not exclusive with evidence indicating that the ligand is expressed on glia (Maciejewski-Lenoir et al., 1999) and the receptor is expressed on neurons (Hughes et al., 2002). The engagement of fractalkine with its receptor decreases microglial activation and inhibits lipopolysaccharide (LPS)-induced proinflammatory cytokine production (Zujovic et al., 2000; Lyons et al., 2009a). Evidence from this laboratory suggested that fractalkine expression was decreased in hippocampal tissue prepared from aged rats in which microglial activation is upregulated, and that the combination of these changes was coupled with a deficit in neuronal plasticity (Lyons et al., 2009a).

Although they were originally identified because of their importance as axon guidance molecules, an immunoregulatory role for some semaphorins has been described (Suzuki et al., 2008). SEMA4D (also referred to as CD100), a transmembrane protein which belongs to class 4 group of the semaphorin family, has been the focus of the studies designed to understand this immunomodulatory role. It is expressed on neurons, though not on microglia (Hirsch et al., 1999), whereas the 2 major receptors for SEMA4D, plexin B1 and CD72 are expressed on microglia (Toguchi et al., 2009). Soluble Sema4D inhibits LPS-induced microglial activation as assessed by a change in cell morphology, nitric oxide (NO) production and cell migration (Toguchi et al., 2009). It also prevents migration of monocytes as a consequence of its interaction with plexin B1 (Chabbert-de Ponnat et al., 2005). However, in complete contrast to these findings, a Sema4D fusion protein has been reported to increase NO production in microglia and this was abolished in cells prepared from plexin B1-deficient mice (Okuno et al., 2010). The possible role of SEMA4D as a regulator of microglial function requires further examination.

3. CD200 and CD200R

3.1 Expression of CD200 and its receptor

Interest in understanding the roles of the NIRegs identified above has been increasing in the past few years and, to date, most emphasis has been placed on evaluating the role of the interaction between CD200 and its receptor on microglial activation. This interaction is recognized as a potent immune suppressor and therefore it is predicted that reduced inhibitory input from CD200 results in dysregulation of microglial function and the risk of inappropriate cellular activation and tissue damage.

CD200, previously known as OX2, is a 41-47 kDa type-1 cell surface glycoprotein with two immunoglobulin domains arranged in a typical V-/C2 set (Clark et al., 1985). The family of IgSF glycoproteins to which CD200 belongs includes neural cell adhesion molecule (NCAM), Thy-1 and L1, which are expressed on both lymphoid tissue and also neuronal tissue; CD200 was originally identified in the thymus and brain (Barclay, 1981) and thereafter in several tissues, and cells including neurons, T cells and astrocytes (Webb and Barclay, 1984, Preston et al., 1997, Wright et al., 2000). Expression of CD200 on vascular endothelium has been described with evidence of more intense staining on veins and venules rather than arteries, although staining in arteries was increased following injection with LPS. Distribution of CD200 in capillaries appears to be tissue-dependent and varies with the type of capillary; thus intense immunoreactivity is observed in continuous endothelia (both fenestrated and non-fenestrated) compared with relatively lower expression on discontinuous endothelia. Interestingly it has been shown that an anti-CD200 antibody blocked the adhesion of T cells to endothelial cells but did not affect the adhesion of macrophages; thus it was suggested that, whereas the primary role of the interaction between CD200 and its receptor may be to reduce activity of macrophages, a second role may be to modulate adhesion and migration of T cells into tissues (Ko et al., 2009). CD200 expression has also been examined on endothelial cells in the brain and it has been reported that expression in the hippocampus was evident only on the luminal surface of endothelial cells that made up the blood brain barrier (BBB), whereas in the area postrema, which lacks a BBB, clear staining was observed on the luminal and abluminal surfaces (Ko et al., 2009).

CD200 expression in brain tissue was found to be widespread with stronger staining in grey matter compared with white matter (Webb and Barclay, 1984). Immunostaining has been reported in the spinal cord, cerebellum and striatum, as well as the hippocampus and parietal cortex, and the evidence suggested that while it was expressed on the cell membrane in most brain areas, there was evidence of CD200 staining in the cytosol in hippocampal neurons. In the spinal cord, axons were CD200-positive whereas myelin did not stain for CD200 (Koning et al., 2009).

CD200 receptor (CD200R), CD200's cognate receptor is also a glycoprotein and, like the ligand, it contains two IgSF domains in a V/C2 set arrangement and cysteine residues in their V-like domains. To date, 5 CD200R family members (R1-R5) have been identified in mice (Gorczynski et al., 2008). The most studied receptor, CD200R1, is expressed primarily on myeloid lineage cells such as microglia and macrophages (Meuth et al., 2008, Masocha, 2009) and also monocytes, granulocytes and dendritic cells (DC) (Wright et al., 2000, Wright et al., 2003). More recent flow cytometry data suggest that CD200R is also expressed on natural killer cells and B cells, as well as on CD4+ T cells which had been reported previously (Wright et al., 2003, Rijkers et al., 2008). It was suggested that CD200 is the natural ligand for only CD200R1 (Wright et al., 2003) although others suggest that this may not be the case (Gorczynski et al., 2004).

3.2 The signaling events induced by CD200R activation

Most inhibitory receptors contain immunoreceptor tyrosine-based inhibitory motifs (ITIM) which enables cell signalling through recruitment of Src homology 2 domain containing phosphatases (SHP), or SHIP, which is an inositol phosphataseSH2-containing inositol phosphatase (SHIP). This is not the case with CD200R; instead, CD200R has a long cytoplasmic tail of 67 amino acids (Figure 1).

This longer cytoplasmic domain on CD200R contrasts with the short intracellular domain of CD200, which contains 19 amino acids and no signalling motifs (Barclay et al., 2002). The cytoplasmic tail of CD200R includes an NPXY signalling motif which interacts with the phosphotyrosine-binding (PTB) domains present in several signalling adaptor molecules (Wright et al., 2000). The NPXY signalling motif contains 3 tyrosine residues, which are phosphorylated following the interaction between CD200 and CD200R (Wright *et al.*, 2000: Snelgrove *et al.*, 2008). This initiates a signaling cascade, which involves recruitment and phosphorylation of adaptor proteins, downstream of tyrosine kinase (Dok) 1 and Dok 2 and the subsequent binding to RasGAP and SHIP (Mihrshahi et al., 2009); the downstream events include inhibition of the Ras/mitogen-activated protein kinase (MAPK) pathway (Zhang et al., 2004). Ultimately this results in a decrease in release of inflammatory cytokines. Thus CD200R agonists inhibited IFNγ-induced release of TNFα from peritoneal macrophages, although no effect on LPS-induced release was observed (Jenmalm et al., 2006). These agonists also increased IFNγ-induced and IL-17-induced release of IL-6, although production of monocyte chemoattractant protein-1 (MCP-1) was unaffected. Tetanus toxin-induced production of IL-5 and IL-13, but not other cytokines, was inhibited by CD200R agonists (Jenmalm et al., 2006). The effects of these agonists were cell-specific; activation of DC by several stimuli, including LPS and inflammatory cytokines, increased numerous markers of cell activation and resulted in release of many cytokines but these changes were resistant to modulation by CD200R agonists.

Recent evidence suggests that Dok 1 negatively regulates Dok 2-induced signalling (Mihrshahi and Brown, 2010) and that the negative regulation induced by CD200R activation is mediated by sequential activation of Dok 2 and RasGAP (Mihrshahi et al., 2009).

3.3 Characteristics of CD200-deficient mice

Deletion of the CD200 gene in mice provided a significant insight into the role of CD200 with the important observation that susceptibility of these mice to autoimmune diseases was markedly increased, with evidence of upregulated inflammatory responses (Hoek et al., 2000). The population of macrophages was increased in these animals and there was evidence of an enhanced activation state, even under resting conditions (Hoek et al., 2000). Specifically, macrophage numbers in the spleen and mesenteric lymph nodes were increased

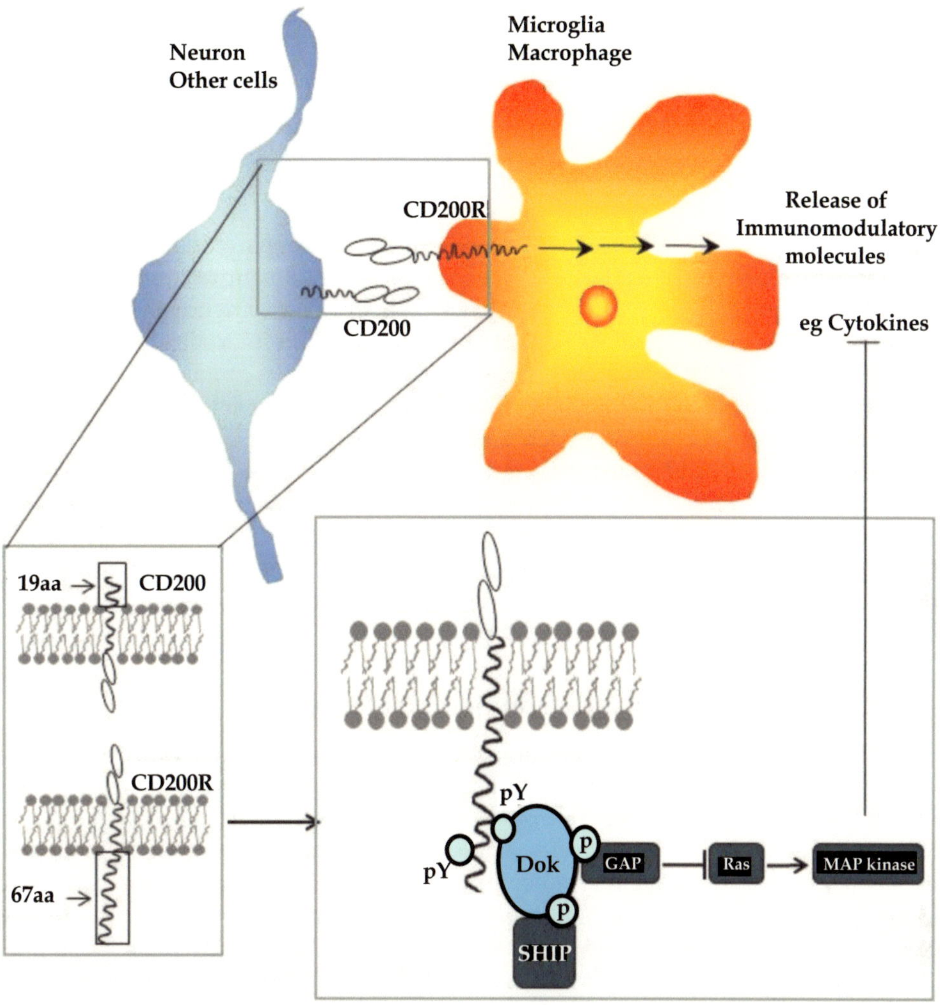

Fig. 1. CD200-induced signalling downregulates glial production of inflammatory cytokines. CD200 is expressed on several cell types including neurons and endothelial cells whereas expression of CD200R is relatively restricted to cells of the myeloid lineage. CD200 has a short cytosolic domain with no signalling capability whereas the signalling motif in the cytosolic domain of CD200R contains 3 tyrosine residues which, when phosphorylated, recruits Dok 1and Dok 2 which leads to activation of SHIP and RasGAP respectively, the latter of which leads to inhibition of MAP kinases thereby permitting increased production of inflammatory cytokines

and a defect in the organization of the mesenteric lymph nodes was described (Barclay et al., 2002). The findings of these studies indicated that CD200R activation provides a mechanism for negatively modulating cell responses and controlling responses of cells to immunological stimuli. An increase in the activation state of microglia was also reported with evidence of increased expression of CD11b and CD45, and the response of microglia to trauma is markedly enhanced in CD200-deficient mice where activated microglia cluster around the lesion area (Hoek et al., 2000). The clustering of activated macrophages or microglia in tissues of CD200-deficient mice has suggested that CD200-CD200R interaction may not simply provide a mechanism by which these myeloid cells are maintained in a relatively quiescent state, but that this interaction may play a key role in controlling migration of cells (Nathan and Muller, 2001). Interestingly, one of the earliest papers on the actions of CD200 suggested that it was expressed on immature (as well as mature) neurons and that it may be involved in migration of these neurons during development of the CNS (Webb and Barclay, 1984).

Symptoms in several models of neurodegenerative and/or neuroinflammatory disease, or the responses to certain infections, or the effects of injury to neurons (detailed in Section 4 below) have been examined in CD200-deficient mice. The evidence consistently shows, across these experiments, that the symptoms are worse, the mortality rate is higher and activation of microglial cells or macrophages is more profound in CD200-deficient, compared with wildtype, mice. Thus CD200-deficient mice exhibit increased sensitivity to infections like influenza where evidence of greater macrophage activity was linked with prolonged symptoms and increased mortality (Snelgrove et al., 2008) and to *Toxoplasma gondii* where the increased macrophage infiltration, accompanied by increased activation of these cells and also microglia, was associated with poorer survival rates (Deckert et al., 2006). In a striking parallel with microglia from CD200-deficient mice, microglia prepared from mice lacking either Dok 1 or Dok 2 also respond more profoundly to LPS than cells from wildtype mice (Shinohara et al., 2005).

4. CD200 functions as a neuroimmunoregulatory protein

4.1 CD200-CD200R interaction maintains microglia in a quiescent state

The findings of several experiments indicate that the interaction between CD200 and CD200R maintains microglia or macrophages in a quiescent state whereas the absence of CD200 is linked with evidence of cell activation and inflammatory changes. Evidence from this laboratory has revealed that co-culture of neurons with mixed glia inhibited LPS-induced increases in release of IL-1β, IL-6 and TNFα. The effect of neurons was blocked when the incubation was carried out in the presence of a blocking anti-CD200 antibody (Lyons et al., 2009b) pinpointing a role for CD200 in modulating cytokine release. Similarly, the Aβ-induced release of IL-1β, IL-6 and TNFα from mixed glia is inhibited when cells are co-cultured with neurons and this effect of neurons is also inhibited by the presence of a blocking anti-CD200 antibody (Lyons et al., 2007a).

One factor which increases CD200 expression is IL-4 and, interestingly, a marked reduction in CD200 expression has been reported on neurons prepared from IL-4-deficient mice (Lyons et al., 2009b). Predictably, therefore, co-incubation of mixed glia with neurons prepared from IL-4-deficient mice did not attenuate Aβ-induced production of inflammatory cytokines (Lyons et al., 2009b), contrasting with the effect of neurons prepared from wildtype mice. As highlighted above, endothelial cells express CD200 and, like neurons, incubation of LPS-treated mixed glia with endothelial cells inhibits the LPS-induced release of IL-1β from mixed glia (Figure 2).

4.2 The age-related increase in microglial activation is associated with decreased CD200 expression

It has been recognized for several years that microglial activation is increased in the brain with age; the evidence suggests that expression of markers of activation, for example MHCII

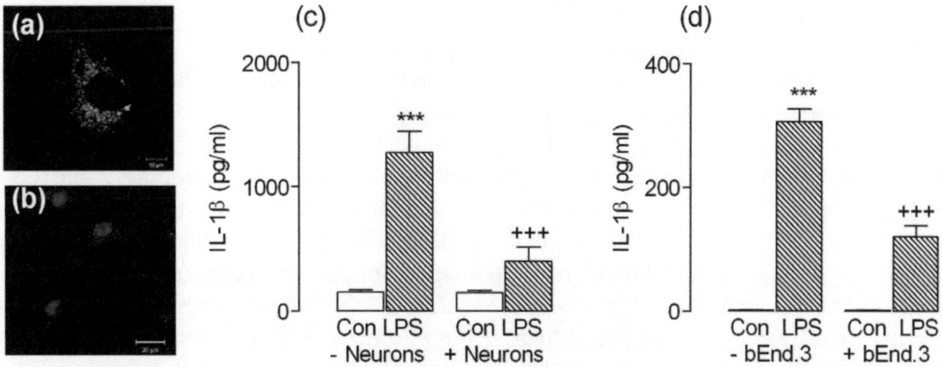

Fig. 2. Endothelial cells, which express CD200, modulate LPS-induced IL-1β production from glia in a manner which resembles the effect of neurons. a,b. Neurons (a) and endothelial cells (b; bEnd.3) express CD200. Mixed glia were incubated in the presence or absence of LPS (100ng/ml), and either neurons (1:2) or endothelial cells (bEnd.3; 1:8) were added. c,d. LPS significantly increased supernatant concentration of IL-1β (***$p < 0.001$; ANOVA) and this was significantly attenuated when mixed glia were co-cultured with either neurons or endothelial cells ($^{+++}p < 0.001$; ANOVA)

and CD11b, are increased in hippocampal and cortical tissue with age and these changes are accompanied by increased expression of inflammatory cytokines (Lynch, 2010). Evidence from this laboratory indicates that CD200 expression is decreased in hippocampal tissue prepared from aged, compared with young, rats. We have proposed that this significantly contributes to the age-related increase in microglial activation (Lyons et al., 2007a) and consequently the age-related decrease in synaptic plasticity, typified by the deficit in long-term potentiation (LTP). Recent evidence has revealed that intracerebroventricular injection of CD200Fc attenuated the age-related deficit in LTP (Cox et al., unpublished). Interestingly, amyloid-β (Aβ), which has been shown to decrease LTP (Lyons et al., 2007a, Lyons et al., 2007b) is associated with increased microglial activation as demonstrated by increased expression of the cell surface markers of microglial activation, MHCII (Lyons et al., 2007a, Lyons et al., 2007b), ICAM and CD86 (Clarke et al., 2007), increased production of inflammatory cytokines, IFNγ and IL-1β (Minogue et al., 2007) and increased production of chemokines MCP-1 and IP-10 (Clarke et al., 2007). Significantly Aβ also decreases CD200 expression *in vitro* while expression of CD200 is also decreased in hippocampal tissue prepared from rats which received an intracerebroventricular injection of Aβ (Lyons et al., 2007a).

4.3 CD200 is a protective molecule during apoptosis

Apoptosis is an ongoing process which is necessary to permit natural cell turnover. It is important to ensure that this occurs without production of inflammatory cytokines which can negatively impact on cells in the microenvironment; a key factor in ensuring maintenance of this steady state is the expression of immunoregulatory signals. Like other peripheral cells, apoptosis of DC occurs on an ongoing basis and, experimentally, apoptosis can be induced by growth factor deprivaton. Recent data have indicated that up to 75% of apoptotic $CD11c^+$ cells express CD200, whereas about one third of non-apoptotic $CD11c^+$ cells express CD200; the evidence indicates that expression of CD200 is p53- and caspase-dependent. Similarly γ-irradiation, which induces apoptosis in C1498 leukemia cells, is associated with increased expression of CD200 (Rosenblum et al., 2004).

It has been proposed that CD200 also plays a role in tolerance. This has been demonstrated in a model of contact hypersensitivity which is induced by 2,4-dinitro-fluorobenzene. In this model, the inflammatory changes which typify contact hypersensitivity are attenuated by prior exposure to low dose ultraviolet light (UVB) and it has been proposed that UVB-induced apoptosis of epidermal DCs is the key to this tolerance. Significantly, and consistent with the findings obtained in vitro, this is dependent on CD200, since tolerance was absent when this experiment was conducted in CD200-deficient mice. The data suggest that CD200-CD200R interaction may be a key event in ensuring that inflammatory changes do not accompany steady-state ongoing apoptosis (Rosenblum et al., 2004). Interestingly several studies have highlighted a role for CD200 in tolerance following transplants (Clark et al., 2008, Gorczynski et al., 2009)

5. The importance of the interaction between CD200 and CD200R in modulating inflammation

CD200-CD200R interaction provides a regulatory signal to macrophages (Broderick *et al.*, 2002) and consequently macrophage numbers in the spleen are increased in CD200$^{-/-}$ mice compared with wildtype mice, while CD200$^{-/-}$ mice also have enlarged lymph nodes (Hoek et al., 2000). A similar regulatory signal modulates microglia and therefore the absence of CD200 is associated with microglial activation. Thus cells prepared from CD200$^{-/-}$ mice exhibited an activated phenotype, and had less ramified morphology and shorter processes, as well as increased expression of cell surface markers, CD11b and CD45, which are indicative of activation (Hoek et al., 2000). Microglia from CD200$^{-/-}$ animals also appeared to form aggregates, which occurs in neuroinflammatory and neurodegenerative, but not under normal, conditions (Hoek et al., 2000). Predictably, cells prepared from CD200$^{-/-}$ mice exhibited a greater response to stimuli including LPS and Aβ (Lyons et al., 2007a). These data indicate that disruption of this interaction between CD200-CD200R results in dysregulation of macrophages and microglia, with cells shifting to a more tonically active state (Hoek *et al.*, 2000).

Evidence from experimental conditions associated with inflammatory changes and microglial activation, adds support to the finding that CD200-CD200R interaction is an important regulator of neuroimmune function. For example, *Toxoplasma gondii*-induced encephalitis is characterized by lymphocytic infiltrates and microglial activation and it has been reported that infection induced a more profound microglial proliferation and greater expression of markers of activation in CD200-deficient, compared with wildtype, mice (Deckert et al., 2006). In addition, nerve injury is associated with microglial activation and it has been reported that facial nerve transaction induced a greater degree of microglial activation in CD200-deficient, compared with wildtype, mice (Hoek et al., 2000). Similarly the neurodegenerative changes that occurred following sciatic nerve crush was associated with a profound loss of CD200 and evidence of macrophage activation (Chang et al., 2011).

5.1 CD200-CD200R interaction in inflammatory diseases and models of disease

One of the most clearcut consequences of the loss of the interaction between CD200 and CD200R is the development of inflammatory changes (Masocha 2009), and therefore, as described above, CD200$^{-/-}$ mice are more susceptible to inflammatory stimuli and exhibit exaggerated symptoms in models of autoimmune diseases (Feuer, 2007). The majority of studies which have examined the role of CD200 as a negative regulator of myeloid cells have focussed on three autoimmune disease models, collagen-induced arthritis (CIA), a model for rheumatoid arthritis, experimental autoimmune uveoretinitis (EAU), a murine model for uveitis and myelin oligodendrocyte glycoprotein (MOG)-induced experimental autoimmune encephalomyelitis (EAE), a model of multiple sclerosis.

5.1.1 CD200-CD200R interaction in CIA

Rheumatoid arthritis is a classical inflammatory disease of the joints, typified by infiltrates of inflammatory cells. The most widely-used model is CIA and the evidence indicates that the symptoms of the disease, including inflammation and joint pathology was much more severe in CD200$^{-/-}$ mice, compared with their wildtype counterparts (Hoek et al., 2000). In contrast, treatment of mice with recombinant CD200 at 3-day intervals, concomitant with collagen immunization, markedly reduced symptoms; this included a reduction in infiltration of inflammatory cells and reduced bone erosion (Melnyk et al., 2011). A similar reduction in the severity of the disease, pathology and production of inflammatory mediators was observed when mice were treated with CD200Fc (Simelyte et al., 2008). These findings suggest that an agonistic antibody to CD200R, as substitute for the CD200-CD200R interaction, might be a useful therapeutic strategy in CIA. Predictably, CD200Fc, an immunoadhensin, produced by fusing the extracellular domains of CD200 to a murine IgG2a Fc construct, decreases TNFα and IFNγ production following collagen injection and halted the progression of symptoms of CIA (Gorczynski et al., 2002).

5.1.2 CD200-CD200R interaction in EAU

EAU, which is induced by immunization with interphotoreceptor retinoid-binding protein, is characterized by destruction of the neuroretina and photoreceptors, and the evidence indicates that this is T cell mediated; the symptoms include leukocyte infiltration of the vitreous and retina, vasculitis and ultimately photoreceptor and ganglion cell death. Symptoms become evident more quickly and are more profound in CD200-/- mice, compared with wildtype animals with significant additional infiltration of CD45+ CD11b+ cells and evidence of photoreceptor death, coupled with increased expression of nitric oxide synthase (NOS)-2 (Broderick et al., 2002). These findings were replicated subsequently and extended to show that the progression of the disease was suppressed by an agonist CD200R antibody (Copland et al., 2007). The modulatory role for CD200 in EAU was also identified in a rat model and, in this case, the evidence indicated that blocking CD200-CD200R interaction by an antibody accelerated the onset and severity of symptoms (Banerjee and Dick, 2004). Experimentally-induced glaucoma, caused by injecting hypertonic saline into the superior episcleral aqueous drainage vein, is another inflammatory and degenerative condition of the eye which is associated with a time-related increase in microglial activation; like EAU a role for CD200-CD200R has been implicated by the finding that the microglial activation is coupled with a decrease in CD200 and evidence of retinal ganglion cell death (Taylor et al., 2011).

5.2 CD200-CD200R interaction and Multiple Sclerosis

Multiple sclerosis is a chronic, progressive, disabling autoimmune disease. The generally-accepted view is that the disease is caused by uncontrolled inflammatory T cell responses to self antigens (myelin) in the brain and spinal cord. This results in a cascade of events which triggers inflammation, as a consequence of microglial and macrophage activation, and is followed by demyelination and degeneration of axons. One of the characteristics of this disease is the presence of inflammatory plaques, which are detected by magnetic resonance imaging (MRI), and post mortem examination has established that the brain lesions are associated with the presence of inflammatory cells (Frohman et al., 2006).

5.2.1 What factors contribute to the pathogenesis of EAE?

A great deal of progress in understanding the mechanisms which precipitate the disease has been made by examining changes which trigger disease symptoms in the widely-used animal model of multiple sclerosis, EAE. EAE is induced by stimulating an immune response directed against CNS antigens, such as myelin basic protein (MBP), proteolipid protein (PLP) and myelin oligodendrocyte glycoprotein (MOG). EAE can be induced by immunisation with these myelin antigens in adjuvant or by adoptive transfer of myelin-specific T cells, both of which result in inflammatory infiltrates into the CNS and demyelination (Stromnes and Goverman, 2006).

Like multiple sclerosis, EAE is characterized by infiltration of macrophages and $CD4^+$ T cells into the CNS, accompanied by microglial activation which, together, are responsible for the temporary paralysis that typifies the disease. The symptoms have been shown to be exaggerated, and the onset of the symptoms is hastened, when CD200-CD200R interaction is attenuated (Hoek et al., 2000, Wright et al., 2000, Meuth et al., 2008). Specifically, initial symptoms following MOG injection appeared 2-3 days earlier in $CD200^{-/-}$ mice than in wildtype mice, and expression of iNOS and CD68 were markedly increased in spinal cord of these mice 7 days after immunization (Hoek et al., 2000), while more severe symptoms were also observed (Wright et al., 2000). Consistently, an anti-CD200R antibody increased the severity of the symptoms and, in parallel, increased T cell infiltration and macrophage numbers in the spinal cord of MOG-treated mice (Meuth et al., 2008). Furthermore, the Wld^s mouse, which exhibits unique protection against neurodegenerative conditions, including EAE, overexpresses CD200 (Chitnis *et al.*, 2007). Interestingly, CD200 expression was reported to be decreased, in parallel with another NIReg, CD47, in laser-dissected active lesions of the post mortem brain of individuals with multiple sclerosis, although CD200R expression was unchanged and there was also no evidence of a change in SIRPα expression (Koning et al., 2007). However more recent studies revealed that CD200 was expressed on astrocytes associated with lesions in multiple sclerosis (Koning et al., 2009).

5.2.2 The development of EAE is associated with altered CD200 expression

MOG-induced EAE is typified by the development of clinical signs which appear initially at about day 7 post-immunization; the well-defined changes progress from the initial flaccid paralysis manifest by a limp tail and developing to paralysis in hindlimbs and ultimately the forelimbs (Stromnes and Goverman, 2006). We have investigated the accompanying changes induced in microglial activation and CD200 in the spinal cord following immunization (Figure 3). CD40 mRNA, which is indicative of microglial activation, increased after immunization whereas CD200 mRNA expression decreased and a significant inverse relationship between the 2 measures was observed. IL-4, which modulates CD200 expression, was decreased at the end of the experiment, paralleling the change in CD200. Similar data were obtained in the hippocampus (not shown).

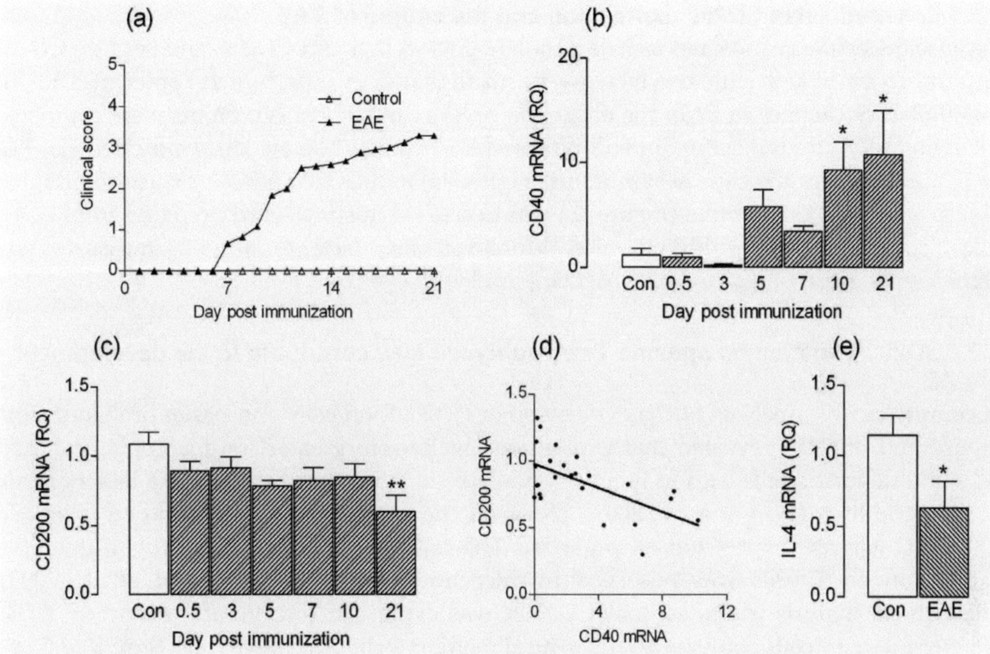

Fig. 3. Immunization with MOG increases microglial activation and decreases CD200 expression. Immunization of mice with MOG induced clinical signs which became evident after 7 days. This was accompanied, in the spinal cord, by a time-related increase in CD40 mRNA, which was significant 10 and 21 days post-immunization (*$p < 0.05$; ANOVA; Figure 3b) and a significant decrease in CD200 mRNA (**$p < 0.01$; ANOVA; Figure 3c). A significant inverse correlation between CD200 mRNA and CD40 mRNA is demonstrated ($p = 0.0017$; Figure 3d). IL-4 mRNA expression was significantly decreased in tissue prepared from animals with EAE (*$p< 0.05$; ANOVA; Figure 3e)

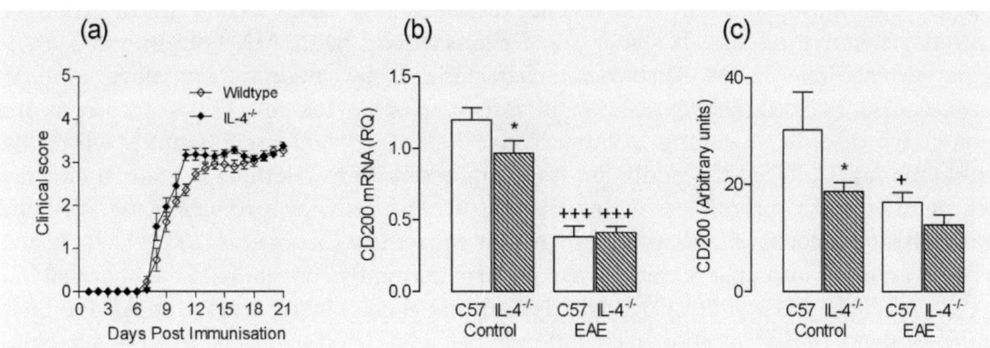

Fig. 4. The loss of IL-4 leads to more profound clinical symptoms of EAE. The symptoms of EAE developed more rapidly in IL-4-deficient mice compared with wildtype mice (Figure 3a). CD200 mRNA (Figure 3b) and CD200 protein (Figure 3c) were both decreased in tissue prepared from mice with EAE at the end of the 21-day experiment ($^+p < 0.05$; $^{+++}p < 0.001$; ANOVA; Figure 3b,c) and a decrease in both was identified in tissue prepared from IL-4-deficient, compared with wildtype, mice (*$p < 0.05$; ANOVA; Figure 3b,c)

5.2.3 IL-4 modulates CD200 expression and the course of EAE

Because the evidence indicates a close parallel between IL-4 and CD200, and because CD200 appears to be linked with the increase in microglial activation which contributes to the inflammatory changes in EAE, the onset and severity of clinical symptoms were compared following MOG immunization in wildtype and IL-4$^{-/-}$ mice. The evidence indicates that loss of IL-4 exacerbates the clinical symptoms (Figure 4a) and CD200 mRNA expression (Figure 4b), as well as CD200 protein (Figure 4c) was decreased in spinal cord prepared from IL-4$^{-/-}$ mice, compared with wildtype mice. Moreover, the decrease in both measures was significantly greater in mice with EAE compared with controls.

5.2.4 CD200R ligation on specific T cell subtypes may contribute to the development of EAE

A comprehensive analysis of the expression of CD200R on cells and tissue prepared from mouse and humans revealed that expression levels were greatest on macrophages, mast cells and dendritic cells, and in lymph nodes, spleen, bone marrow and, to a lesser extent, in lung and liver (Wright et al., 2003). However the receptor was also found on polarized Th2 cells, whereas expression on polarized Th1 cells was markedly less; this differential expression on T cells was observed in mice and human cells (Wright et al., 2003). Subsequent analysis indicated that CD200R was expressed to a greater extent on CD4$^+$ effector memory cells compared with central memory cells and naïve cells. Similarly CD8$^+$ central memory cells had higher expression than naïve cells (Rijkers et al., 2008). Clearly these findings suggest that CD200R ligation can modulate T cell function in addition to myeloid cell function; this may contribute to the exaggerated symptoms in autoimmune diseases, for example EAE.

6. Evidence of a role for CD200-CD200R interaction in other neurodegenerative diseases

6.1 Parkinson's Disease

PD is the most common movement disorder and the second most common neurodegenerative disease. It shares some characteristics with AD. Both are, at least to some extent, age-related disorders, characterized by neuroinflammatory changes accompanied by increased expression of inflammatory cytokines. PD is a chronic and progressive disorder, resulting in the selective loss of dopaminergic neurons within the substantia nigra (SN) of the midbrain. As the disease progresses there is gradual circuitry degeneration and neuronal loss within the nigrostriatal pathway, producing cognitive and psychiatric symptoms, as well as disturbances in movement (Braak et al, 2003). Cytoplasmic accumulations of insoluble proteins are likely to significantly contribute to the neuronal loss apparent in both AD and PD. Cognitive dysfunction is particularly marked in AD but there is also evidence of deterioration in cognition in PD. It has been suggested that the microglial activation which is prevalent in hippocampus and parahippocampal regions, coupled with the decrease in hippocampal volume (Laakso et al., 1996) and associated neuronal loss in the limbic areas (Emre, 2003a, b) may account for the cognitive dysfunction in PD. Although clinical trials have failed to show that NSAIDs are effective in treating AD or PD, epidemiological studies have suggested that chronic treatment with NSAIDs reduces the risk of both diseases suggesting that inflammatory changes may contribute to the progression of the diseases. Interestingly, the protective effects in AD may be confined to particular subpopulations. Recent retrospective studies indicated that statin therapy reduced the risk of developing PD and AD.

It is unclear whether microglial activation directly contributes to neuronal loss in PD (or indeed AD) but post mortem examination has established that activated microglia are clustered at high density in the SN (McGeer et al., 1988), the most vulnerable area of the brain in PD due to the low intracellular glutathione concentration and high iron level within nigrostriatal dopaminergic neurons (Sian et al., 1994). Indeed dopaminergic neurons are especially vulnerable to LPS-induced neurodegeneration (Smidt, 2009). Interestingly the number of MHCII-positive cells in this area increases in parallel with neuronal loss (Imamura *et al.* 2003). Similarly, an inverse relationship between ^{11}C-(R)-PK11195 binding (which is indicative of microglial activation) in the midbrain and binding of [^{11}C]CFT to the dopamine transporter (which reflects the viability of presynaptic dopaminergic neurons) in the putamen has been described. It has been reported that the combination of binding of these 2 tracers positively correlates with motor deficits in early PD (Ouchi *et al.* 2009). The correlative changes suggest a role for microglial activation in the pathogenesis of PD but do not address the question whether microglial activation plays an explicit role in dopaminergic cell death; animal models have been used to explore this. Environmental factors including pesticides have been implicated in the aetiology of PD and therefore experimental models of the disease include those in which animals are treated with rotenone or paraquat (Cicchetti et al., 2009); the loss of dopaminergic neurons in these models appears to be mediated by microglia since the superoxide which is considered to be pivotal to inducing cell damage was generated from microglia (Gao et al., 2002, Wu et al., 2005). Another animal model of PD involves prenatal exposure to LPS, which ultimately causes protracted inflammation and loss of dopaminergic neurons which progresses with subsequent insults; data from this model suggests that the priming of microglia is responsible for the ongoing degeneration and has led to the development of the 'multiple hit' hypothesis (Ling *et al.* 2006). An important tenet of this theory is that prolonged inflammation, rather than an acute inflammatory response, is responsible for the progressive neuronal loss (Park *et al.* 2009, Long-Smith et al. 2009). Interestingly, an age-related increase in microglial-activation in the SN has been reported (Beach et al., 2007) and the suggestion is that this 'priming' may contribute to development of the disease.

The most commonly-used models of PD which lead to neurodegeneration of dopaminergic neurons and induce Parkinson-like symptoms involve injection of rotenone or 6-hydroxydopamine (6-OHDA). It has recently been reported that rotenone+iron-induced dopaminergic neurotoxicity is mediated by microglia and that the toxicity is enhanced by a CD200R blocking antibody (Wang et al., 2011). The evidence indicated that microglia were the source of superoxide, that production was enhanced by the antibody and that inhibiting CD200R activation in microglia has detrimental effects on neuronal function. In addition to the Parkinson-like symptoms, injection of 6-OHDA also induces marked microglial activation (Long-Smith et al., 2009). These findings and the observations of other groups over many years (Chen et al., 1998, Le et al., 2001, Liu and Hong, 2003, Kim and Joh, 2006, Purisai et al., 2007) have provided significant support for the thesis that activated microglia play an important part in the onset and/or progression of PD.

In an effort to further address this question, and specifically to evaluate whether CD200 may play a role in modulating microglial activation which accompanies the loss of dopaminergic neurons following 6-OHDA injection, we examined the expression of CD200 in the ipsilateral and contralateral SN of rats following unilateral injection of 6-OHDA into the medial forebrain bundle. Immunocytochemical analysis of sections prepared from these animals revealed that there was marked dopaminergic cell loss in the side of the brain in which the 6-OHDA injection was made, as shown by decreased expression of tyrosine hydroxylase (Figure 5d), but that there was no evidence of cell loss on the contralateral side (Figure 5c). No cell loss was evident on either the ipsilateral or contralateral side of sham-treated rats Figure 5a,b). The data show that the marked 6-OHDA-induced dopaminergic cell loss in the ipsilateral SN was coupled with a marked decrease in CD200 expression (Figure 5d) whereas there was no discernible loss in the contralateral side of 6-OHDA-injected animals (Figure 5c) or the ipsilateral or contralateral side of sham-treated rats (Figure 5a,b). The loss of dopaminergic neurons was also associated with marked microglial activation as indicated by increased OX42 staining (red; Figure 5h); this is consistent with previous evidence indicating that loss of CD200 is linked with microglial activation (Lyons et al., 2007a). There was no evidence of microglial staining in sections prepared from the contralateral side of 6-OHDA-injected animals (Figure 5g) or the ipsilateral or contralateral side of sham-treated rats (Figure 5e,f).

6.2 Alzheimer's Disease

Despite an enormous effort, the molecular/cellular events which trigger AD remain unknown. It is undoubtedly the case that neuroinflammatory changes characterize the disease with evidence of profound microglial activation and, specifically, activated microglia and astrocytes clustered around Aβ-containing plaques (Xiang et al., 2006) and blood vessels (McGeer and McGeer, 2003) where amyloid deposits are also observed. As indicated above, several reports suggest that NSAID treatment reduces the risk of developing AD (McGeer and McGeer, 1999, Szekely et al., 2008, Vlad et al., 2008, Breitner et al., 2009) but NSAIDs are of little value in treating the disease. One possible explanation for this might be that inflammatory changes occur very early in the disease, prior to development of symptoms, and that preventing or delaying inflammation is beneficial because it is factor which contributes to the later neurodegenerative changes. A corollary to this previously-rehearsed proposal is that anti-inflammatory agents will not be beneficial once neurodegenerative changes are advanced. In support of this view, it has been consistently shown that inflammatory cytokines like IL-1β, IL-6 and TNFα negatively impact on neuronal and synaptic function (Lynch, 2010), and that these cytokines can contribute to neuronal cell death (Thornton et al., 2008, Long-Smith et al., 2010). Since activated glia, particularly microglia, are responsible for releasing these cytokines, it could be argued that targeting these cells might be a reasonable strategy for the treatment of AD, at least in its very early stages. This argument has been advanced by Walker and colleagues, who reported that CD200 expression was decreased in brains of individuals with AD. Thus sections prepared from inferior temporal gyrus of non-demented individuals exhibited colocalization of CD200 with NeuN but a marked loss of CD200 immunoreactivity was observed in sections prepared from post-mortem brains of AD patients. An AD-associated decrease in CD200R was also observed. Furthermore, the evidence suggested that the plaque density, and also the neurofibrillary tangle score, was inversely related to CD200R expression (Walker et al., 2009).

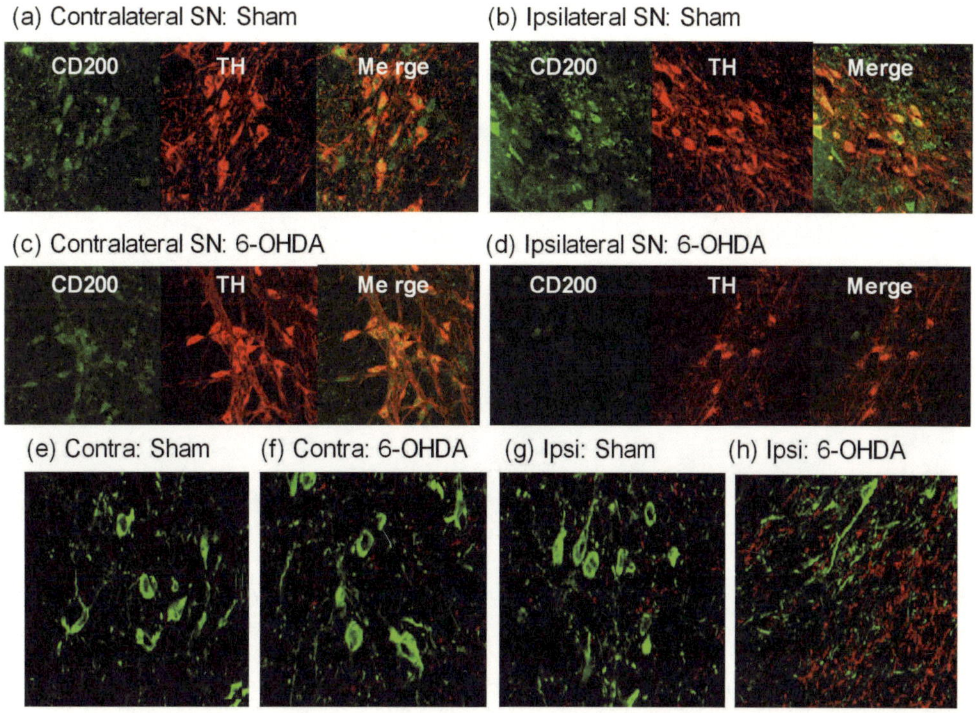

Fig. 5. 6-OHDA injection leads to dopaminergic cell loss and a marked reduction in CD200 immunoreactivity, coupled with microglial activation. Rats were anaesthetized with equal amounts of xylazine hydrochloride and ketamine hydrochloride (0.2ml/100g body weight; 1.5 ml of each compound dissolved in 7 ml PBS). Rats received a single injection of 6-OHDA (2μg/μl) into the medial forebrain bundle (AP -2.2 mm, ML + 1.5 mm from bregma; depth 7.8 mm). Rats were killed 10 days later. a-d: CD200 immunoreactivity (green) and tyrosine hydroxylase (TH) immunoreactivity was evident in contralateral and ipsilateral SN and there was clear evidence of co-localization indicating the presence of CD200 on dopaminergic neurons. There was a marked decrease in TH immunoreactivity in sections prepared from the ipsilateral SN of rats which received 6-OHDA, indicative of substantial dopaminergic cell loss but no changes were observed in the other treatment groups. TH loss was accompanied by a loss in CD200 immunoreactivity. e-h: TH expression (green) was similar in the contralateral SN obtained from sham- or 6-OHDA-treated rats and in the ipsilateral side of sham-treated rats. In contrast, a marked change in morphology indicative of dopaminergic cell loss was observed in sections prepared from the ipsilateral SN of rats which received 6-OHDA. Microglial activation was assessed by evaluating OX42 immunoreactivity (red staining); marked staining was observed in sections prepared from the ipsilateral SN of rats which received 6-OHDA but in none of the other groups

6.3 Stroke

Ischaemia induces a profound disturbance in homeostasis and significant pathology in the brain. Among the earliest changes is infiltration of neutrophils into the brain parenchyma and the evidence indicates that, in the endothelin model of stroke, these cells accumulated in the core of the lesion 2 weeks after injection and correlated with the infarct volume (Weston

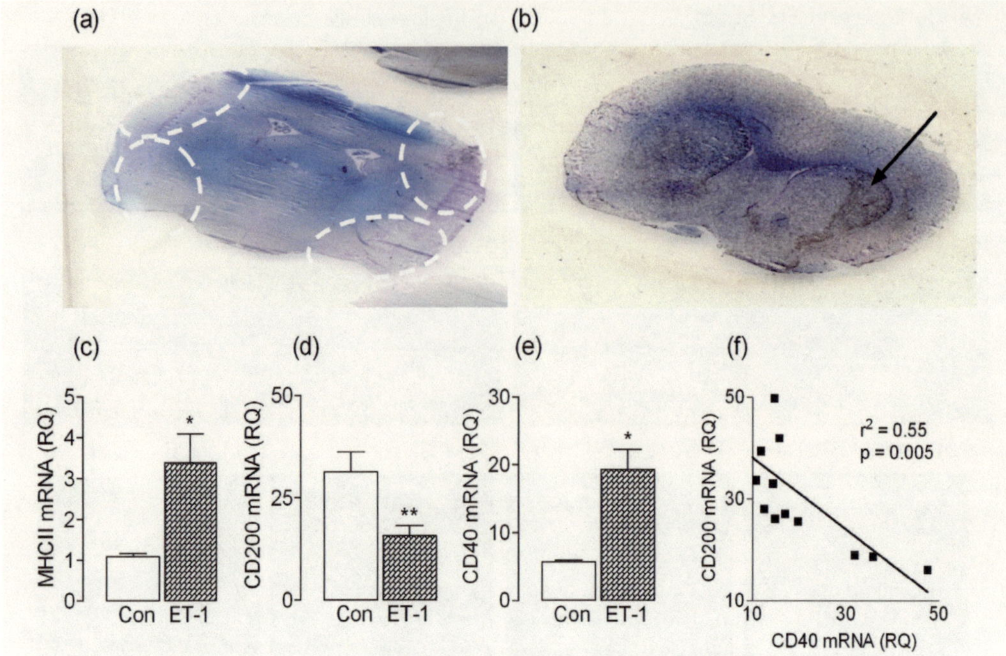

Fig. 6. CD40 mRNA is increased and CD200 mRNA is decreased in striatum following endothelin injection. Male Wistar rats (3 months; 270-350g; BioResources Unit, Trinity College, Dublin, Ireland) were anaesthetized with isofluorane (5% in O_2), placed in a stereotaxic frame and injected with endothelin-1 (ET-1; 600pmol; 3 μl), delivered through a drill hole (0.52 cm lateral to midline, 0.05 cm posterior to bregma; depth 0.05cm from the base of the skull) (Moyanova et al., 2003). Animals were killed and brain tissue harvested 7 days after injection. Cryostat sections were prepared from part of the brain and striatum was taken from the remaining brain tissue to analyse expression of CD40 and CD200 mRNA. Endothelin induced significant neuronal loss (Figure 1a) and microglial activation, as assessed by OX6 staining, particularly in striatum (Figure 1b). Analysis of striatal tissue indicated that MHCII mRNA and CD40 mRNA were significantly increased in tissue prepared from endothelin-1-injected animals (*$p < 0.05$; student's t test for independent means; Figure 1c,d) whereas CD200 mRNA was significantly decreased (**$p < 0.01$; student's t test for independent means; Figure 1e); a significant inverse relationship between CD40 mRNA and CD200 mRNA was observed ($p = 0.0039$; Figure 1f)

et al., 2007). Neutrophils have also been shown to contribute to the increase in BBB permeability following stroke (McColl et al., 2007). Neutrophils release inflammatory cytokines, chemokines and reactive oxygen species, all of which contribute to the pathology, and also recruitment of immune cells (Denes et al., 2010). However microglia can also act similarly and the evidence has indicated that microglial activation is increased following ischaemia but the effect of this activation remains unclear. On the one hand, these cells may contribute to the cell damage because of their ability to secrete inflammatory molecules but their reparative role has also been clearly identified (Denes et al., 2010). It has been known for almost 2 decades that release of the inflammatory cytokine, IL-1β, was increased following ischaemia and that the endogenous antagonist, IL-1 receptor antagonist (IL-1ra) reduced the associated neurodegenerative changes (Relton and Rothwell, 1992). However, more recent findings have indicated that the reduction in synaptic responses following ischaemia, and the decrease in LTP, were partially reversed following intra-arterial injection of microglia into rats (Hayashi et al., 2006). Thus microglia exert both a positive and negative impact.

We investigated microglial activation 7 days after endothelin-1 injection and demonstrate that markers of activation were increased while CD200 was decreased. Thus staining of the tissue revealed that there was marked cell loss (Figure 6a) and extensive OX6 staining (Figure 6b), with particularly marked staining in the striatum. PCR analysis revealed that there was a significant increase in expression of MHCII mRNA (Figure 6c) as well as another marker of microglial activation, CD40 mRNA (Figure 6e), in striatal tissue prepared from endothelin 1-treated rats compared with controls (*$p < 0.05$). CD200 mRNA was markedly decreased in striatal tissue prepared from endothelin-1-injected animals and, interestingly, there was a significant inverse relationship between these CD200 mRNA and CD40 mRNA ($p = 0.0039$; Figure 6f). These findings indicate that there is a persistent increase in microglial activation following ischaemia which has been reported previously (Denes et al., 2010). The underlying cause of this increase has not been fully explained. The present results suggest that the decrease in CD200, which might be anticipated to accompany the loss of neurons, may be a contributory factor.

6.4 Conclusions

In the past decade or so, it has become clear that microglia are maintained in a non-activated state by soluble factors including growth factors and anti-inflammatory cytokines, as well as cell-cell interactions. Among the ligand-receptor pairs which play a key role in modulating microglial activation is CD200-CD200R and the evidence indicates that when CD200R activation is disrupted, for example in CD200-deficient mice, the result is activation of microglia and macrophages, accompanied by inflammatory changes, and exacerbation of changes in models of autoimmune disease. The experimental evidence certainly suggests that targeting the interaction between CD200 and its receptor is a powerful weapon in attenuating inflammation and there is a growing body of evidence suggesting that disruption of the interaction, in combination with microglial and/or macrophage activation occurs in

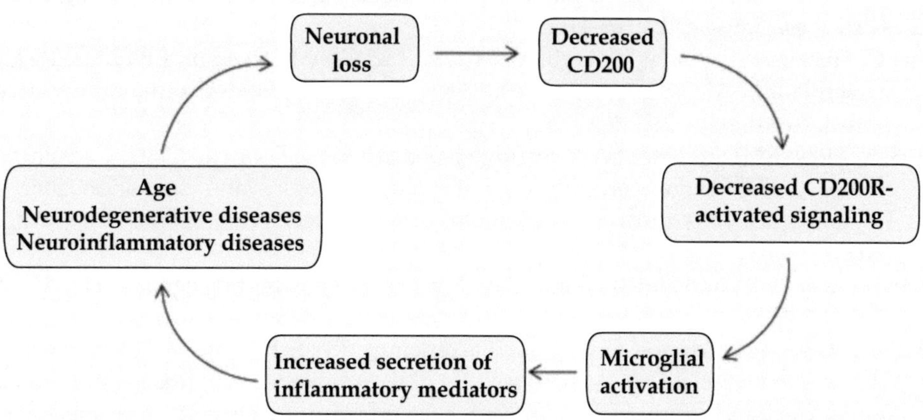

Fig. 7. Proposed role for CD200-CD200R interaction in neurodegenerative changes

models of neurodegenerative diseases. Figure 7 presents a schematic diagram which suggests that CD200R activation plays a pivotal role in modulating microglial activation. It is proposed that the secretion of immunomodulatory molecules from activated microglia contributes to the development of neurodegenerative changes which characterize neurodegenerative and neuroinflammatory diseases, and which also occur with age, these changes are inextricably linked with neuronal loss and consequently CD200 expression is decreased resulting in a decrease in signalling through CD200R, completing the continuing cycle of events.

7. Acknowledgements

Funding was obtained from Science Foundation Ireland and the Health Research Board (Ireland).

8. References

Banerjee D, Dick AD (2004) Blocking CD200-CD200 receptor axis augments NOS-2 expression and aggravates experimental autoimmune uveoretinitis in Lewis rats. Ocul Immunol Inflamm 12:115-125.

Barclay AN (1981) The localization of populations of lymphocytes defined by monoclonal antibodies in rat lymphoid tissues. Immunology 42:593-600.

Barclay AN, Wright GJ, Brooke G, Brown MH (2002) CD200 and membrane protein interactions in the control of myeloid cells. Trends Immunol 23:285-290.

Bazan JF, Bacon KB, Hardiman G, Wang W, Soo K, Rossi D, Greaves DR, Zlotnik A, Schall TJ (1997) A new class of membrane-bound chemokine with a CX3C motif. Nature 385:640-644.

Beach TG, Sue LI, Walker DG, Lue LF, Connor DJ, Caviness JN, Sabbagh MN, Adler CH (2007) Marked microglial reaction in normal aging human substantia nigra: correlation with extraneuronal neuromelanin pigment deposits. Acta Neuropathol 114:419-424.

Blasko I, Stampfer-Kountchev M, Robatscher P, Veerhuis R, Eikelenboom P, Grubeck-Loebenstein B (2004) How chronic inflammation can affect the brain and support the development of Alzheimer's disease in old age: the role of microglia and astrocytes. Aging cell 3:169-176.

Breitner JC, Haneuse SJ, Walker R, Dublin S, Crane PK, Gray SL, Larson EB (2009) Risk of dementia and AD with prior exposure to NSAIDs in an elderly community-based cohort. Neurology 72:1899-1905.

Broderick C, Hoek RM, Forrester JV, Liversidge J, Sedgwick JD, Dick AD (2002) Constitutive retinal CD200 expression regulates resident microglia and activation state of inflammatory cells during experimental autoimmune uveoretinitis. Am J Pathol 161:1669-1677.

Brown EJ, Frazier WA (2001) Integrin-associated protein (CD47) and its ligands. Trends Cell Biol 11:130-135.

Chabbert-de Ponnat I, Marie-Cardine A, Pasterkamp RJ, Schiavon V, Tamagnone L, Thomasset N, Bensussan A, Boumsell L (2005) Soluble CD100 functions on human monocytes and immature dendritic cells require plexin C1 and plexin B1, respectively. Int Immunol 17:439-447.

Chang CY, Lee YH, Jiang-Shieh YF, Chien HF, Pai MH, Chen HM, Fong TH, Wu CH (2011) Novel distribution of cluster of differentiation 200 adhesion molecule in glial cells of the peripheral nervous system of rats and its modulation after nerve injury. Neuroscience 183:32-46.

Chen S, Le WD, Xie WJ, Alexianu ME, Engelhardt JI, Siklos L, Appel SH (1998) Experimental destruction of substantia nigra initiated by Parkinson disease immunoglobulins. Arch Neurol 55:1075-1080.

Cicchetti F, Drouin-Ouellet J, Gross RE (2009) Environmental toxins and Parkinson's disease: what have we learned from pesticide-induced animal models? Trends Pharmacol Sci 30:475-483.

Clark DA, Gorczynski RM, Blajchman MA (2008) Transfusion-related immunomodulation due to peripheral blood dendritic cells expressing the CD200 tolerance signaling molecule and alloantigen. Transfusion 48:814-821.

Clark MJ, Gagnon J, Williams AF, Barclay AN (1985) MRC OX-2 antigen: a lymphoid/neuronal membrane glycoprotein with a structure like a single immunoglobulin light chain. EMBO J 4:113-118.

Clarke RM, O'Connell F, Lyons A, Lynch MA (2007) The HMG-CoA reductase inhibitor, atorvastatin, attenuates the effects of acute administration of amyloid-beta1-42 in the rat hippocampus in vivo. Neuropharmacology 52:136-145.

Copland DA, Calder CJ, Raveney BJ, Nicholson LB, Phillips J, Cherwinski H, Jenmalm M, Sedgwick JD, Dick AD (2007) Monoclonal antibody-mediated CD200 receptor signaling suppresses macrophage activation and tissue damage in experimental autoimmune uveoretinitis. Am J Pathol 171:580-588.

Deckert M, Sedgwick JD, Fischer E, Schluter D (2006) Regulation of microglial cell responses in murine Toxoplasma encephalitis by CD200/CD200 receptor interaction. Acta Neuropathol (Berl) 111:548-558.

Denes A, Thornton P, Rothwell NJ, Allan SM (2010) Inflammation and brain injury: acute cerebral ischaemia, peripheral and central inflammation. Brain Behav Immun 24:708-723.

Emre M (2003a) Dementia associated with Parkinson's disease. Lancet Neurol 2:229-237.

Emre M (2003b) What causes mental dysfunction in Parkinson's disease? Mov Disord 18 Suppl 6:S63-71.

Frohman EM, Racke MK, Raine CS (2006) Multiple sclerosis--the plaque and its pathogenesis. N Engl J Med 354:942-955.

Gao HM, Hong JS, Zhang W, Liu B (2002) Distinct role for microglia in rotenone-induced degeneration of dopaminergic neurons. J Neurosci 22:782-790.

Gorczynski R, Boudakov I, Khatri I (2008) Peptides of CD200 modulate LPS-induced TNF-alpha induction and mortality in vivo. J Surg Res 145:87-96.

Gorczynski R, Chen Z, Kai Y, Lee L, Wong S, Marsden PA (2004) CD200 is a ligand for all members of the CD200R family of immunoregulatory molecules. J Immunol 172:7744-7749.

Gorczynski RM, Chen Z, He W, Khatri I, Sun Y, Yu K, Boudakov I (2009) Expression of a CD200 transgene is necessary for induction but not maintenance of tolerance to cardiac and skin allografts. J Immunol 183:1560-1568.

Gorczynski RM, Chen Z, Lee L, Yu K, Hu J (2002) Anti-CD200R ameliorates collagen-induced arthritis in mice. Clin Immunol 104:256-264.

Gordon S (2003) Alternative activation of macrophages. Nat Rev Immunol 3:23-35.

Griffiths MR, Gasque P, Neal JW (2010) The regulation of the CNS innate immune response is vital for the restoration of tissue homeostasis (repair) after acute brain injury: a brief review. Int J Inflam 2010:151097.

Haag MD, Hofman A, Koudstaal PJ, Stricker BH, Breteler MM (2009) Statins are associated with a reduced risk of Alzheimer disease regardless of lipophilicity. The Rotterdam Study. J Neurol Neurosurg Psychiatry 80:13-17.

Harrison JK, Jiang Y, Chen S, Xia Y, Maciejewski D, McNamara RK, Streit WJ, Salafranca MN, Adhikari S, Thompson DA, Botti P, Bacon KB, Feng L (1998) Role for neuronally derived fractalkine in mediating interactions between neurons and CX3CR1-expressing microglia. Proc Natl Acad Sci U S A 95:10896-10901.

Hatherley D, Graham SC, Harlos K, Stuart DI, Barclay AN (2009) Structure of signal-regulatory protein alpha: a link to antigen receptor evolution. J Biol Chem 284:26613-26619.

Hayashi Y, Tomimatsu Y, Suzuki H, Yamada J, Wu Z, Yao H, Kagamiishi Y, Tateishi N, Sawada M, Nakanishi H (2006) The intra-arterial injection of microglia protects hippocampal CA1 neurons against global ischemia-induced functional deficits in rats. Neuroscience 142:87-96.

Hirsch E, Hu LJ, Prigent A, Constantin B, Agid Y, Drabkin H, Roche J (1999) Distribution of semaphorin IV in adult human brain. Brain Res 823:67-79.

Hoek RM, Ruuls SR, Murphy CA, Wright GJ, Goddard R, Zurawski SM, Blom B, Homola ME, Streit WJ, Brown MH, Barclay AN, Sedgwick JD (2000) Down-regulation of the macrophage lineage through interaction with OX2 (CD200). Science 290:1768-1771.

Hughes PM, Botham MS, Frentzel S, Mir A, Perry VH (2002) Expression of fractalkine (CX3CL1) and its receptor, CX3CR1, during acute and chronic inflammation in the rodent CNS. Glia 37:314-327.

Jenmalm MC, Cherwinski H, Bowman EP, Phillips JH, Sedgwick JD (2006) Regulation of myeloid cell function through the CD200 receptor. J Immunol 176:191-199.

Kim YS, Joh TH (2006) Microglia, major player in the brain inflammation: their roles in the pathogenesis of Parkinson's disease. Exp Mol Med 38:333-347.

Ko YC, Chien HF, Jiang-Shieh YF, Chang CY, Pai MH, Huang JP, Chen HM, Wu CH (2009) Endothelial CD200 is heterogeneously distributed, regulated and involved in immune cell-endothelium interactions. J Anat 214:183-195.

Koenigsknecht J, Landreth G (2004) Microglial phagocytosis of fibrillar beta-amyloid through a beta1 integrin-dependent mechanism. J Neurosci 24:9838-9846.

Koning N, Bo L, Hoek RM, Huitinga I (2007) Downregulation of macrophage inhibitory molecules in multiple sclerosis lesions. Ann Neurol 62:504-514.

Koning N, Swaab DF, Hoek RM, Huitinga I (2009) Distribution of the immune inhibitory molecules CD200 and CD200R in the normal central nervous system and multiple sclerosis lesions suggests neuron-glia and glia-glia interactions. J Neuropathol Exp Neurol 68:159-167.

Laakso MP, Partanen K, Riekkinen P, Lehtovirta M, Helkala EL, Hallikainen M, Hanninen T, Vainio P, Soininen H (1996) Hippocampal volumes in Alzheimer's disease, Parkinson's disease with and without dementia, and in vascular dementia: An MRI study. Neurology 46:678-681.

Lamy L, Foussat A, Brown EJ, Bornstein P, Ticchioni M, Bernard A (2007) Interactions between CD47 and thrombospondin reduce inflammation. J Immunol 178:5930-5939.

Le W, Rowe D, Xie W, Ortiz I, He Y, Appel SH (2001) Microglial activation and dopaminergic cell injury: an in vitro model relevant to Parkinson's disease. J Neurosci 21:8447-8455.

Liu B, Hong JS (2003) Role of microglia in inflammation-mediated neurodegenerative diseases: mechanisms and strategies for therapeutic intervention. J Pharmacol Exp Ther 304:1-7.

Long-Smith CM, Collins L, Toulouse A, Sullivan AM, Nolan YM (2010) Interleukin-1beta contributes to dopaminergic neuronal death induced by lipopolysaccharide-stimulated rat glia in vitro. J Neuroimmunol 226:20-26.

Long-Smith CM, Sullivan AM, Nolan YM (2009) The influence of microglia on the pathogenesis of Parkinson's disease. Prog Neurobiol 89:277-287.

Lynch MA (2010) Age-related neuroinflammatory changes negatively impact on neuronal function. Front Aging Neurosci 1:6.

Lyons A, Downer EJ, Crotty S, Nolan YM, Mills KH, Lynch MA (2007a) CD200 ligand receptor interaction modulates microglial activation in vivo and in vitro: a role for IL-4. J Neurosci 27:8309-8313.

Lyons A, Griffin RJ, Costelloe CE, Clarke RM, Lynch MA (2007b) IL-4 attenuates the neuroinflammation induced by amyloid-beta in vivo and in vitro. J Neurochem 101:771-781.

Lyons A, Lynch AM, Downer EJ, Hanley R, O'Sullivan JB, Smith A, Lynch MA (2009a) Fractalkine-induced activation of the phosphatidylinositol-3 kinase pathway attentuates microglial activation in vivo and in vitro. J Neurochem 110:1547-1556.

Lyons A, McQuillan K, Deighan BF, O'Reilly JA, Downer EJ, Murphy AC, Watson M, Piazza A, O'Connell F, Griffin R, Mills KH, Lynch MA (2009b) Decreased neuronal CD200 expression in IL-4-deficient mice results in increased neuroinflammation in response to lipopolysaccharide. Brain Behav Immun.

Maciejewski-Lenoir D, Chen S, Feng L, Maki R, Bacon KB (1999) Characterization of fractalkine in rat brain cells: migratory and activation signals for CX3CR-1-expressing microglia. J Immunol 163:1628-1635.

Masocha W (2009) Systemic lipopolysaccharide (LPS)-induced microglial activation results in different temporal reduction of CD200 and CD200 receptor gene expression in the brain. J Neuroimmunol 214:78-82.

McColl BW, Allan SM, Rothwell NJ (2007) Systemic inflammation and stroke: aetiology, pathology and targets for therapy. Biochem Soc Trans 35:1163-1165.

McGeer EG, McGeer PL (2003) Inflammatory processes in Alzheimer's disease. Prog Neuropsychopharmacol Biol Psychiatry 27:741-749.

McGeer PL, Itagaki S, Boyes BE, McGeer EG (1988) Reactive microglia are positive for HLA-DR in the substantia nigra of Parkinson's and Alzheimer's disease brains. Neurology 38:1285-1291.

McGeer PL, McGeer EG (1999) Inflammation of the brain in Alzheimer's disease: implications for therapy. J Leukoc Biol 65:409-415.

Melnyk M, Shalev I, Zhang J, Bartczak A, Gorczynski R, Selzner N, Inman R, Marsden P, Phillips M, Clark D, Levy G (2011) The prothrombinase activity of FGL2 contributes to the pathogenesis of experimental arthritis. Scand J Rheumatol.

Meuth SG, Simon OJ, Grimm A, Melzer N, Herrmann AM, Spitzer P, Landgraf P, Wiendl H (2008) CNS inflammation and neuronal degeneration is aggravated by impaired CD200-CD200R-mediated macrophage silencing. J Neuroimmunol 194:62-69.

Mihrshahi R, Barclay AN, Brown MH (2009) Essential roles for Dok2 and RasGAP in CD200 receptor-mediated regulation of human myeloid cells. J Immunol 183:4879-4886.

Mihrshahi R, Brown MH (2010) Downstream of tyrosine kinase 1 and 2 play opposing roles in CD200 receptor signaling. J Immunol 185:7216-7222.

Minogue AM, Lynch AM, Loane DJ, Herron CE, Lynch MA (2007) Modulation of amyloid-beta-induced and age-associated changes in rat hippocampus by eicosapentaenoic acid. J Neurochem 103:914-926.

Mott RT, Ait-Ghezala G, Town T, Mori T, Vendrame M, Zeng J, Ehrhart J, Mullan M, Tan J (2004) Neuronal expression of CD22: novel mechanism for inhibiting microglial proinflammatory cytokine production. Glia 46:369-379.

Moyanova S, Kirov R, Kortenska L (2003) Multi-unit activity suppression and sensorimotor deficits after endothelin-1-induced middle cerebral artery occlusion in conscious rats. J Neurol Sci 212:59-67.

Mutez E, Duhamel A, Defebvre L, Bordet R, Destee A, Kreisler A (2009) Lipid-lowering drugs are associated with delayed onset and slower course of Parkinson's disease. Pharmacol Res 60:41-45.

Nathan C, Muller WA (2001) Putting the brakes on innate immunity: a regulatory role for CD200? Nat Immunol 2:17-19.

Okuno T, Nakatsuji Y, Moriya M, Takamatsu H, Nojima S, Takegahara N, Toyofuku T, Nakagawa Y, Kang S, Friedel RH, Sakoda S, Kikutani H, Kumanogoh A (2010) Roles of Sema4D-plexin-B1 interactions in the central nervous system for pathogenesis of experimental autoimmune encephalomyelitis. J Immunol 184:1499-1506.

Preston S, Wright GJ, Starr K, Barclay AN, Brown MH (1997) The leukocyte/neuron cell surface antigen OX2 binds to a ligand on macrophages. Eur J Immunol 27:1911-1918.

Purisai MG, McCormack AL, Cumine S, Li J, Isla MZ, Di Monte DA (2007) Microglial activation as a priming event leading to paraquat-induced dopaminergic cell degeneration. Neurobiol Dis 25:392-400.

Reinhold MI, Lindberg FP, Plas D, Reynolds S, Peters MG, Brown EJ (1995) In vivo expression of alternatively spliced forms of integrin-associated protein (CD47). J Cell Sci 108 (Pt 11):3419-3425.

Relton JK, Rothwell NJ (1992) Interleukin-1 receptor antagonist inhibits ischaemic and excitotoxic neuronal damage in the rat. Brain Res Bull 29:243-246.

Rijkers ES, de Ruiter T, Baridi A, Veninga H, Hoek RM, Meyaard L (2008) The inhibitory CD200R is differentially expressed on human and mouse T and B lymphocytes. Mol Immunol 45:1126-1135.

Rosenblum MD, Olasz E, Woodliff JE, Johnson BD, Konkol MC, Gerber KA, Orentas RJ, Sandford G, Truitt RL (2004) CD200 is a novel p53-target gene involved in apoptosis-associated immune tolerance. Blood 103:2691-2698.

Shinohara H, Inoue A, Toyama-Sorimachi N, Nagai Y, Yasuda T, Suzuki H, Horai R, Iwakura Y, Yamamoto T, Karasuyama H, Miyake K, Yamanashi Y (2005) Dok-1 and Dok-2 are negative regulators of lipopolysaccharide-induced signaling. J Exp Med 201:333-339.

Sian J, Dexter DT, Lees AJ, Daniel S, Agid Y, Javoy-Agid F, Jenner P, Marsden CD (1994) Alterations in glutathione levels in Parkinson's disease and other neurodegenerative disorders affecting basal ganglia. Ann Neurol 36:348-355.

Simelyte E, Criado G, Essex D, Uger RA, Feldmann M, Williams RO (2008) CD200-Fc, a novel antiarthritic biologic agent that targets proinflammatory cytokine expression in the joints of mice with collagen-induced arthritis. Arthritis Rheum 58:1038-1043.

Smidt MP (2009) Specific vulnerability of substantia nigra compacta neurons. J Neural Transm Suppl 39-47.

Snelgrove RJ, Goulding J, Didierlaurent AM, Lyonga D, Vekaria S, Edwards L, Gwyer E, Sedgwick JD, Barclay AN, Hussell T (2008) A critical function for CD200 in lung immune homeostasis and the severity of influenza infection. Nat Immunol 9:1074-1083.

Stamenkovic I, Sgroi D, Aruffo A, Sy MS, Anderson T (1991) The B lymphocyte adhesion molecule CD22 interacts with leukocyte common antigen CD45RO on T cells and alpha 2-6 sialyltransferase, CD75, on B cells. Cell 66:1133-1144.

Stromnes IM, Goverman JM (2006) Active induction of experimental allergic encephalomyelitis. Nat Protoc 1:1810-1819.

Suzuki K, Kumanogoh A, Kikutani H (2008) Semaphorins and their receptors in immune cell interactions. Nat Immunol 9:17-23.

Szekely CA, Breitner JC, Fitzpatrick AL, Rea TD, Psaty BM, Kuller LH, Zandi PP (2008) NSAID use and dementia risk in the Cardiovascular Health Study: role of APOE and NSAID type. Neurology 70:17-24.

Tan J, Town T, Mullan M (2000) CD45 inhibits CD40L-induced microglial activation via negative regulation of the Src/p44/42 MAPK pathway. J Biol Chem 275:37224-37231.

Taylor S, Calder CJ, Albon J, Erichsen JT, Boulton ME, Morgan JE (2011) Involvement of the CD200 receptor complex in microglia activation in experimental glaucoma. Exp Eye Res 92:338-343.

Thornton P, Pinteaux E, Allan SM, Rothwell NJ (2008) Matrix metalloproteinase-9 and urokinase plasminogen activator mediate interleukin-1-induced neurotoxicity. Mol Cell Neurosci 37:135-142.

Toguchi M, Gonzalez D, Furukawa S, Inagaki S (2009) Involvement of Sema4D in the control of microglia activation. Neurochem Int 55:573-580.

Ton TG, Heckbert SR, Longstreth WT, Jr., Rossing MA, Kukull WA, Franklin GM, Swanson PD, Smith-Weller T, Checkoway H (2006) Nonsteroidal anti-inflammatory drugs and risk of Parkinson's disease. Mov Disord 21:964-969.

Vlad SC, Miller DR, Kowall NW, Felson DT (2008) Protective effects of NSAIDs on the development of Alzheimer disease. Neurology 70:1672-1677.

Walker DG, Dalsing-Hernandez JE, Campbell NA, Lue LF (2009) Decreased expression of CD200 and CD200 receptor in Alzheimer's disease: a potential mechanism leading to chronic inflammation. Exp Neurol 215:5-19.

Wang XJ, Zhang S, Yan ZQ, Zhao YX, Zhou HY, Wang Y, Lu GQ, Zhang JD (2011) Impaired CD200-CD200R-mediated microglia silencing enhances midbrain dopaminergic neurodegeneration: roles of aging, superoxide, NADPH oxidase, and p38 MAPK. Free Radic Biol Med 50:1094-1106.

Webb M, Barclay AN (1984) Localisation of the MRC OX-2 glycoprotein on the surfaces of neurones. J Neurochem 43:1061-1067.

Weston RM, Jones NM, Jarrott B, Callaway JK (2007) Inflammatory cell infiltration after endothelin-1-induced cerebral ischemia: histochemical and myeloperoxidase correlation with temporal changes in brain injury. J Cereb Blood Flow Metab 27:100-114.

Wright GJ, Cherwinski H, Foster-Cuevas M, Brooke G, Puklavec MJ, Bigler M, Song Y, Jenmalm M, Gorman D, McClanahan T, Liu MR, Brown MH, Sedgwick JD, Phillips JH, Barclay AN (2003) Characterization of the CD200 receptor family in mice and humans and their interactions with CD200. J Immunol 171:3034-3046.

Wright GJ, Puklavec MJ, Willis AC, Hoek RM, Sedgwick JD, Brown MH, Barclay AN (2000) Lymphoid/neuronal cell surface OX2 glycoprotein recognizes a novel receptor on macrophages implicated in the control of their function. Immunity 13:233-242.

Wu XF, Block ML, Zhang W, Qin L, Wilson B, Zhang WQ, Veronesi B, Hong JS (2005) The role of microglia in paraquat-induced dopaminergic neurotoxicity. Antioxid Redox Signal 7:654-661.

Xiang Z, Haroutunian V, Ho L, Purohit D, Pasinetti GM (2006) Microglia activation in the brain as inflammatory biomarker of Alzheimer's disease neuropathology and clinical dementia. Dis Markers 22:95-102.

Zhang S, Cherwinski H, Sedgwick JD, Phillips JH (2004) Molecular mechanisms of CD200 inhibition of mast cell activation. J Immunol 173:6786-6793.

Zujovic V, Benavides J, Vige X, Carter C, Taupin V (2000) Fractalkine modulates TNF-alpha secretion and neurotoxicity induced by microglial activation. Glia 29:305-315.

Part 5

Hormonal Control and Metabolism in Neurodegeneration

15

Hormonal Signaling Systems of the Brain in Diabetes Mellitus

Alexander Shpakov, Oksana Chistyakova,
Kira Derkach and Vera Bondareva
Sechenov Institute of Evolutionary Physiology and Biochemistry
Russia

1. Introduction

Diabetes mellitus (DM) is nowadays a major global health problem affecting more than 200 million people worldwide. It is one of the most severe metabolic disorders in humans characterized by hyperglycemia due to a relative or an absolute lack of insulin or the action of insulin on its target tissue or both. Many neurodegenerative disorders, such as diabetic encephalopathy and Alzheimer's disease (AD), are associated with the type 1, insulin-dependent, and the type 2, non-insulin-dependent, diabetes mellitus (DM1 and DM2). Manifestations of these disorders in diabetic patients include alterations in neurotransmission, electrophysiological abnormalities, structural changes and cognitive deficit (Biessels et al., 2001). In the recent time attention to the neurological consequences of DM in the CNS has increased considerably.

Many approaches and tools have been used to study etiology and pathogenesis of DM and DM-associated neurodegenerative disorders, and their diagnostics and treatment. The most perspective approaches are based on a combined use of the methods of biochemistry, molecular biology and physiology, they include clinical investigations of diabetic patients and the experimental models of DM and their complications, such as the model of DM1 induced by streptozotocin (STZ) treatment of young or adult rodents, the neonatal model of DM2 induced by the STZ treatment of newborn rats, and also the models of spontaneous DM and nutritional background causing DM2, as well as the models produced by transgenic manipulations or gene knockout techniques are all successfully used to study the molecular, cellular and morphological changes in diabetic brain (Shafrir, 2010).

A severe hyperglycemia in DM1, mild hyperglycemia typical of DM2, and recurrent hypoglycemia induced by inadequate insulin therapy are the major factors responsible for the development of CNS complications in DM. The brain is mainly a glucose-dependent organ, which can be damaged by hyper- as well as by hypoglycemia (Scheen, 2010). Being a major problem in clinical practice, hypoglycemia unawareness is associated with an increased risk of coma. Note that low blood glucose level induces negative mood states, primarily self-reported "nervousness" (Boyle & Zrebiec, 2007). Moreover, patients with a history of severe hypoglycemia show a much higher level of anxiety compared to other DM patients (Wredling, 1992). The prolonged influence of mild hypoglycemia on the brain leads to deregulation of many processes in CNS, which underlines the importance of scrupulously avoiding even mild hypoglycemic episodes in patients with DM. Hypoglycemia induces progressive reduction in cerebral glycogen and glucose, which is due to an increase in gene expression of GLUT3, the glucose transporter rather abundant in the brain (Antony et al., 2010b). Alteration of expression of GLUT3 in the cerebral cortex in hypoglycemia is the evidence for impairment of neuronal glucose transport during glucose deprivation. The impaired transport and utilization of neuronal glucose in hypoglycemia is likely to be an important factor contributing to an increase of neuronal vulnerability. The disturbances of neuronal glucose transport and metabolism in hyperglycemia are similar to those in hypoglycemia and also induce neuronal damages and CNS disorders. For example, chronic diabetic encephalopathy leading to cognitive dysfunctions and dementia may be the result of recurrent hypoglycaemia and/or chronic hyperglycaemia, both inducing cerebral vascular damages (Scheen, 2010).

A new view of the nature and pathogenesis of DM-induced cerebral complications shared by many specialists nowadays has been prompted by the results of study of functional activity of hormonal signaling systems regulated by insulin, insulin-like growth factor-1 (IGF-1), leptin, biogenic amines, purines, glutamate, and peptide hormones controlling the fundamental processes in the neuronal and glial cells. The data were obtained showing that the alterations and abnormalities of hormonal signaling systems regulated by these hormones and the changes in expression of hormones and signal proteins, the components of these systems, induce disturbances of growth, differentiation, metabolism and apoptosis in neuronal cells and contribute to triggering and development of neurodegenerative processes in the diabetic brain. The present review is devoted to the achievements in the study of the functional state of hormone-sensitive signaling systems of the brain in human and experimental DM, to the alterations and abnormalities in these systems, and to the search of new approaches in the therapy of cerebral complications of DM based on restoration of normal functioning of some signaling systems and overall integrative signaling network in the diabetic brain.

2. Insulin, insulin-like growth factor-1 and leptin in the diabetic brain

Polypeptide hormones insulin, IGF-1 and leptin, the principal players responsible for pathogenesis of DM and its central and peripheral complications, are to a large extent affected in the diabetic brain. The abnormalities in numerous signaling pathways regulated by insulin, IGF-1 and leptin lead to disturbances of the biochemical and physiological functions of the neuronal and glial cells. It was shown by many investigators that the level of these hormones in the brain is decreased in DM, and the signaling pathways regulated by insulin, IGF-1 and leptin and involving a large number of effector proteins, such as insulin receptor substrate (IRS) proteins, phosphatidylinositol 3-kinase (PI 3-kinase), protein phosphotyrosine phosphatases, AKT kinase, ERK1/ERK2 kinases and glycogen synthase kinase 3β (GSK3β), are impaired (Fig. 1). Therefore, the treatment of diabetic patients with insulin, IGF-1 and leptin, and the restoration of activity of the signaling pathways they regulate are a reliable approach in the therapy of central and neuroendocrine dysfunctions in DM.

2.1 Insulin and insulin-like growth factor-1

Insulin and IGF-1 are genetically related polypeptides with similar three-dimensional and primary structures. Insulin is synthesized predominantly in pancreatic β-cells, while IGF-1 is synthesized primarily in the liver and also in the brain. Peripheral insulin penetrates the blood-brain barrier (BBB) and binds to brain insulin receptors (IRs), which leads to the triggering of their intrinsic tyrosine kinase activity and, as a result, to tyrosine phosphorylation and activation of IRS proteins (Boura-Halfon & Zick, 2009). Phosphorylated IRS proteins then activate p110/p85 heterodimeric PI 3-kinase, protein phosphotyrosine phosphatase and adaptor Shc/GRB2 dimer complex, which triggers the intracellular signaling cascades controlling the gene expression and, thus, regulating growth,

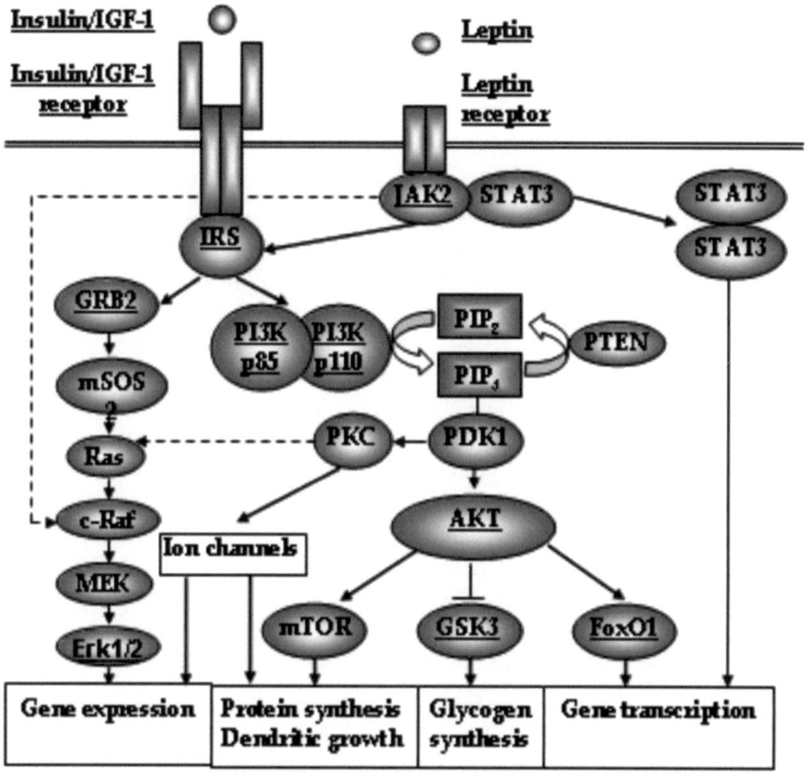

Fig. 1. Critical nodes in the insulin/IGF-1 and leptin signaling systems. The signal components of the systems whose expression and functional activity are significantly changed in DM are underlined. These changes are brain area-specific, they depend on the type of human DM, its severity and duration, DM-induced complications, and on the model of experimental DM. Abbreviations: IRS, insulin receptor substrate proteins; GRB2, growth-factor-receptor-bound protein-2; mSOS, mammalian *son of sevenless* nucleotide exchange factor; Ras, small G protein of Ras family; c-Raf, cytoplasmic serine/threonine-specific protein kinase Raf; MEK, mitogene-activated protein kinase; ERK1/2, extracellular signal-regulated kinases 1 and 2; p85/p110 PI 3K, heterodimeric p85/p110 phosphatidylinositol 3-kinase; PTEN, phosphatase and tensin homologue; PDK1, phosphoinositide-dependent kinase 1; PKC, protein kinase C; AKT, protein kinase B; mTOR, mammalian target of rapamycin; GSK3, glycogen synthase kinase 3; FoxO1, forkhead box O1 protein; JAK2, Janus kinase-2; STAT3, signal transducer and activator of transcription of the type 3; PIP_2 and PIP_3, phosphatidylinositol 3,4-diphosphate and phosphatidylinositol 3,4,5-triphosphate, respectively

differentiation and the other processes in neuronal cells. The activation of PI 3-kinase leads to phosphorylation and activation of AKT kinase that regulates the metabolism and cell survival via numerous downstream proteins in the peripheral insulin-sensitive tissues as well as in the CNS, primarily in hypothalamic neurons (Iskandar et al., 2010). AKT kinase partly facilitates signal transduction via phosphorylation and cytoplasmic sequestering of forkhead-box protein O1, a negative regulator of insulin signaling, whose nuclear translocation is associated with obesity and hyperphagia (Kitamura et al., 2006). The same signaling network is regulated by IGF-1 that specifically binds with cognate IGF-1 receptor demonstrating a close structural homology and sequence identity with IR and also possessing the tyrosine kinase activity and triggerring IRS-dependent signaling pathways.

Both IRs and IGF-1 receptors are widely expressed in the brain and are localized preferably in neuron rich structures in many brain areas, such as the granule cell layers of the olfactory bulb, hippocampal formation and cerebral cortex. The fact that these receptors are localized in the brain accounts for the role of insulin and IGF-1 in CNS functioning. Since the main function of insulin is to regulate glucose homeostasis, central insulin and brain IRs specifically recognizing the hormone modulate the energy, glucose and fat homeostasis in the brain, being involved, in addition, in the regulation of metabolism in the peripheral tissues. However, in the brain insulin performs some other functions specific of the CNS. Interacting with the other regulatory peptides and neurotransmitters, central insulin participates in controlling the feeding behavior, learning and memory, and is involved in the intercellular communication within brain structures, the hypothalamus and the limbic system in particular (Gerozissis, 2008). IGF-1 is involved in neuronal development, stimulates neurogenesis and synaptogenesis, facilitates oligodendrocyte development, promotes neuron and oligodendrocyte survival, and stimulates myelination. All this speaks about a very important role it has in preserving the integrity of neuronal cells and in protecting the brain structures from damages and injury (D'Ercole et al., 2002).

The alterations of proteins, the components of brain insulin- and IGF-1-regulated signaling cascades, typical of DM and pre-diabetic states, are the causes of the DM-associated neurodegenerative diseases. It should be emphasized that the abnormalities in brain insulin/IGF-1 signaling can be provoked by DM, being a result of the systemic changes of integral signaling network in the diabetic brain, and, on the other hand, the disturbances of the functioning of insulin/IGF-1 signaling systems of the brain induced by neurodegenerative disorders can also lead to DM. In the latter case we can talk about the central genesis of DM.

The initial component of insulin/IGF-1-regulated cascades is a hormonal molecule, insulin or IGF-1, whose brain concentrations are significantly reduced in DM (Gelling et al., 2006). A significant decrease of the IGF-1 level was found in the cerebellum of insulin-deficient rats with STZ-induced DM with poorly controlled glycemia, whereas there were no changes in cerebellar IGF-1 mRNA level, which indicates the abnormalities of hormone processing and secretion in the diabetic brain (Busiguina et al., 1996). The appropriate glycemic control with insulin completely restored IGF-1 concentration in the cerebellum (D'Ercole et al., 2002). Since IGF-1, the same as insulin, crosses the BBB, a decrease of serum IGF-1 in human DM1 and STZ-induced DM also contributes to brain IGF-1 deficit leading to attenuation of IGF-1 signaling (Busiguina et al., 2000). The children with DM1 had a 50% decrease of peripheral IGF-1 level compared with control group, and in diabetic children with poor glucose control it was decreased even more compared with moderate metabolic control. In the patients with DM2 the peripheral level of IGF-1 at the early stages of the disease did not change significantly, but began to decline markedly in prolonged DM2 and in long-term hyperglycemia (Clauson et al., 1998). It indicates the temporal dynamics of a decrease of IGF-1 and the impairments of its signaling in the diabetic brain, correlating with an increase of neurological disorders in prolonged uncontrolled DM2.

Central administration of insulin and IGF-1 restores to a great extent the function of the CNS, being in some cases the most effective co-administration of insulin and IGF-1, the latter refers mostly to the cases of much lower concentrations. It is shown that in DM1, in the case of insulin deficit, a concomitant decrease of insulin and IGF-1 levels in the brain leads to atrophy of some brain areas inducing impaired learning and memory. A combined infusion for 12 weeks of insulin and IGF-1 into the brain lateral ventricles of STZ rats prevents a decrease of the brain weight, and leads to normalization of the level of DNA and the content of proteins associated with neurons and glial cells, whose level and activity are significantly decreased in the diabetic brain. As a result, the brain DNA loss in DM1 is prevented (Serbedzija et al., 2009). The administration of IGF-1 to STZ rats prevents irrespective of the severity of hyperglycemia IGF-1 reduction in the brain and the DM-associated cognitive disturbances (Lupien et al., 2003). Anti-IGF-1 antibody infused into the lateral ventricles led, on the contrary, to deterioration of learning and memory functions of diabetic as well as non-diabetic rats. Quite often DM and its complications in human are associated with the changes in IGF-1 binding proteins, which contribute to the concentration of peripheral and central IGF-1 (Busiguina et al., 2000). The alterations of the content of these proteins are responsible for a decline in memory and for many DM-associated neurodegenerative disorders, such as AD and vascular dementia (Zhu et al., 2005).

The second component of insulin/IGF-1 signaling is IR or IGF-1 receptor. According to some reports, mice with a neuron-specific disruption of the IR gene increased food intake and diet-sensitive obesity with an increase in body fat, mild insulin resistance, elevated plasma insulin and leptin levels, and hypertriglyceridemia typical of DM2 (Bruning et al., 2000). These mutant mice also exhibited impaired spermatogenesis and ovarian follicle maturation due to deregulation of luteinizing hormone-releasing factor secretion caused by attenuation of insulin signaling in the hypothalamus. The restoration of IRs in the brain of these mice maintained energy homeostasis, improved functions of the CNS and prevented DM (Okamoto et al., 2004). The expression of IRs in the brain of mice lacking the genes encoding IR and the glucose transporter GLUT4 also improved their survival, but did not completely eliminate the symptoms of DM2 due to dysfunction of GLUT4 (H.V. Lin & Accili, 2011). The study of expression of IRs and IGF-1 receptors in the frontal cortices of 8-month-old diabetic rats with spontaneous onset of DM1 and DM2 showed that the IR expression was decreased in DM1 only, whereas IGF-1 receptor expression was decreased in both models (Z.G. Li et al., 2007). The disruption of IR expression in discrete hypothalamic nuclei led to hyperphagia and increased fat mass, which was a result of disturbances of regulation of hepatic glucose production by central insulin (Obici et al., 2002). The mice lacking the brain IR had severe hypoleptinemia as well as more severe hyperinsulinemia and hyperglycemia than the mice lacking the receptor in the peripheral tissues, which demonstrates the major role of central insulin in regulating white adipose tissue mass and glucose metabolism in the liver (Koch et al., 2008). Both neuron-specific IR knockout (NIRKO) mice and the rats with spontaneous DM exhibited a complete loss of insulin-mediated activation of PI 3-kinase and inhibition of neuronal apoptosis, and had markedly reduced phosphorylation of AKT kinase and GSK3β, leading to substantially increased phosphorylation of the microtubule-associated Tau protein at sites associated with neurodegenerative diseases (Z.G. Li et al., 2007; Koch et al., 2008). This is one of the molecular mechanisms responsible for the altered insulin signaling and insulin resistance in the brain to be predisposed for the development of neurodegeneration, creating a clinical link between DM2 and AD and other CNS dysfunctions (Schubert et al., 2004).

The third component of insulin/IGF-1 signaling is IRS proteins. They have a key role in linking IR and IGF-1 receptor to the intracellular signaling cascades and in coordinating signals from these receptors with those generated by other neurotransmitters, peptide hormones, pro-inflammatory cytokines and nutrients. The alterations of the IRS protein functions are responsible for the failure of insulin/IGF-1 signaling not only in the peripheral tissues, but also in neuronal cells, they induce insulin resistance and, finally, cause DM and neurodegenerative diseases associated with it (Lee & White, 2004). The deletion of gene encoding IRS-2 protein leads to the weakening of hypothalamic insulin signaling and increases both food intake and hepatic glucose production (X. Lin et al., 2004). Conversely, over expression of IRS-2 in the mediobasal hypothalamus was found to significantly enhance the glycemic response to systemic insulin treatment in STZ rats (Gelling et al., 2006). It was shown that in *Irs2* gene knockout mice the embryonic brain size is 55% of that in normal animals due to the reduced neuronal proliferation in the course of development, indicating IRS-2 to be involved in the brain growth. It seems likely that IRS-2 are involved in neuroprotective effects of insulin and IGF-1, because in the hippocampus of old *Irs2* knockout mice there are formed neurofibrillary tangles containing phosphorylated Tau protein, a hallmark of neurodegenerative processes (Schubert et al., 2003). No direct evidence for IRS-2 being involved in human brain growth and differentiation is available, but breaks at the distal end of human chromosome 13 (13q) near the *Irs2* gene between micro satellites D13S285 and D13S1295 are frequently associated with microcephaly, while very distal deletions between D13S274 and D13S1311 with microcephaly and neural tube defects, suggesting a possible contribution of partial *Irs2* deficiency to microcephaly (J. Luo et al., 2000). Based on these data, the conclusion was made that the regulation of activity of IRS-1 and IRS-2 controlling the growth, metabolism and survival of neuronal cells is a new strategy aimed at prevention or cure of DM and its CNS complications. However, according to the recently obtained data, the deletion of gene encoding IRS-2 improves the functioning of the brain of mutant mice, because IRS-2 act as negative regulators of memory formation by restricting dendritic spine generation (Irvine et al., 2011). The above may be due to the fact that various groups of scientists are engaged in the study of mutant lines of animals with a large number of alterations of insulin/IGF-1 signaling, and these alterations induce different changes in the brain signaling network. With this in mind, it is clear why the functions of IRS-2 can be redistributed among the other types of IRS proteins or described as depending on the activity of upstream or downstream signal proteins interacting with IRS-2.

The downstream components of insulin/IGF-1 signaling, such as PI 3-kinase, AKT kinase and protein phosphotyrosine phosphatase 2A (PP2A) are also changed in DM and greatly contribute in etiology and pathogenesis of DM-induced neurodegenerative diseases. The main molecular mechanism in this case is a rapid and significant increase of phosphorylation of Tau protein (Clodfelder-Miller et al., 2006). The hyperphosphorylation of Tau was detected in the mouse cerebral cortex and hippocampus within 3 days after STZ treatment and can be rapidly reversed by peripheral insulin administration. The increase of Tau phosphorylation in the brain in DM partly depends on the fact that the activity of PP2A, the major protein phosphatase acting on Tau, was decreased by 44% in the cerebral cortex and by 55% in the hippocampus. This indicates that a significant decrease in PP2A activity is likely to account for a majority of cases of a significant increase in Tau phosphorylation caused by STZ treatment. The decreased PP2A activity and Tau hyperphosphorylation on the background of insulin deficiency may increase the susceptibility of the diabetic brain to insults associated with AD, thereby contributing to the relationship between DM and heightened susceptibility to AD (Clodfelder-Miller et al., 2006).

To study the role of PI 3-kinase in the diabetic brain, it was shown by making i.c.v. infusion of LY294002, a specific inhibitor of the enzyme, into the 3rd cerebral ventricle of STZ rats that the inhibition of PI 3-kinase activity and downstream effector AKT kinase in this case leads to attenuation of the glycemic response to systemic insulin treatment (Gelling et al., 2006). The glucose-lowering effect of insulin in STZ rats after adenovirus delivery of *Irs-2* gene into the hypothalamic arcuate nucleus was increased 2-fold compared to diabetic rats receiving a control adenovirus. The same results were obtained after injection of adenovirus encoding a constitutively active AKT kinase. These findings indicate that the response to adenovirus encoding IRS-2 involves signal transduction via PI 3-kinase and AKT kinase, and the increased hypothalamic signaling either upstream or downstream of PI 3-kinase is sufficient to enhance insulin-induced glucose lowering in diabetic rats (Gelling et al., 2006). Hence, being the most insulin-responsive brain area, the hypothalamus contributes to whole-body glucose homeostasis via IRS–PI 3-kinase signaling.

The prime function of the other mechanism of neuroprotective action of insulin and IGF-1 realized via PI 3-kinase is to control the oxidative stress and susceptibility of the brain endothelium, the important contributing factors in the development of CNS disorders in DM (Okouchi et al., 2006). It was found that chronic hyperglycemia exacerbated apoptosis of human brain endothelial cells in accordance with exaggerated cytosolic and mitochondrial glutathione and protein-thiol redox imbalance. Insulin activates the PI 3-kinase/AKT kinase/mTOR kinase cascade, increases serine phosphorylation and nuclear translocation of nuclear NF-E2-related factor 2 (Nrf2), and enhances the expression of catalytic subunit of Nrf2-dependent glutamate-L-cysteine ligase, a heterodimeric enzyme participating in glutathione metabolism, and, hence, attenuates hyperglycemia-induced apoptosis via the restored cytosolic and mitochondrial redox balance. Inhibitors of IR tyrosine kinase, PI 3-kinase, AKT kinase and mTOR kinase abrogate insulin-induced Nrf2-mediated glutamate-L-cysteine ligase expression, redox balance, and the survival of human brain endothelial cells (Okouchi et al., 2006). Insulin-regulated PI 3-kinase-dependent pathways are involved in the prevention of endoplasmic reticulum stress that contributes to DM and neurodegenerative disorders (Hosoi et al., 2007). It was found that PI 3-kinase regulates the expression of CHOP protein, an endoplasmic reticulum stress-induced transcription factor involved in control of neuronal cell survival.

The important role in regulation of insulin level in the diabetic brain belongs to the insulin-degrading enzyme (IDE). In addition to insulin, it also degrades β-amyloid peptide. Thus, in the case of hyperinsulinemia in DM2, insulin competes with β-amyloid peptide for IDE and this leads to an increase in β-amyloid peptide concentration and provokes neurodegenerative processes and the development of AD (Qiu & Folstein, 2006). The genetic studies indicate that *IDE* gene variations are associated with the clinical symptoms of AD as well as with the risk of DM2. In DM1 it was shown that the activity of IDE and the level of mRNA encoding IDE were significantly decreased in the temporal cortex of STZ rats. Since the activity of two other β-amyloid peptide-degrading enzymes, neprilysin and endothelin-converting enzyme 1, was also decreased though to a different extent in the brain of diabetic rats, the level of the β-amyloid peptide 1–40 was markedly elevated, which induced DM-associated AD and other abnormalities of CNS (Y. Liu et al., 2011). The other authors reported a significant reduction of IDE expression in the brain of STZ mice after 9 weeks of hyperglycemia (Jolivalt et al., 2008). The treatment with insulin partially restored phosphorylation of IR and downstream components of insulin signaling system and led to restoration of IDE activity. Based on these data the conclusion was made that in both types of DM the level of β-amyloid peptides was increased, although the molecular mechanisms and the role of IDE in this case may be different.

2.2 Leptin

Leptin, the product of the *ob* gene, is mainly secreted by peripheral adipocytes, it regulates energy metabolism and body weight. Leptin deficiency in rodents and humans leads to severe obesity. Leptin penetrates into the brain through the BBB as a result of receptor-mediated endocytosis, binds to the leptin receptors located on neurons in the hypothalamus, where the density of receptors is high, and in some extrahypothalamic regions including the cortex, thalamus, cerebellum, choroid plexus and olfactory bulb (Mutze et al., 2006, Marino et al., 2011). The leptin receptor belonging to the cytokine family receptors has several isoforms, but only the full-length isoform generates an intracellular signal. Activated leptin receptors trigger the stimulation of JAK2 tyrosine kinase that phosphorylates the intracellular domain of the receptor to create a binding site for IRS proteins activating PI 3-kinase and the MEK/ERK signaling pathway (Hegyi et al, 2004). JAK2 kinase also activates the transcription factor STAT3, and the JAK/STAT pathway plays the major role in leptin signaling via the membrane receptors (Mutze et al., 2006).

Central leptin interacts with the hypothalamic nuclei and regulates energy expenditure and food intake through production of agouti-related protein (AgRP), the antagonist of melanocotin receptors (MCRs), and neuropeptide Y (NPY), and α-melanocyte-stimulating hormone (α-MSH) (M.W. Schwartz et al. 2000; Signore et al., 2008). Leptin, like insulin, is involved in the control of the excitability of hypothalamic neurons, modulates the synaptic plasticity and promotes the learning and cognition. Leptin facilitates the presynaptic transmitter release and postsynaptic sensitivity to the transmitters in the hippocampal neurons and regulates hippocampal synaptic plasticity and neuronal development. The rodents with dysfunction of leptin signaling display impaired hippocampal synaptic plasticity, and the application of leptin restores the functions of hippocampus (X.L. Li et al, 2002). In neuronal cells leptin activates JAK/STAT, MEK/ERK and PI 3-kinase signaling pathways and functions as the antiapoptotic factor regulating cell survival. The central effects of leptin are mainly mediated via PI 3-kinase and AKT kinase (Morton et al., 2005). Leptin also serves as neurotrophic factor, because it reverses the loss of dopaminergic neurons and dopamine (DA)-mediated behavior induced by the toxin destroying these neurons (Weng et al., 2007). Therefore, leptin not only protects the rescuing dopaminergic neurons from toxicity, but also preserves the DA-regulated signaling network in neurodegenerative diseases, which might prove useful in the treatment of DM-associated neurodegenerative diseases.

Some time ago in the CA1 hippocampal region of leptin receptor-deficient rodents (Zucker *fa/fa* rats and *db/db* mice) the impairments of hippocampal long-term potentiation (LTP) and long-term depression (LTD) were detected (X.L. Li et al., 2002). The animals showed deficiencies in neuronal and behavioral plasticity and, as demonstrated by the impairment of spatial memory in the Morris water-maze test, had memory deficit due, at least in part, to a deficiency in leptin receptors. The leptin administration gave no results probably because of insensitivity of the hippocampus to the hormone. Since the deficiency in hippocampal plasticity in diabetic patients and STZ-treated animals is independent of insulin level, it can be assumed that the cause for these abnormalities is the concert functioning of leptin and insulin signaling systems and their ability to modulate other neuronal systems regulated by γ-aminobutyric acid (GABA), DA and melanocortin (Van der Heide et al., 2005). A close interrelation between the signaling pathways controlled by leptin and the dopaminergic and peptidergic signaling systems is supported by the following data obtained with experimental DM and obesity. The leptin deficiency in the obese mice lacking leptin (*$Lep^{ob/ob}$* mice) led to a decrease in the content of somatodendritic vesicular DA and the amount of DA to be released (Roseberry et al., 2007). One possible cause is related to a decrease of the number of functionally active DA transporters controlling the synaptic level of DA. I.c.v. and parenchymal hypothalamic administration of leptin into MKR mice, a model of non-obese DM2, lacking IGF-1 receptor and having hyperglycemia, hyperinsulinemia, and hyperlipidemia, significantly increased the rate of disappearance of glucose. These effects were mediated by brain MCRs, as central administration of SHU9119, the antagonist of MCRs of the types 3 and 4 (MC_3R and MC_4R), blocked the ability of hypothalamic leptin to increase skeletal muscle glucose metabolism, glucose uptake and fat oxidation, while in the presence of the agonists of the receptors the anti-diabetic effects of leptin were retained and intensified even more (Toda et al., 2009). The involvement of hypothalamic signaling systems regulated by neurotransmitters in the regulatory effects of central leptin on the energy balance and peripheral glucose homeostasis is supported by the results of the study of non-obese diabetic MKR mice, where i.c.v. administration of leptin dramatically improved insulin sensitivity both via the hypothalamus and direct contact with the peripheral tissues (X. Li et al., 2011).

Studying the action of i.c.v. administered leptin on metabolic imbalance caused by experimental DM1 it was found that leptin normalizes the glucose homeostasis and ameliorates the functioning of CNS in STZ-treated rodents (Kojima et al., 2009; Wang et al., 2010). I.c.v. infusion of leptin reversed lethality and greatly improved hyperglycemia, hyperglucagonemia, hyperketonemia, and polyuria in STZ mice. The leptin therapy improved the expression of the metabolically relevant hypothalamic neuropeptides pro-opiomelanocortin (POMC) and NPY, and also the expression of AgRP in the brain of diabetic mice and restored their signaling cascades impaired in DM1. For the effects of leptin to be long-term, the technique of i.c.v. administration of recombinant adeno-associated virus vector (*rAAV*) encoding leptin gene (*rAAV-lep*) was developed and used in adult STZ-treated mice. The injection of *rAAV-lep* gene markedly increased the level of hypothalamic leptin, rescued the STZ mice from early mortality, gradually decreased hyperphagia to normalize food intake by the 20th week, and maintained body weight within significantly lower than the control range. The blood levels of glucose in these mice started to recede dramatically by the 2nd-3rd week to normalize by the 8th week, and euglycemia was sustained during 52 weeks of experiment. *rAAV-lep* gene injected mice did not exhibit any discernible untoward behavioral changes, nor diabetic complications (Kojima et al., 2009).

The addition of low-dose insulin to the leptin therapy provides physiological insulin level for the peripheral targets of STZ rats and leptin in this case suppresses the hyperglucagonemia, avoiding high doses of insulin required to decrease the elevated glucagon level (Wang et al., 2010). Thus, leptin administration has multiple short- and long-term advantages over insulin monotherapy of DM1, and the combined application of leptin and insulin can be recommended for the treatment of human DM1. A high efficiency of the combined action of insulin and leptin suggests that the brain signaling systems sensitive to these hormones have the common components enabling their interaction which takes place in the hypothalamus or the other brain areas sensitive to insulin and leptin. This view finds support in the fact that leptin directly governs glucose homeostasis via activation of leptin receptors in neurons within the hypothalamic arcuate nucleus enriched by IRs (Huo et al., 2009). Summing up, the brain is a critical site for mediating leptin metabolic-improving actions in DM and the action of central leptin is in concert with the action of insulin and, probably of IGF-1.

3. Neurotransmitter signaling systems in the diabetic brain

The various neurotransmitter systems, including dopaminergic, serotonergic, cholinergic, glutamatergic, and GABAergic, undergo a significant change in DM (Jackson & Paulose, 1999; Gireesh et al., 2008; Antony et al., 2010a; Anu et al., 2010; T.P. Kumar et al., 2010) (Fig. 2). The well-coordinated activation and inhibition of different neurotransmitter systems in normal brain are disrupted in DM-associated hyper- and hypoglycemia and in the case of insulin and leptin deficit. The synergistic effect of alterations of neurotransmitter receptors leads to neurodegenerative changes in different brain areas and to the development of CNS disorders and dysfunctions.

3.1 Dopamine signaling

DA is the predominant catecholamine neurotransmitter in the brain of mammals, where it controls a variety of functions including locomotor activity, cognition, emotion, positive reinforcement, food intake, and endocrine regulation. DA also plays multiple roles in the periphery as a modulator of cardiovascular function, catecholamine release, hormone secretion, vascular tone, and gastrointestinal motility. The results obtained with diabetic animals and the clinical study of patients with DM2 showed that reduced dopaminergic activity in the brain is involved in the pathogenesis of DM2 and metabolic syndrome and is responsible for DM-induced changes in the CNS (Pijl & Edo, 2002).

The treatment of diabetic patients with selective ligands of dopamine receptors (DARs) is a promising approach to improve the functions of CNS in DM. In the recent years a selective D_2-DAR agonist bromocriptine, an ergot derivative, has been widely used in the treatment of DM, especially DM2, and obesity. Bromocriptine acts on a central target in the brain, mainly in hypothalamus, and reduces ventromedial, arcuate and paraventricular hypothalamic drive for increased hepatic glucose production, lipid synthesis and mobilization, and insulin resistance, which decreases the risk of damage of neuronal cells and the cardiovascular system in patients with DM2 (Scranton et al., 2007). It is very important that bromocriptine reduces fasting and postprandial glucose without increasing insulin level and its therapeutic effects are not associated with weight gain or hypoglycemia. The main mechanism of action of bromocriptine is based on its ability to bind with D_2-DAR coupled with the adenylyl cyclase (AC) via G_i protein, which provides the utility in resetting hypothalamic circadian organization of monoamine neuronal activities in patients with DM2. The other mechanisms include the influence of bromocriptine on signaling pathways regulated by α-adrenergic ligands and prolactin, as well as its inhibitory effect on serotonin (5-hydroxytryptamine, 5-HT) turnover in the CNS, and may also be involved in glucose-lowering effects of bromocriptine (Kerr et al., 2010).

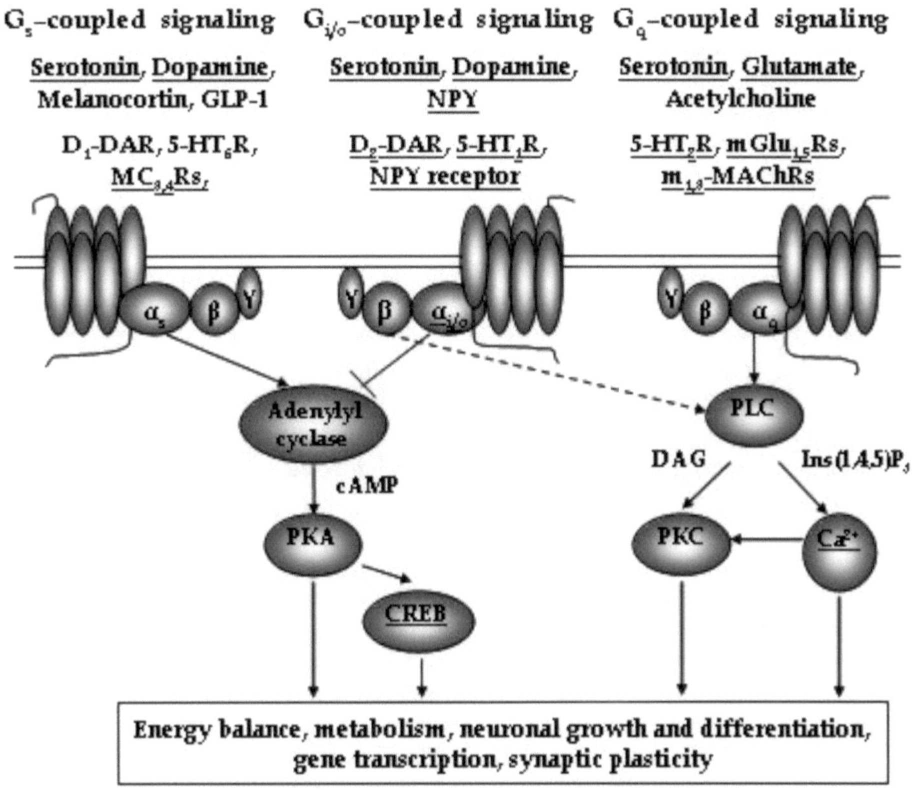

Fig. 2. G_s-, $G_{i/o}$- and G_q-coupled signaling pathways including the receptors of the serpentine type regulated by biogenic amines, glutamate, acetylcholine and peptide hormones. The signal components whose activity and expression are significantly altered in DM are underlined. Abbreviations: NPY, neuropeptide Y; GLP-1, glucagon-like peptide-1; $D_{1,2}DARs$, dopamine receptors of the types 1 and 2; 5-$HT_{1,2,6}Rs$, 5-hydroxytryptamine receptors of the types 1, 2 and 6; $MC_{3,4}Rs$, melanocortin receptors of the types 3 and 4; $mGlu_{1,5}Rs$, metabotropic glutamate receptors of the types 1 and 5; $m_{1,3}$-MAChRs, muscarinic acetylcholine receptors of the types 1 and 3; $\alpha_{s,i/o,q}\beta\gamma$, heterotrimeric G_s-, $G_{i/o}$- and G_q-proteins; PKA, protein kinase A; CREB, cAMP response element-binding; PLC, phosphoinositide-specific phospholipase C; PKC, protein kinase C; cAMP, 3′,5′-cyclic adenosine monophosphate; DAG, diacylglycerol; $Ins(1,4,5)P_3$, phosphatidylinositol 1,4,5-triphosphate

The treatment with bromocriptine can reverse the metabolic abnormalities in humans with DM2 and obesity and in obese experimental animals. Using 22 obese patients with DM2 it was found that bromocriptine significantly reduces both glycosylated hemoglobin level and fasting and postprandial plasma glucose concentrations, it decreases the mean plasma glucose concentration during oral glucose tolerance test, which indicates the improvement in glucose tolerance (Pijl et al., 2000). There are also reports that administration of Cycloset (bromocriptine mesylate) either as monotherapy or adjunctive therapy to sulfonylurea or insulin markedly reduces glycosylated hemoglobin, plasma triglycerides and free fatty acid levels (Scranton et al., 2007). The effects of once-daily morning Cycloset therapy on glycemic control and plasma lipids are demonstrable throughout the diurnal portion of the day (7 a.m. to 7 p.m.) across postprandial time points. Recently it was shown that the bromocriptine therapy of 4328 patients with DM2 during 6–24 weeks leads to a significant decrease of glycosylated hemoglobin and plasma glucose levels (Kerr et al., 2010).

Bromocriptine improved the functional state of obese glucose-intolerant Syrian hamsters, inducing a decrease in their insulin resistance and markedly lowering the plasma levels of insulin and free fatty acids (S. Luo et al., 2000). These anti-diabetic effects of bromocriptine are associated with its influence on the daily rhythms of metabolic hormones and daily monoamine profiles within the hypothalamic suprachiasmatic nuclei that modulate circadian neuroendocrine activities and, thus, regulate metabolism of seasonal animals. The bromocriptine significantly reduced DA turnover during the light period and shifted daily peaks of the content of 5-HT and 5-hydroxy-indoleacetic acid (5-HIAA), the main metabolite of 5-HT, by 12 h from the light to the dark period of the day within the hypothalamic suprachiasmatic nuclei, it also increased extracellular 5-HIAA in the brain of diabetic hamsters during the dark phase toward levels observed in normal glucose-tolerant animals.

Using animal models it was found that a combined administration of agonists of D_1- and D_2-DARs is a successful approach for decreasing appetite in both STZ rats and ob/ob mice (Bina & Cincotta, 2000; Kuo, 2006). The anorectic response induced by D_1/D_2 agonists is due to their antagonistic action on hypothalamic neurons containing NPY, the most potent appetite transducer in the CNS, and on NPY-dependent signaling. In DM the NPY system is up-regulated due to increased expression of both NPY and its receptor and to enhanced release of NPY. The co-administration of D_1/D_2 agonists normalized the elevated NPY content and hyperphagic effect observed in STZ rats and *ob/ob* mice (Bina & Cincotta, 2000; Kuo, 2006). However, the response of D_1/D_2 agonist-induced appetite suppression was attenuated in diabetic rats compared to normal animals, which can be ascribed both to a decreased inhibitory action of central dopaminergic system and to enhanced activity of hypothalamic NPY neurons in DM. The insulin treatment in DM normalized the response to D_1/D_2 agonists owing to the restoration of NPY content in the hypothalamus and DA signaling.

The reduction of activity of the brain dopaminergic system in DM is mainly due to changes of the initial stages of DA-induced signal transduction which involves DARs, G_i or G_s proteins and effectors, AC and phospholipase C (PLC), generating second messengers. In many brain regions the activity of DARs and signal proteins coupled to them has DAR-specific differential alterations. The studies in this area are mostly devoted to the functional state of DARs in DM. In the early 1980s it was found that the binding of $[^3H]$-spiperone, antagonist of D_2-DAR, to striatal membranes is significantly increased in rats with DM induced by alloxan or STZ treatment, and insulin therapy leads to normalization of functioning of central dopaminergic system (Lozovsky et al., 1981). Recently it was shown that the expression of D_1- and D_2-DARs and total DAR binding (B_{max}) are increased in the cerebral cortex of STZ rats (T.P. Kumar et al., 2010). In the cerebellum D_1-DAR was down regulated and D_2-DAR up regulated, a total number of DARs being however decreased. The treatment with insulin or curcumin, an active component in rhizome of *Curcuma longa*, reduced DM-induced alteration of D_1- and D_2-DARs in the cerebral cortex and increased D_1-DAR expression in the cerebellum to near control, thereby improving the cognitive and emotional functions associated with these regions. In the hypothalamus and brainstem of STZ rats a significant decrease in the DA content and the number of D_2-DARs, and an increase in affinity of the latter were found, and the insulin therapy did not completely reverse the DM-induced changes of D_2-DAR functions (Shankar et al., 2007). The hypothalamus and brainstem are two parts of the brain very important for monitoring the glucose status and the regulation of feeding. The hypothalamus, in addition, controls the release of pituitary hormones having a key role in regulation of the CNS and the periphery. These data indicate that the activity of the dopaminergic system in different areas of the diabetic brain either increases or decreases, which must be taken into consideration in clinic practice for successful management of DM and its cerebral complications.

The alteration of DA-regulated signaling cascades in DM is associated with their downstream components, such as the transcription factor CREB playing a pivotal role in DAR-mediated nuclear signaling and neuroplasticity (Finkbeiner, 2000) and D_1-DAR-coupled PLC involved in the neuromodulation of hippocampal LTD (J. Liu et al., 2009). It was found that STZ-induced DM produces a significant attenuation of functional activity of CREB and PLC in the cerebral cortex and cerebellum of diabetic rats and these alterations are largely eliminated by the treatment with insulin and curcumin (T.P. Kumar et al., 2010).

We showed that in the brain of rats with STZ-induced DM1, duration one month, as well as with neonatal model of DM2, duration 3 to 6 months, the sensitivity of AC to regulatory action of bromocriptine was decreased (Shpakov et al., 2006, 2007a). The inhibitory effect of bromocriptine on forskolin-stimulated AC activity and its stimulating effect on GppNHp binding of G_i proteins in synaptosomal membranes of diabetic rats were significantly decreased, predominantly in DM1. As the binding characteristics of DARs and the catalytic activity of AC did not change essentially, a suggestion was made that the impairment of bromocriptine-induced signaling in the diabetic brain was due to the reduced function of G_i proteins (Shpakov et al., 2007b). This view finds support in the fact that the regulatory effects of somatostatin and 5-HT_1R agonists acting, like bromocryptine, on AC via G_i protein-coupled receptors were decreased in the brain of diabetic rats (Shpakov et al., 2007a). The attenuation of D_2 agonist-induced suppression of appetite in STZ rats (Kuo, 2006) is also likely to be the result of reduction of G_i protein activity in the diabetic brain.

Another cause why the activity of dopaminergic system in the diabetic brain is decreased is the reduction in DA uptake and the DA transporter (DAT) expression that depend on the activity of PI 3-kinase and AKT kinase (Garcia et al., 2005). The uptake by DAT is the primary pathway for the clearance of extracellular DA and hence for regulating the magnitude and duration of dopaminergic signaling. Insulin activates PI 3-kinase and AKT kinase, increases DA uptake and blocks the amphetamine-induced DAT intracellular accumulation leading to a decrease of the number of active transporters. In DM1, which is characterized by hypoinsulinemia, the available cell surface DATs are reduced, and this leads to decrease of synaptic DA level. As a result, the DM-induced alterations in DA uptake and transport induce attenuation of synaptic DA signaling. Actually, the impairment of DA uptake and transport systems in the hippocampus of both STZ and spontaneously diabetic *WBN/Kob* rats leads to a significant decrease in the basal level of DA (Yamato et al., 2004).

3.2 Serotonin signaling

The brain serotonergic system regulates several behaviors (e.g., feeding, locomotion, reproduction, sleep, pain, aggression and stress responses) as well as some autonomic functions (e.g., thermogenesis, cardiovascular control, circadian rhythm and pancreatic function). The changes of serotonergic transmission in the diabetic brain provoke disturbances in neuronal processing and the altered plasticity of neurotransmission, and play an important role in DM-induced behavioral abnormalities. This is due first of all to the alteration of the brain sensitivity to 5-HT, which depends on the functioning of 5-HT-regulated signaling pathways and the disturbances in the biochemical conversion, reuptake and transport of 5-HT and its metabolites. These changes cause a distorted response of neuronal cells and the CNS as a whole to 5-HT and its analogs, as well as to the drugs that increase the level of central 5-HT.

Selective 5-HT reuptake inhibitors are widely used in the pharmacological treatment of depression typical of both DM1 and DM2 and have a significant effect on the course and outcome of this medical illness (Lustman & Clouse, 2005). The 5-HT reuptake inhibitors contribute to lowering the level of hyperglycemia, decrease the rate of hemoglobin glycosylation, improve metabolic control through their positive effect on weight loss, thereby improving insulin resistance, and restore cognitive functions impaired in DM (Van Tilburg et al., 2001). It was shown that the treatment of 60 patients with depression associated with DM1 and DM2 by fluoxetine, selective 5-HT reuptake inhibitor, significantly reduces depressive symptoms and increases the sensitivity of the brain and the peripheral tissues to insulin (Lustman et al., 2000). Consequently, the approach leading to an increase of the brain 5-HT level and, thus, improving 5-HTR signaling in the CNS is a successful strategy to treat DM (Zhou et al., 2007).

In the late 1970s, it was shown that STZ-induced DM and hyperglycemia have a significant influence on the brain tryptophan (Trp) and 5-HT metabolism (MacKenzie & Trulson, 1978). The content of 5-HT and 5-hydroxyindoleacetic acid (5-HIAA), the main metabolite of 5-HT, as well as 5-HT turnover (5-HIAA/5-HT) is decreased in different brain areas of STZ rats with long-term hyperglycemia and in the hippocampus of spontaneously diabetic *WBN/Kob* rats (Sandirini et al., 1997; Jackson & Paulose, 1999; Yamato et al., 2004). A decrease in 5-HT level is due to the decreased uptake of Trp, the precursor of 5-HT, by the brain (Mackenzie & Trulson, 1978). An increase in the level of insulin can result in decreased plasma concentrations of large neutral amino acids (phenylalanine, valine, leucine, isoleucine, tyrosine) competing with Trp for uptake by the brain, which accounts for a low availability of plasma Trp. The other cause of a decrease of the biosynthesis of 5-HT is a long-lasting inhibition of the rate-limiting enzyme tryptophan-5-hydroxylase 2 (Herrera et al., 2005). It was shown that the Trp level and the free/total Trp ratio in the plasma and in the brain of children and adolescents with DM1 and in women with DM2 were also significantly decreased (Manjarrez-Gutierrez et al., 2009). Free fraction and free fraction/total Trp ratio were also decreased in adolescents with metabolic syndrome, although to a small extent (Herrera-Marquez et al., 2011). In the case of diabetic adolescents two groups of patients, with and without depression, were studied and it was shown that diabetic patients with depression had a lower level of Trp compared with diabetic adolescents without depression (Manjarrez-Gutierrez et al., 2009). Diabetic patients with depression had the most expressed hypoinsulinemia and more extended episodes of hyperglycemia than patients without depression. These results indicate that the degree of disturbances of brain serotonergic activity is likely to correlate with the degree of metabolic disturbances induced by DM1.

Hypoglycemia caused by fasting or by treatment of diabetic patients with peripheral insulin, like hyperglycemia associated with STZ DM, leads to disturbances in serotoninergic system of the brain (Das, 2010). Hypoglycemia increases turnover of 5-HT and decreases the level of 5-HT precursor 5-HIAA in both ventromedial and lateral hypothalamic areas, which induces a decrease of central 5-HT concentration (Shimizu & Bray, 1990). At the same time, i.c.v. administered insulin at doses 50 and 100 µUnits, which induced minimal hypoglycemia, increased 5-HT concentration in the midbrain and ponsmedulla oblongata of hyperglycemic rats with alloxan DM and partially restored 5-HT-regulated functions of the CNS (Bhattacharya & Saraswati, 1991). It indicates the importance of the appropriate glycemic control for restoration of 5-HT metabolism in the diabetic brain.

With a decrease of concentration of 5-HT and 5-HIAA in the diabetic brain the number of different types of 5-HTRs and their affinity to available 5-HT increases inducing alteration of 5-HT neurotransmission. Thus, in the frontal cortex of STZ rats the density of $5\text{-HT}_{2A}R$, coupled to PLC via G_q proteins, was significantly higher than in control group of animals (Sandrini et al., 1997). An increase in affinity of $5\text{-HT}_{2A}Rs$ in the cerebral cortex without any change in the number of receptors, and a significant increase in B_{max} for these receptors in the brainstem with a decrease in affinity during STZ-induced DM were also shown (Jackson & Paulose, 1999). The alterations of $5\text{-HT}_{2A}R$ in the cerebral cortex and brainstem are a compensatory mechanism responsible for a decrease of 5-HT level in these brain areas in DM. All these parameters returned to normal level by insulin therapy. It seems likely that up-regulation of the $5\text{-HT}_{2A}R$ may have a role in the regulation of insulin secretion from pancreatic islets. As is known, the increased activity of $5\text{-HT}_{2A}R$ in the cerebral cortex and brainstem can increase the sympathetic nerve discharge, thereby increasing the levels of circulating norepinephrine and epinephrine, which leads to inhibition of insulin release from the pancreas. In addition to insulin regulation, an increase in affinity and the number of $5\text{-HT}_{2A}Rs$ has a role in pathogenesis of depression and cognitive deficit in DM.

In our view, being a compensatory response of the brain to lower levels of 5-HT and its precursors, the increase of the number of 5-HTRs is also a reaction to the weakening of signal transduction through these receptors. The latter may be associated with a decreased expression or the functions of signal proteins, the components of 5-HT-regulated signaling pathways. It was shown that one week after STZ treatment the flat body posture induced by $5\text{-HT}_{1A}R$ agonist 8-hydroxy-2-(dipropylamino)tetralin hydrobromide (8-OH-DPAT) and head twitching induced by $5\text{-HT}_{2A}R$ agonist 2,5-dimethoxy-4-iodoamphetamine hydrochloride (DOI) were markedly reduced in the diabetic rats compared with control animals, which indicates that STZ-induced DM profoundly affects the sensitivity to drugs acting at 5-HT_{1A}- and $5\text{-HT}_{2A}Rs$ (J.X. Li & France, 2008). Insulin treatment during one week restored 8-OH-DPAT and DOI-induced behavioral effects. We found no alteration of the sensitivity of AC signaling system in the brain of STZ rats to selective agonists of 5-HT_6R coupled with G_s proteins, while the sensitivity of this system to agonists of $5\text{-HT}_{1A}R$ and $5\text{-HT}_{1B}R$ coupled with G_i proteins was significantly decreased (Shpakov et al., 2007a). We consider the weakening of 5-HT_1R-mediated signaling to be associated with decreased expression and activity of G_i proteins because, as mentioned above, a decrease in activity of the other G_i protein-coupled cascades regulated by somatostatin and DA was also detected in the brain in DM. Note that in the diabetic brain the signaling pathways involving G_s proteins were either unchanged or changed very little (Shpakov et al., 2007b). The impairment of response of the diabetic brain to 5-HT was made evident in the recent clinic study where citalopram, a selective 5-HT reuptake inhibitor, was used in the treatment of patients with DM2. It was shown that citalopram is less effective in diabetic patients compared with healthy individuals (Trento et al., 2010). The appropriate control of glucose and insulin plasma level in patients with DM2 makes it possible to increase the efficiency of citalopram treatment and the response of the hypothalamic-pituitary-adrenal axis to this drug, and to improve the clinical as well as cognitive and emotional variables.

Dysfunctions of the serotonergic system of the brain can be the result of DM, but on the other hand, they can be the cause of DM. The attenuation of 5-HT signaling in the brain induces hyperphagia and other disturbances of feeding behavior, which, in turn, leads to the obesity and DM2 (Heisler et al., 2002). The cause of this is in that the central 5-HT activates, via 5-HT_{2C}Rs expressed on POMC neurons, signaling pathways regulated by melanocortin and its analogs via MC_4R/MC_3R located on the same neurons in the arcuate nucleus of the hypothalamus (Zhou et al., 2007; Nonogaki et al., 2008). It follows, these neurons are a potential target for 5-HT_{2C}R agonists because they receive direct input from 5-HT dorsal raphe nucleus neurons and project to the regions associated with energy regulation. 5-HT_{2C}R agonists significantly improved glucose tolerance and reduced plasma insulin in animals with obesity and DM2. 5-HT_{2C}R agonist-induced improvements in glucose homeostasis occurred at concentrations of agonist that had no effect on feeding behavior, energy expenditure, locomotor activity, body weight, and fat mass (Zhou et al., 2007). These data are supported by the results of genetic studies. It was revealed in the murine knockout studies that only deletion of the gene encoding the 5-HT_{2C} receptor produces insulin resistance and DM2 with antecedent hyperphagia and obesity, which demonstrates that 5-HT_{2C}Rs are critical for energy homeostasis (Bonasera & Tecott, 2000). It was found that three loci of single nucleotide substitution ($G \rightarrow A$ at -995, $C \rightarrow T$ at -759, $G \rightarrow C$ at -697) and $(GT)_n$ dinucleotide repeat polymorphism in the upstream region (promoter) of the 5-HT_{2C}R gene are involved in the development of obesity and DM2 in human (Yuan et al., 2000). The haplotypes containing the nucleotide substitutions are associated with higher transcription levels of the gene and thereby with resistance to obesity and DM2.

3.3 Glutamate signaling

Glutamate is the major excitatory neurotransmitter in the CNS. It exerts action via ionotropic glutamate receptors (iGluRs) - AMPA and NMDA receptors, and via metabotropic glutamate receptors (mGluRs). mGluRs are predominantly found in pre- and post-synaptic neurons in synapses of the hippocampus, cerebellum and cerebral cortex but are also present in other parts of the brain and in the peripheral tissues. mGluR subtypes are critical in gating the plasticity and memory formation. mGluRs interact with iGluRs, ion channels and membrane-associated enzymes, the generators of second messengers, that modulate the cellular response involved in the processes of differentiation and degeneration of neuronal cells. The activation of $mGlu_1R$ and $mGlu_5R$, belonging to group I of mGluRs, enhances phosphoinositide hydrolysis and mobilization of intracellular Ca^{2+} due to stimulation of PLC, induces the activation of Na^+ and K^+ channels, modulates voltage-dependent Ca^{2+} channels and inhibits glutamate release, all this being of great importance in the regulation of cascades of biochemical reactions resulting in death of neuronal cells (N.E. Schwartz & Alford, 2000). The iGluRs are ligand-gated nonselective cation channels allowing the flow of K^+, Na^+ and Ca^{2+} in response to glutamate binding. These receptors, like mGluRs, have influence on synaptic plasticity and are of prime importance in excitotoxicity. An increase or a decrease of the number of iGluRs on post-synaptic neurons leads to LTP or LTD of neuronal cell, respectively. The activation of NMDA receptors in post-synaptic neurons increases Ca^{2+} influx, leading to phospholipase A_2-mediated arachidonic acid release and neuronal injury by inhibiting the Na^+-channels.

Glutamate is essential for synaptic communication in the CNS, but inadequate increase of extracellular glutamate and excessive activation of GluRs causes toxicity in the brain leading to neurodegenerative disorders (Trudeau et al., 2004). Excessive glutamate over-activates the cognate receptors, specifically NMDA receptors, which gives the influx of high level of Ca^{2+} in the post-synaptic cell. In the diabetic brain the glutamate level and the number of

GluRs are significantly increased, which is the main cause of neurodegenerative changes in DM (N. Li et al., 1999; Tomiyama et al., 2005; Joseph et al., 2008; Anu et al., 2010) (Fig. 3).

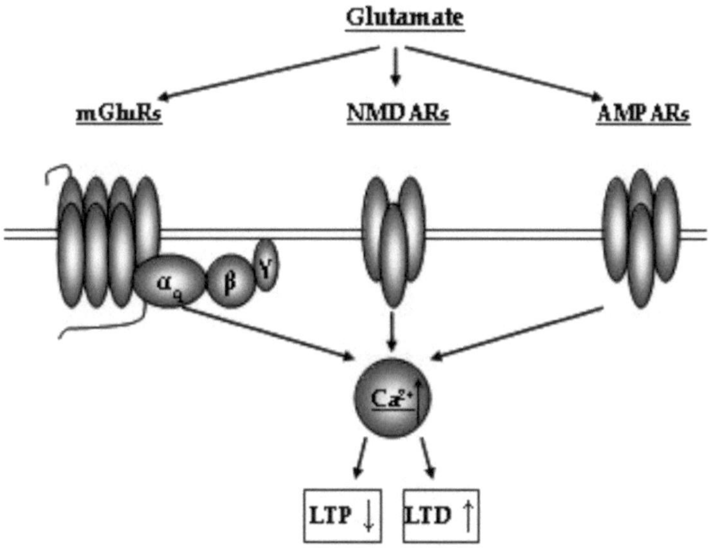

Fig. 3. Signaling pathways responsible for glutamate toxicity

Abbreviations: mGluRs, metabotropic glutamate receptors; NMDARs and AMPARs, ionotropic glutamate receptors of NMDA and AMPA types; $\alpha_q\beta\gamma$, heterotrimeric G_q-protein; LTP and LTD, long-term potentiation and long-term depression, respectively.

The synaptic level of glutamate in the brain depends on the high-affinity glutamate transporter GLAST, the major component of synaptic glutamate reuptake system, that plays an important role in the termination of glutamatergic neurotransmission and prevention of excitotoxicity, it also depends on the activity of GluRs regulating synaptic glutamate release (Danbolt, 2001). In nerve terminals specific vesicular transporters GluT1-3 allow incorporation of glutamate into synaptic vesicles. These transporters have an essential role in glutamate recycling and homeostasis in the CNS and the abnormalities of this functioning are responsible for development of neurological disorders (Benarroch, 2010). Synaptic release of endogenous glutamate is mediated with the voltage-dependent N-, L- and P/Q-type Ca^{2+} channels controlling the entry of Ca^{2+} into nerve terminals. In the diabetic brain the content of glutamate transporters and the α_{1A} subunit of P/Q type Ca^{2+} channels are changed. In the cerebellum of STZ rats the expression of the glutamate transporter GLAST gene was decreased, which indicates a decrease of glutamate reuptake (Anu et al., 2010). In the hippocampus a decrease of the level of glutamate transporters was transient, being evident mainly at the early stages of DM. This suggests that after the initial stress induced by DM the hippocampus was somehow able to respond to DM-induced stress, and after two weeks of DM the level of glutamate transporters recovered so that the values remained under control longer. After eight weeks of DM, the levels of glutamate transporters and P/Q-type Ca^{2+} channels did not change but the basal release of glutamate was significantly increased in hippocampal synaptosomes, which may underlie alterations in synaptic transmission at the later stages of DM (Baptista et al., 2011).

In the cerebral synaptosomes from STZ mice the K^+- and 4-aminopyridine-evoked Ca^{2+}-dependent glutamate release was significantly increased. The treatment of synaptosomes with a combination of ω-agatoxin IVA (a P-type Ca^{2+} channel blocker) and ω-conotoxin GVIA (an N-type Ca^{2+} channel blocker) completely inhibited K^+- or 4-aminopyridine-induced increase in glutamate release and prevented glutamate toxicity typical of the diabetic brain (Satoh & Takahashi, 2008). It means that STZ-induced DM enhanced a depolarization-evoked Ca^{2+}-dependent glutamate release in cerebral synaptosomes by stimulating Ca^{2+} entry through both P- and N-type Ca^{2+} channels. It was also shown that voltage-dependent Ca^{2+} currents through N-, P- and L-type Ca^{2+} channels were enhanced in dorsal root ganglion neurons of STZ rats and Bio Bred/Worchester diabetic rats, which directly mediated the increase of glutamate exocytosis and induced DM-associated excitotoxicity (Voitenko et al., 2000; Hall et al., 2001). These data allow the selective blockers of the Ca^{2+} channels to be considered possible drugs for the treatment of diabetic patients with neuronal disorders associated with an increased level of synaptic glutamate.

In the cerebral cortex and cerebellum of STZ rats and hypoglycemic diabetic rats the expression of NR1 and NR2B receptor subunits and $mGlu_5R$ genes and the number of the receptors were increased (Joseph et al., 2008). The activity of $mGlu_5R$ was increased, which led to stimulation of the activity of PLC coupled with $mGlu_5R$ via G_q protein and to an increase of the content of intracellular inositol 1,4,5-triphosphate receptors interacting with the second messenger phosphatidyl inositol 1,4,5-triphosphate generated by PLC. The increase of activity of NMDA receptors and the $mGlu_5R$-associated stimulation of PLC activity mediated Ca^{2+} overload in cells causing neuronal cell damage and neurodegeneration in the diabetic brain, affecting as it did the motor learning and memory ability (Anu et al., 2010). In the dorsal horn of the lumbar spinal cord of STZ rats the levels of mRNAs coding several AMPA receptor subunits (GluR1, GluR2, and GluR3), NMDA receptor subunits (NR2A and NR2B), as well as $mGlu_1R$ and $mGlu_5R$ were also up regulated (Tomiyama et al., 2005). In the deep dorsal horn of STZ rats the level of NMDA receptors with high affinity for glutamate, namely NR1/NR2A or NR1/NR2B receptors, was the highest. Also increased was the number of NMDA and AMPA receptors in the gray matter of the spinal cord of the *ob/ob* mice responsible for pain, sensory perception and muscle control (N. Li et al., 1999). Thus, the elevated level of specific GluRs/GluR subunits in the spinal cord is a precondition for the pathogenesis of sensory impairment leading to diabetic neuropathy in DM. The use of GluRs antagonists decreasing enhanced activity of these receptors in the diabetic brain significantly ameliorated hyperalgesia and allodynia in experimental DM1 (Malcangio & Tomlinson, 1998; Calcutt & Chaplan, 1997), which suggests that increased excitatory tone in the spinal cord plays an important role in the development of diabetic neuropathy. It should be pointed out that NR2B-selective antagonists are effective in suppressing hyperalgesia in STZ rats with neuropathic pain at doses devoid of negative side effects, which indicates their suitability for control of sensory symptoms induced by DM (Tomiyama et al., 2005). It is worth mentioning that some antagonists of GluRs, e.g. the NMDA receptor antagonists dextromethorphan and amantadine, are used in clinical practice in the treatment of diabetic patients and markedly ameliorate the neuropathic pain in some patients (Nelson et al., 1997; Amin & Sturrock, 2003).

3.4 GABA signaling

GABAergic inhibitory function in the cerebral cortex is of great importance in the regulation of excitability and responsiveness of cortical neurons. GABA inhibition is mediated both by

$GABA_A$ receptors, which open membrane chloride channels and stabilize the membrane potential below firing threshold, and $GABA_B$ receptors, which act via G proteins to reduce transmitter release from presynaptic terminals. The inhibitory GABA-releasing interneurons mediate the function of excitatory glutamatergic neurons in the brain regions, which contributes significantly to the control of glutamate content in brain regions and prevents glutamate toxicity induced in the brain of hypo- and hyperglycemic diabetic rats. Disruption of GABAergic inhibition induces seizures leading to neuronal damage and, therefore, the pathophysiology of many seizure disorders is the result of alteration of GABA receptor function (Antony et al., 2010a).

It was shown that the synaptic level of GABA and its release in the diabetic brain are slightly changed or remain unchanged. The extracellular basal level of GABA at dentate gyrus of STZ rats 12 weeks after the induction of DM showed no changes (Reisi et al., 2009). The content of vesicular GABA transporter was significantly decreased in hippocampal synaptosomal membranes in two week DM, although only minor changes in the release of GABA and in the loading capacity of GABA transporters were found (Baptista et al., 2011). This indicates that the alterations of GABA signaling, typical of the diabetic brain, are due to the changes in the level and functional activity of GABA receptors and down-stream signal components of GABA-regulated intracellular cascades.

Actually, the GABA binding and the gene expression of the subunits of $GABA_{A\alpha1}$ and $GABA_B$ receptors were decreased in the cerebral cortex of diabetic rats compared to control animals. In the diabetic hypoglycemic rats having two episodes of insulin-induced hypoglycemia in the course of 10 days GABA binding and expression of GABA receptor subunits were reduced to a greater extent in comparison with diabetic hyper/euglycemic animals. This is the evidence that hypoglycemia amplifies the adverse effects of hyperglycemia on GABAergic system, and the impairments of functions of GABAergic neurons in the diabetic cerebral cortex are intensified in hypoglycemia. The expression of glutamate decarboxylase, the rate-limiting enzyme of GABA synthesis, which is used as a marker of GABAergic activity, was also significantly down regulated in DM and hypoglycemia exacerbated the altered expression (Antony et al., 2010a). The same picture is found in the cerebellum, where GABA receptors are involved in control of coordination and motor learning and, like in the cerebral cortex, play a critical role in neuronal excitability and modulation of synaptic neurotransmission (Luján, 2007). In the cerebellum of STZ rats with hyperglycemia the gene expression of $GABA_{A\alpha1}$ subunit and glutamate decarboxylase was decreased and these molecular alterations were exacerbated by recurrent hypoglycemia (Sherin et al., 2010). The gene expression of CREB, a stimulus-inducible transcription activator implicated in the activation of protein synthesis required for long-term memory and seizure formation, was significantly down regulated in DM and recurrent hypoglycemia. Since CREB up-regulates endogenous $GABA_{A\alpha1}$ transcription, the decreased expression of CREB in the cerebellum of hypoglycemic and hyperglycemic rats led to the attenuation of GABAergic system and, as a result, to excitotoxic damage of neuronal cells (Sherin et al., 2010). It follows that hypo- and hyperglycemia in DM both decrease GABAergic neuroprotective function in the cerebral cortex and cerebellum, which accounts for increased vulnerability of these brain areas to subsequent neuronal damage.

3.5 Acetylcholine signaling

In the brain acetylcholine functions either as a neuromodulator, or as a neutotransmitter, activating via metabotropic muscarinic acetylcholine receptors (MAChRs) a multitude of signaling pathways important for modulating neuronal excitability, synaptic plasticity and feedback regulation of acetylcholine release and, thus, controls the functional, behavioral and pathological states of the CNS (Dani, 2001). Acetylcholine also activates ionotropic nicotinic acetylcholine receptors that form ligand-gated ion channels in the plasma membranes of the neurons and on the postsynaptic side of the neuromuscular junction. The activation of nicotinic receptors in the CNS induces depolarization of the plasma membrane, culminating in an excitatory postsynaptic potential in neuron, the activation of voltage-gated ion channels and the increase of calcium permeability. The changes in the number and activity of the metabotropic and ionotropic acetylcholine receptors have been implicated in the pathophysiology of many diseases of the CNS, including cognitive impairment.

It was shown that in the cerebral cortex, hypothalamus and brainstem of STZ rats the number of G_q-coupled m_1-MAChRs and the expression of genes encoding m_1-MAChR were decreased with an increase in affinity of the receptor to agonists, and the binding parameters of the m_1-MAChR were reversed to near control by the treatment with insulin (Gireesh et al., 2008; Peeyush Kumar et al., 2011). In the cerebral cortex of the diabetic and control rats with insulin-induced long-term hypoglycemia the maximal binding of m_1-MAChRs and their expression were reduced to a greater extent compared with diabetic animals with hyperglycemia (Sherin et al., 2011). At the same time, in the cerebellum and corpus striatum of both diabetic rats and hypoglycemic diabetic and control rats the binding parameters and gene expression of m_1-MAChRs was, on the contrary, increased (Antony et al., 2010b). This indicates that the alterations in the initial steps of m_1-MAChR signaling in the diabetic brain are area-specific.

The STZ-induced DM and insulin-induced hypoglycemia both lead to a significant increase of the binding of another G_q-coupled m_3-MAChR in the cerebral cortex and cerebellum but the extent of changes induced by hypoglycemia was significantly higher compared to DM, which indicates the detrimental effect of recurrent hypoglycemia on cholinergic system in the brain (Antony et al., 2010b; Peeyush Kumar et al., 2011; Sherin et al., 2011). This allows a conclusion that the imbalance in glucose homeostasis affects acetylcholine metabolism and cholinergic muscarinic neurotransmission in the brain, and changes the expression and function of cholinergic receptors. The study of 7-week- and 90-week-old STZ rats showed that in the brainstem of both groups of animals the number of m_1-MAChRs was significantly decreased whereas the number of m_3-MAChRs greatly increased compared to their respective controls, and the insulin treatment reversed the binding parameters of m_1- and m_3-MAChRs to near control level (Balakrishnan et al., 2009). In the cerebral cortex of 7-week-old STZ rats the number of m_1-MAChRs decreased by 28 %, while the number of m_3-MAChRs increased by 30 %. In the cerebral cortex of 90-week-old diabetic rats the number of m_1- and m_3-MAChRs increased by 43 and 23 %, respectively, and the level of acetylcholine was significantly increased compared to control (Savitha et al., 2010). These alterations of m_1- and m_3-MAChR expression correlate with cholinergic hypofunction in short-term and prolonged STZ-induced DM. It should be noted that m_1- and m_3-MAChRs are abundantly expressed in the brain regions involved in cognition, including the cerebral cortex, hippocampus and striatum (Porter et al., 2002).

As a rule, most animal models of obesity and hyperinsulinemia are associated with increased vagal cholinergic activity that is strongly associated with the m_3-MAChR expressed in the brain and the peripheral tissues (Gautam et al., 2008). The absence of m_3-MAChR protects the animals against experimentally or genetically induced obesity and obesity-associated metabolic deficit and greatly ameliorates the impairments in glucose homeostasis and insulin sensitivity. The m_3-MAChR-deficient mice are largely protected against obesity-associated glucose intolerance, insulin resistance, hyperinsulinemia, and hyperglycemia triggered by a high-fat diet, chemical disruption of hypothalamic neurons by gold-thioglucose, and genetic disruption of the leptin gene. These data favor the fact that the m_3-MAChR and other subtypes of MAChRs can represent a potential pharmacologic target for the treatment of DM, obesity and associated neurological disorders.

Along with insulin, some substances, vitamin D_3 and curcumin in particular, which differ in the chemical nature and the mechanism of action are also capable of restoring the functions of cholinergic system in the diabetic brain. Vitamin D_3, as well as insulin, markedly recovers the altered gene expression of m_1- and m_3-MAChRs in the cerebral cortex and cerebellum of STZ rats and binding parameters of these receptors to near control (P.T. Kumar et al., 2011). Vitamin D_3-induced improvement of the cholinergic system and glucose homeostasis in the diabetic brain is due to the influence of vitamin D_3 on activity of pancreatic m_3-MAChR followed by enhanced synthesis and secretion of insulin and reduction of the neuronal disorders in DM (P.T. Kumar et al., 2011). It was found, in addition, that vitamin D_3 restores the disrupted expression of IR in the cerebral cortex of diabetic rats. Curcumin possesses powerful anti-diabetic properties and has the ability to modulate MAChRs thereby ameliorating the impaired cognitive functions in DM (Peeyush Kumar et al., 2011).

Ionotropic nicotine acetylcholine receptors are also involved in the pathogenesis of neurodegenerative processes in DM. Note that the stimulation of nicotinic acetylcholine receptors and MAChRs provokes opposing physiological and behavioral responses, which is due to the existence of multiple nicotinic and muscarinic receptor subtypes and their different anatomical distributions in the CNS. For example, nicotine administration inhibits food intake, increases metabolic rate, and leads to reduced adiposity (M.D. Li et al., 2003), while the activation of m_3-MAChRs induces hyperphagia and obesity (Gautam et al., 2008).

α7-Nicotinic receptors highly expressed in the course of brain development are implicated in memory, attention and information processing (Picciotto et al., 2000). In the cortex of STZ rats the expression of α7-nicotinic receptors was markedly increased. The receptors significantly influenced the activity within the cortex circuitry, and DM-associated deregulation of this activity could contribute to disorders involving the cerebral cortex (Peeyush Kumar et al., 2011). Alongside with the increase in α7-nicotinic receptors expression, in the cerebral cortex of diabetic rats were revealed the increased acetylcholine esterase and the decreased choline acetyl transferase mRNA levels, which indicates fast acetylcholine degradation and a subsequent down stimulation of acetylcholine receptors causing undesirable effects on cognitive functions. These changes in the expression of acetylcholine esterase and choline acetyl transferase in DM led to a reduction of cholinergic neurotransmission efficiency due to a decrease in acetylcholine levels in the synaptic cleft, thus contributing to progressive cognitive impairment and other neurological dysfunctions in DM. Insulin therapy and curcumin substantially regularize the increased expression of acetylcholine esterase and choline acetyl transferase, and significantly revert up-regulation of α7-nicotinic receptor in the cortex of STZ rats improving the cognitive functions, such as learning and memory.

4. Peptide hormones in the diabetic brain

4.1 Melanocortin signaling

The DM2 and obesity of humans and animals are strongly associated with variations in a gene encoding MC_4R coupled with AC via G_s proteins (Farooqi et al., 2003) (Fig. 2). MC_4R

expression is restricted primarily to the brain, where it is widely expressed. MC_4R agonists α-MSH, a product of POMC, and melanotan II promote a negative energy balance by decreasing the food intake and increasing the CNS activity and energy expenditure, whereas hypothalamic AgRP, MC_4R antagonist, on the contrary, increases food intake (Balthasar et al., 2005). MC_4R pathways also regulate glucose metabolism and insulin sensitivity (Fan et al., 2000; Obici et al., 2001; Nogueiras et al., 2007). Central injection of the MC_4R agonist reduces insulin secretion, while administration of the MC_4R antagonist increases serum insulin levels. Furthermore, elevated plasma insulin level was detected in the young lean MC_4R knockout mice, and impaired insulin tolerance before the onset of detectable hyperphagia or obesity (Fan et al., 2000; Haskell-Luevano et al., 2009). The mice with functionally inactive MC_4R had obesity strikingly reminiscent of the agouti syndrome, which indicates that the disturbances in MC_4R signaling pathways were the primary cause of the agouti obesity. The available data indicate that hypothalamic melanocortin system controls adiposity levels rapidly and perhaps more efficiently than the other CNS signaling pathways (Nogueiras et al., 2007). It should be emphasized that the hypothalamic melanocortin system is regulated by leptin. It must be really so because the conditions associated with low leptin levels, such as fasting or genetic leptin deficiency, provide for decreased hypothalamic POMC mRNA level as well as increased expression of AgRP (Havel et al., 2000). Leptin infusion is followed by an increase in POMC mRNA level as well as in MC_4R mRNA level and inhibits the production of AgRP (Gout et al., 2008).

Despite the lack of data on the relationship between neurodegenerative diseases and the alterations of the hypothalamic melanocotrin system in obesity and DM, a suggestion was made that a decreased activity of this system and increased expression of AgRP are the prime causes of neurodegenerative processes in the diabetic brain. As is known, MC_4R-mediated improvement of cognitive functions involves neuroprotective action, regenerative trophic effects, promotion of adaptive plasticity, and suppression of damage pathways triggered by apoptotic and inflammatory factors (Tatro, 2006). The treatment with Nle^4,D-Phe^7-MSH, a selective MC_4R agonist, reduced postischemic tissue injury and improved the recovery of behavioral functions even when the treatment began as late as 9 hours after ischemia. The neuroprotective effect of Nle^4,D-Phe^7-MSH was prevented by MC_4R antagonists (Giuliani et al., 2006). The treatment blocked the ischemia-induced impairment of spatial learning and memory for at least 12 days due to the MC_4R-mediated reduction of death of hippocampal cells. Because a very high dose of MC_4R agonists actually enhanced learning, it was assumed that their effect is likely to have involved neurotrophic action of melanocortin, including promotion of neurite sprouting and functional recovery from nerve injury. The regulatory effects of α-MSH and selective MC_4R agonists on neuronal plasticity and survival could be mediated by their influence on neuronal signaling pathways regulated by other neurotransmitters. It was shown that MC_4R activation by agonists exerts the inhibitory effect on hypothalamic neurons through inhibition of neuronal firing rate and facilitation of GABA transmission (Nargund et al., 2006). This suggests the central melanocortin system to be responsible for a large number of neurodegenerative processes in the CNS previously associated with the other signaling systems of the brain.

Studying the activity of antibodies against extracellular loops of MC_3R and MC_4R strong evidence was obtained for the involvement of central melanocortin system in DM and obesity. Hofbauer and coworkers immunized the rats with peptides corresponding to the N-terminal extracellular domain MC_4R and to the first and third extracellular loops of MC_3R (Hofbauer et al., 2008; Peter et al., 2010). The antibodies to the N-terminal domain of MC_4R

acted as partial agonists and decreased the level of cAMP in cell cultures. In rats injected with peptide corresponding to the N-terminal domain of MC_4R, like in the case of blockade of hypothalamic MCRs, the food intake, body weight, plasma insulin and triglycerides levels increased significantly (Hofbauer et al., 2008). Antibodies against peptide derived from the first loop of MC_3R amplified AC stimulating effect of α-MSH; contrary to this, antibodies against the peptide derivatives of the third loop of the same receptor reduced the effect of hormone, acting as non-competitive antagonist. In rats injected with peptide derived from the third loop of MC_3R, the body weight and blood pressure were increased and motor activity was decreased. In plasma the levels of triglycerides, insulin and leptin were significantly increased compared with control. At the same time, the rats injected with peptide derived from the first loop had no changes of physiological and biochemical parameters (Peter et al., 2010). These data indicate that peptides derived from the MCRs and the antibodies to them directly influence melanocortin signaling pathways and cause changes in brain signaling, their action being receptor- and site-specific, i.e. depends on the antigenic determinants they correspond to, and can either inhibit or enhance signal transduction via the cognate receptor. This is in good agreement with the results obtained with other peptides, the derivatives of extracellular and intracellular regions of G protein-coupled receptors (Shpakov, 2011). Thus, peptides derived from the extracellular loops of MCRs and the other receptors involved in the functioning of the brain are a promising tool in the study of pathogenesis of DM and its CNS complications and give a perspective approach to develop new models of DM and obesity based on antibody-induced deregulation of the central signaling network controlled by hormones of different nature.

4.2 Neuropeptide Y signaling

NPY, a 36-amino acid peptide, stimulates feeding and decreases energy expenditure. NPY, one of the most abundant brain peptides in the paraventricular and arcuate nuclei and in the other regions of the hypothalamus is implicated in regulation of the feeding behavior, energy balance, and pituitary secretion. Disruptions in NPY signaling due to high or low abundance of NPY and cognate receptors deregulate the homeostatic milieu to promote hyperinsulinemia, hyperglycemia, fat accrual, and overt DM. In STZ rats the activity of hypothalamic NPY neurons was significantly increased, and induced marked hyperphagia (Sindelar et al., 2002; Kuo et al., 2006). STZ rats between 3 and 14 weeks after induction of DM1 had a significant increase (35–200 %) of NPY concentration in the paraventricular and the ventromedial nuclei and lateral hypothalamic area of hypothalamus, the major appetite-regulating areas sensitive to hyperphagic and polydipsic action of NPY. The concentration of NPY was also increased in the arcuate nucleus and medial preoptic area, the regions involved in modulating hormone secretion. A significant increase of NPY level was found in the hypothalamic sites of diabetic rats 6 months after STZ treatment, and insulin therapy for 3 months completely prevented the STZ-induced increments in NPY levels in all hypothalamic sites (Sahu et al., 1990).

In the rats with DM2 the level of NPY and the activity of arcuate nucleus NPY neurons were also increased, which led to hyperphagia and obesity, and may have contributed to hyperinsulinemia and altered pituitary secretion, and the insulin treatment returned the activity of NPY system (Maekawa et al., 2006). The level of mRNA encoding NPY was increased in cells of the arcuate nucleus of young 11-week-old Goto-Kakizaki rats having hyperphagia associated with leptin resistance. Following i.c.v. injection of the NPY-Y1 receptor antagonist 1229U91, the amount of food intake in Goto-Kakizaki rats was indistinguishable from that in Wistar rats, thus eliminating hyperphagia. Note that in NPY-deficient diabetic mice the mean daily food intake did not change, while in wild diabetic mice it increased two-fold. Alongside, in NPY-deficient mice the level of mRNA encoding POMC was decreased by as little as 11%, but in wild diabetic mice by 65%. Proceeding from these results, the conclusion was made that NPY is required both for an increase of food intake and for a decrease of POMC gene expression in DM (Sindelar et al., 2002).

The NPY signaling system is tightly associated with dopaminergic, melanocortin and leptin systems of the brain. The increased content of hypothalamic NPY plays a major role in attenuating the anorectic response of D_1/D_2-DARs agonists in STZ rats (Bina, Cincotta, 2000; Kuo, 2006). Leptin directly restrains the release of NPY and cohorts from the hypothalamic NPY neuronal network, and the complete absence of leptin or hypothalamic leptin receptors induces up-regulation of NPY signaling, which promotes unabated hyperphagia and fat storage (Kalra, 2008). The NPY and melanocortin signaling systems in the arcuate nucleus, where NPY and α-MSH are expressed, act in concert but have opposite functions. Hypothalamic NPY pathways favor anabolic processes and increase the food intake, whereas POMC neurons do the reverse. As a result, in hypothalamus signaling systems both form a complex network integrating hormonal (e.g., insulin and leptin) and metabolic (e.g., glucose) signals of energy homeostasis and initiating the adaptive responses of the diabetic brain (Fioramonti et al., 2007).

4.3 Glucagon-like peptide-1 signaling

Glucagon-like peptide-1 (GLP-1), a 30-amino-acid peptide hormone, is responsible for modulating blood glucose concentrations by stimulating glucose-dependent insulin secretion and by activating β-cell proliferation. GLP-1 is effective in restoring first-phase insulin response and lowering hyperglycemia in DM2 (Doyle & Egan, 2007). GLP1 also functions in the brain as a neurotransmitter, has the growth factor-like properties and protects neurons from neurotoxic influence, controlling learning behavior, memory and synaptic plasticity (Hamilton & Holscher, 2009; Hamilton et al., 2011). The action of GLP-1 is realized via GLP-1 receptors that in the brain affect neuronal activity through regulation of intracellular cAMP-dependent pathways, modulation of Ca^{2+} channels, activation of ERK1/ERK2 kinases and other second messenger systems involved in transmitter vesicle release (Gilman et al., 2003) (Fig. 2).

GLP-1 receptor agonists, exendin-4 and Liraglutide, like the inhibitors of GLP-1 degradation (dipeptidylpeptidase IV inhibitors), have been approved for treatment of DM2 (Lovshin & Drucker, 2009; Holst et al., 2011). Note that Liraglutide, analog of human GLP-1 with prolonged half life having a fatty acid palmitoyl group conjugated to the side-chain of Lys^{26} and an Arg^{34}Ser substitution, is now widely used in DM2 therapy (Lovshin, Drucker, 2009). Exendin-4 and Liraglutide injected subcutaneously for 4, 6, or 10 weeks once daily in *ob/ob, db/db* and high-fat-diet-fed mice enhanced proliferation rate of progenitor cells by 100–150 % and stimulated differentiation into neurons in the dentate gyrus (Hamilton et al., 2011). The GLP-1 receptor antagonist exendin(9–36) significantly reduced progenitor cell proliferation in these mice. Exendin-4 and Liraglutide enhanced LTP in the brain and once-daily injection of the GLP-1 analog with Ala^{8}Val substitution enhanced LTP in the brain and reduced the number of amyloid dense-core plaques in mice with insulin resistance and in patients with DM-associated obesity and AD (McClean et al., 2010). These results demonstrate that the

GLP-1 analogs show promise in the treatment of neurodegenerative diseases induced by DM, because they cross the BBB and increase neuroneogenesis. The GLP-1 analogs, such as GLP-1 with the substitution of $Ala^8$2-aminobutyric acid, with the increased stability to dipeptidyl peptidase IV elicit the insulinotropic activity and improve the central and peripheral symptoms of DM2 (Green & Flatt, 2007). The dipeptidyl peptidase-stable analogs of GLP-1 stimulate AC activity in neuronal cells and the AC stimulating effect correlates with their neuroprotective properties.

5. Conclusion

The data presented in this review suggest that alterations and disturbances occurring in a majority of hormonal signaling systems in the diabetic brain are responsible for the functioning of the CNS, the central regulation of peripheral functions as well as for memory, cognitive processes, emotion, and social behavior. These alterations leading to the DM-associated CNS disorders and centrally induced diseases of the peripheral systems are likely to develop via several mechanisms.

The first mechanism is associated with the appearance of damages in one of the signaling systems that may be caused by alterations in the expression or functional activity of sensory, adaptor or effector protein, a component of this system, and also by a deficit or, on the contrary, an excess of hormonal or hormone-like molecules that specifically regulate the system. The damages may be a result of hyperactivation, weakening or modification of the functions of signal protein due to mutations in the translated region of the gene encoding this protein or in the untranslated regions responsible for gene transcription, or else be induced by gene polymorphism in human DM. The other causes are the gene knockout and the mutations leading to gain, loss or modification of the function of signal proteins in experimental models of DM. The changes in concentration and availability of signal molecules can be ascribed to abnormalities in the systems responsible for their synthesis, transport and degradation. In the case of insulin and IGF-1 that penetrate the BBB, a decrease or increase of their level in plasma induces the corresponding alterations of insulin and IGF-1 levels in the brain, which directly affects the functioning of the signaling pathways regulated by these hormones. DM1 gives rise to peripheral hypoinsulinemia which leads to insulin deficiency in the brain, and DM2 to moderate hyperinsulinemia which leads to an increase of central insulin concentration. The abnormalities in one single signaling system influence the activity of the other signaling cascades coupled with and depending on it and induce changes in their functional activity which is a compensatory response of the brain to the primary local dysfunction of hormonal signaling. If the abnormalities are not eliminated, then the changes of brain signaling will amplify and cause deregulation of a comprehensive neuronal signaling network, which resembles "a domino effect". As a result, the disturbances are systemic and irreversible; they have influence on the signal transduction pathways regulated by insulin, IGF-1, leptin, biogenic amines, glutamate, and neuropeptides.

The second mechanism is based on the systemic response of the hormonal signaling systems in the brain to significant and prolonged changes of cerebral glucose homeostasis, the state of recurrent hypoglycemia and severe long-term hyperglycemia. This causes alterations in the energy balance in the neuronal and glial cells, inducing different compensatory changes in the signal network to allow maintaining the activity of the brain in the case of inadequate glucose concentrations. The short-term fluctuations in cerebral glucose level cause temporary changes in brain signaling, they are reversible and do not significantly affect the physiological functions of the brain, but the long-term alterations of the level and its large amplitude provoke dramatic and irreversible changes and cause the neurodegenerative disorders. For example, a prolonged and untreated DM1 with markedly expressed hyperglycemia as well as DM1 with intensive therapy using high doses of insulin and inadequate control of glucose plasma level, leading to recurrent hypoglycemia, are the major factors causing abnormalities in several signaling systems in parallel including the glutamatergic system responsible for development of glutamate excitotoxicity and CNS disorders.

Until recently, it was generally accepted that abnormalities and alterations in the neurotransmitter systems of the brain and the associated neurodegenerative disorders are the complications of DM and their role in the etiology of this disease is not very important. In the last few years, however, the conception of central genesis of DM has been significantly extended (Cole et al., 2007; de la Monte, 2009). According to this conception, there are cases when the abnormalities in the hormonal signaling systems of the brain will trigger the mechanism leading to insulin resistance or insulin deficiency and, as a result, to the development of DM and its central and peripheral complications. The following factors contribute to DM, a dysfunction in the leptin and the melanocortin systems (leptin and melanocortin model of DM2), and alterations in the 5-HT_{2C}R-coupled serotonergic and the D_2R-coupled dopaminergic systems (Bonasera & Tecott, 2000; Heisler et al., 2002; Zhou et al., 2007; Hofbauer et al., 2008; Toda et al., 2009; Peter et al., 2010). In the years to come, this list will, no doubt, be extended with the results of study of the forms of DM with central genesis. Some neurodegenerative diseases are considered to be pre-diabetes or specific forms of earlier DM, e.g. AD is referred to as the third type of DM (de la Monte, 2009).

The etiology of DM should be studied in order to find the most optimal strategy for adequate therapy and clinical management of DM and its CNS complications. The neuronal abnormalities precede DM as its causal factors; therefore it seems appropriate to eliminate the changes in the central signaling systems responsible for these abnormalities, and then to use the effective treatment of DM without high doses of insulin causing dangerous hypoglycemic episodes. A high efficiency has been shown in the case of combined use of insulin and IGF-1 and the drugs that improve the function of dopaminergic, serotonergic, melanocortin, GABAergic and glutamatergic systems. The approaches based on restoration of the functioning of a comprehensive signaling network of the brain are a new avenue of the treatment of DM of both central and peripheral genesis. This will allow avoiding many side effects of insulin monotherapy negatively affecting the CNS in diabetic patients.

6. Acknowledgment

This work was supported by Grant No. 09-04-00746 from the Russian Foundation of Basic Research and Program of the Russian Academy of Sciences "Fundamental Sciences – Medicine" (2009–2011). We express our thanks to *Inga Menina* for linguistic assistance.

7. References

Amin, P. & Sturrock, N.D. (2003). A pilot study of the beneficial effects of amantadine in the treatment of painful diabetic peripheral neuropathy. *Diabetes Medicine,* Vol.20, No2, (August 2002), pp. 114–118, ISSN 0742-3071

Antony, S.; Kumar, T.P.; Kuruvilla, K.P.; George, N. & Paulose, C.S. (2010a). Decreased GABA receptor binding in the cerebral cortex of insulin induced hypoglycemic and streptozotocin induced diabetic rats. *Neurochemical research,* Vol.35, No.10, (June 2010), pp. 1516-1521, ISSN 0364-3190

Antony, S.; Kumar, T.P.; Mathew, J.; Anju, T.R. & Paulose, C. (2010b). Hypoglycemia induced changes in cholinergic receptor expression in the cerebellum of diabetic rats. *Journal of biomedical science,* Vol.17, No.1, (February 2010), pp. 7-15, ISSN 1021-7770

Anu, J.; Peeyush Kumar, T.; Nandhu, M.S. & Paulose, C. (2010). Enhanced NMDAR1, $NMDA_{2B}$ and $mGlu_5$ receptors gene expression in the cerebellum of insulin induced hypoglycaemic and streptozotocin induced diabetic rats. *European journal of pharmacology,* Vol.630, No.1-3, (December 2009), pp. 61-68, ISSN 0014-2999

Balakrishnan, S.; Mathew, J.; Antony, S. & Paulose, C.S. (2009). Muscarinic M_1, M_3 receptors function in the brainstem of streptozotocin induced diabetic rats: their role in insulin secretion from the pancreatic islets as a function of age. *European journal of pharmacology,* Vol.608, No.1-3, (April 2009), pp.14-22, ISSN 0014-2999

Balthasar, N.; Dalgaard, L.T.; Lee, C.E.; Yu, J.; Funahashi, H.; Williams, T.; Ferreira, M.; Tang, V.; McGovern, R.A,; Kenny, C.D.; Christiansen, L.M.; Edelstein, E.; Choi, B.; Boss, O.; Aschkenasi, C.; Zhang, C.Y.; Mountjoy, K.; Kishi, T.; Elmquist, J.K. & Lowell, B.B. (2005). Divergence of melanocortin pathways in the control of food intake and energy expenditure. *Cell,* Vol.123, No.3, (November 2005), pp. 493–505, ISSN 0092-8674

Baptista, F.I.; Gaspar, J.M.; Cristóvão, A.; Santos, P.F.; Köfalvi, A. & Ambrósio, A.F. (2011). Diabetes induces early transient changes in the content of vesicular transporters and no major effects in neurotransmitter release in hippocampus and retina. *Brain Research,* Vol.1383, (January 2011), pp. 257-269, ISSN 0006-8993

Benarroch, E.E. (2010). Glutamate transporters: diversity, function, and involvement in neurologic disease. *Neurology,* Vol.74, No.3, (January 2010), pp. 259–264, ISSN 0028-3878

Bhattacharya, S.K. & Saraswati, M. (1991). Effect of intracerebroventricularly administered insulin on brain monoamines and acetylcholine in euglycaemic and alloxan-induced hyperglycaemic rats. *Indian journal of experimental biology,* Vol.29, No.12, (December 1991), pp. 1095–1100, ISSN 0019-5189

Biessels, G.J.; Smale, S.; Duis, S.E.; Kamal, A. & Gispen, W.H. (2001). The effect of γ-linolenic acid-α-lipoic acid on functional deficits in the peripheral and central nervous system of streptozotocin-diabetic rats. *Journal of the neurological sciences,* Vol.182, No.2 , (January 2001), pp. 99–106, ISSN 0022-510X

Bina, K.G. & Cincotta, A.H. (2000). Dopaminergic agonists normalize elevated hypothalamic neuropeptide Y and corticotropin-releasing hormone, body weight gain, and hyperglycemia in ob/ob mice. *Neuroendocrinology,* Vol.71, No.1, (January 2000), pp. 68–78, ISSN 0028-3835

Bonasera, S.J. & Tecott, L.H. (2000). Mouse models of serotonin receptor function: toward a genetic dissection of serotonin systems. *Pharmacology & therapeutics,* Vol.88, No.2, (November 2000), pp. 133–142, ISSN 0163-7258

Boura-Halfon, S. & Zick, Y. (2009). Phosphorylation of IRS proteins, insulin action, and insulin resistance. *American journal of physiology. Endocrinology and metabolis,*. Vol.296, No.4, (August 2008), pp. E581–591, ISSN 0193-1849

Boyle, P.J. & Zrebiec, J. (2007). Physiological and behavioral aspects of glycemic control and hypoglycemia in diabetes. *Southern medical journal*, Vol.100, No.2, (February 2007), pp. 175–182, ISSN 0038-4348

Brüning, J.C.; Gautam, D.; Burks, D.J.; Gillette, J.; Schubert, M.; Orban, P.C.; Klein, R.; Krone, W.; Müller-Wieland, D. & Kahn, CR. (2000). Role of brain insulin receptor in control of body weight and reproduction. *Science*, Vol.289, No.5487, (September 2000), pp. 2122-2125, ISSN 0036-8075

Busiguina, S.; Chowen, J.A.; Argente, J. & Torres-Aleman, I. (1996). Specific alterations of the insulin-like growth factor I system in the cerebellum of diabetic rats. *Endocrinology*, Vol.137, No.11, (November 1996), pp. 4980-4987, ISSN 0013-7227

Busiguina, S.; Fernandez, A.M.; Barrios, V.; Clark, R.; Tolbert, D.L.; Berciano, J. & Torres-Aleman, I. (2000). Neurodegeneration is associated to changes in serum insulin-like growth factors. *Neurobiology of disease*, Vol.7, No.6 Pt B, (December 2000), pp. 657-665, ISSN 0969-9961

Calcutt. N.A. & Chaplan, S.R. (1997). Spinal pharmacology of tactile allodynia in diabetic rats, *British journal of pharmacology*, Vol.122, No.7, (December 1997), pp. 1478–1482, ISSN 0007-1188

Clauson, P.G.; Brismar Hall, K.; Linnarsson, R. & Grill, V. (1998). Insulin-like growth factor-I and insulin-like growth factor binding protein-1 in a representative population of type 2 diabetic patients in Sweden. *Scandinavian journal of clinical and laboratory investigation*, Vol.58, No.4, (July 1998), pp. 353-360, ISSN 0036-5513

Clodfelder-Miller, B.J.; Zmijewska, A.A.; Johnson, G.V. & Jope, RS. (2006). Tau is hyperphosphorylated at multiple sites in mouse brain in vivo after streptozotocin-induced insulin deficiency. *Diabetes*, Vol.55, No.12, (December 2006), pp. 3320-3325, ISSN 0012-1797

Cole, A.R.; Astell, A.; Green, C. & Sutherland, C. (2007). Molecular connexions between dementia and diabetes. *Neuroscience and biobehavioral reviews*, Vol.31, No.7, (April 2007.), pp. 1046-1063, ISSN 0149-7634

Danbolt, N.C. (2001). Glutamate uptake. *Progress in neurobiology*, Vol.65, No.1, (May 2001), pp. 1–105, ISSN 0301-0082

Dani, J.A. (2001). Overview of nicotinic receptors and their roles in the central nervous system. *Biological psychiatry*, Vol.49, No.3, (February 2001), pp. 166–174. ISSN 0006-3223

Das, U.N. (2010). Hypothesis: Intensive insulin therapy-induced mortality is due to excessive serotonin autoinhibition and autonomic dysregulation. *World journal of diabetes*, Vol.1, No.4, (September 2010), pp. 101-108, ISSN 1948-9358

de la Monte, S.M. (2009). Insulin resistance and Alzheimer's disease. *BMB reports*, Vol.42, No.8, (August 2009), pp. 475-481, ISSN 1976-6696

D'Ercole, A.J.; Ye, P. & O'Kusky, J.R. (2002). Mutant mouse models of insulin-like growth factor actions in the central nervous system. *Neuropeptides*, Vol.36, No.2-3, (April-June 2002), pp. 209-220, ISSN 0143-4179

Doyle, M.E. & Egan, J.M. (2007). Mechanisms of action of glucagon-like peptide 1 in the pancreas. *Pharmacology & Therapeutics,* Vol.113, No.3, (March 2007), pp. 546–593, ISSN 0163-7258

Fan, W.; Dinulescu, D.M.; Butler, A.A.; Zhou, J.; Marks, D.L. & Cone, R.D. (2000). The central melanocortin system can directly regulate serum insulin levels. *Endocrinology,* Vol.141, No.9, (September 2000), pp. 3072–3079, ISSN 0013-7227

Farooqi, I.S.; Keogh, J.M.; Yeo, G.S.; Lank, E.J.; Cheetham, T. & O'Rahilly, S. (2003) . Clinical spectrum of obesity and mutations in the melanocortin 4 receptor gene. *The New England journal of medicine,* Vol.348, No.12, (March 2003), pp.1085–1095, ISSN 0028-4793

Finkbeiner, S. (2000). CREB couples neurotrophin signals to survival messages. *Neuron,* Vol.25, No.1, (January 2000), pp. 11-14, ISSN 0896-6273

Fioramonti, X.; Contie, S.; Song, Z.; Routh, V.H.; Lorsignol, A. & Penicaud, L. (2007). Characterization of glucosensing neuron subpopulations in the arcuate nucleus: integration in neuropeptide Y and pro-opio melanocortin networks? *Diabetes,* Vol.56, No.6, (May 2007), pp. 1219-1227, ISSN 0012-1797

Garcia, B.G.; Wei, Y.; Moron, J.A.; Lin, R.Z.; Javitch, J.A. & Galli, A. (2005). .Akt is essential for insulin modulation of amphetamine-induced human dopamine transporter cell-surface redistribution. *Molecular pharmacology,* Vol.68, No.1, (July 2005), pp. 102-109, ISSN 0026-895X

Gautam, D.; Jeon, J.; Li, J.H.; Han, S.J.; Hamdan, F.F.; Cui, Y.; Lu, H.; Deng, C.; Gavrilova, O. & Wess, J. (2008). Metabolic roles of the M_3 muscarinic acetylcholine receptor studied with M_3 receptor mutant mice: a review. *Journal of receptor and signal transduction research,* Vol. 28, No.1-2, pp. 93-108, ISSN 1532-4281

Gelling, R.W.; Morton, G.J.; Morrison, C.D.; Niswender, K.D.; Myers, M.G. Jr.; Rhodes, C.J. & Schwartz, M.W. (2006). Insulin action in the brain contributes to glucose lowering during insulin treatment of diabetes. *Cell metabolism,* Vol.3, No.1, (January 2006), pp. 67–73, ISSN 1550-4131

Gerozissis, K. (2008). Brain insulin, energy and glucose homeostasis; genes, environment and metabolic pathologies. *European journal of pharmacology,* Vol.585, No.1, (May 2008), pp.38-49, ISSN 0014-2999

Gilman, C.P.; Perry, T.; Furukawa, K.; Grieg, N.H.; Egan, J.M. & Mattson, M.P. (2003). Glucagon-like peptide 1 modulates calcium responses to glutamate and membrane depolarization in hippocampal neurons. *Journal of neurochemistry,* Vol.87, No.5 (December 2003), pp. 1137–1144, ISSN 0022-3042

Gireesh, G.; Kaimal, S.B.; Kumar, T.P. & Paulose, C.S. (2008). Decreased muscarinic M_1 receptor gene expression in the hypothalamus, brainstem, and pancreatic islets of streptozotocin-induced diabetic rats. *Journal of neuroscience research,* Vol.86, No.4, (March 2008), pp. 947-953, ISSN 0360-4012

Giuliani, D.; Mioni, C.; Altavilla, D.; Leone, S.; Bazzani, C.; Minutoli, L.; Bitto, A.; Cainazzo, M-M.; Marini, H.; Zaffe, D.; Botticelli, A.R.; Pizzala, R.; Savio, M.; Necchi, D.; Schiöth, H.B.; Bertolini, A.; Squadrito, F. & Guarini, S. (2006). Both early and delayed treatment with melanocortin 4 receptor-stimulating melanocortins produces neuroprotection in cerebral ischemia. *Endocrinology,* Vol.147, No.3, (March 2006), pp. 1126–1135, ISSN 0013-7227

Gout, J.; Sarafian, D.; Tirard, J.; Blondet, A.; Vigier, M.; Rajas, F.; Mithieux, G.; Begeot, M. & Naville, D. (2008). Leptin infusion and obesity in mouse cause alterations in the hypothalamic melanocortin system. *Obesity (Silver Spring),* Vol.16, No.8, (August 2008), pp. 1763-1769, ISSN 1930-7381

Green, B.D. & Flatt, P.R. (2007) Incretin hormone mimetics and analogues in diabetes therapeutics. *Best practice & research. Clinical endocrinology & metabolism,* Vol.21, No.4, (December 2007), pp. 497–516, ISSN 1521-690X

Hall, K.E.; Liu, J.; Sima A.A.F. & Wiley, J.W. (2001). Impaired inhibitory G-protein function contributes to increased calcium currents in rats with diabetic neuropathy, *Journal of neurophysiology*, Vol.86, No.2, (August 2001), pp. 760–770, ISSN 0022-3077

Hamilton, A. & Holscher, C. (2009). Receptors for the insulin-like peptide GLP-1 are expressed on neurons in the CNS. *Neuroreport*, Vol.20, No.13, (August 2009), pp. 1161–1166, ISSN 0959-4965

Hamilton, A.; Patterson, S.; Porter, D.; Gault, V.A. & Holscher, C. (2011). Novel GLP-1 mimetics developed to treat type 2 diabetes promote progenitor cell proliferation in the brain. *Journal of neuroscience research,* Vol.89, No.4, (April 2011), pp. 481-489, ISSN 0360-4012

Haskell-Luevano, C.; Schaub, J.W.; Andreasen, A.; Haskell, K.R.; Moore, M.C.; Koerper, L.M.; Rouzaud, F.; Baker, H.V.; Millard, W.J.; Walter, G.; Litherland, S.A. & Xiang, Z. (2009). Voluntary exercise prevents the obese and diabetic metabolic syndrome of the melanocortin-4 receptor knockout mouse. *The FASEB journal*, Vol.23, No.2, (February 2009), pp. 642-655, ISSN 0892-6638

Havel, P.J.; Hahn, T.M.; Sindelar, D.K.; Baskin, D.G.; Dallman, M.F.; Weigle, D.S. & Schwartz, M.W. (2000). Effects of STZ-induced diabetes and insulin treatment on the hypothalamic melanocortin system and muscle uncoupling protein 3 expression in rats. *Diabetes*, Vol.49, No.2, (February 2000), pp. 44-52, ISSN 0012-1797

Heisler, L.K.; Cowley, M.A.; Tecott, L.H.; Fan, W.; Low, M.J.; Smart, J.L.; Rubinstein, M.; Tatro, J.B.; Marcus, J.N.; Holstege, H.; Lee, C.E.,; Cone, R.D. & Elmquist, J.K. (2002). Activation of central melanocortin pathways by fenfluramine. *Science,* Vol.297, No.5581, (July 2002), pp. 609–611, ISSN 0036-8075

Hegyi, K.; Fulop, K.; Kovacs, K.; Toth, S. & Falus, A. (2004). Leptin-induced signal transduction pathways. *Cell biology international,* Vol.28, No.3, (March 2004), pp. 159-169, ISSN 1065-6995

Herrera, R.; Manjarrez, G. & Hernandez, J. (2005). Inhibition and kinetic changes of brain tryptophan-5-hydroxylase during insulin-dependent diabetes mellitus in the rat. *Nutritional neuroscience*, Vol.8, No.1, (February 2005), pp. 57-62, ISSN 1028-415X

Herrera-Marquez, R.; Hernandez-Rodriguez, J.; Medina-Serrano, J.; Boyzo-Montes de Oca, A. & Manjarrez-Gutierrez, G. (2011). Association of metabolic syndrome with reduced central serotonergic activity. *Metabolic brain disease*, Vol.26, No.1, (March 2011), pp. 29-35, ISSN 0885-7490

Hofbauer, K.G.; Lecourt, A.C. & Peter, J.C. (2008). Antibodies as pharmacologic tools for studies on the regulation of energy balance. *Nutrition*, Vol.24, No.9, (July 2008), pp. 791-797, ISSN 0899-9007

Holst, J.J.; Burcelin, R. & Nathanson, E. (2001). Neuroprotective properties of GLP-1: theoretical and practical applications. *Current medical research and opinion*, Vol.27, No.3, (March 2011), pp. 547-558, ISSN 0300-7995

Hosoi, T.; Hyoda, K.; Okuma, Y.; Nomura, Y. & Ozawa, K. (2007). Inhibitory effect of 4-(2-aminoethyl)-benzenesulfonyl fluoride, a serine protease inhibitor, on PI3K inhibitor-induced CHOP expression. *European journal of pharmacology*, Vol.554, No.1, (January 2007), pp. 8-11, ISSN 0014-2999

Huo, L.; Gamber, K.; Greeley, S.; Silva, J.; Huntoon, N.; Leng, X.H. & Bjørbaek, C. (2009). Leptin-dependent control of glucose balance and locomotor activity by POMC neurons. *Cell metabolism*, Vol.9, No.6, (June 2009), pp. 537-547, ISSN 1550-4131

Irvine, E.E.; Drinkwater, L.; Radwanska, K.; Al-Qassab, H.; Smith, M.A.; O'Brien, M.; Kielar, C.; Choudhury, A.I.; Krauss, S.; Cooper, J.D.; Withers, D.J. & Giese, K.P.(2011). Insulin receptor substrate 2 is a negative regulator of memory formation. *Learning & memory*, Vol.18, No.6, (May 2011), pp. 375-383, ISSN 1072-0502

Iskandar, K.; Cao, Y.; Hayashi, Y.; Nakata, M.; Takano, E.; Yada, T.; Zhang, C.; Ogawa, W.; Oki, M.; Chua, S Jr.; Itoh, H.; Noda, T.; Kasuga, M. & Nakae, J. (2010). PDK-1/FoxO1 pathway in POMC neurons regulates Pomc expression and food intake. *American journal of physiology*, Vol.298, No.4, (January 2010), pp. 787–798, ISSN 0193-1849

Jackson, J. & Paulose, C.S. (1999). Enhancement of [*m*-methoxy ^{3}H]MDL100907 binding to $5HT_{2A}$ receptors in cerebral cortex and brain stem of streptozotocin induced diabetic rats. *Molecular and cellular biochemisty*, Vol.199, No.1-2, (September 1999), pp. 81-85, ISSN 0300-8177

Jolivalt, C.G.; Lee, C.A.; Beiswenger, K.K.; Smith, J.L.; Orlov, M.; Torrance, M.A. & Masliah, E. (2008). Defective insulin signaling pathway and increased glycogen synthase kinase-3 activity in the brain of diabetic mice: parallels with Alzheimer's disease and correction by insulin. *Journal of neuroscience research*, Vol.86, No.15, (November 2008), pp. 3265-3274, ISSN 0360-4012

Joseph, A.; Antony, S. & Paulose, C.S. (2008). Increased glutamate receptor gene expression in the cerebral cortex of insulin induced hypoglycemic and streptozotocin-induced diabetic rats. *Neuroscience*, Vol.156, No.2, (October 2008), pp. 298-304, ISSN 0306-4522

Kalra, S.P. (2008). Disruption in the leptin-NPY link underlies the pandemic of diabetes and metabolic syndrome: new therapeutic approaches. *Nutrition*, Vol.24, No.9, (September 2008), pp. 820-826, ISSN 0899-9007

Kerr, J.L.; Timpe, E.M. & Petkewicz, K.A. (2010). Bromocriptine mesylate for glycemic management in type 2 diabetes mellitus. *Annals of pharmacotherapy*, Vol.44, No.11, (November 2010), pp. 1777-1785, ISSN 1060-0280

Kitamura, T.; Feng, Y.; Kitamura, Y.I.; Chua, S.C. Jr.; Xu, A.W.; Barsh, G.S.; Rossetti, L. & Accili, D. (2006). Forkhead protein FoxO1 mediates Agrp-dependent effects of leptin on food intake. *Nature medicine*, Vol.12, No.5, (April 2006), pp. 534–540, ISSN 1078-8956

Koch, L.; Wunderlich, F.T.; Seibler, J.; Könner, A.C.; Hampel, B.; Irlenbusch, S.; Brabant, G.; Kahn, C.R.; Schwenk, F. & Brüning, J.C. (2008). Central insulin action regulates peripheral glucose and fat metabolism in mice, *The Journal of clinical investigation*, Vol.118, No.6, (May 2008), pp. 2132–2147, ISSN 0021-9738

Kojima, S.; Asakawa, A.; Amitani, H.; Sakoguchi, T.; Ueno, N.; Inui, A. & Kalra, S.P. (2009). Central leptin gene therapy, a substitute for insulin therapy to ameliorate hyperglycemia and hyperphagia, and promote survival in insulin-deficient diabetic mice. *Peptides*, Vol.30, No.5, (January 2009), pp. 962-966, ISSN 0196-9781

Kumar, T.P.; Antony, S.; Gireesh, G.; George, N. & Paulose, C.S. (2010). Curcumin modulates dopaminergic receptor, CREB and phospholipase C gene expression in the cerebral cortex and cerebellum of streptozotocin induced diabetic rats. *Journal of biomedical science*, Vol.17, No.1, (May 2010), pp. 43-53, ISSN 1021-7770

Kumar, P.T.; Antony, S.; Nandhu, M.S.; Sadanandan, J.; Naijil, G. & Paulose, C.S. (2011). Vitamin D_3 restores altered cholinergic and insulin receptor expression in the cerebral cortex and muscarinic M_3 receptor expression in pancreatic islets of streptozotocin induced diabetic rats. *The Journal of nutritional biochemistry*, Vol.22, No.5, (May 2011), pp. 418-425, ISSN 0955-2863

Kuo, D.Y. (2006). Hypothalamic neuropeptide Y (NPY) and the attenuation of hyperphagia in streptozotocin diabetic rats treated with dopamine D1/D2 agonists. *British journal of pharmacology*, Vol.148, No.5, (July 2006), pp. 640-647, ISSN 0007-1188

Lee, Y.H. & White, M.F. (2004). Insulin receptor substrate proteins and diabetes. *Archives of pharmacal research*, Vol.27, No.4, (April 2004), pp. 361-370, ISSN 0253-6269

Li, X.L.; Aou, S.; Oomura, Y.; Hori, N.; Fukunaga, K. & Hori, T. (2002). Impairment of long-term potentiation and spatial memory in leptin receptor-deficient rodents. *Neuroscience*, Vol.113, No.3, (August 2002), pp. 607–615, ISSN 0306-4522

Li, X.; Wu, X.; Camacho, R.; Schwartz, G.J. & LeRoith, D. (2011). Intracerebroventricular leptin infusion improves glucose homeostasis in lean type 2 diabetic MKR mice via hepatic vagal and non-vagal mechanisms. *PloS one [electronic resource]*, Vol.6, No.2, (February 2011), p. e17058, ISSN 1932-6203

Li, J.X. & France, C.P. (2008). Food restriction and streptozotocin treatment decrease 5-HT1A and 5-HT2A receptor-mediated behavioral effects in rats. *Behavioural pharmacology*, Vol.19, No.4, (July 2008), pp. 292-297, ISSN 0955-8810

Li, M.D.; Kane, J.K. & Konu, O. (2003). Nicotine, body weight and potential implications in the treatment of obesity. *Current topics in medicinal chemistry*, Vol.3, No.8, (August 2003), pp. 899–919, ISSN 1568-0266

Li, N.; Young, M.M.; Bailey, C.J. & Smith, M.E. (1999). NMDA and AMPA glutamate receptor subtypes in the thoracic spinal cord in lean and obese-diabetic *ob/ob* mice. *Brain research*, Vol.849, No.1-2, (December 1999), pp. 34–44, ISSN 0006-8993

Li, Z.G.; Zhang, W. & Sima, A.A. (2007). Alzheimer-like changes in rat models of spontaneous diabetes. *Diabetes*, Vol.56, No.7, (July 2007), pp. 1817-1824, ISSN 0012-1797

Lin, H.V. & Accili, D. (2011). Reconstitution of insulin action in muscle, white adipose tissue, and brain of insulin receptor knock-out mice fails to rescue diabetes. *The Journal of biological chemistry*, Vol.286, No.11, (March 2011), pp. 9797-9804, ISSN 0021-9258

Lin, X.; Taguchi, A.; Park, S.; Kushner, J.A.; Li, F.; Li, Y. & White, M.F. (2004). Dysregulation of insulin receptor substrate 2 in β cells and brain causes obesity and diabetes. *The Journal of clinical investigation*, Vol.114, No.7, (October 2004), pp. 908–916, ISSN 0021-9738

Liu, J.; Wang, W.; Wang, F.; Cai, F.; Hu, Z.L.; Yang, Y.J.; Chen, J. & Chen, J.G. (2009). Phosphatidylinositol-linked novel D_1 dopamine receptor facilitates long-term depression in rat hippocampal CA1 synapses. *Neuropharmacology*, Vol.57, No.2, (August 2009), pp. 164-171, ISSN 0028-3908

Liu, Y.; Liu, L.; Lu, S.; Wang, D.; Liu, X.; Xie, L. & Wang, G. (2011). Impaired amyloid β-degrading enzymes in brain of streptozotocin-induced diabetic rats. *Journal of endocrinological investigation,* Vol.34, No.1, (January 2011), pp. 26-31, ISSN 0391-4097

Lozovsky, D.; Saller, C.F. & Kopin, I.J. (1981). Dopamine receptor binding is increased in diabetic rats. *Science,* Vol.214, No.4524, (November 1981), pp. 1031-1033, ISSN 0036-8075

Lovshin, J.A.& Drucker, D.J. (2009). Incretin-based therapies for type 2 diabetes mellitus. *Nature reviews. Endocrinology,* Vol.5, No.5, (May 2009), pp. 262–269, ISSN 1759-5029

Luján R., (2007). Subcellular regulation of metabotropic GABA receptors in the developing cerebellum, *The cerebellum,* Vol.6, No.2, pp. 123–129, ISSN 1473-4222

Luo, J.; Balkin, N.; Stewart, J.; Sarwark, J.; Charrow, J. & Nye, J. (2000). Neural tube defects and the 13q deletion syndrome: evidence for a critical region in 13q33-34. *American journal of medical genetics,* Vol.91, No.3, (March 2000), pp. 227-230, ISSN 0148-7299

Luo, S.; Luo, J. & Cincotta, A.H. (2000). Association of the antidiabetic effects of bromocriptine with a shift in the daily rhythm of monoamine metabolism within the suprachiasmatic nuclei of the Syrian hamster. *Chronobiology international,* Vol.17, No.2, (March 2000), pp. 155-172, ISSN 0742-0528

Lupien, S.B.; Bluhm, E.J. & Ishii, D.N. (2003). Systemic insulin-like growth factor-I administration prevents cognitive impairment in diabetic rats, and brain IGF regulates learning/memory in normal adult rats. *Journal of neuroscience research,* Vol.74, No.4, (November 2003), pp. 512-523, ISSN 0360-4012

Lustman, P.J.; Freedland, K.E.; Griffith, L.S. & Clouse, R.E. (2000). Fluoxetine for depression in diabetes: a randomized double-blind placebo-controlled trial. *Diabetes Care,* Vol.23, No.5, (May 2000), pp. 618–623, ISSN 0149-5992

Lustman, P.J. & Clouse, R.E. (2005). Depression in diabetic patients: the relationship between mood and glycemic control. *Journal of diabetes and its complications,* Vol.19, No.2, (March-April 2005), pp. 113-122, ISSN 1056-8727

Mackenzie, R.G. & Trulson, M.E. (1978). Effects of insulin and streptozotocin-induced diabetes on brain tryptophan and serotonin metabolism in rats. *Journal of neurochemistry,* Vol.30, N0.1, (January 1978), pp. 205–211, ISSN 0022-3042

Maekawa, F.; Fujiwara, K.; Kohno, D.; Kuramochi, M.; Kurita, H. & Yada, T. (2006). Young adult-specific hyperphagia in diabetic Goto-kakizaki rats is associated with leptin resistance and elevation of neuropeptide Y mRNA in the arcuate nucleus. *Journal of neuroendocrinology,* Vol.18, No.10, (October 2006), pp. 748-756, ISSN 0953-8194

Malcangio, M. & Tomlinson, D.R. (1998). A pharmacologic analysis of mechanical hyperalgesia in streptozotocin/diabetic rats. *Pain,* Vol.76, No.1-2, (May 1998), pp. 151–157, ISSN 0304-3959

Manjarrez-Gutierrez, G.; Marquez, R.H.; Mejenes-Alvarez, S.A.; Godinez-Lopez, T. & Hernandez, R.J. (2009). Functional change of the auditory cortex related to brain serotonergic neurotransmission in type 1 diabetic adolescents with and without depression. *World J Biol Psychiatry,* Vol.4, No.10(4 Pt 3), pp. 877-883, ISSN 1562-2975

Marino, J.S.; Xu, Y. & Hill, J.W. (2011). Central insulin and leptin-mediated autonomic control of glucose homeostasis. *Trends in endocrinology and metabolism : TEM,* Vol.22, No.7, (July 2011), pp. 275-285, ISSN 1043-2760

McClean P.L.; Gault, V.A.; Harriott, P. & Hölscher, C. (2010). Glucagon-like peptide-1 analogues enhance synaptic plasticity in the brain: a link between diabetes and Alzheimer's disease. *European journal of pharmacology*, Vol.630, No.1-3, (March 2010), pp. 158-162, ISSN 0014-2999

Morton, G.J.; Gelling, R.W.; Niswender, K.D.; Morrison, C.D.; Rhodes, C.J. & Schwartz, M.W. (2005). Leptin regulates insulin sensitivity via phosphatidylinositol-3-OH kinase signaling in mediobasal hypothalamic neurons, *Cell metabolism*, Vol.2, No.6, (December 2005), pp. 411–420, ISSN 1550-4131

Mutze, J.; Roth, J.; Gersberg, M.; Matsumura, K. & Hubschle, T. (2006). Immunohistocemical evidence of functional leptin receptor expression in neuronal and endothelial cells of the brain. *Neuroscience letters*, Vol..394, No.2, (November 2005), pp. 105-110, ISSN 0304-3940

Nargund, R.P.; Strack, A.M. & Fong, T.M. (2006). Melanocortin-4 receptor (MC4R) agonists for the treatment of obesity. *Journal of medicinal chemistry*, Vol.49, No.14, (July 2006), pp. 4035-4043, ISSN 0022-2623

Nelson, K.A.; Park, K.M.; Robinovitz, E.; Tsigos, C. & Max, M.B. (1997). High-dose oral dextromethorphan versus placebo in painful diabetic neuropathy and postherpetic neuralgia, *Neurology*, Vol.48, No.5, (May 1997), pp. 1212–1218, ISSN 0028-3878

Nogueiras, R.; Wiedmer, P.; Perez-Tilve, D.; Veyrat-Durebex, C.; Keogh, J.M.; Sutton, G.M.; Pfluger, P.T.; Castanada, T.R.; Neschen, S. & Hofmann, S.M. (2007). The central melanocortin system directly controls peripheral lipid metabolism. *The Journal of clinical investigation*, Vol.117, No.11, (November 2007), pp. 3475–3488, ISSN 0021-9738

Nonogaki, K.; Ohba, Y.; Sumii, M.; & Oka, Y. (2008). Serotonin systems upregulate the expression of hypothalamic NUCB2 via 5-HT2C receptors and induce anorexia via a leptin-independent pathway in mice. *Biochemical and biophysical research communications*, Vol.372, No.1, (July 2008), pp. 186-190, ISSN 0006-291X

Obici, S.; Feng, Z.; Karkanias, G.; Baskin, D.G. & Rossetti, L. (2002). Decreasing hypothalamic insulin receptors causes hyperphagia and insulin resistance in rats, *Nature neuroscience*, Vol.5, No.6, (June 2002), pp. 566–572, ISSN 1097-6256

Obici, S.; Feng, Z.; Tan, J.; Liu, L.; Karkanias, G. & Rossetti, L. (2001). Central melanocortin receptors regulate insulin action. *The Journal of clinical investigation*, Vol.108, No.7, (October 2001), pp. 1079–1085, ISSN 0021-9738

Okamoto, H.; Nakae, J.; Kitamura, T.; Park, B.C.; Dragatsis, I. & Accili, D. (2004). Transgenic rescue of insulin receptor-deficient mice. *The Journal of clinical investigation*, Vol.114, No.2, (July 2004), pp. 214-223, ISSN 0021-9738

Okouchi, M.; Okayama, N.; Alexander, J.S. & Aw, T.Y. (2006). NRF2-dependent glutamate-L- cysteine ligase catalytic subunit expression mediates insulin protection against hyperglycemia- induced brain endothelial cell apoptosis. *Current neurovascular research*, Vol.3, No.4, (November 2006), pp. 249-261, ISSN 1567-2026

Peeyush Kumar, T.; Antony, S.; Soman, S.; Kuruvilla, K.P.; George, N. & Paulose, C.S. (2011). Role of curcumin in the prevention of cholinergic mediated cortical dysfunctions in streptozotocin-induced diabetic rats. *Molecular and cellular endocrinology*, Vol.331, No.1, (January 2011), pp. 1-10, ISSN 0303-7207

Peter, J.C.; Zipfel, G.; Lecourt, A.C.; Bekel, A. & Hofbauer, K.G. (2010). Antibodies raised against different extracellular loops of the melanocortin-3 receptor affect energy balance and autonomic function in rats. *Journal of receptor and signal transduction research,* Vol.30, No.6, (December 2010), pp. 444-453, ISSN 1532-4281

Picciotto, M.R,; Caldarone, B.J.; King, S.L. & Zachariou, V. (2000). Nicotinic receptors in the brain. Links between molecular biology and behavior, *Neuropsychopharmacology,* Vol.22, No. 22, (May 2000), pp. 451–465, ISSN 0893-133X

Pijl, H. & Edo, A.M. (2002). Modulation of monoaminergic neural circuits: potential for the treatment of type 2 diabetes mellitus. *Treatments in endocrinology,* Vol.1, No.2, (April 2002), pp. 71-78, ISSN 1175-6349

Pijl, H.; Ohashi, S.; Matsuda, M.; Miyazaki, Y.; Mahankali, A.; Kumar, V.; Pipek, R.; Iozzo, P.; Lancaster, J.L.; Cincotta, A.H. & DeFronzo, R.A..(2000). Bromocriptine: a novel approach to the treatment of type 2 diabetes. *Diabetes care,* Vol.23, No.8, (August 2000), pp. 1154-1161, ISSN 0149-5992

Porter, A.C.; Bymaster, F.P.; DeLapp, N.W.; Yamada, M.; Wess, J.; Hamilton, S.E.; Nathanson, N.M. & Felder, C.C. (2002). M_1 muscarinic receptor signaling in mouse hippocampus and cortex. *Brain research,* Vol.944, No.1-2, (July 2002), pp. 82-89, ISSN 0006-8993

Qiu, W.Q. & Folstein, M.F. (2006). Insulin, insulin-degrading enzyme and amyloid-beta peptide in Alzheimer's disease: review and hypothesis. *Neurobiology of aging,* Vol.27, No.2, (February 2006), pp. 190-198, ISSN 0197-4580

Reisi, P.; Alaei, H.; Babri, S.; Sharifi, M.R.; Mohaddes, G. & Soleimannejad, E. (2009). Determination of the extracellular basal levels of glutamate and GABA at dentate gyrus of streptozotocin-induced diabetic rats, *Pathophysiology,* Vol.16, No.1, (June 2009), pp. 63-66, ISSN 0928-4680

Roseberry, A.G.; Painter, T.; Mark, G.P. & Williams, J.T. (2007). Decreased vesicular somatodendritic dopamine stores in leptin-deficient mice. *The Journal of neuroscience,* Vol.27, No.26, (June 2007), pp. 7021-7027, ISSN 0270-6474

Sahu, A.; Sninsky, C.A.; Kalra, P.S. & Kalra, S.P. (1990). Neuropeptide-Y concentration in microdissected hypothalamic regions and *in vitro* release from the medial basal hypothalamus-preoptic area of streptozotocin-diabetic rats with and without insulin substitution therapy. *Endocrinology,* Vol.126, No.1, (January 1990), pp. 192-198, ISSN 0013-7227

Sandrini, M.; Vitale, G.; Vergoni, A.V.; Ottani, A. & Bertolini, A. (1997). Streptozotocin-induced diabetes provokes changes in serotonin concentration and on 5-HT_{1A} and 5-HT_{2A} receptor in rat brain, *Life sciences,* Vol.60, No.16, (March 1997), pp. 1393-1397, ISSN 0024-3205

Satoh, E. & Takahashi, A. (2008). Experimental diabetes enhances Ca2+ mobilization and glutamate exocytosis in cerebral synaptosomes from mice. *Diabetes research and clinical practice,* Vol.81, No.2, (August 2008), pp. e14-e17, ISSN 0168-8227

Savitha, B.; Joseph, B.; Peeyush Kumar, T. & Paulose, C.S. (2010). Acetylcholine and muscarinic receptor function in cerebral cortex of diabetic young and old male Wistar rats and the role of muscarinic receptors in calcium release from pancreatic islets. *Biogerontology,* Vol.11, No.2, (April 2010), pp. 151-166, ISSN 1389-5729

Scheen, A.J. (2010). Central nervous system: a conductor orchestrating metabolic regulations harmed by both hyperglycaemia and hypoglycaemia. *Diabetes & metabolism,* Vol.36, Suppl.3, (October 2010), pp. 31-38, ISSN 1262-3636

Schubert, M.; Brazil, D.P.; Burks, D.J.; Kushner, J.A.; Ye, J.; Flint, C.L.; Farhang-Fallah, J.; Dikkes, P.; Warot, X.M.; Rio, C.; Corfas, G. & White, M.F. (2003). Insulin receptor substrate-2 deficiency impairs brain growth and promotes tau phosphorylation. *The Journal of neuroscience*, Vol.23, No.18, (August 2003), pp. 7084-7092, ISSN 0270-6474

Schubert, M.; Gautam, D.; Surjo, D.; Ueki, K.; Baudler, S.; Schubert, D.; Kondo, T.; Alber, J.; Galldiks, N.; Küstermann, E.; Arndt, S.; Jacobs, A.H.; Krone, W.; Kahn, C.R. & Brüning, J.C. (2004). Role for neuronal insulin resistance in neurodegenerative diseases. *Proceedings of the National Academy of Sciences of the U SA,* Vol.101, No.9, (March 2004), pp. 3100-3105, ISSN 0027-8424

Schwartz, N.E. & Alford, S. (2000). Physiological activation of presynaptic metabotropic glutamate receptors increases intracellular calcium and glutamate release. *Journal of neurophysiology*, Vol.84, No.1, (July 2000), pp. 415-427, ISSN 0022-3077

Schwartz, M.W.; Woods, S.C.; Porte, DJr.; Seeley, R.J. & Baskin, D.G. (2000). Central nervous system control of food intake. *Nature*, Vol.404, No.6778, (April 2000), pp. 661-671, ISSN 0028-0836

Scranton, R.E.; Gaziano, J.M.; Rutty, D.; Ezrokhi, M. & Cincotta, A. (2007). A randomized, double-blind, placebo-controlled trial to assess safety and tolerability during treatment of type 2 diabetes with usual diabetes therapy and either Cycloset or placebo. *BMC endocrine disorders [electronic resource],* Vol.7, No.3 (June 2007), pp. 7, ISSN 1472-6823

Serbedzija, P.; Madl, J.E. & Ishii, D.N. (2009). Insulin and IGF-I prevent brain atrophy and DNA loss in diabetes. *Brain research*, Vol.1303, (September 2009), pp. 179-194, ISSN 0006-8993

Shafrir, E. (2010). Contribution of animal models to the research of the causes of diabetes. *World journal of diabetes,* Vol.1, No.5, (November 2010), pp. 137-140, ISSN 1948-9358

Shankar, P.N.; Joseph, A. & Paulose, C.S. (2007). Decreased [3H] YM-09151-2 binding to dopamine D2 receptors in the hypothalamus, brainstem and pancreatic islets of streptozotocin-induced diabetic rats. *European journal of pharmacology,* Vol.557, No.2-3, (February 2007), pp. 99–105, ISSN 0014-2999

Sherin, A.; Peeyush, K.T.; Naijil, G.; Chinthu, R. & Paulose, C.S. (2010). Hypoglycemia induced behavioural deficit and decreased GABA receptor, CREB expression in the cerebellum of streptozotocin induced diabetic rats. *Brain research bulletin,* Vol.83, No.6, (November 2010), pp. 360-366, ISSN 0361-9230

Sherin, A.; Peeyush, K.T.; Naijil, G.; Nandhu, M.S.; Jayanarayanan, S.; Jes, P. & Paulose, C.S. (2011). The effects of abnormalities of glucose homeostasis on the expression and binding of muscarinic receptors in cerebral cortex of rats. *European journal of pharmacology*, Vol.65, No.1-3, (January 2011), pp. 128-136, ISSN 0014-2999

Shimizu, H. & Bray, G.A. (1990). Effects of insulin on hypothalamic monoamine metabolism. *Brain research,* Vol.510, No.2, (March 1990), pp.251–258, ISSN 0006-8993

Shpakov, A.O. (2011). GPCR-based peptides: structure, mechanisms of action and application. *Global Journal of Biochemistry*, Vol.2, No.2, (June 2011), pp. 96–123, ISSN 2229 – 709X

Shpakov, A.O.; Kuznetsova, L.A.; Plesneva, S.A.; Bondareva, V.M.; Guryanov, I.A.; Vlasov, G.P. & Pertseva M.N. (2006). Decrease in functional activity of G-proteins hormone-sensitive adenylate cyclase signaling system, during experimental type II diabetes mellitus. *Bulletin of experimental biology and medicine*, Vol.142, No.6, (December 2006), pp. 685-689, ISSN 0007-4888

Shpakov, A.O.; Kuznetsova, L.A.; Plesneva, S.A.; Gurianov, I.A.; Vlasov, G.P. & Pertseva, M.N. (2007a). The identification of disturbances in hormone-sensitive AC system in rat tissues in types 1 and 2 diabetes mellitus with using functional probes and synthetic peptides. *Tekhnologii zhivykh system*, Vol.4, No.2, (March 2007), pp. 96-108, (in Russian), ISSN 2070-0997

Shpakov, A.O.; Kuznetsova, L.A.; Plesneva, S.A. & Pertseva, M.N. (2007b). The disturbance of the transduction of adenylyl cyclase inhibiting hormonal signal in myocardium and brain of rats with experimental type II diabetes. *Tsitologiia*, Vol.49, No.6, (June 2007), pp. 442-450 (in Russian), ISSN 0041-3771

Signore, A.P.; Zhang, F.; Weng1, Z.; Gao, Y.Q. & Chen, J. (2008). Leptin neuroprotection in the CNS: mechanisms and therapeutic potentials. *Journal of neurochemistry*, Vol.106, No.5, (September 2008), pp. 1977–1990, ISSN 0022-3042

Sindelar, D.K.; Mystkowski, P.; Marsh, D.J.; Palmiter, R.D. & Schwartz, M.W. (2002). Attenuation of diabetic hyperphagia in neuropeptide Y--deficient mice. *Diabetes*, Vol.51, No.3, (March 2002), pp. 778–783, ISSN 0012-1797

Tatro, J.B. (2006). Melanocortins defend their territory: multifaceted neuroprotection in cerebral ischemia. *Endocrinology*, Vol.147, No.3, (March 2006), pp. 1122-1125, ISSN 0013-7227

Toda, C.; Shiuchi, T.; Lee, S.; Yamato-Esaki, M.; Fujino, Y.; Suzuki, A.; Okamoto, S. & Minokoshi, Y. (2009). Distinct effects of leptin and a melanocortin receptor agonist injected into medial hypothalamic nuclei on glucose uptake in peripheral tissues. *Diabetes*, Vol.58, No.12, (December 2009), pp. 2757-2765, ISSN 0012-1797

Tomiyama, M.; Furusawa, K.; Kamijo, M.; Kimura, T.; Matsunaga, M. & Baba, M. (2005). Upregulation of mRNAs coding for AMPA and NMDA receptor subunits and metabotropic glutamate receptors in the dorsal horn of the spinal cord in a rat model of diabetes mellitus. *Brain research*, Vol.138, No.1-2, (May 2005), pp. 275–281, ISSN 0169-328X

Trento, M.; Kucich, C.; Tibaldi, P.; Gennari, S.; Tedesco, S.; Balbo, M.; Arvat, E.; Cavallo, F.; Ghigo, E. & Porta, M. (2010). A study of central serotoninergic activity in healthy subjects and patients with Type 2 diabetes treated by traditional one-to-one care or Group Care. *Journal of endocrinological investigation*, Vol.33, No.9, (October 2010), pp. 624-628, ISSN 0391-4097

Trudeau, F.; Gagnon, S. & Massicotte, G. (2004). Hippocampal synaptic plasticity and glutamate receptor regulation: influences of diabetes mellitus. *European journal of pharmacology*, Vol.490, No.1–3, (April 2004), pp. 177–186, ISSN 0014-2999

Van der Heide, L.P.; Kamal, A.; Artola, A.; Gispen, W.H. & Ramakers, G.M. (2005). Insulin modulates hippocampal activity-dependent synaptic plasticity in N-methyl-D-aspartate receptor and phosphatidyl-inositol-3-kinase-dependent manner. *Journal of neurochemistry*, Vol.94, No.4, (August 2005), pp. 1158-1166, ISSN 0022-3042

Van Tilburg, M.A.; McCaskill, C.C.; Lane, J.D.; Edwards, C.L.; Bethel, A.; Feinglos, M.N. & Surwit, R.S. (2001). Depressed mood is a factor in glycemic control in type 1 diabetes. *Psychosomatic medicine*, Vol.63, No.4, (July-August 2001), pp. 551–555, ISSN 0033-3174

Voitenko, N.V.; Kruglikov, I.A.; Kostyuk, E.P. & Kostyuk, P.G. (2000). Effect of STZ-induced diabetes on the activity of calcium channels in rat dorsal horn neurons. *Neuroscience,* Vol.95, No.2, (February 2000), pp. 519–524, ISSN 0306-4522

Wang, M.Y.; Chen, L.; Clark, G.O.; Lee, Y.; Stevens, R.D.; Ilkayeva, O.R.; Wenner, B.R.; Bain, J.R.; Charron, M.J.; Newgard, C.B. & Unger, R.H. (2010). Leptin therapy in insulin-deficient type I diabetes. *Proceedings of the National Academy of Sciences USA,* Vol.107, No.11, (March 2010), pp. 4813-48199, ISSN 0027-8424

Weng, Z.; Signore, A.P.; Gao, Y.; Wang, S.; Zhang, F.; Hastings, T.; Yin, X.M. & Chen, J. (2007). Leptin protects against 6-hydroxydopamine-induced dopaminergic cell death via mitogen-activated protein kinase signaling. *The Journal of biological chemistry,* Vol.282, No.47, (September 2007), pp. 34479-34491, ISSN 0021-9258

Wredling, R.A.; Theorell, P.G.; Roll, H.M.; Lins, P.E. & Adamson, U.K. (1992). Psychosocial state of patients with IDDM prone to recurrent episodes of severe hypoglycemia, *Diabetes care,* Vol.15, No.4, (April 1992), pp. 518–521, ISSN 0149-5992

Yamato, T.; Misumi, Y.; Yamasaki, S.; Kino, M. & Aomine, M. (2004). Diabetes mellitus decreases hippocampal release of neurotransmitters: an in vivo microdialysis study of awake, freely moving rats. *Diabetes, nutrition & metabolism,* Vol.17, No.3, (June 2004), pp. 128–136, ISSN 0394-3402

Yuan, X.; Yamada, K.; Ishiyama-Shigemoto, S.; Koyama, W. & Nonaka, K. (2000). Identification of polymorphic loci in the promoter region of the serotonin 5-HT2C receptor gene and their association with obesity and type II diabetes. *Diabetologia,* Vol.43, No.3, (March 2000), pp. 373-376, ISSN 0012-186X

Zhou, L.; Sutton, G.M.; Rochford, J.J.; Semple, R.K.; Lam, D.D.; Oksanen, L.J.; Thornton-Jones, Z.D.; Clifton, P.G.; Yueh, C.Y.; Evans, M.L.; McCrimmon, R.J.; Elmquist, J.K.; Butler, A.A. & Heisler, L.K. (2007). Serotonin 2C receptor agonists improve type 2 diabetes via melanocortin-4 receptor signaling pathways. *Cell metabolism,* Vol.6, No.5, (November 2007), pp. 398-405, ISSN 1550-4131

Zhu, X.; Perry, G. & Smith, M.A. (2005). Insulin signaling, diabetes mellitus and risk of Alzheimer disease. *Journal of Alzheimer's disease,* Vol.7, No.1, (February 2005), pp. 81-84, ISSN 1387-2877

16

Can VEGF-B Be Used to Treat Neurodegenerative Diseases?

Xuri Li, Anil Kumar, Chunsik Lee, Zhongshu Tang, Yang Li, Pachiappan Arjunan, Xu Hou and Fan Zhang
National Eye Institute, National Institutes of Health, Rockville, Maryland United States of America

1. Introduction

Studies on vascular endothelial growth factor B (VEGF-B) during the past decade or so have shown that VEGF-B appears to be a mysterious molecule with obscure, if not controversial, functions. When VEGF-B was initially discovered (Grimmond et al., 1996; Olofsson et al., 1996a), it was naturally believed to be an angiogenic factor, due to its high sequence homology and similar receptor binding pattern to VEGF, the prototypic angiogenic molecule. Much of our research effort was focused on this speculated angiogenic activity of VEGF-B for a long time. However, studies into this aspect, most of the time, turned out to be disappointing because of the negative findings. Unlike VEGF-A, VEGF-B did not seem to play a significant role in inducing blood vessel growth or vascular permeability, etc (Li et al., 2009). In addition, VEGF-B deficiency in mice did not seem to matter greatly, since VEGF-B-null mice appeared largely healthy (Aase et al., 2001; Bellomo et al., 2000; Louzier et al., 2003; Reichelt et al., 2003), in contrast to the early embryonic lethality of VEGF-A null mice (Carmeliet et al., 1996; Ferrara et al., 1996). Based on the negative findings, we had once suspected that VEGF-B might be a redundant molecule. In recent years, VEGF-B has been shown to be a potent neuroprotective factor and an apoptosis inhibitor (Li et al., 2009; Li et al., 2008b; Poesen et al., 2008; Sun et al., 2004; Sun et al., 2006), opening up a new research avenue in VEGF-B biology.

Thus far, there are five members within the VEGF family, VEGF-A, VEGF-B, PlGF, VEGF-C and VEGF-D (Li and Eriksson, 2001; Lohela et al., 2009). As a prototypic angiogenic factor, VEGF-A has a potent and "universal" angiogenic effect under most physiological and pathological conditions (Carmeliet & Jain, 2000; Ferrara & Kerbel, 2005; Folkman, 2007). The placenta growth factor (PlGF) is required for pathological angiogenesis (Luttun et al., 2002). However, when PlGF-1 is produced in the same population of cells with VEGF-A, it can also act as a natural antagonist of VEGF-A (Cao, 2009; Eriksson et al., 2002). VEGF-C and VEGF-D are important players in lymphangiogenesis (Alitalo et al., 2005; Lohela et al., 2009). Remarkably, the biological function of VEGF-B has remained less studied. VEGF-B displays a high degree of sequence homology to VEGF-A and PlGF, and also binds to the tyrosine kinase VEGF receptor-1 (VEGFR-1) and neuropilin-1 (NP-1), like VEGF-A and PlGF (Olofsson et al., 1998; Olofsson et al., 1996a). VEGF-B is abundantly expressed in most tissues and organs (Aase et al., 1999; Li et al., 2001; Olofsson et al., 1996a). However, VEGF-B under most conditions appeared to be "redundant" or "inert" with no obvious function. The *in vivo* role of VEGF-B therefore remained enigmatic for a long time. In this review, we summarize the recent advances on VEGF-B biology, with a particular interest in its neuroprotective/survival effect on neuronal and vascular cells (Claesson-Welsh, 2008; Karpanen et al., 2008; Lahteenvuo et al., 2009; Li et al., 2008a; Li et al., 2008b; Poesen et al., 2008; Zhang et al., 2009), and further discuss the therapeutic potential of VEGF-B in treating different types of neurodegenerative diseases.

2. VEGF-B is a neuronal protective factor

VEGF-B is highly expressed in different types of neural tissues, such as the brain (Li et al., 2001; Sun et al., 2004), retina (Li et al., 2008b), spinal cord (Poesen et al., 2008), etc.

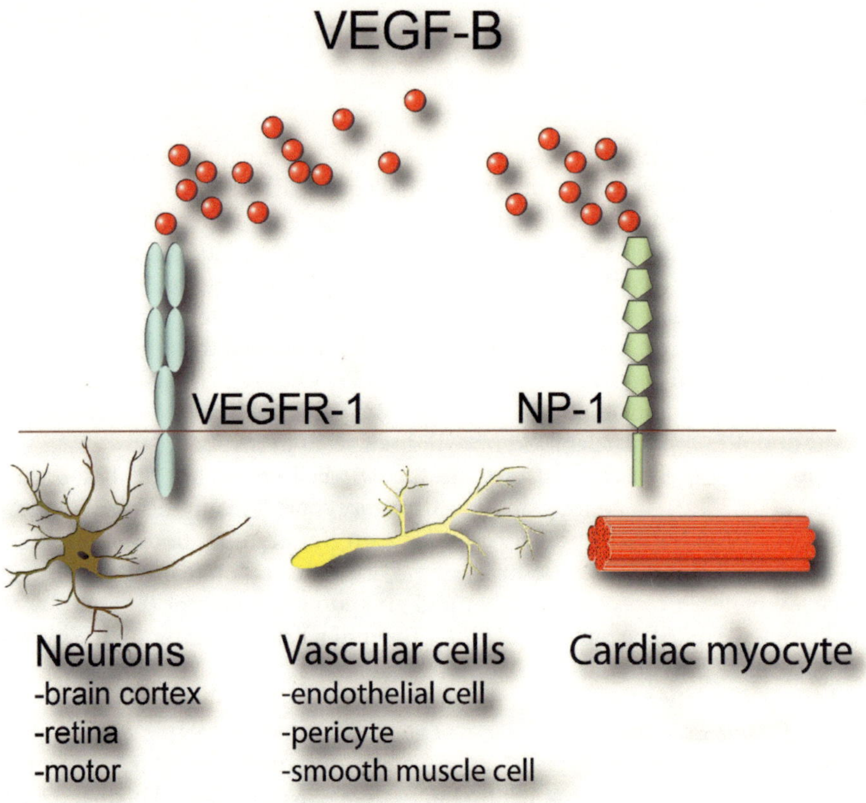

Fig. 1. Pleiotropic protective/survival effect of VEGF-B on multiple cell types. Both *in vitro* data derived from cultured neurons and *in vivo* work using different types of animal models have shown that VEGF-B is a critical protective/survival factor for different types of neurons, including cortical, retinal, and spinal cord motor neurons. In addition, VEGF-B is also a potent protective/survival factor for different types of vascular cells, including vascular endothelial cells, smooth muscle cells and pericytes. Moreover, VEGF-B has also been reported to be a protective factor for cardiac myocytes

We and others have shown that VEGF-B is a potent protective/survival factor for different types of neurons, including brain cortical neurons (Li et al., 2008b; Sun et al., 2004), retinal neurons (Li et al., 2008b), and motor neurons in the spinal cord (Poesen et al., 2008). *In vitro,* VEGF-B protein treatment dose-dependently increased the survival of cultured primary brain cortex neurons (Li et al., 2008b; Sun et al., 2004). *In vivo,* VEGF-B treatment inhibited apoptosis of brain cortical neurons and reduced stroke volume in a middle cerebral artery ligation-induced brain stroke model (Li et al., 2008b). In the retina, we have shown that VEGF-B treatment protected different types of retinal neurons from apoptosis under different pathological conditions. In an optic nerve crush injury model, VEGF-B treatment increased the survival of retinal ganglion cells. In a NMDA-induced retinal neuron apoptosis model, VEGF-B treatment protected retinal neurons in the ganglion cell layer, inner nuclear layer, and outer nuclear layer (Li et al., 2008b). Moreover, Poesen, K *et al* recently showed that VEGF-B treatment protected cultured primary motor neurons from apoptosis (Poesen et al., 2008). Indeed, the neuroprotective effect of VEGF-B was further confirmed using mice in which VEGF-B was genetically deleted. VEGF-B deficiency led to more severe strokes in an experimental stroke model, and exacerbated retinal ganglion cell death in an optic nerve crush injury model (Li et al., 2008b). Moreover, VEGF-B deficient mice developed a more severe form of motor neuron degeneration when intercrossed with the mutant SOD1 mice, whereas VEGF-B intracerebroventricular injection prolonged the survival of mutant SOD1 rats (Poesen et al., 2008). Taken together, both *in vitro* data derived from cultured neurons and *in vivo* work obtained using different animal models showed that VEGF-B is a critical survival factor for different types of neurons (Fig. 1).

3. VEGF-B is a vascular survival factor

VEGF-B and its receptors are expressed by different types of vascular cells (Aase et al., 1999; Li et al., 2008a; Zhang et al., 2009). We recently found that VEGF-B is a potent survival factor for multiple types of vascular cells, including vascular endothelial cells (EC), pericytes (PC), and smooth muscle cells (SMC) (Li et al., 2009; Zhang et al., 2009). *In vitro,* in both cultured primary vascular cells and established vascular cell lines, VEGF-B treatment increased the survival of not only ECs, but also that of PCs and SMCs (Zhang et al., 2009). In contrast, VEGF-B inhibition by shRNA treatment led to apoptosis in the ECs and PCs. Moreover, increased apoptosis was found in VEGF-B deficient ECs and SMCs isolated from VEGF-B null mice, when the cells were cultured in serum-free medium or under H_2O_2-induced oxidative stress (Zhang et al., 2009). *In vivo,* VEGF-B deficiency led to poorer blood vessel survival in the cornea after withdrawal of the implanted growth factors, fewer surviving hyaloid vessels in postnatal mouse eyes, and greater oxygen-induced retinal blood vessel degeneration in neonatal mice (Zhang et al., 2009). Thus, both gain- and loss-of-function analyses showed that VEGF-B is required for the survival of multiple types of vascular cells, especially, under pathological conditions (Fig. 1).

4. VEGF-B promotes energy metabolism

The human brain weighs only about 2% of the total body weight. However, it consumes about 20% of the total energy produced in the body, demonstrating the importance of energy metabolism to the neural systems. Indeed, numerous reports have shown that energy deficit is involved in various neurodegenerative disorders, such as Alzheimer's disease (AD) (Beal, 2007), Huntington's Disease (HD) (Browne and Beal, 2004), Parkinson's disease (PD) (Elstner et al., 2011) and Amyotrophic lateral sclerosis (ALS) (D'Alessandro et al., 2011). In addition, dysregulation of lipid pathways has been implicated in AD (Di Paolo and Kim, 2011). These findings thus warrant investigating and developing therapeutic reagents that can regulate neuronal bioenergetic pathways. Recently, VEGF-B has been shown to be involved in energy metabolism, where it facilitates fatty acid uptake from circulation and transfer to metabolically active tissues (Hagberg et al., 2010). We have also seen that VEGF-B upregulated the expression of a number of key enzymes that are involved in lipid and glucose metabolism in cultured cells (our own unpublished data). Based on the above findings, VEGF-B might be an important molecule that could be used to regulate neuronal bioenergetic pathways. Further studies are needed to verify this.

5. VEGF-B does not induce blood vessel permeability

It is known that all the other VEGF family members, VEGF-A (Dvorak et al., 1995), PlGF (Carmeliet et al., 2001), VEGF-C (Joukov et al., 1997), VEGF-D (Rissanen et al., 2003) and VEGF-E (Ogawa et al., 1998), induce blood vessel permeability. However, numerous studies using different models and approaches, such as VEGF-B deficient and transgenic mice, recombinant protein or gene transfer, have shown that VEGF-B does not affect blood vessel permeability (Aase et al., 2001; Mould et al., 2005; Reichelt et al., 2003) (Fig. 2). Intradermal injection of VEGF-A_{165}, VEGF-A_{121}, and VEGF-C in mice ears increased vascular permeability, while VEGF-B administration had no such effect (Brkovic & Sirois, 2007). VEGF-B_{167} recombinant protein injection into mouse brain or eye did not induce blood vessel permeability (Li et al., 2008b). In preserved lung grafts, VEGF-A and VEGF-C, but not VEGF-B mediate increased vascular permeability (Abraham et al., 2002). Indeed, when overexpressed in the lung by adenoviral gene transfer, VEGF-B had no effect on blood vessel permeability (Louzier et al., 2003). Adenoviruses expressing VEGF-A and VEGF-D delivered into rabbit hind limb skeletal muscles induced vascular permeability, while adenovirus encoding VEGF-B did not affect blood vessel permeability when administered into skeletal muscles (Rissanen et al., 2003). Thus, data derived from different model systems showed that VEGF-B is the only member of the VEGF family that does not have a significant role in inducing blood vessel permeability

6. Minimum side effect of VEGF-B and its negligible role in angiogenesis

Due to its high sequence homology and similar receptor binding patterns to VEGF-A (Li and Eriksson, 2001; Nash et al., 2006), VEGF-B was initially believed to be an angiogenic factor. However, studies along this line using VEGF-B deficient and transgenic mice and gene transfer approaches have, most of the time, led to negative findings (Fig. 2).

VEGF-A or VEGF-C deficiency caused embryonic lethality in mice (Carmeliet et al., 1996; Ferrara et al., 1996; Karkkainen et al., 2004). VEGF-B deficient mice, however, are largely healthy with normal physiological angiogenesis (Aase et al., 2001; Bellomo et al., 2000; Louzier et al., 2003; Reichelt et al., 2003). PlGF deficient mice display impaired pathological angiogenesis (Carmeliet et al., 2001; Luttun et al., 2002). VEGF-B deficiency, however, does not affect pathological angiogenesis in most organs studied, such as the wounded skin, hypoxic lung, ischemic retina and limb (Li et al., 2008a). Even though one study reported a role of VEGF-B in pathological (inflammatory) angiogenesis using arthritis models (Mould et al., 2003), we did not observe such an effect in our study (unpublished observation). In contrast to VEGF-A and PlGF, VEGF-B is not required for neovessel formation in proliferative retinopathy (Reichelt et al., 2003) or blood vessel remodeling in pulmonary hypertension (Louzier et al., 2003).

Transgenic expression of all the other VEGF family members, such as VEGF-A (Detmar et al., 1998; Larcher et al., 1998; Xia et al., 2003), PlGF (Odorisio et al., 2002), VEGF-C (Jeltsch et al., 1997), VEGF-D (Karkkainen et al., 2009) or VEGF-E (Kiba et al., 2003) induced either angiogenesis or lymphangiogenesis. VEGF-B is the only member of the VEGF family, transgenic overexpression of which in different organs did not induce angiogenesis or lymphangiogenesis (Karpanen et al., 2008; Mould et al., 2005). VEGF-B overexpression in cardiac myocytes under the alpha-myosin heavy chain promoter did not induce angiogenesis in the heart (Karpanen et al., 2008). Instead, blood vessel density was decreased in the hearts overexpressing VEGF-B (Karpanen et al., 2008). In addition, VEGF-B

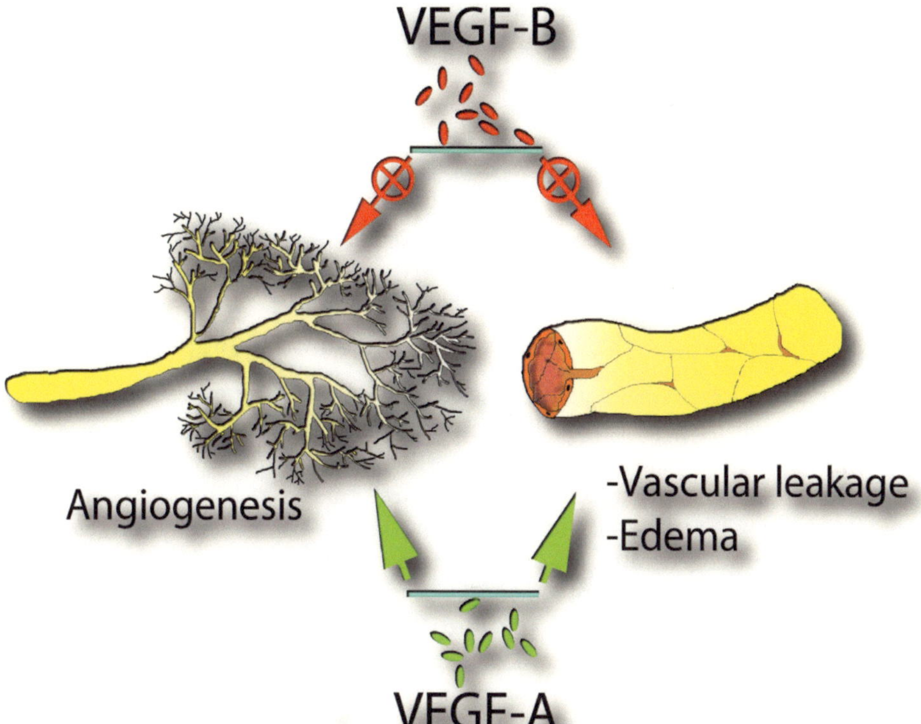

Fig. 2. VEGF-B does not induce blood vessel permeability and is minimally angiogenic. Adenoviral gene transfer of the other VEGF family members, such as VEGF-A, VEGF-C and VEGF-D, into rabbit hindlimb skeletal muscles induced strong angiogenesis, vascular permeability, or lymphangiogenesis (Rissanen et al., 2003). VEGF-B adenoviral gene transfer, however, did not induce angiogenesis or lymphangiogenesis in the same model system (Rissanen et al., 2003). Similarly, adenoviral gene transfer of VEGF-A and VEGF-D to rabbit carotid arteries induced robust adventitial angiogenesis, whereas VEGF-B adenoviral gene transfer failed to do so (Bhardwaj et al., 2003, 2005). Another study also showed that VEGF-B_{167} gene delivery to the mouse skin or ischemic limb did not induce blood vessel growth (Li et al., 2008a)

transgenic expression in endothelial cells under Tie2 promoter did not induce angiogenesis in different types of organs (liver, heart, kidney, etc) (Mould et al., 2005), and VEGF-B transgenic expression in the skin under keratin-14 promoter only marginal potentiated angiogenesis (Karpanen et al., 2008).

Studies using VEGF-B protein treatment also showed a minimum side effect of VEGF-B and a negligible role in angiogenesis. VEGF-B_{167} recombinant protein injection into adult mouse eyes at a dose effective for retinal neuron survival did not induce ocular angiogenesis (Li et al., 2008b). Poesen, K., *et al* has also shown that intracerebroventricular injection of the VEGF-B_{186} recombinant protein did not cause any blood vessel growth or blood-brain barrier leakage (Poesen et al., 2008).

VEGF-B is most abundantly expressed in the heart (Li et al., 2001; Olofsson et al., 1996a). Using a cardiac ischemia model, we found that VEGF-B has a restricted role in the revascularization of ischemic myocardium (Claesson-Welsh, 2008; Li et al., 2008a). Indeed, this observation was also reported by another study demonstrating that in pigs and rabbits, VEGF-B_{186} gene transfer induced myocardium-specific angiogenesis and arteriogenesis (Lahteenvuo et al., 2009). Thus, ours and others' work have shown that in most organs, VEGF-B is dispensable for blood vessel growth in development, normal physiology, and many pathological conditions but with a selective angiogenic activity in the ischemic heart. Taken together, compared with the other VEGF family members, VEGF-B appears to have a unique safety profile that is highly desirable as a potential therapeutic reagent to treat human diseases.

7. Therapeutic potential of VEGF-B in treating neurodegenerative diseases

Currently, for most neurodegenerative diseases, there are no effective treatments. Although novel remedies such as gene or cell therapies are being explored intensively, few have proved to be clinically beneficial. Neurodegenerative diseases often involve complex multi-etiological aspects. Neuronal apoptosis is a central characteristic of neurodegenerative diseases. In addition, blood vessel degeneration in the relevant neural system is often seen in many of the neurodegenerative disorders. Therefore, therapeutic reagents targeting one pathway only will most likely not be sufficient to cure the disease. Reagents that can improve multiple pathological aspects are more desirable. Based on our recent findings that VEGF-B is a potent protective/survival factor for both the neuronal and vascular systems, which are two critical components in most neurodegenerative disorders, we hypothesize that VEGF-B may have therapeutic implications in treating various types of neurodegenerative diseases, such as Alzheimer's disease (AD), Parkinson's disease (PD), Huntington's disease (HD), amyotrophic lateral sclerosis (ALS) stroke, retinitis pigmentosa (RP), glaucoma, diabetic retinopathy (DR) and atrophic age-related macular degeneration (AMD). Below, we discuss the therapeutic potential of VEGF-B in relation to these pathologies.

7.1 Alzheimer's Disease

Alzheimer's Disease (AD) is a major contributor to dementia in the elderly, and affects about 2% of the population in developed countries. The total number of AD patients is estimated to increase significantly in the near future due to the growing aging population (Mattson, 2004). In AD patients, plaques containing the beta-amyloid protein deposit extracellularly, and neurofibrillary tangles of hyperphosphorylated tau protein accumulate intracellularly in the brain, leading to the degeneration of synapses and neurons, and eventually the loss of memory and cognitive ability (Mattson, 2004). Both genetic and environmental factors contribute to the development of AD. Several drugs are currently available for AD treatment, such as tacrine, donepezil, rivastigmine tartrate and galantamine hydrobromide. These drugs can sometimes relieve the symptoms of early stage AD patients. However, they cannot stop or reverse the progression of the illness, and the effects of these drugs are often inconsistent and diminished over time. Therefore, more effective treatments are still needed. Many new reagents have been tested in preclinical or clinical studies, such as intravenous immunoglobulin (Relkin et al., 2008), γ-secretase inhibitors (Siemers et al., 2006; Wilcock et al., 2008), blockers of the receptor for advanced glycation end product (Chen et al., 2007), Dimebon (Doody et al., 2008), etc. However, their therapeutic efficacies are yet to be proven. It is noteworthy that in recent years, AD has been considered more as a vascular, rather than a neural disease based on clinical imaging, epidemiological, pharmacotherapy and histopathological evidence (Chow et al., 2007; de la Torre, 2002; de la Torre, 2004; Kalaria and Hedera, 1995). Indeed, vascular degeneration has been observed in different experimental Alzheimer's disease models (Girouard and Iadecola, 2006; Wu et al., 2005)·(Hsu et al., 2007). In addition, it has been known that the functional relationships among neuronal, glial, and vascular cells within the so-called neurovascular unit is compromised in Alzheimer's disease (Salmina, 2009). Thus, mounting evidence indicates that vascular abnormalities, such as capillary degeneration, are important factors that can initiate Alzheimer's disease. Due to the potent survival effect of VEGF-B on both neuronal and vascular cells, VEGF-B may have a therapeutic potential in the prevention and treatment of Alzheimer's disease. Further studies are needed to verify this.

7.2 Parkinson's Disease

Parkinson's Disease (PD) is the second most prevalent neurodegenerative disease following AD. PD is characterized by the age-related progressive loss of dopaminergic neurotransmission in the basal ganglia (Nutt and Wooten, 2005). The etiology of PD is complicated and involves multiple factors and mechanisms. PD patients suffer from severe motor symptoms, including uncontrollable resting tremor, bradykinesia, rigidity and postural imbalance. Current treatment for PD can only attenuate the symptoms. There is no effective drug that can stop the neuronal death in PD patients. Levodopa, in combination with a peripheral dopa decarboxylase inhibitor, is the most effective therapy thus far (Lees et al., 2009). However, levodopa motor and nonmotor complications are challenging issues to overcome clinically (Jankovic, 2005). Dopamine agonists and monoamine oxidase-B inhibitors can reduce the symptoms either as a monotherapy or in combination with levodopa (Jankovic, 2006). However, even though the symptoms may be controlled after the administration of these drugs, at least following the initial treatment, the death of the dopaminergic neurons persists and the disease continues to progress.

Neuroprotection is at the forefront of PD research, and many neuroprotective reagents have been investigated (Bonuccelli and Del Dotto, 2006; Djaldetti and Melamed, 2002). The glial cell derived neurotrophic factor (GDNF) has been shown to enhance the survival of midbrain dopaminergic neurons *in vitro* and rescued degenerating neurons *in vivo* (Love et al., 2005). However, a multicenter clinical trial showed no clinical benefit (Lang et al., 2006), and GDNF antibody development was observed in some PD patients (Sherer et al., 2006).

Indeed, in a rat α-synuclein PD model, overexpression of GDNF failed to exert effective neuroprotection (Decressac et al., 2011). The vascular endothelial growth factor–A (VEGF-A) has been shown to induce neuroprotection in a PD model of the 6-hydroxydopamine (6-OHDA) lesioned rats (Yasuhara et al., 2004). However unwarranted side effect of VEGF-A proved to be detrimental to the brain, since VEGF-A also induced edema and undesired angiogenesis in the brain (Yasuhara et al., 2005). In addition, it has also been reported that VEGF-A induces astrogliosis, microgliosis and disrupts the blood-brain barrier (Rite et al., 2007). Thus, new and better neuroprotective reagents are still needed.

Apart from neuronal death, normal contact between nigral neurons and capillaries is often impaired in the brains of PD patients. Capillary basement membrane thickening and collagen accumulation are often seen in PD patients, suggesting that capillary dysfunction may play an important role in PD development (Farkas et al., 2000; Faucheux et al., 1999). Indeed, it is believed that markers of cerebrovascular disease may predict the development of different types of dementia, including PD (Staekenborg et al., 2009). Recent work has shown that VEGF-B expression was upregulated by neurodegenerative challenges in the midbrain, and exogenous application of VEGF-B has a neuroprotective effect in a culture model of PD (Falk et al., 2009). In another study, VEGF-B_{186} was used to test its neuroprotective effect in a PD model since it is more diffusable and hardly binds to extracellular matrix than VEGF-B_{167} (Olofsson et al., 1996b; Poesen et al., 2008). In this study, a single dose of VEGF-B_{186} (3μg/rat) rescued dopaminergic neurons from death in the caudal sub region of substantia nigra in rats (Falk et al., 2011). Thus, as a potent neuronal and vascular protective factor, VEGF-B may have therapeutic implications in PD treatment. Future investigations are needed to investigate into this.

7.3 Amyotrophic lateral sclerosis

Amyotrophic lateral sclerosis (ALS) is a devastating adult-onset neurodegenerative disorder characterized by progressive loss of motoneurons in the primary motor cortex, corticospinal tracts, brainstem and spinal cord, leading to muscular paralysis and eventually death (Wijesekera and Leigh, 2009). The pathogenesis of familial ALS is unclear. Sporadic ALS is believed to be related to superoxide dismutase (SOD) 1 mutation in about 20-30% of the patients (Yamamoto et al., 2008). Although many drug candidates have been tested, such as antioxidants, neurotrophic factors, anti-apoptotic, anti-inflammatory and anti-aggregation reagents, the only drug currently available for ALS patients is Riluzole, a glutamate antagonist (Traynor et al., 2006; Yamamoto et al., 2008). Recently, it is believed that vascular defect may be a critical contributor to the pathogenesis of ALS. In the amyotrophic lateral sclerosis-linked SOD1 mutant mice, vascular endothelial damage accumulates before motor neuron degeneration and plays a central role in ALS initiation (Segura et al., 2009). The therapeutic promise of VEGF-B in ALS treatment has been shown by Poesen et al. VEGF-B_{186} protected cultured primary motor neurons against degeneration (Poesen et al., 2008). *In vivo*, VEGF-B treatment protected motor neurons from degeneration in several experimental ALS models (Poesen et al., 2008). In the future, it will be exciting to see whether this effect of VEGF-B holds true in ALS patients.

7.4 Stroke

Ischemic stroke due to sudden loss of blood supply in the brain is a leading cause of morbidity and mortality in the United States. Currently, there is no satisfying therapy for stroke patients despite extensive effort on identifying better interventions. Since early 1990s, neuroprotection as a potential therapeutic strategy for stroke treatment has received much attention (Ginsberg, 2008). During the past decade or so, about 160 clinical trials on neuroprotection for ischemic stroke treatment have been conducted (Ginsberg, 2008). However, no effective neuroprotective drug has been identified. The potential therapeutic value of VEGF-B for stroke treatment has been supported by several studies. It has been shown that VEGF-B is a potent survival factor for cortical neurons. VEGF-B deficiency in mouse increased stroke volume by about 40% in an experimental stroke model, and led to more severe neurologic impairment (Sun et al., 2004). Indeed, VEGF-B protein treatment protected cultured cerebral cortical neurons from hypoxic injury, demonstrating a direct survival effect of VEGF-B on neurons (Sun et al., 2004). Furthermore, intraventricular administration of VEGF-B decreased stroke volume (Li et al., 2008b) and restored neurogenesis to normal level in VEGF-B deficient mice (Sun et al., 2006). Mechanistically, we have shown that VEGF-B exerts its neuronal survival effect by inhibiting the expression of many proapoptotic BH3-only protein genes (Li et al., 2008b). In summary, both *in vitro* and *in vivo* data from several groups have suggested a therapeutic potential of VEGF-B in stroke treatment and warrant further studies to investigate into this.

7.5 Huntington's Disease

Huntington's Disease (HD) is a hereditary autosomal dominant neurodegenerative disorder characterized by the selective degeneration of striatal projection neurons that are responsible for choreic movements, resulting in progressive movement disorder, cognitive decline and psychiatric disturbances. Over the course of HD, the mutated huntingtin protein leads to intracellular dysfunctions and neuronal death in the striatum, selected layers of the cerebral cortex, as well as other brain regions (Gil and Rego, 2008). Currently, no effective therapy exists for HD. Pharmacological treatment may ameliorate hyperkinesis and psychiatric symptoms, but neuropsychological deficits and dementia remain untreatable. The apoptotic cascade is believed to be a possible cause of neurodegeneration in HD (Pattison et al., 2006). The therapeutic potential of some neuroprotective reagents in HD treatment, such as GDNF, coenzyme Q10, minocycline and unsaturated fatty acids, has been investigated (Alberch et al., 2002; Bonelli and Hofmann, 2007). Since VEGF-B is a potent apoptosis inhibitor (Li et al., 2008b), it will be interesting to test whether VEGF-B could slow down, if not stop, neuronal degeneration in HD.

7.6 Retinal degenerative diseases

Retinal degenerative diseases are a group of disorders involving degeneration of the retina. Progressive loss of retinal neurons is a common characteristic of such disorders and the major reason for vision impair or loss. Further, blood vessel deterioration is often seen in many of the retinal degenerative diseases. Unfortunately, thus far, there is no efficacious treatment for most of the retinal degenerative diseases.

7.6.1 Retinitis pigmentosa (RP)

Retinitis pigmentosa (RP) is a heterogeneous retinal dystrophy characterized by the progressive loss of photoreceptors and subsequent degeneration of retinal pigmented epithelial (RPE) cells (Hartong et al., 2006). RP is the leading cause of blindness in inherited retinal degeneration-associated diseases world-wide. The first symptom of RP is often night blindness, followed by the gradual loss of peripheral visual field, and ultimately blindness. Apart from the photoreceptor dystrophy, retinal arterioles are attenuated in RP, leading to poor oxygenation of rods and cones and increased apoptosis in the neural retina. It is known that about 45 genes/loci are involved in this pathology. Due to the large number of genes and mutations implicated, correcting the defective genes/mutations represents an overwhelming challenge. The current available therapies are vitamin supplement and sunlight protection, which can only slow down the degenerative process (Hamel, 2006). There is no treatment that can stop the progress of the disease or restore vision in RP patients. Since VEGF-B can protect both neuronal and vascular cells from apoptosis, VEGF-B administration may preserve both the photoreceptors and blood vessels in RP. Future studies are needed to verify this.

7.6.2 Glaucoma

Glaucoma is the most prevalent form of adult optic neuropathies affecting approximately 2% of the population over the age of 40 (Levin, 2005; Marcic et al., 2003). Glaucoma is characterized by the increased apoptosis of retinal ganglion cells, loss of optic nerve fibers, and, if uncontrolled, impair or loss of vision (Weinreb, 2005). Apoptosis of retinal ganglion cells is believed to be an early event in glaucoma (Cheung et al., 2008). The number of glaucoma patients is significantly increasing because of the growing ageing population and other factors (Morley and Murdoch, 2006). Currently, there is no general treatment effective for all glaucoma patients. Recent years have seen increasing evidence showing that glaucoma is, to a large extent, a neurodegenerative disease similar to other neurodegenerative disorders in the central nervous system, such as Alzheimer's disease (Cheung et al., 2008). Traditionally, lowering the intraocular pressure (IOP) has been a major therapeutic goal in glaucoma treatment. However, such therapeutic approaches have not been effective in preventing many patients from progressive vision loss. Thus, the fact that retinal ganglion cells (RGC) continue to die in some glaucoma patients with normal or even lower IOP has changed the research focus to neuroprotection for glaucoma treatment in recent years. Therefore, neuroprotective reagents used to treat other neurodegenerative diseases have been under considerable investigation for glaucoma treatment, and neuroprotection in glaucoma treatment has gained more and more attention. However, the number of effective neuroprotective reagents is limited. We have recently revealed that VEGF-B is expressed in normal retinal ganglion cells (Li et al., 2008b). Importantly, the expression of VEGF-B is up-regulated after optic nerve crush injury in the retina (Li et al., 2008b), suggesting a role of VEGF-B in retinal ganglion cell function. Indeed, VEGF-B inhibits the expression of many apoptotic genes in the retina and protected retinal ganglion cells from axotomy-induced apoptosis (Li et al., 2008b). These data have provided evidence that VEGF-B may be a promising drug candidate for glaucoma treatment as a neuroprotective factor. Further studies are warranted to investigate this.

7.6.3 Diabetic retinopathy

Diabetic retinopathy (DR) is a common complication of diabetes. About 50-75% of diabetic patients develop DR. In the United States, DR is the leading cause of legal blindness in the 20 to 74 year-old population (Imai et al., 2009). Conventionally, DR is believed mainly to be a microvascular disease. However, it is now considered to be also a neurodegenerative disease involving functional and structural defects of different types of neurons in the retina (Imai et al., 2009). Indeed, neuronal apoptosis has been found to be an early event in a rat model of diabetes (Barber et al., 1998). Four months after the onset of diabetes, there were only about 50% of total neurons left in the retinae of the rats (Barber et al., 1998), and the number of retinal ganglion cells (RGC) and the thickness of the inner retina layer were significantly reduced (Barber et al., 1998). In diabetic patients, increased apoptosis was also observed in the retina (Imai et al., 2009). Moreover, significant nerve fibre loss in the superior segment of the retina was observed in type 1 diabetic patients, suggesting RGC loss (Kern and Barber, 2008; Lopes de Faria et al., 2002). In addition, thinning of the inner retinal layer was observed in early stage of type 1 diabetic patients (van Dijk et al., 2009). It is reported that the mitochondria- and caspase-dependent cell-death pathways are involved in the neuronal degeneration in diabetic retinopathy (Oshitari et al., 2008). The potential role of VEGF-B in diabetic retinopathy has not been investigated thus far. However, given that VEGF-B is a potent apoptosis inhibitor and has a strong protective effect on both retinal ganglion cells and different types of vascular cells, it is reasonable to speculate that VEGF-B could be used to rescue the chronic retinal degeneration in DR. However, further investigation and research into this aspect are still needed.

7.6.4 Atrophic AMD

Age-related macular degeneration (AMD) is the most common cause of blindness in developed countries. Atrophic (dry) AMD is a late-onset, multifactorial, slowly progressing retinal neurodegenerative disease caused by the degeneration of retinal pigment epithelium (RPE) that lies beneath the photoreceptor cells in the retina. Although RPE is a central element in the pathogenesis of age-related macular degeneration, RPE dysfunction results in the secondary death of macular rods and cones due to abnormal metabolic support from the RPE, eventually leading to irreversible vision loss (de Jong, 2006). Drusen formation, oxidative stress, accumulation of lipofuscin, local inflammation and reactive gliosis are believed to be involved in the pathogenesis of atrophic AMD (Petrukhin, 2007). Currently, there is no effective treatment for atrophic AMD. There are reports showing that antioxidants supplement can provide protection against age-related macular degeneration. A high dietary intake of beta carotene, vitamin C, vitamin E, and zinc may reduce the risk of AMD in elderly people substantially (Johnson, 2009; van Leeuwen et al., 2005). Compared with the other types of retinal degenerative diseases, neuroprotection as a potential therapeutic strategy has been less studied in atrophic AMD. Our recent findings showed that VEGF-B is a potent apoptosis inhibitor. Moreover, the anti-apoptotic property of VEGF-B is likely a general effect on many different types of cells, including RPE cells (Li et al., 2009; Li et al., 2008b; Zhang et al., 2009). VEGF-B therefore might potentially be used to enhance RPE survival for AMD treatment.

8. Conclusion

In summary, despite the complex etiology of different types of neurodegenerative diseases, one common characteristic of them is the apoptotic neuronal death. In addition, degeneration of the blood vessels is often seen in many of the neurodegenerative diseases. Thus, combination therapy acting on both aspects is highly desirable. We and others have recently shown that VEGF-B appears to be a multi-functional molecule with a potent protective/survival effect on both the neuronal and vascular systems. Importantly, the protective/survival effect of VEGF-B is accompanied by a unique and rare safety profile, since VEGF-B under most conditions appears to be inert, but acts only when there is a pathological challenge. Thus, VEGF-B may have important therapeutic values in treating different types of neurodegenerative diseases by preserving both the endangered neurons and blood vessels, and, possibly, other cell types as well.

9. Acknowledgment

This research was supported in part by the Macular Degeneration Research, a program of the American Health Assistance Foundation, and the Intramural Research Program of the NIH, National Eye Institute.

10. References

Aase, K.; Lymboussaki, A.; Kaipainen, A.; Olofsson, B.; Alitalo, K. & Eriksson, U. (1999). Localization of VEGF-B in the mouse embryo suggests a paracrine role of the growth factor in the developing vasculature. *Developmental Dynamics*. 215:12-25.

Aase, K.; von Euler, G.; Li, X.; Ponten, A.; Thoren, P.; Cao, R.; Cao, Y.; Olofsson, B.; Gebre-Medhin, S.; Pekny, M.; Alitalo, K.; Betsholtz, C. & Eriksson, U. (2001). Vascular Endothelial Growth Factor-B-Deficient Mice Display an Atrial Conduction Defect. *Circulation*. 104:358-364.

Abraham, D.; Taghavi, S.; Riml, P.; Paulus, P.; Hofmann, M.; Baumann, C.; Kocher, A.; Klepetko, W. & Aharinejad, S. (2002). VEGF-A and -C but not -B mediate increased vascular permeability in preserved lung grafts. *Transplantation*. 73:1703-1706.

Alberch, J.; Perez-Navarro, E. &. Canals, J.M. (2002). Neuroprotection by neurotrophins and GDNF family members in the excitotoxic model of Huntington's disease. *Brain Res Bull*. 57:817-822.

Alitalo, K.; Tammela, T. & Petrova, T.V. (2005). Lymphangiogenesis in development and human disease. *Nature*. 438:946-953.

Barber, A.J.; Lieth, E.; Khin, S.A.; Antonetti, D.A.; Buchanan, A.G. & Gardner, T.W. (1998). Neural apoptosis in the retina during experimental and human diabetes. Early onset and effect of insulin. *J Clin Invest*. 102:783-791.

Beal, M.F. (2007). Mitochondria and neurodegeneration. *Novartis Found Symp*. 287:183-92; discussion 192-196.

Bellomo, D.; Headrick, J.P.; Silins, G.U.; Paterson, C.A.; Thomas, P.S.; Gartside, M.; Mould, A.; Cahill, M.M.; Tonks, I.D. ; Grimmond, S.M.; Townson, S.; Wells, C.; Little, M.; Cummings, M.C.; Hayward N.K. & Kay, G.F. (2000). Mice lacking the vascular endothelial growth factor-B gene (Vegfb) have smaller hearts, dysfunctional coronary vasculature, and impaired recovery from cardiac ischemia. *Circulation Research*. 86:E29-E35.

Bhardwaj, S.; Roy, H.; Gruchala, M.; Viita, H.; Kholova, I.; Kokina, I.; Achen, M.G.; Stacker, S.A.; Hedman, M.; Alitalo, K. & Yla-Herttuala, S. (2003). Angiogenic responses of vascular endothelial growth factors in periadventitial tissue. *Hum Gene Ther*. 14:1451-1462.

Bhardwaj, S.; Roy, H.; Heikura, T. & Yla-Herttuala, S. (2005). VEGF-A, VEGF-D and VEGF-D induced intimal hyperplasia in carotid arteries. *Eur J Clin Invest.* 35:669-676.

Bonelli, R.M. & Hofmann, P. (2007). A systematic review of the treatment studies in Huntington's disease since 1990. *Expert Opin Pharmacother.* 8:141-153.

Bonuccelli, U. & Del Dotto, P. (2006). New pharmacologic horizons in the treatment of Parkinson disease. *Neurology.* 67:S30-38.

Brkovic, A. & Sirois, M.G. (2007). Vascular permeability induced by VEGF family members in vivo: Role of endogenous PAF and NO synthesis. *J Cell Biochem.* 100:727-737.

Browne, S.E. & Beal, M.F. (2004). The energetics of Huntington's disease. *Neurochem Res.* 29:531-546.

Cao, Y. (2009). Positive and negative modulation of angiogenesis by VEGFR1 ligands. *Sci Signal.* 2:re1.

Carmeliet, P.; Ferreira, V.; Breier, G.; Pollefeyt, S.; Kieckens, L.; Gertsenstein, M.; Fahrig, M.; Vandenhoeck, A.; Harpal, K.; Eberhardt, C.; Declercq, C.; Pawling, J.; Moons, L.; Collen, D.; Risau, W. & Nagy, A. (1996). Abnormal blood vessel development and lethality in embryos lacking a single VEGF allele. *Nature.* 380:435-439.

Carmeliet, P. & Jain, R.K. (2000). Angiogenesis in cancer and other diseases. *Nature.* 407:249-257.

Carmeliet, P.; Moons, L.; Luttun, A.; Vincenti, V.; Compernolle, V.; De Mol, M.; Wu, Y.; Bono, F.; Devy, L.; Beck, H.; Scholz, D.; Acker, T.; DiPalma, T.; Dewerchin, M.; Noel, A.; Stalmans, I.; Barra, A.; Blacher, S.; Vandendriessche, T.; Ponten, A.; Eriksson, U.; Plate, K.H.; Foidart, J.M.; Schaper, W.;. Charnock-Jones, D.S.; Hicklin, D.J.; Herbert, J.M.; Collen, D. & Persico, M.G. (2001). Synergism between vascular endothelial growth factor and placental growth factor contributes to angiogenesis and plasma extravasation in pathological conditions. *Nat Med.* 7:575-583.

Chen, X.; Walker, D.G.; Schmidt, A.M.; Arancio, O.; Lue, L.F. & Yan, S.D. (2007). RAGE: a potential target for Abeta-mediated cellular perturbation in Alzheimer's disease. *Curr Mol Med.* 7:735-742.

Cheung, W.; Guo, L. & Cordeiro, M.F. (2008). Neuroprotection in glaucoma: drug-based approaches. *Optom Vis Sci.* 85:406-416.

Chow, N.; Bell, R.D.; Deane, R.; Streb, J.W.; Chen, J.; Brooks, A.; Van Nostrand, W.; Miano, J.M. & Zlokovic, B.V. (2007). Serum response factor and myocardin mediate arterial hypercontractility and cerebral blood flow dysregulation in Alzheimer's phenotype. *Proc Natl Acad Sci U S A.* 104:823-828.

Claesson-Welsh, L. (2008). VEGF-B taken to our hearts: specific effect of VEGF-B in myocardial ischemia. *Arterioscler Thromb Vasc Biol.* 28:1575-1576.

D'Alessandro, G.; Calcagno, E.; Tartari, S.; Rizzardini, M.; Invernizzi, R.W. & Cantoni, L. (2011). Glutamate and glutathione interplay in a motor neuronal model of amyotrophic lateral sclerosis reveals altered energy metabolism. *Neurobiol Dis.* 43:346-355.

de Jong, P.T. (2006). Age-related macular degeneration. *N Engl J Med.* 355:1474-1485.

de la Torre, J.C. (2002). Alzheimer disease as a vascular disorder: nosological evidence. *Stroke.* 33:1152-1162.

de la Torre, J.C. (2004). Is Alzheimer's disease a neurodegenerative or a vascular disorder? Data, dogma, and dialectics. *Lancet Neurol.* 3:184-190.

Decressac, M.; Ulusoy, A.; Mattsson, B.; Georgievska, B.; Romero-Ramos, M.; Kirik, D. & Bjorklund, A. (2011). GDNF fails to exert neuroprotection in a rat {alpha}-synuclein model of Parkinson's disease. *Brain*. [Epub ahead of print]

Detmar, M.; Brown, L.F.; Schon, M.P.; Elicker, B.M.; Velasco, P.; Richard, L.; Fukumura, D.; Monsky, W.; Claffey, K.P. & Jain, R.K. (1998). Increased microvascular density and enhanced leukocyte rolling and adhesion in the skin of VEGF transgenic mice. *J Invest Dermatol*. 111:1-6.

Di Paolo, G. & Kim, T.W. (2011). Linking lipids to Alzheimer's disease: cholesterol and beyond. *Nat Rev Neurosci*. 12:284-296.

Djaldetti, R. & Melamed, E. (2002). New drugs in the future treatment of Parkinson's disease. *J Neurol*. 249 Suppl 2:II30-35.

Doody, R.S.; Gavrilova, S.I.; Sano, M.; Thomas, R.G.; Aisen, P.S.; Bachurin, S.O.; Seely, L. & Hung, D. (2008). Effect of dimebon on cognition, activities of daily living, behaviour, and global function in patients with mild-to-moderate Alzheimer's disease: a randomised, double-blind, placebo-controlled study. *Lancet*. 372:207-215.

Dvorak, H.F.; Brown, L.F.; Detmar, M. & Dvorak, A.M. (1995). Vascular permeability factor/vascular endothelial growth factor, microvascular hyperpermeability, and angiogenesis. *Am J Pathol*. 146:1029-1039.

Elstner, M.; Morris, C.M.; Heim, K.; Bender, A.; Mehta, D.; Jaros, E.; Klopstock, T.; Meitinger, T.; Turnbull, D.M. & Prokisch, H. (2011). Expression analysis of dopaminergic neurons in Parkinson's disease and aging links transcriptional dysregulation of energy metabolism to cell death. *Acta Neuropathol*. 122:75-86.

Eriksson, A.; Cao, R.; Pawliuk, R.; Berg, S.M.; Tsang, M.; Zhou, D.; Fleet, C.; Tritsaris, K.; Dissing, S.; Leboulch, P.& Cao, Y. (2002). Placenta Growth Factor-1 antagonizes VEGF-induced angiogenesis and tumor growth by the formation of functionally inactive PlGF-1/VEGF heterodimers. *Cancer Cell*. 1:99-108.

Falk, T.; Yue, X.; Zhang, S.; McCourt, A.D.; Yee, B.J.; Gonzalez, R.T. & Sherman S.J. (2011). Vascular endothelial growth factor-B is neuroprotective in an in vivo rat model of Parkinson's disease. *Neurosci Lett*. 496:43-47.

Falk, T.; Zhang, S. & Sherman, S.J. (2009). Vascular endothelial growth factor B (VEGF-B) is up-regulated and exogenous VEGF-B is neuroprotective in a culture model of Parkinson's disease. *Mol Neurodegener*. 4:49.

Farkas, E.; De Jong, G.I.; de Vos, R.A.; Jansen Steur, E.N. & Luiten, P.G. (2000). Pathological features of cerebral cortical capillaries are doubled in Alzheimer's disease and Parkinson's disease. *Acta Neuropathol*. 100:395-402.

Faucheux, B.A.; Bonnet, A.M.; Agid Y. & Hirsch, E.C. (1999). Blood vessels change in the mesencephalon of patients with Parkinson's disease. *Lancet*. 353:981-982.

Ferrara, N.; Carver-Moore, K.; Chen, H.; Dowd, M.; Lu, L.; O'Shea, K.S.; Powell-Braxton, L.; Hillan, K.J. & Moore, M.W. (1996). Heterozygous embryonic lethality induced by targeted inactivation of the VEGF gene. *Nature*. 380:439-442.

Ferrara, N. & Kerbel, R.S. (2005). Angiogenesis as a therapeutic target. *Nature*. 438:967-974.

Folkman, J. 2007. Angiogenesis: an organizing principle for drug discovery? *Nat Rev Drug Discov*. 6:273-286.

Gil, J.M. & Rego, A.C. (2008). Mechanisms of neurodegeneration in Huntington's disease. *Eur J Neurosci*. 27:2803-2820.

Ginsberg, M.D. (2008). Neuroprotection for ischemic stroke: past, present and future. *Neuropharmacology*. 55:363-389.

Girouard, H. & Iadecola, C. (2006). Neurovascular coupling in the normal brain and in hypertension, stroke, and Alzheimer disease. *J Appl Physiol*. 100:328-335.

Grimmond, S.; Lagercrantz, J.; Drinkwater, C.; Silins, G.; Townson, S.; Pollock, P.; Gotley, D.; Carson, E.; Rakar, S.; Nordenskjold, M.; Ward, L.; Hayward, N. & Weber, G. (1996). Cloning and characterization of a novel human gene related to vascular endothelial growth factor. *Genome Res*. 6:124-131.

Hagberg, C.E.; Falkevall, A.; Wang, X.; Larsson, E.; Huusko, J.; Nilsson, I.; van Meeteren, L.A.; Samen, E.; Lu, L.; Vanwildemeersch, M.; Klar, J.; Genove, G.; Pietras, K.; Stone-Elander, S.; Claesson-Welsh, L.; Yla-Herttuala, S.; Lindahl, P. & Eriksson, U. (2010). Vascular endothelial growth factor B controls endothelial fatty acid uptake. *Nature*. 464:917-921.

Hamel, C. (2006). Retinitis pigmentosa. *Orphanet J Rare Dis*. 1:40.

Hartong, D.T.; Berson, E.L. & Dryja, T.P. (2006). Retinitis pigmentosa. *Lancet*. 368:1795-809.

Hsu, M.J.; Hsu, C.Y.; Chen, B.C.; Chen, M.C.; Ou, G. & Lin, C.H. (2007). Apoptosis signal-regulating kinase 1 in amyloid beta peptide-induced cerebral endothelial cell apoptosis. *J Neurosci*. 27:5719-5729.

Imai, H.; Singh, R.S.; Fort, P.E. & Gardner, T.W. (2009). Neuroprotection for diabetic retinopathy. *Dev Ophthalmol*. 44:56-68.

Jankovic, J. (2005). Motor fluctuations and dyskinesias in Parkinson's disease: clinical manifestations. *Mov Disord*. 20 Suppl 11:S11-16.

Jankovic, J. (2006). An update on the treatment of Parkinson's disease. *Mt Sinai J Med*. 73:682-689.

Jeltsch, M.; Kaipainen, A.; Joukov, V.; Meng, X.; Lakso, M.; Rauvala, H.; Swartz, M.; Fukumura, D.; Jain, R.K. & Alitalo, K. (1997). Hyperplasia of lymphatic vessels in VEGF-C transgenic mice. *Science*. 276:1423-1425.

Johnson, E.J. (2010). Age-related macular degeneration and antioxidant vitamins: recent findings. *Curr Opin Clin Nutr Metab Care*. 13(1):28-33.

Joukov, V.; Sorsa, T.; Kumar, V.; Jeltsch, M.; Claesson-Welsh, L.; Cao, Y.; Saksela, O.; Kalkkinen, N. & Alitalo, K. (1997). Proteolytic processing regulates receptor specificity and activity of VEGF-C. *Embo J*. 16:3898-3911.

Kalaria, R.N. & Hedera, P. (1995). Differential degeneration of the cerebral microvasculature in Alzheimer's disease. *Neuroreport*. 6:477-480.

Karkkainen, A.M.; Kotimaa, A.; Huusko, J.; Kholova, I.; Heinonen, S.E.; Stefanska, A.; Dijkstra, M.H.; Purhonen, H.; Hamalainen, E.; Makinen, P.I.; Turunen, M.P. & Yla-Herttuala, S. (2009). Vascular endothelial growth factor-D transgenic mice show enhanced blood capillary density, improved postischemic muscle regeneration, and increased susceptibility to tumor formation. *Blood*. 113:4468-4475.

Karkkainen, M.J.; Haiko, P.; Sainio, K.; Partanen, J.; Taipale, J.; Petrova, T.V.; Jeltsch, M.; Jackson, D.G.; Talikka, M.; Rauvala, H.; Betsholtz, C. & Alitalo, K. (2004). Vascular endothelial growth factor C is required for sprouting of the first lymphatic vessels from embryonic veins. *Nat Immunol*. 5:74-80.

Karpanen, T.; Bry, M.; Ollila, H.M.; Seppanen-Laakso, T.; Liimatta, E.; Leskinen, H.; Kivela, R.; Helkamaa, T.; Merentie, M.; Jeltsch, M.; Paavonen, K.; Andersson, L.C.;

Mervaala E.; Hassinen, I.E.; Yla-Herttuala, S.; Oresic, M. & Alitalo, K. (2008). Overexpression of vascular endothelial growth factor-B in mouse heart alters cardiac lipid metabolism and induces myocardial hypertrophy. *Circ Res*. 103:1018-1026.

Kern, T.S. & Barber, A.J. (2008). Retinal ganglion cells in diabetes. *J Physiol*. 586:4401-8.

Kiba, A.; Sagara, H.; Hara, T. & Shibuya, M. (2003). VEGFR-2-specific ligand VEGF-E induces non-edematous hyper-vascularization in mice. *Biochem Biophys Res Commun*. 301:371-7.

Lahteenvuo, J.E.; Lahteenvuo, M.T.; Kivela, A.; Rosenlew, C.; Falkevall, A.; Klar, J.; Heikura, T.; Rissanen, T.T.; Vahakangas, E.; Korpisalo, P.; Enholm, B.; Carmeliet, P.; Alitalo K.; Eriksson, U & Yla-Herttuala, S. (2009). Vascular endothelial growth factor-B induces myocardium-specific angiogenesis and arteriogenesis via vascular endothelial growth factor receptor-1- and neuropilin receptor-1-dependent mechanisms. *Circulation*. 119:845-856.

Lang, A.E.; Gill, S.; Patel, N.K.; Lozano, A.; Nutt, J.G.; Penn, R.; Brooks, D.J.; Hotton, G.; Moro, E.; Heywood, P.; Brodsky, M.A.; Burchiel, K.; Kelly, P.; Dalvi, A.; Scott, B.; Stacy, M.; Turner, D.;. Wooten, V.G.; Elias, W.J.; Laws, E.R.; Dhawan, V.; Stoessl, A.J.; Matcham, J.; Coffey, R.J. & Traub, M. (2006). Randomized controlled trial of intraputamenal glial cell line-derived neurotrophic factor infusion in Parkinson disease. *Ann Neurol*. 59:459-466.

Larcher, F.; Murillas, R.; Bolontrade, M.; Conti, C.J. & Jorcano, J.L. (1998). VEGF/VPF overexpression in skin of transgenic mice induces angiogenesis, vascular hyperpermeability and accelerated tumor development. *Oncogene*. 17:303-311.

Lees, A.J.; Hardy, J. & Revesz, T. (2009). Parkinson's disease. *Lancet*. 373:2055-2066.

Levin, L.A. (2005). Neuroprotection and regeneration in glaucoma. *Ophthalmol Clin North Am*. 18:585-596, vii.

Li, X.; Aase, K.; Li, H.; von Euler, G.& Eriksson, U. (2001). Isoform-specific expression of VEGF-B in normal tissues and tumors. *Growth Factors*. 19:49-59.

Li, X. & Eriksson, U. (2001). Novel VEGF family members: VEGF-B, VEGF-C and VEGF-D. *Int J Biochem Cell Biol*. 33:421-426.

Li, X.; Lee, C.; Tang, Z.; Zhang, F.; Arjunan, P.; Li, Y.; Hou, X.; Kumar, A. & L. Dong. (2009). VEGF-B: a survival, or an angiogenic factor? *Cell Adh Migr*. 3:322-327.

Li, X.; Tjwa, M.; Van Hove, I.; Enholm, B.; Neven, E.; Paavonen, K.; Jeltsch, M.; Juan, T.D.; Sievers, R.E.; Chorianopoulos, E.; Wada, H.; Vanwildemeersch, M.; Noel, A.; Foidart, J.M.; Springer, M.L.; von Degenfeld, G.; Dewerchin, M.; Blau, H.M.; Alitalo, K.; Eriksson, U.; Carmeliet, P. & Moons, L. (2008a). Reevaluation of the role of VEGF-B suggests a restricted role in the revascularization of the ischemic myocardium. *Arterioscler Thromb Vasc Biol*. 28:1614-1620.

Li, Y.; Zhang, F.; Nagai, N.; Tang, Z.; Zhang, S.; Scotney, P.; Lennartsson, J.; Zhu, C.; Qu, Y.; Fang, C.; Hua, J.; Matsuo, O.; Fong, G.H.; Ding, H.; Cao, Y.; Becker, K.G.; Nash, A.; Heldin, C.H.& Li, X. (2008b). VEGF-B inhibits apoptosis via VEGFR-1-mediated suppression of the expression of BH3-only protein genes in mice and rats. *J Clin Invest*. 118:913-923.

Lohela, M.; Bry, M.; Tammela, T. & Alitalo, K. (2009). VEGFs and receptors involved in angiogenesis versus lymphangiogenesis. *Curr Opin Cell Biol*. 21:154-165.

Lopes de Faria, J.M.; Russ, H. & Costa, V.P. (2002). Retinal nerve fibre layer loss in patients with type 1 diabetes mellitus without retinopathy. *Br J Ophthalmol.* 86:725-728.

Louzier, V.; Raffestin, B.; Leroux, A.; Branellec, D.; Caillaud, J.M.; Levame, M.; Eddahibi, S. & Adnot, S. (2003). Role of VEGF-B in the lung during development of chronic hypoxic pulmonary hypertension. *Am J Physiol Lung Cell Mol Physiol.* 284:L926-L937.

Love, S.; Plaha, P.; Patel, N.K.; Hotton, G.R.; Brooks, D.J. & Gill, S.S. (2005). Glial cell line-derived neurotrophic factor induces neuronal sprouting in human brain. *Nat Med.* 11:703-704.

Luttun, A.; Tjwa, M.; Moons, L.; Wu, Y.; Angelillo-Scherrer, A.; Liao, F.; Nagy, J.A.; Hooper, A.; Priller, J.; De Klerck, B.; Compernolle, V.; Daci, E.; Bohlen, P.; Dewerchin, M.; Herbert, J.M.; Fava, R.; Matthys, P.; Carmeliet, G.; Collen, D.; Dvorak, H.F.; Hicklin, D.J. & Carmeliet, P. (2002). Revascularization of ischemic tissues by PlGF treatment, and inhibition of tumor angiogenesis, arthritis and atherosclerosis by anti-Flt1. *Nat Med.* 1:1.

Marcic, T.S.; Belyea, D.A. & Katz, B. (2003). Neuroprotection in glaucoma: a model for neuroprotection in optic neuropathies. *Curr Opin Ophthalmol.* 14:353-356.

Mattson, M.P. (2004). Pathways towards and away from Alzheimer's disease. *Nature.* 430:631-639.

Morley, A.M. & Murdoch, I. (2006). The future of glaucoma clinics. *Br J Ophthalmol.* 90:640-645.

Mould, A.W.; Greco, S.A.; Cahill, M.M.; Tonks, I.D.; Bellomo, D.; Patterson, C.; Zournazi, A.; Nash, A.; Scotney, P.; Hayward, N.K. & Kay, G.F. (2005). Transgenic overexpression of vascular endothelial growth factor-B isoforms by endothelial cells potentiates postnatal vessel growth in vivo and in vitro. *Circ Res.* 97:e60-70.

Mould, A.W.; Tonks, I.D.; Cahill, M.M.; Pettit, A.R.; Thomas, R.; Hayward, N.K. & Kay, G.F. (2003). Vegfb gene knockout mice display reduced pathology and synovial angiogenesis in both antigen-induced and collagen-induced models of arthritis. *Arthritis Rheum.* 48:2660-2669.

Nash, A.D.; Baca, M.; Wright, C. & Scotney, P.D. (2006). The biology of vascular endothelial growth factor-B (VEGF-B). *Pulm Pharmacol Ther.* 19:61-69.

Nutt, J.G. & Wooten, G.F. (2005). Clinical practice. Diagnosis and initial management of Parkinson's disease. *N Engl J Med.* 353:1021-1027.

Odorisio, T.; Schietroma, C.; Zaccaria, M.L.; Cianfarani, F.; Tiveron, C.; Tatangelo, L.; Failla, C.M. & Zambruno, G. (2002). Mice overexpressing placenta growth factor exhibit increased vascularization and vessel permeability. *J Cell Sci.* 115:2559-2567.

Ogawa, S.; Oku, A.; Sawano, A.; Yamaguchi, S.; Yazaki, Y. & Shibuya, M. (1998). A novel type of vascular endothelial growth factor, VEGF-E (NZ-7 VEGF), preferentially utilizes KDR/Flk-1 receptor and carries a potent mitotic activity without heparin-binding domain. *J Biol Chem.* 273:31273-1282.

Olofsson, B.; Korpelainen, E.; Pepper, M.S.; Mandriota, S.J.; Aase, K.; Kumar, V.; Gunji, Y.; Jeltsch, M.M.; Shibuya, M.; Alitalo, K. & Eriksson, U. (1998). Vascular endothelial growth factor B (VEGF-B) binds to VEGF receptor-1 and regulates plasminogen activator activity in endothelial cells. *Proc Natl Acad Sci U S A.* 95:11709-11714.

Olofsson, B.; Pajusola, K.; Kaipainen, A.; von Euler, G.; Joukov, V.; Saksela, O.; Orpana, A.; Pettersson, R.F.; Alitalo, K. & Eriksson, U. (1996a). Vascular endothelial growth factor B, a novel growth factor for endothelial cells. *Proc Natl Acad Sci U S A.* 93:2576-2581.

Olofsson, B.; Pajusola, K.; von Euler, G.; Chilov, D.; Alitalo, K. & Eriksson, U. (1996b). Genomic organization of the mouse and human genes for vascular endothelial growth factor B (VEGF-B) and characterization of a second splice isoform. *J Biol Chem.* 271:19310-19317.

Oshitari, T.; Yamamoto, S.; Hata, N. & Roy. S. (2008). Mitochondria- and caspase-dependent cell death pathway involved in neuronal degeneration in diabetic retinopathy. *Br J Ophthalmol.* 92:552-556.

Pattison, L.R.; Kotter, M.R.; Fraga, D. & Bonelli, R.M. (2006). Apoptotic cascades as possible targets for inhibiting cell death in Huntington's disease. *J Neurol.* 253:1137-1142.

Petrukhin, K. (2007). New therapeutic targets in atrophic age-related macular degeneration. *Expert Opin Ther Targets.* 11:625-639.

Poesen, K.; Lambrechts, D.; Van Damme, P.; Dhondt, J.; Bender, F.; Frank, N.; Bogaert, E.; Claes, B.; Heylen, L.; Verheyen, A.; Raes, K.; Tjwa, M.; Eriksson, U.; Shibuya, M.; Nuydens, R.; Van Den Bosch, L.; Meert, T.; D'Hooge, R.; Sendtner, M.; Robberecht, W. & Carmeliet, P. (2008). Novel role for vascular endothelial growth factor (VEGF) receptor-1 and its Ligand VEGF-B in motor neuron degeneration. *J Neurosci.* 28:10451-10459.

Reichelt, M.; Shi, S.; Hayes, M.; Kay, G.; Batch, J.; Gole, G.A. & Browning, J. (2003). Vascular endothelial growth factor-B and retinal vascular development in the mouse. *Clin Experiment Ophthalmol.* 31:61-65.

Relkin, N.R.; Szabo, P.; Adamiak, B.; Burgut, T.; Monthe, C.; Lent, R.W.; Younkin, S.; Younkin, L.; Schiff, R. & Weksler, M.E. (2008). 18-Month study of intravenous immunoglobulin for treatment of mild Alzheimer disease. *Neurobiol Aging.* 30(11):1728-1736.

Rissanen, T.T.; Markkanen, J.E.; Gruchala, M.; Heikura, T.; Puranen, A.; Kettunen, M.I.; Kholova, I.; Kauppinen, R.A.; Achen, M.G.; Stacker, S.A.; Alitalo, K. & Yla-Herttuala, S. (2003). VEGF-D is the strongest angiogenic and lymphangiogenic effector among VEGFs delivered into skeletal muscle via adenoviruses. *Circ Res.* 92:1098-1106.

Rite, I..; Machado, A.; Cano, J. & Vener,. J.L. (2007). Blood-brain barrier disruption induces in vivo degeneration of nigral dopaminergic neurons. *J Neurochem.* 101:1567-1582.

Salmina, A.B. (2009). Neuron-glia interactions as therapeutic targets in neurodegeneration. *J Alzheimers Dis.* 16:485-502.

Segura, I., De Smet, F.; Hohensinner, P.J.; Almodovar, C.R. & Carmeliet, P. (2009). The neurovascular link in health and disease: an update. *Trends Mol Med.* 15:439-451.

Sherer, T.B.; Fiske, B.K.; Svendsen, C.N.; Lang, A.E. & Langston, J.W. (2006). Crossroads in GDNF therapy for Parkinson's disease. *Mov Disord.* 21:136-141.

Siemers, E.R.; Quinn, J.F.; Kaye, J.; Farlow, M.R.; Porsteinsson, A.; Tariot, P.; Zoulnouni, P.; Galvin, J.E.; Holtzman, D.M.; Knopman, D.S.; Satterwhite, J.; Gonzales, C.; Dean,

R.A. & May, P.C. (2006). Effects of a gamma-secretase inhibitor in a randomized study of patients with Alzheimer disease. *Neurology*. 66:602-604.

Staekenborg, S.S.; Koedam, E.L.; Henneman, W.J.; Stokman, P.; Barkhof, F.; Scheltens, P. & van der Flier, W.M. (2009). Progression of mild cognitive impairment to dementia: contribution of cerebrovascular disease compared with medial temporal lobe atrophy. *Stroke*. 40:1269-1274.

Sun, Y.; Jin, K.; Childs, J.T.; Xie, L.; Mao, X.O. & Greenberg, D.A. (2004). Increased severity of cerebral ischemic injury in vascular endothelial growth factor-B-deficient mice. *J Cereb Blood Flow Metab*. 24:1146-1152.

Sun, Y.; Jin, K.; Childs, J.T.; Xie, L.; Mao, X.O. & Greenberg, D.A. (2006). Vascular endothelial growth factor-B (VEGFB) stimulates neurogenesis: evidence from knockout mice and growth factor administration. *Dev Biol*. 289:329-335.

Traynor, B.J.; Bruijn, L.; Conwit, R.; Beal, F.; O'Neill, G.; Fagan, S.C. & Cudkowicz, M.E. (2006). Neuroprotective agents for clinical trials in ALS: a systematic assessment. *Neurology*. 67:20-27.

van Dijk, H.W.; Kok, P.H.; Garvin, M.; Sonka, M.; Devries, J.H.; Michels, R.P.; van Velthoven, M.E.; Schlingemann, R.O.; Verbraak, F.D. & Abramoff, M.D. (2009). Selective loss of inner retinal layer thickness in type 1 diabetic patients with minimal diabetic retinopathy. *Invest Ophthalmol Vis Sci*. 50:3404-3409.

van Leeuwen, R.; Boekhoorn, S.; Vingerling, J.R.; Witteman, J.C.; Klaver, C.C.; Hofman, A. & de Jong, P.T. (2005). Dietary intake of antioxidants and risk of age-related macular degeneration. *Jama*. 294:3101-107.

Weinreb, R.N. (2005). Clinical trials of neuroprotective agents in glaucoma. *Retina*. 25:S78-S79.

Wijesekera, L.C. & Leigh, P.N. (2009). Amyotrophic lateral sclerosis. *Orphanet J Rare Dis*. 4:3.

Wilcock, G.K.; Black, S.E.; Hendrix, S.B.; Zavitz, K.H.; Swabb, E.A. & Laughlin, M.A. (2008). Efficacy and safety of tarenflurbil in mild to moderate Alzheimer's disease: a randomised phase II trial. *Lancet Neurol*. 7:483-493.

Wu, Z.; Guo, H.; Chow, N.; Sallstrom, J.; Bell, R.D.; Deane, R.; Brooks, A.I.; Kanagala, S.; Rubio, A.; Sagare, A.; Liu, D.; Li, F.; Armstrong, D.; Gasiewicz, T.; Zidovetzki, R.; Song, X.; Hofman, F. & Zlokovic, B.V. (2005). Role of the MEOX2 homeobox gene in neurovascular dysfunction in Alzheimer disease. *Nat Med*. 11:959-965.

Xia, Y.P.; Li, B.; Hylton, D.; Detmar, M.; Yancopoulos, G.D. & Rudge, J.S. (2003). Transgenic delivery of VEGF to mouse skin leads to an inflammatory condition resembling human psoriasis. *Blood*. 102:161-168.

Yamamoto, M.; Tanaka, F.; Tatsumi, H. & Sobue, G. (2008). A strategy for developing effective amyotropic lateral sclerosis pharmacotherapy: from clinical trials to novel pharmacotherapeutic strategies. *Expert Opin Pharmacother*. 9:1845-1857.

Yasuhara, T.; Shingo, T.; Kobayashi, K.; Takeuchi, A.; Yano, A.; Muraoka, K.; Matsui, T.; Miyoshi, Y.; Hamada, H. & Date. I. (2004). Neuroprotective effects of vascular endothelial growth factor (VEGF) upon dopaminergic neurons in a rat model of Parkinson's disease. *Eur J Neurosci*. 19:1494-1504.

Yasuhara, T.; Shingo, T.; Muraoka, K.; wen Ji, Y.; Kameda, M.; Takeuchi, A.; Yano, A.; Nishio, S.; Matsui, T.; Miyoshi, Y.; Hamada, H. & Date. I. (2005). The differences between high and low-dose administration of VEGF to dopaminergic neurons of in vitro and in vivo Parkinson's disease model. *Brain Res*. 1038:1-10.

Zhang, F.; Tang, Z.; Hou, X.; Lennartsson, J.; Li, Y.; Koch, A.W.; Scotney, P.; Lee, C.; Arjunan, P.; Dong, L.; Kumar, A.; Rissanen, T.T.; Wang, B.; Nagai, N.; Fons, P.; Fariss, R.; Zhang, Y.; Wawrousek, E.; Tansey, G.; Raber, J.; Fong, G.H.; Ding, H.; Greenberg, D.A.; Becker, K.G.; Herbert, J.M.; Nash, A.; Yla-Herttuala, S.; Cao, Y.; Watts, R.J. & Li, X. (2009). VEGF-B is dispensable for blood vessel growth but critical for their survival, and VEGF-B targeting inhibits pathological angiogenesis. *Proc Natl Acad Sci U S A*. 106:6152-6157.

17

Power of a Metabonomic Approach to Investigate an Unknown Nervous Disease

Céline Domange[1], Alain Paris[2], Henri Schroeder[3] and Nathalie Priymenko[1,4]
[1]*Toulouse Nationale Veterinary School, Alimentation & Botanics, Toulouse*
[2]*INRA - Mét@risk Unit, AgroParisTech, Paris*
[3]*UR AFPA, INRA UC340, Nancy University, Faculty of Sciences & Technologies, Nancy*
[4]*UMR 1331 ToxAlim INRA INP, Toulouse*
France

1. Introduction

The field of neurological disorders becomes now one of the most important investigation areas in clinical medicine, whatever the toxicological, genetic, degenerative or environmental aetiology they have. Because it involves the main complex organ as target tissue, because also of the intrinsic specificity of the biological network of the nervous system, or the technical difficulty to access such a composite organ, the nervous diseases remain particularly difficult to study. Certainly, the rapid development of transgenic animal models of neurological diseases and the expanding growth of imaging techniques to functionally and non-invasively access some specific brain regions constitute a favourable situation to study the basis and the progression of some nervous diseases. However, the use of such transgenic animals or spontaneous animal models needs that the clinical symptoms are reproducible and that a *prior* knowledge of the aetiopathology of these diseases may exist. These latter conditions are not always available, especially concerning toxicology. In this case, how can both pathophysiology and therapies be investigated? Indeed, classically, when considering a toxicological approach, clinical signs, similar to those ascribed on the target species, need to be reproduced on the animal model. But how to do with disease displaying no known aetiology or with an animal model, on which it is impossible to reproduce, at least partially, some clinical signs of the target species? Furthermore, because of evident ethical reasons added to practical ones, some neurological disorders in humans or in large animals remain scarcely explored. "Omics" approaches seem to be a good alternative in the clinical medical research, enabling to take advantage of the global living system and, simultaneously of the control of the toxicological factor. To illustrate such an original approach, a neurological horse disease, Australian stringhalt, which has been described for several centuries, but for which aetiology is still only partially known, was reassessed using metabonomics in combination with other classical techniques. This has led to show how powerful this method may stand for in clinical medical research and, particularly in neurological studies.

2. Current neurological investigations: Advantages and limits of routinely used approaches and techniques

2.1 Limits of classical studies

Up to now, the neurological investigations tended to reproduce a human disease using a convenient animal model. However, they laboured to give results. In fact, it may appear surprising to recreate all the metabolic complexity prevailing in the genesis of a given disease and, to work on it, before having any knowledge of the specifically involved metabolic pathways specifically involved. Before considering an animal model as a convenient model of a human disease, it seems more consistent to record and describe all the putative impacts of a controlled *stimulus* on a living system without any *a priori* hypothesis because of our ignorance of the inherent metabolic disruptions involved. Indeed, this may help to efficiently tackle a neurological disease.

2.2 Behavioural approaches

The use of animal models of human diseases, on which some behavioural tests are carried out, is fundamental to investigate nervous disorders. The field of psychopharmacology or behavioural pharmacology enables to test and to measure effects of drugs on behaviour. The toxicological studies test the short- or long-term exposure, the acute intoxication or the chronic effects following administration of subclinical doses and the associated effects of chemical compounds or contaminants. Each behavioural manifestation in animal model tends to reflect a specific human behavioural alteration or cognitive effect like depression, anxiety, fear or schizophrenia. This may be susceptible to reveal a disruption in some mean way of neurological transduction involving, for example, dopamine, acetylcholine, amphetamine or catecholamine's impairments. However, this approach has some limits. In case of the lack of any behavioural manifestation in animals, the conclusion isn't that there is a lack of effect but only that there is an impossibility to give an interpretation of this lack of effect because of an inadequate "observation window" as in delayed toxicity of some contaminants for example. Moreover, the putative link between a visible behavioural impairment and a putative mechanistic explanation requires going back to the cerebral metabolism to translate the observed behavioural variance and to confirm the pertinence of metabolic pathways specifically involved. Most of the time, such behavioural approaches are hardly self-sufficient; they need to be completed by other studies such as metabolic, histological, anatomical or immunologic ones.

2.3 Imaging techniques

A wide range of imaging techniques provides powerful tools for studying tumours (Cooper et al., 2011), congenital diseases (Toga et al., 2006), metabolic and infectious diseases (Kastrup et al., 2005), development of organisms (Davis et al., 2011) and for realizing preclinical or clinical studies, or for measuring a treatment effect (Song et al., 2011). These techniques can also be used in neurotoxicology (Pogge and Slikker, 2004) or for exploring neurodegenerative or psychiatric disorders (Masdeu, 2011; Stoessl, 2011). The choice of one of these techniques is made according to some awaited answers to a specific anatomical, metabolic or functional information question, some of imaging techniques being able to perform several specific assessments. They are well adapted to describe functions in the frame of non-invasive *in vivo* studies, some being planned with a longitudinal follow-up. Concerning some specific tissues analyses, some compromises have to be done between the spatial or the temporal resolution according to what it has to be focussed on. Among these different techniques, anatomic or functional imaging techniques have to be distinguished. The first ones, tomodensitometry and magnetic resonance imaging or MRI (Griffith et al., 2007) provide highly detailed anatomic information. Their ability to give an access to *in vivo* biological information acquired non-invasively or to define a seemingly normal body composition and its perturbation in response to a pharmacological or a pathological event may facilitate exploration of nervous diseases (Frisoni and Filippi, 2005; Griffith et al., 2007; Tartaglia and Arnold, 2006). In parallel with the description of novel biomarkers coming from transgenic animal models developed for studying neurodegenerative diseases and more efficient therapies, the use of MRI and magnetic resonance spectroscopy (MRS) provide new information for *in vivo* neurochemistry, such as neuronal apoptosis, osmoregulation, energy metabolism, membrane function or signalling disruptions (Choi et al., 2007; Ross and Sachdev, 2004; Ross and Bluml, 2001). Most of clinical researches are based on the metabolites that are detectable using proton spectroscopy (Figure 1), which can quantify them in localized volumes in brain.

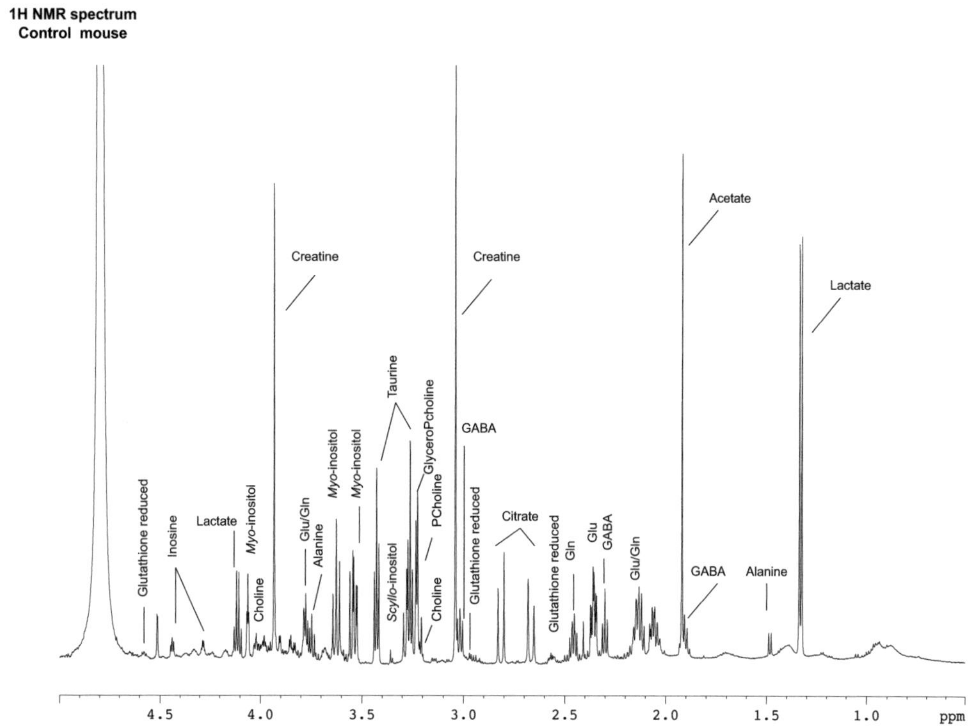

Fig. 1. 600.13 MHz ^{1}H NMR spectra from aqueous extracts of brain in mouse (control animal) (from Domange, 2008)

Nuclear magnetic resonance (or NMR) methods (MRI or MRS) can be successfully used to reveal neurological markers like N-acetyl-aspartate (a neuronal and axonal marker associated with neuronal viability), *myo*-inositol (a cerebral osmolyte and an astrocytic marker), glutamate and glutamine (the first is a major excitatory neurotransmitter and the second can restore it), creatine (which plays a crucial role in ATP biosynthesis in astrocytes), choline (its increased concentration theoretically means an alteration of myelin) and gamma-amino butyric acid (a main inhibitory neurotransmitter) (Martin, 2007). But MRS can also record intrinsic containing metabolites containing other atoms, as phosphorus, sodium, potassium, carbon, nitrogen and fluorine (this last atom often being a constituent of many drugs). Among the functional imaging techniques, positron emission tomography (PET) is a three-dimensional diagnostic imaging technology used in nuclear medicine that measures physiological function by looking at various functions of the body. It is a non-invasive diagnostic imaging tool enabling to follow some chemical neurotransmitters like dopamine in Parkinson's disease. Whatever the technique used to cover a specific neurological question, most of the time, it often requires laboratory animal and more particularly animal models of given human diseases.

2.4 Laboratory animals model contribution

The use of animal models in clinical research is crucial. As models, they usually display the same features and clinical signs as those observed in humans. So, they enable to establish some comparisons and extrapolations with the human physiology, to give access putative metabolic mechanisms involved in the progression of the disease and, hence, to identify biomarkers. A wide range of animal models has been used according to their origin. Animal models can be spontaneous, namely "mutant". Therefore, identification and characterization of novel laboratory animal lines carrying an interesting mutation combined with genotype-driven approaches are useful approaches to investigate some specific mechanistically-related molecules, to give new information about the function of the mammalian nervous system (Banks et al., 2011) or to study how genetic, environmental, toxicological or dietary factors can explain aetiology of a given disease. Animal models can also be created, using surgery, pharmacology or genetic interventions. These models are used to identify aetiological markers of disease or drug target and to test some new therapeutic drugs. The first cases have traditionally been induced by neurotoxins, acting selectively on neurons affected by human diseases. They are particularly useful for the study of the pathogenetic mechanism or to test new therapies for human neurological disorders (psychiatric or motor disorders) like obsessive-compulsive disorder or Parkinson's disease (Nowak et al., 2011). In parallel, the knockout technique, in which a gene is made inoperative leading to animals deficient in one specific gene, enables to evaluate the effects of the depletion of one protein in all the series of biological reactions within an organism and the putative followed consequences (Berman et al., 2011). More recently, the use of transgenic animals, constructed by inserting a human gene downstream into promoter, followed by microinjection in animal, ensures to indicate whether an over- or under-expression of a gene in one or several tissues should be susceptible to promote the pathogenesis and the development of a disease (Liu et al., 2011). The common point of all these animal models is the necessity of having some preliminary knowledge concerning a disease or the deleterious effect of a given xenobiotic. However, this information is not always available. Therefore, researchers have apace become aware of the necessity to access a wider range of knowledge in a living system and not only a specific molecular entity.

3. "Omics" approaches and their interest in clinical research

3.1 "Omics" approaches presentation

Similarly to imaging techniques, omics-based approaches appeared to be used according to the biological pool they consider (genes, proteins, lipids, metabolites) and the nature of target they have to reach (gene, enzymatic mechanism, biomarker). The full range of metabolites synthesized by a given biological system corresponds to its metabolome. In the same way, the full range of genes is contained in the term genome, the mRNA and the proteins ones, respectively, in the terms transcriptome and proteome (Figure 2). All these systems can be defined according to the level of biological organization, *i.e.* organism, organ, tissue, and cell. Related to these biological levels, omics-based approaches, mainly genomics, transcriptomics, proteomics (Colucci-D'Amato et al., 2011), lipidomics (Li et al., 2007), and metabolomics are terms standing for various global molecular-oriented approaches to better understand the underlying mechanisms, as the physiological regulations and the networks involved on all levels of gene products (mRNA, proteins, metabolites) in their respective systems and, if possible, between different sub-networks. Indeed, the observable property of organisms, *i.e.* their phenotype, is issued from genotype submitted to the concomitantly interactive action of the environment. Most of the time, the association between some of these approaches can be beneficial, enabling to understand the temporal progression of a pathophysiological state or the functioning of metabolic networks (Fiehn, 2001). Interest of these methods is to apply a controlled disruption to a biological system, whatever its nature (genetic, toxicological, pathophysiological, dietary), under some

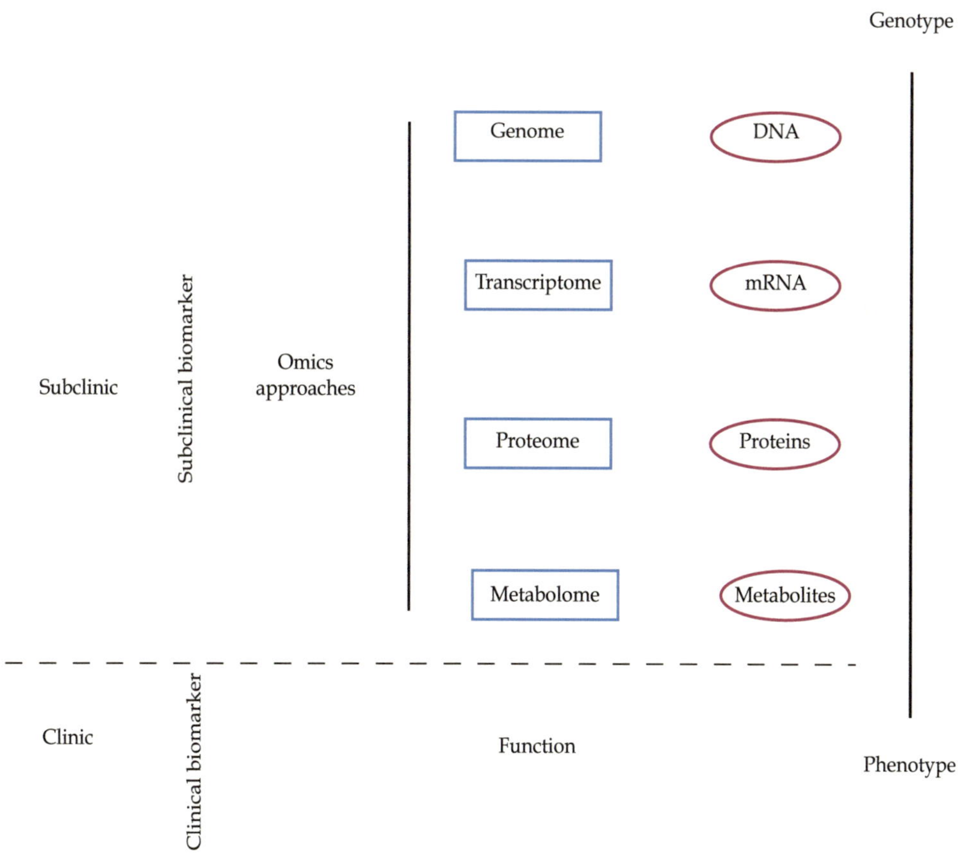

Fig. 2. "Omics" approaches and their different levels of biological living systems investigation

specific conditions (most of the time, the investigation is focused on an animal model), and to consider the subclinical consequences of such a disruptive perturbation. Therefore, "omics" approaches are widely used in biomedical research to make easier the understanding of disease mechanisms and to give access target tissues, to make easier the identification of biomarkers useful for therapeutic and diagnostic development and to predict clinical responses to treatments. The large amount of acquired data is as much an advantage as a hindrance. Indeed, the challenging subtlety is that all this information needs to be explored without any *a priori* hypothesis but by extracting only the interesting data. This fact partially explains why the real capacity of "omics" technologies stays in some instances rather limited because of the necessary requirement of some specific bioinformatics tools to efficiently mine multidimensional data but also the requirement of some specific analytical database to identify the candidate biomarkers at the gene, mRNA, enzyme, protein, or metabolite level. Moreover, transcriptomic studies require high-cost technologies and so, are less used than proteomic ones, which are based on two-dimensional gel-electrophoresis, which is cheaper and can be more easily used in many laboratories. However, analytical techniques related to the detection of large arrays of metabolites seem more robust, the resulting information being often easier to interpret because of the lower number of molecular entities, even though a rigorous identification of new metabolites still remains particularly fussy. According to the aim of studies and considering an increasing level of complexity of the analytical strategy used, investigation of metabolites may require either a metabolic profiling approach, which is focused on a small number of known metabolites (targeted metabolic profiling), or metabolomics including investigation of several classes of compounds (open metabolic profiling) or functional genomics, also called metabolic fingerprinting or metabonomics. This latter one is based on classification of samples according to their biological relevance to the studied disruption event and on identification of the fully informative markers detected at the statistical and functional sides and measured within the analyzed biological matrices.

Therefore, among these omics-based approaches, metabonomics stands for one of the most used holistic methods. Its emergence and its development mainly come from pioneering works of Pr J. Nicholson from the Imperial College of London. Because metabonomics enables to identify and quantify simultaneously low molecular weight compounds (metabolites) using spectroscopic methods such as nuclear magnetic resonance (NMR) or mass spectroscopy (MS), it gives access to a molecular level and may define the quantitative measurement of multiparametric metabolic responses of living system to pathophysiological stimuli. This can bring to the determination of some comprehensive metabolic signatures of biological matrices (Nicholson et al., 1999; Robertson, 2005). Metabonomics approach can be divided into successive steps. After the crucial step concerning the development of the experimental design, the choice of the animal model, the choice of the instrumentation used to quantitatively generate the metabolic information, the choice of samples of interest to be collected during the animal or the human experiment (biofluids such as plasma, urine, cerebral spinal fluid, saliva or faeces, tissues or organs), these biological samples are treated using appropriate analytical techniques. These latter ones enable to establish a metabolic fingerprint through the spectrum recording for every sample. All these fingerprints are summed up into datasets, in which metabolic information is subdivided and identified through coding variables. Each of them stands for either an integration bucket in NMR spectra corresponding to a defined chemical shift, or a relative or an absolute intensity of the ionic current measured at a specific mass to charge ratio in MS. Datasets are then treated using sophisticated statistical tools, *i.e.* multivariate or multidimensional statistical analysis tools, to access the most suitable model able to discriminate the different groups of samples according to the studied factors and to reveal main variables explaining this segregation. These variables can be considered at this step as many putative biomarkers, which need to be fully characterized by convenient structural identification methods. Finally, a detailed map of regulation and interaction between identified metabolites, their disruptions and the putative explanation of the pathophysiological state according to all involved factors may be suggested. Among analytical techniques mainly used in metabolomics, MS spectroscopy coupled to liquid (LC-MS) or gas chromatography (GC-MS) and NMR spectroscopy are the most appropriate ones concerning analysis of biofluids or liquid samples, whereas high resolution magic angle spinning (HR-MAS) NMR and MRS are adapted to solid samples like tissue or to achieve *in vivo* studies, respectively.

3.2 An integrated and functional approach

As previously mentioned above, the major constraint the "omics" approaches have to answer to, is to give access to a global pool of information belonging to the living system without focusing on a specific molecular entity. Indeed, one of the main assets of these approaches is the property of data integration necessary to render it as functionally understandable as possible. These features can be revealed through three complementary characteristics, namely *i)* the global nature of living systems underlined by homeostasis, *ii)* the multifactorial nature of diseases with both intrinsic and extrinsic factors, and *iii)* the ability to access multiple biological levels in living systems, and then to compile them to reveal one of the most realistic progressions of a disruption within a complex organism. Let's go into details of these three points. i) Contrary to classical biochemical approaches, which are set out to study only a single or few metabolites or metabolic reactions at the same time, metabolomics provides quantitative data on a wide range of known and unknown metabolites. It enables to visualize an overall pattern comprehensively linked to a set of interactions between metabolites or metabolic pathways and, hence, to an intrinsic homeostasis defined in these specific conditions (Kaddurah-Daouk et al., 2008). Indeed, whatever the stress applied on living systems, some allostatic changes, defined as an adaptive process, lead to short-term corrective changes of the different relevant regulatory systems to maintain a metabolic homeostasis. Concept of homeostasis is fundamental in biology and in clinical medicine to understand pathophysiological processes. The current clinical medicine tends now to come back to a more global view and, at the same time, on a more individualized approach of every patient because each of them differently answers to the environment according to their own homeostatic specificity. Clinical and subclinical signs give personalized information for every subject and, hence, physiological "means" used to adapt for everybody the set of parameters of homeostatic control in response to a disruptive stimulus and so to avoid falling down in a pathological state. The understanding of overall adaptation requires a good knowledge of metabolic pathways and related biochemical networks involved in the efficient control of homeostasis. For example, the knowledge of the glucose metabolism and the different ways by which homeostatic control of the circulating glucose concentration is achieved is crucial in the investigation of the Type 2 diabetes (Fiehn et al., 2010). ii) From global approaches can emerge a more accurate understanding of a given disease considering it is not only a single functional entity which is concerned, that is not only the consequence of a single causative explanation with a single mechanism involved in a single cell type in a given condition. Indeed, most of the pathophysiological disorders are not unique functional events but are resulting from complex interactions. These latter ones involve different concomitant actions in different biological compartments leading to different disruptions, which can be categorized according to the environmental conditions encountered and the inherent variability of subjects. Becoming aware of the importance of the environment and, more particularly, of the multifactorial nature of most of the disruptive events displayed by a living system is among the first pillars of the concept of global approach used in biological research in clinical medicine or in toxicology. iii) Finally, as a microscope could do it, omics-based approaches enable to focus on a specific level of a living system depending on the available analytical techniques used to generate data, but also to statistically integrate data coming from complementary fingerprinting techniques by using canonical analyses.

3.3 A metabolomic-based approach to reveal subclinical metabolic disruptions: A powerful tool in investigation of biomarkers

Besides the ability to define and to understand the aetiology of a disease, the discovery of novel biomarkers stands for a fundamental step to characterize and to manage it, especially to spot the homeostatic break down before appearance of the first clinical signs. Biomarkers, which are relevant indicators of disrupted biological processes in a given pathophysiological context, have to disclose features of disease (Moore et al., 2007; Nicholson and Lindon, 2008). The metabonomic approach is particularly interesting to explore subclinical disruptions of a living system before the outset of manifest clinical signs, and to identify biomarkers of disease risk and, if possible, to initiate prevention like in cancer (Roberts et al., 2011), diabetes (Wang et al., 2011), or nervous system illnesses (Kaddurah-Daouk and Krishnan, 2009; Nicholson and Lindon, 2008; Quinones and Kaddurah-Daouk, 2009). The identification of the metabolites requires the use of up-to-date structural databases of metabolites and metabolic pathway resources (Kouskoumvekaki and Panagiotou, 2011). As it has been previously mentioned, the use of complementary approaches stands for a wise way search of biomarkers displayed at different levels, namely biochemical, neuroanatomical, metabolic, genetic and neuropsychological ones, as it can be reported in the case of Alzheimer's disease investigation (Wattamwar and Mathuranath, 2010).

3.4 Examples of "omics" approaches in neurological investigation area

Use of metabolomics in neurological studies has been reported in many reviews (Choi et al., 2003; Rudkin and Arnold, 1999). It has been applied to a variety of biological samples for a better understanding of pathogenesis. This approach, because of its integrated and functional nature, stands for a powerful tool to study normal or pathological living systems, especially in central nervous system disorders through the use of specific animal models (Pears et al., 2005). Thus, it allows the identification of biomarkers of such diseases, but also of illness progression or response to therapy. In the drug discovery process, metabolomics brings some biochemical information about drug candidates, their mechanism of action and their therapeutic potential. In the field of neurosciences, the use of metabolomic approach can generate some questionings. Contrary to other organs in mammals, brain is isolated from the rest of organism by the blood-brain barrier, with consequences on the passage of some metabolites. Therefore, a metabolic fingerprint of brain predicted from a blood or

urine metabolomic analysis is not prone to reflect the real state of the subject, contrary to data coming from other organs like liver and kidney. Nevertheless, some first encouraging studies on neurological disorders performed using metabolomics have confirmed the interest of application of this approach in the field of neuroscience (Griffin and Salek, 2007). Analysis of blood or urine gives access to putative cerebral disruptions and can help to successfully reveal some biomarkers, as in the case of the manganese neurotoxicity, which is a significant public health concern (Dorman et al., 2008). So, because it reflects the presence of both extrinsic and intrinsic disruptive factors, metabonomics can define accurate biomarkers in neurology. Moreover, some specific metabolic pathways or some biological disruptions can be particularly interesting to study, because of their central or ubiquitous role in many pathological states. One example is the oxidative stress, leading to neuronal death, a mechanism that is found in early stages but also in secondary manifestations of many neurodegenerative states like Alzheimer's, Parkinson's and Huntington's diseases, amyotrophic lateral sclerosis, and neuroinflammatory disorders (Sayre et al., 2008). Because of the pivotal role of a metabolite in many biological functions, a
better understanding of some metabolic pathways like the biosynthesis of the amino acid L-serine can be interesting to investigate (Tabatabaie et al., 2010). Metabolic profiles acquired on human or animal biofluids like urine, cerebrospinal fluid (Lutz et al., 2007b), plasma, serum or tissue extracts, using either NMR or MS techniques, can give some precious information concerning neurological disorders (Sinclair et al., 2009). For example, ultra performance liquid chromatography/mass spectroscopy (UPLC/MS) metabolic profiles from serum collected on cerebral infarction patients have been analyzed using a metabonomic approach (Jiang et al., 2011). Quantitative analysis of human cerebrospinal fluid using NMR spectroscopy has been performed in multiple sclerosis (Lutz et al., 2007a), to identify biomarkers in the early stages of the amyotrophic lateral sclerosis (Blasco et al., 2010). Plasmatic metabolic disruptions between healthy and old persons with Alzheimer's disease were investigated using UPLC/MS-based metabonomic approach (Li et al., 2010). CRND8 transgenic mouse, model of this disease, enabled to analyze brain extracts using ^{1}H NMR spectroscopy (Salek et al., 2010). The interest of brain extracts coming from an animal model has been also illustrated to investigate epilepsy, for which the pharmacologically-induced animal model was obtained using pentylenetetrazole, a drug that induces seizures (Carmody and Brennan, 2010). Plasma from an experimental animal model of the spinal cord injury (Blasco et al., 2010) has been analyzed by ^{1}H NMR to get fingerprint profiles of this pathology (Jiang et al., 2010). Other cerebral alterations like brain tumors (Tate et al., 1996; Tate et al., 1998), schizophrenia and meningitis (Holmes et al., 2006; Lutz et al., 2007a) have also been investigated.

Beyond the use of a unique "omics" approach, it seems that it is all the more interesting and powerful to call for several complementary approaches and to tend to integrate so-generated data to yield a more comprehensive understanding of many diseases. In this way, Caudle et al. have used "omics" to characterize and identify some biomarkers of Parkinson's disease (Caudle et al., 2010). As an example, the following part illustrates the power of such a use, in a rodent model, of a neuro-intoxication caused in the horse by a plant, *Hypochoeris radicata* (L.). Indeed, because of the lack of knowledge about a neurological disease described only in the horse, we have tempted to use a laboratory animal model of this intoxication by applying metabonomics combined to imaging or behavioural experiments to reveal, in brain, candidate biomarkers of this pathology.

4. Example of a metabonomic approach of a neurological horse disease, the Australian stringhalt or how to address a toxicological issue on a seemingly non-target species without referring to a known toxic molecule

4.1 Problem for studying such an animal disease

Australian stringhalt is the name of a horse disease described since the middle of the 19th century in Australia (Robertson-Smith et al., 1985). It is defined as a syndrome characterized by an abnormal gait and an involuntary hyperflexion of both hind limbs during movement (Figure 3).

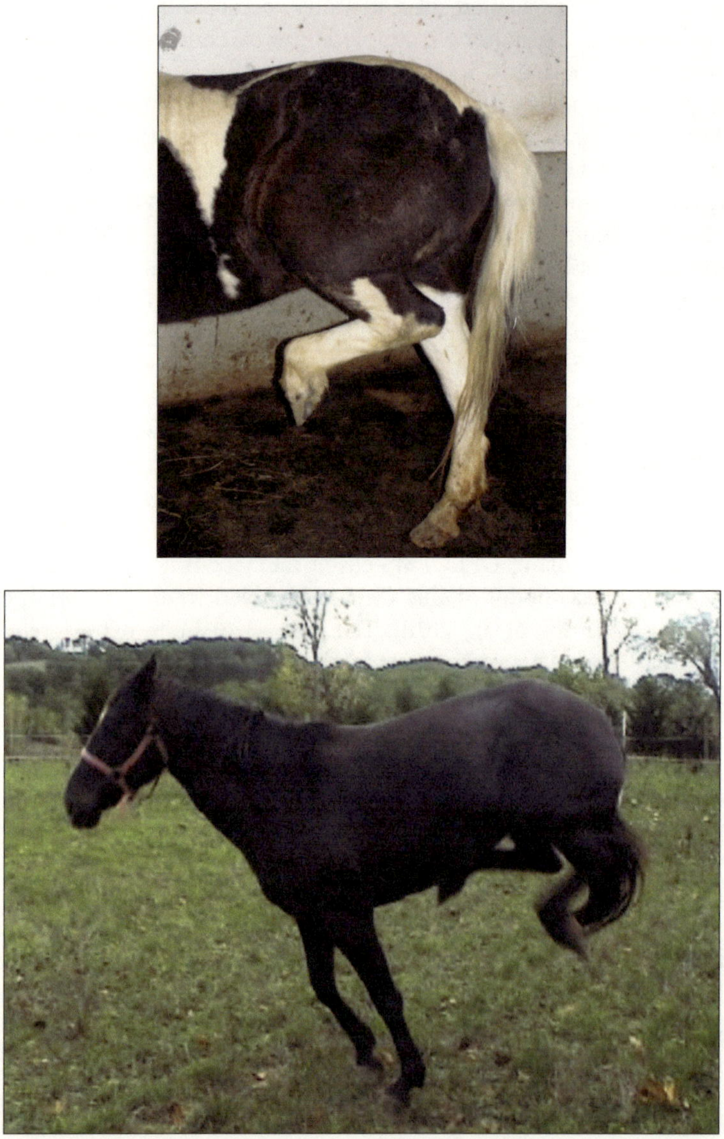

Fig. 3. Horses displaying clinical signs of Australian stringhalt (grade IV on the left, grade V on the right) (from (Collignon, 2007))

Since this time, several other outbreaks had been reported in many countries such as New Zealand (Cahill et al., 1985; Cahill et al., 1986; Cahill and Goulden, 1992), Chile (Araya et al., 1998), United States (Gay et al., 1993; Huntington et al., 1989; Robertson-Smith et al., 1985; Slocombe et al., 1992), Italy (Torre, 2005), Brasil (Araujo), more recently in France (Domange et al., 2010; Gouy et al., 2005) and were suspected in Japan (Takahashi et al., 2002). According to most of the authors, a plant of the Asteraceae family (formerly Compositeae family), *Hypochoeris radicata* L. also named cat's ear, flatweed or capeweed was suspected to be responsible for this disease (Araujo et al., 2008; Gardner et al., 2005; Gay et al., 1993; Gouy et al., 2005). This rosette-forming herb with a yellow terminal flower has a deep taproot, giving it resistance to drought. This explains a growth achieved preferentially on poor-quality pastures after a prolonged dry period, mainly in late summer and early autumn. Such climatic conditions, associated with the aggressiveness and the dominance of *Hypochoeris radicata* L. on other species, enable it to colonize pastures and to become the major plant available as herbivore feeding. These favouring factors, in aggravation for many years because of the global change in climatic conditions, appeared particularly marked in 2003 in France, after a blistering and dry summer, leading to an epizooty with a few tens of recorded intoxicated horses (Domange et al., 2010; Gouy et al., 2005). These latter's showed a wide range of symptoms but mainly dominated by several severity degrees from grade I to grade V, (Huntington et al., 1989) with an involuntary exaggerated hyperflexion of hind limbs and a delayed extension of hocks during forward movement. A marked atrophy of the hind limbs musculature, especially in the distal muscles, is often associated with this gait in the most affected animals. Most of the time, this amyotrophy is related to neurological lesions of the hind limbs with a proximal-to-distal gradient in the intensity, *i.e.* a loss of fibres, a decrease of the number of large myelinated nerve fibres, in agreement with the supposed pathogenesis described as a distal axonopathy (Cahill et al., 1986; Domange et al., 2010). However, in spite of these rare epidemiological and pathological data, the link between this horse disease and the toxicity of *Hypochoeris radicata* (HR) has been poorly investigated in spite of a recent study, which tended to reproduce the disease on animals after a 50-day HR treatment (9.8 kg HR/animal/day) (Araujo et al., 2008). The lack of investigation of such a disease is further partially explained by the critical approach of the nervous system, especially the peripheral nervous system and by the only target species. Besides, we need to consider ethical and financial issues. Moreover, as Araujo and colleagues underlined, the plant material is susceptible to differ in toxicity depending on several factors, one being the geographical location (Araujo et al., 2008).

4.2 Concept of orthology and interest in metabonomics

Most of the time, investigating a disease often requires a convenient laboratory animal model enabling to reproduce clinical symptoms, to access pharmacological data, to reveal some biomarkers of the disease and, in the best cases, to suggest some therapeutic treatments. Because of the nervous nature of Australian stringhalt, the fact that this illness was only described in target species, and the difficulties to link the supposed plant (more particularly if a specific secondary metabolite present in the plant would be involved) to the pathogenesis, the assessment of such an induced intoxication using a "classical" neurological approach seemed not efficient enough to reveal valuable biomarkers. Data obtained until recently remained too scarce. The "omics" approach, more particularly metabonomics, appears to be the most suitable mean to obtain some pertinent information about the target organs and candidate metabolic biomarkers by using an *a priori* "metabolically competent" animal model. The orthologous hypothesis considered in the case of an induction of a metabolic disruption in a rodent animal model of another animal species, here horse species, is crucial in characterizing a set of candidate metabolic biomarkers. Even though clinical signs may strikingly differ between the two species, some metabolic similarities may exist between their metabolic networks, particularly in their ability to be similarly disrupted by one or few toxicants. Among these latter's, plant secondary metabolites, for which nothing is known at the chemical and pharmacological sides, can be studied.

4.3 Use of complementary approaches: ^{1}H NMR-based metabonomics, MRI and behavioural tests

4.3.1 Metabolic fingerprints on biofluids and tissue extracts

Using the orthologous metabolic disruption assumption existing between two species, horse and mouse in the present case, metabonomics was used to investigate at the metabolic side this orphan neurological disease, Australian stringhalt. The purpose was to combine it with MRI as published elsewhere (Griffith et al., 2007) and with behavioural tests to improve the functional understanding of the metabolic data. Based on the orthologous hypothesis previously mentioned, the mouse was chosen as a "metabolically competent" laboratory animal model of horse intoxicated by HR, even though this rodent model of exposure to HR does not display any observable clinical sign. In a first time, metabonomic studies using male and female C57BL/6J mice fed for 21 days a diet containing 3 or 9% HR had been performed (Domange et al., 2008). ^{1}H NMR spectroscopy analyses have been done on weekly collected urine samples but also on tissue extracts prepared from liver and brain tissues collected at 0, 8, 15 and 21 days of treatment, after sacrifice of a subpopulation of the animals included in the experimental design. Urine and liver analyses were performed to detect the putative systemic disruption after the HR ingestion, and the brain analysis to access the nervous system disruption. All ^{1}H NMR spectra were acquired at 300 K on a Bruker DRX-600 Avance NMR spectrometer operating at 600.13 MHz for ^{1}H resonance frequency, using a cryoprobe and the 1D "Improved Watergate" sequence for suppression of water resonance. Multidimensional statistical analyses of fingerprint data were achieved on log-transformed variables. After removing redundant variables, linear discriminant analyses and partial least-squares regression-based discriminant analyses (PLS-DA) were performed on NMR data to maximize the groups' separation on a factorial map. Projection of these groups on every factorial axis enables to associate canonical ^{1}H NMR variables to the axis construction revealing thus the respective influence of the different factors of interest (gender, intoxication duration, toxicant dose). Therefore, the main part of the metabolic information related to urine ^{1}H NMR data and enabling the discrimination between the different groups of animals can be summed up in a factorial map (Figure 4). On this map, appears the temporal evolution between day 0 and day 21 of the metabolism of animals. This latter depends significantly on the gender of mice, through the 1st axis (this factor contains the main part of the variance explained by the statistical model used) and on the diet factor, through the second axis, covering from the bottom part of the factorial map diets without HR (named "control") to the middle part, diets with 3% HR (named "3%HR"), then to the top part, diets with 9% HR (named "9%HR"). By searching the first variables involved in the second axis construction, we reached the main metabolites, the concentration of which was influenced by a HR-induced metabolic disruption (Domange et al., 2008).

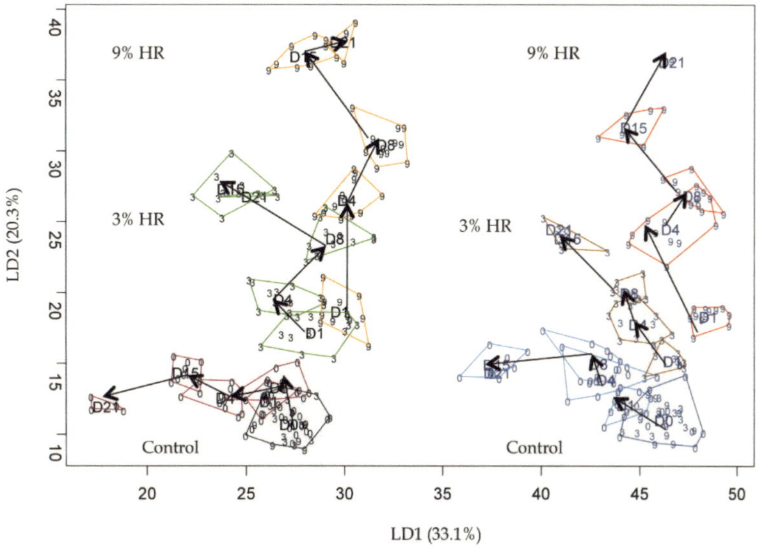

Fig. 4. LDA performed on 150 metabolic variables selected from fingerprints obtained by ^{1}H NMR performed at 600.13 MHz on 332 urinary samples (from Domange et al., 2008). The dummy variable selected is the « group » factor. A 61.5% amount of the total metabolic information is projected on the factorial plan LD1 x LD2. Arrows stand for metabolic trajectories throughout the study followed by every group fed either a control or a 3 or 9% HR diet. Barycenters give the dates of urine collection and correspond to the duration of HR intoxication (d8, day 8; d15, day 15; d21, day 21)

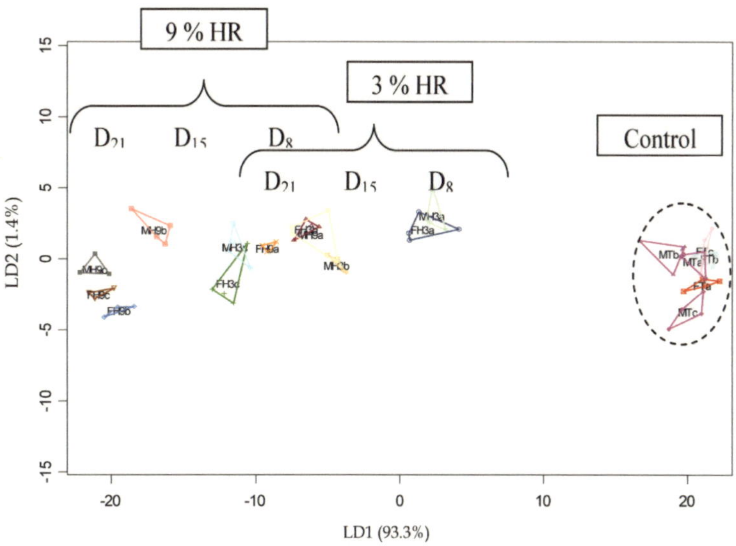

Fig. 5. LDA performed on 20 variables filtered from 600.13 MHz ^{1}H NMR data of brain aqueous extracts from male and female mice according to groups and in agreement with the two first components (from Domange, 2008). Barycenters give the date of brain collection and correspond to the duration of HR intoxication (d8, day 8; d15, day 15; d21, day 21)

In a same way, the main part of metabolic information contained in ^{1}H NMR data characterizing liver and brain hydrosoluble extracts and enabling the discrimination between the different groups of animals during the experiment could be summed up into a more complex factorial map (Figure 5). Firstly, is displayed the temporal evolution of the brain metabolism of mice orally exposed or not to HR, which holds almost all the part of the variance explained by the statistical model with, respectively from the right to the left side, a projection of the cerebral metabolisms of control animals, then the 3%HR-treated mice, and finally, the 9%HR-treated ones (Domange, 2008). The factor "time" is clearly revealed through every HR treatment with, respectively, from the right to the left side, an emphasis of the disrupted metabolism in a given direction all along the experiment duration. Given the fact that the two matrices of ^{1}H NMR fingerprinting data obtained on hydrosoluble brain and liver extracts were issued from the same individuals, a global correlation using a canonical analysis (PLS2 here) have been performed between them. A significant correlation between the two first PLS2 components has been revealed (Figure 6), in which, the gender factor is orthogonally projected to the diet one. Concerning the projection of variables involved in the variance calculation, *i.e.* the information explaining this construction, on the same plot, we can show that liver and brain ^{1}H NMR fingerprint data display close

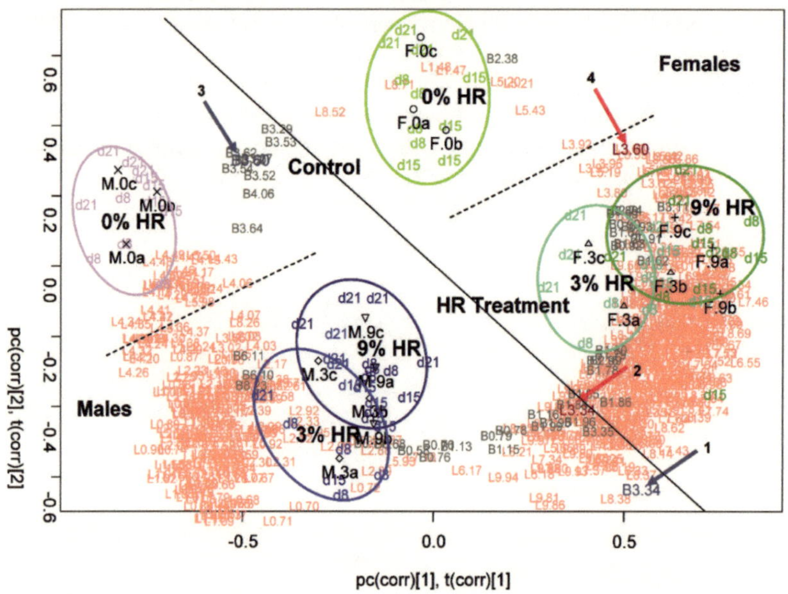

Fig. 6. Resulting biplot performed on the two first PLS2 components calculated between the hydrosoluble liver and brain extracts (from (Domange et al., 2008). Only the projection of the variables with contribution is above 0.5 is displayed (in grey for brain variables, in pink for the liver ones). Most of the variables containing the variance explained by the statistical model is spread according to the gender factor for the liver and according to the diet concerning the brain. The brain variable named B3.34 (arrow numbered 1) and the corresponding liver variable named L3.34 (arrow numbered 2) stand for the *scyllo*-inositol, detected at δ = 3.34 ppm. The brain variable named B3.60 (arrow numbered 3) and the corresponding liver variable named L3.60 (arrow numbered 4) stand for the *myo*-inositol detected at δ = 3.60 ppm

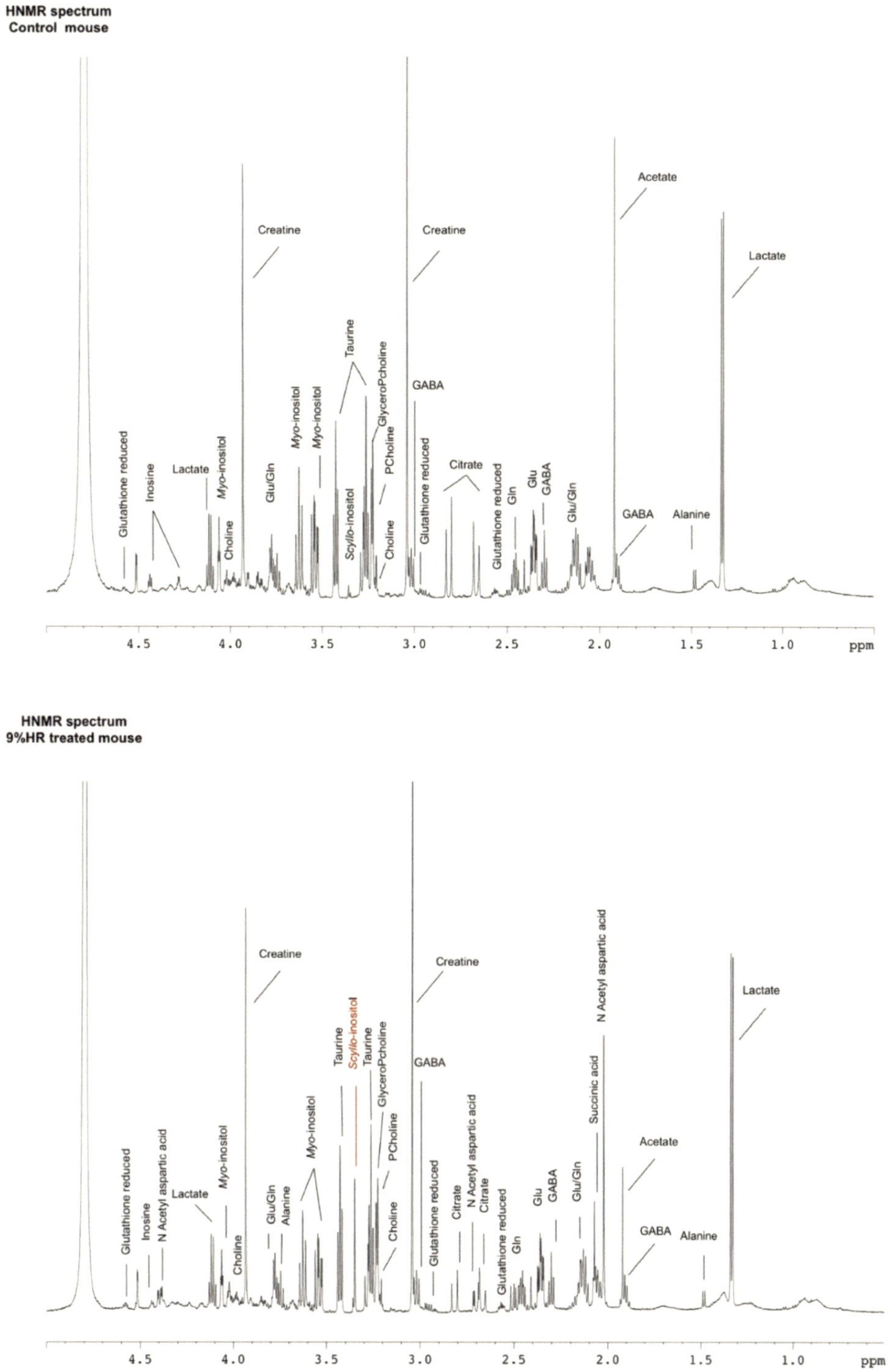

Fig. 7. 600.13 MHz ^{1}H NMR spectra from aqueous extracts of brain in 9% HR-treated mouse and control mouse (from Domange, 2008)

information. Among the main variables involved in the segregation of the groups of animals, *i.e.* which are related to the HR-treatment factor, and whatever the biological matrix analysed, the first identified variables correspond to the chemical shifts of the *scyllo*-inositol (δ = 3.35 or 3.36 ppm in urine and in liver extract fingerprints, δ = 3.34 ppm in cerebral and liver fingerprints), which are positively correlated to HR-treatment, when the *myo*-inositol ones (δ = 3.60 ppm) are negatively correlated to HR-treatment (Figures 7 and 8). Moreover, the comparison between ^{1}H-NMR metabolic fingerprints in control and HR-fed laboratory animals revealed a dose-dependent increase of the ratio *scyllo*-inositol/*myo*-inositol in urine, plasma, and hydrosoluble extracts of liver and brain of the HR-treated animals, enabling us to reveal some putative candidate metabolic biomarker(s) even though no aetiological factor was characterized, and no requirement of the target species was performed in this toxicological exploration.

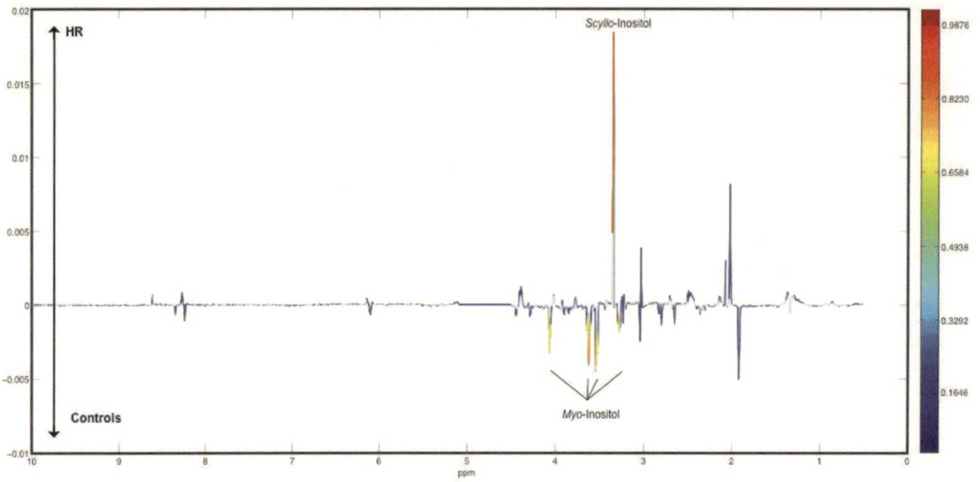

Fig. 8. Loading plot from O-PLS models performed from the aqueous extracts of brain in 9% HR-treated mice

4.3.2 Magnetic resonance imaging

To get access *in situ* to some potent cerebral metabolic changes thanks to a second spectroscopic technique, ^{1}H NMR localized spectroscopy, six male mice given a 9% HR diet and six control mice were used for *in vivo* metabolite quantification. All experiments were performed at 9.4 T on a Bruker Avance DRX 400 microimaging system with a wide-bore vertical magnet and a Micro 2.5 gradient system (Bruker Ettlingen, Germany). Because a preliminary experiment performed on a spectroscopic volume of interest (VOI) positioned in the cortex of mice was inconclusive, spectra have been performed from ^{1}H NMR data acquired by *in vivo* MRI using a VOI positioned in the thalamus of control and 9% HR-treated male mice (Figure 9.a). In this region, only the 9% HR-treated mice displayed a significant although minor signal found at δ = 3.34 ppm corresponding to *scyllo*-inositol (Figure 9.b). A one-way ANOVA performed for every other identified variables quantified at the same time from raw integrated spectra coming from *in vivo* MRI enables us to give significant results only for *scyllo*-inositol (p = 0.0013). As it could be described above, and as one of the interests of metabonomic approach is to combine data generated by different techniques to get more powerful biomarkers, a PLS2-based canonical regression between the set of brain metabolites issued by *in vivo* MRI and the ^{1}H NMR fingerprints of hydrosoluble brain extracts performed on the same animals has been obtained after correction of the two data sets by an OSC-PLS-driven correction procedure. The canonical analysis obtained by the PLS2 analysis between these two corrected data sets showed that the ^{1}H NMR variable called B3.34, namely *scyllo*-inositol, was projected in the region where scores of HR-treated animals were also projected (Figure 9.c). Moreover, the relative contents of *N*-acetyl-aspartate (NAA), lactate and choline were increased ($p < 10^{-5}$, $p = 0.02$ and $p = 0.03$, respectively) whereas the glutamine one was decreased ($p = 0.04$) in response to the 9% HR treatment. MRI studies were also conducted in poisoned living mice and corroborated the abnormal higher presence of *scyllo*-inositol in the thalamus of poisoned animals. Even this result was unable to explain the exact pathophysiological mechanism involved and the outset of the illness, it confirmed that *scyllo*-inositol was a biomarker of interest in the central nervous system, particularly when it is related to some brain metabolic disturbances (Griffith et al., 2007; Jenkins et al., 1993; Viola et al., 2004). The increase in NAA, which has been previously revealed following MRI and ^{1}H NMR spectroscopy of hydrosoluble brain extracts was suggested to be linked to the enhanced locomotor activity observed in 9% HR-treated mice. Besides, NAA has been reported in epileptic seizures cases (Akimitsu et al., 2000).

This accumulation of NAA has also been shown in a rat model of the Canavan's disease, suggesting that NAA increase in brain should be linked to neuroexcitation and neurodegeneration (Kitada et al., 2000).

4.3.3 Behavioural testing

The two previous exploratory studies led us to consider in more details the role of inositols in the development of the Australian stringhalt. The location of such metabolic disturbances, the current knowledge of the metabolism and the pathways involved, such as neurotransmission, signalling system and regulation of many cellular functions, depending on the balance between *scyllo* and *myo* inositol needed to be rounded out by a complementary functional assessment as a large extent behavioural testing of HR-treated animals can provide it. Indeed, the administration of inositol (*myo*-inositol) is used as a therapeutic molecule in depression (Einat et al., 1999), panic disorder, obsessive-compulsive disorder (Cohen et al., 1997; Levine, 1997). It partially explains an enhanced locomotion (Kofman et al., 1998) and may be linked to a putative anxiolytic effect (Kofman et al., 2000) with possible involvement of serotoninergic (5-HT_2) receptors (Einat et al., 2001). Therefore, to investigate the functional consequences of such previous disrupted metabolic events, various behavioural aspects of C57BL/6J mice orally exposed to 9% HR for 3 weeks were performed in parallel with the ^{1}H NMR metabolomic exploration of the brain. Several behavioural tests related to locomotor activity (open-field test), motor coordination (Locotronic® apparatus, Wespoc test), learning and memory [Y maze, (Hughes, 2004), Figure 10.a and Morris water maze], anxiety [elevated plus maze, (Rodgers and Johnson, 1995), hole board (do-Rego et al., 2006; Takeda et al., 1998), Figure 10.b], and depression forced swimming test or test of Porsolt (Porsolt et al., 1977; Porsolt et al., 1979), social interaction (resident/intruder model), and addiction (place preference test) were carried out (Domange et al., submitted).

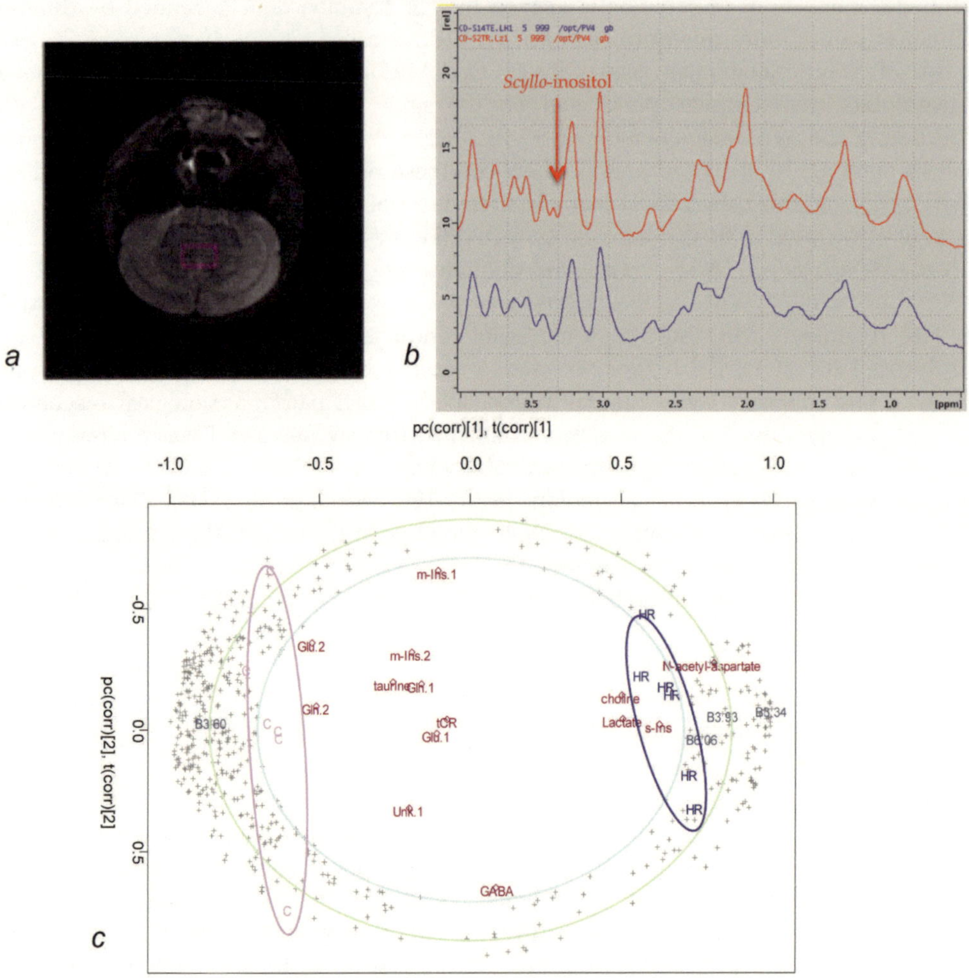

Fig. 9. a) MRI performed at 9.4 T on a Bruker Avance DRX 400 microimaging system positioned in the thalamus region with an *in vivo* parallel metabolite quantification using ^{1}H NMR localized spectroscopy (VOI, 12 mm^3). b) Spectrum comparison between the sum of six ^{1}H NMR spectra acquired on control male mice and the sum of six ^{1}H NMR spectra acquired on 9%HR-treated male mice with the presence of *scyllo*-inositol (chemical shift detected at $\delta = 3.34$ ppm). c) PLS2 between MRI quantitative data and ^{1}H NMR data. A loading projection is given for metabonomic variables having a norm above 0.5 (pale blue circle) or above 0.75 (pale green circle). The purple and the dark-blue ellipses, respectively, correspond to the scores of control and 9% HR-treated mice. Among the main MRI loadings having a positive correlation with HR treatment are *scyllo*-inositol (*s*-Ins), *N*-acetyl-aspartate, lactate and choline. For MRI variables having a negative correlation with HR treatment are glutamate (Glu.2, second chemical shift) and glutamine (Gln.2, second chemical shift). Uninformative MRI loadings: *myo*-inositol (*m*-Ins), glutamate, first chemical shift (Glu.1), glutamine, first chemical shift (Gln.1), GABA, taurine and unknown 1 are projected in the centre of the biplot (from Domange et al., 2008)

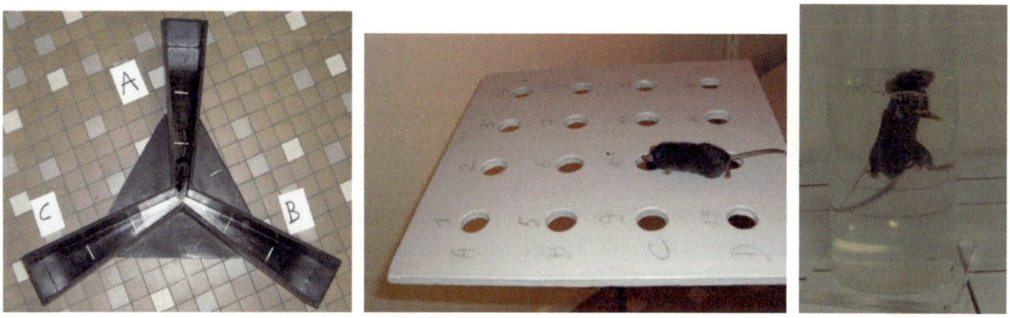

(a) (b) (c)

Fig. 10. Examples of behavioural tests used in mice: a) Y-maze or Y-maze spontaneous alternation that estimates the immediate working memory performance. b) Hole board test that evaluates the exploratory rate and the anxiety level. c) Forced swimming test defined to visualize a depression state (from Domange et al., submitted)

Although the lack of motor coordination impairment is commonly observed in the sick horses, 9% HR-treated mice displayed a motor hyperactivity, which is reflected by the decrease of immobility time in the forced swimming test, and the increased numbers of head dipping in the hole board test, of arms visited in Y-maze and of the number of entries in the upper quarter of the maze in the Morris water maze (Domange et al., submitted). This increased activity of treated mice, which is clearly observable at the end of tests, could be linked to a decrease in the resignation state or an enhanced motivation. Moreover, the 9% HR-contaminated mice seem to be addicted to the plant as indicated by results obtained in the place preference test. A regularized canonical analyses performed using mixOmics, an R package (Le Cao et al., 2009) to establish a canonical link between the two multidimensional data sets, *i.e.* the one containing the ^{1}H NMR fingerprints of hydrosoluble brain extracts and the one corresponding to the behavioural data set, which comprises nearly 100 variables, has revealed a clear relationship between some behavioural impairment variables (the motor hyperactivity and the addiction for the plant) and the main metabolic disruptions, *i.e.* the increase in *scyllo*-inositol in the brain of HR-treated mice and the relative decrease in *myo*-inositol. These results underlie the interest of such a dual and combined approach to characterize the functional end-points of a pathophysiological model of the horse Australian stringhalt in a seemingly metabolically orthologous murine species.

5. Conclusion

In this chapter, we underlined the interest of "omics" approaches and their recent introduction in the field of neuro-toxicological research. Indeed, metabonomics can especially be considered as a potentially powerful mean to explore the subclinical disruptions of an organism before the outset of clinical signs, and would particularly be useful in discovery markers of disease risk. This approach would help to prevent some risks in spite of the difficulty to detect some minor metabolites or molecules in tiny doses or mixtures, with the ability to access and explore some isolated and intricate tissues (like brain) *via* the general metabolism (urine, plasma) and to link statistically these subclinical metabolic changes with complementary data coming from other phenotyping approaches and across multiple physiological levels. Besides, these combined techniques have been applied in some toxico-environmental assessments possibly aetiologically linked to some neuro-physiological diseases. Thus, coupling metabolomic and behavioural studies may help to functionally describe neurotoxicity resulting from ingestion of milk of lactating goats fed a hay contaminated with various persistent organic pollutants (POPs) like Polycyclic Aromatic Hydrocarbons (PAHs), PolyChloroDibenzo-p-Dioxins (PCDDs), PolyChloroDibenzoFurans (PCDFs) and PolyChloroBiphenyls (PCBs) (Schroeder et al., in preparation). Nevertheless, these "omics" technologies required new specific bioinformatics tools to mine multifactorial data and, in the case of metabolomics, some well-documented analytical databases to structurally characterize metabolites revealed as candidate biomarkers. Therefore, further progress needs to be obtained to improve at the statistical side these integration strategies and to reduce some still existing drawbacks. Nonetheless, such techniques have also the outstanding capacity to give some interpretation of the results in a larger biological perspective, given that this holistic approach stands for an emerging level of knowledge in clinical medical research.

6. Acknowledgment

We gratefully acknowledge the excellent technical support and the contribution in the animal experimentation of Florence Blas Y Estrada and Raymond Gazel (INRA Toulouse, INP, UMR1331 ToxAlim) during metabonomic studies, Amidou Traoré, Guy Biélicki and Cécile Keller (INRA Clermont-Ferrand/Theix, QuaPA STIM, F-63122 St Genès Champanelle) during MRI experiments and Nicolas Violle and Julie Peiffer (UR AFPA, INRA UC340, Nancy University) during behavioural tests.

7. References

Akimitsu, T., Kurisu, K., Hanaya, R., Iida, K., Kiura, Y., Arita, K., Matsubayashi, H., Ishihara, K., Kitada, K., Serikawa, T., Sasa, M., 2000. Epileptic seizures induced by N-acetyl-L-aspartate in rats: in vivo and in vitro studies. *Brain Research*. Vol.861, pp. 143-150.

Araujo, J.A., Curcio, B., Alda, J., Medeiros, R.M., Riet-Correa, F., 2008. Stringhalt in Brazilian horses caused by Hypochaeris radicata. *Toxicon*. Vol.52, pp. 190-193.

Araya, O., Krause, A., Solis de Ovando, M., 1998. Outbreaks of stringhalt in southern Chile. *The Veterinary Record*. Vol.142, pp 462-463.

Banks, G.T., Haas, M.A., Line, S., Shepherd, H.L., Alqatari, M., Stewart, S., Rishal, I., Philpott, A., Kalmar, B., Kuta, A., Groves, M., Parkinson, N., Acevedo-Arozena, A., Brandner, S., Bannerman, D., Greensmith, L., Hafezparast, M., Koltzenburg, M., Deacon, R., Fainzilber, M., Fisher, E.M., 2011. Behavioral and other phenotypes in a cytoplasmic Dynein light intermediate chain 1 mutant mouse. *Journal of Neurosciences*. Vol.31, pp. 5483-5494.

Berman, A.E., Chan, W.Y., Brennan, A.M., Reyes, R.C., Adler, B.L., Suh, S.W., Kauppinen, T.M., Edling, Y., Swanson, R.A., 2011. N-acetylcysteine prevents loss of dopaminergic neurons in the EAAC1-/- mouse. *Annals of Neurology*. Vol.69, pp. 509-520.

Blasco, H., Corcia, P., Moreau, C., Veau, S., Fournier, C., Vourc'h, P., Emond, P., Gordon, P., Pradat, P.F., Praline, J., Devos, D., Nadal-Desbarats, L., Andres, C.R., 2010. 1H-

NMR-based metabolomic profiling of CSF in early amyotrophic lateral sclerosis. *PLoS One*. Vol.5, e13223.
Cahill, J.I., Goulden, B.E., Pearce, H.G., 1985. A review and some observations on stringhalt. *New Zealand Veterinarian Journal*. Vol.33, pp. 101-104.
Cahill, J.I., Goulden, B.E., Jolly, R.D., 1986. Stringhalt in horses: a distal axonopathy. *Neuropathology Applied Neurobiolology*. Vol.12, pp 459-475.
Cahill, J.I., Goulden, B.E., 1992. Stringhalt--current thoughts on aetiology and pathogenesis. *Equine Veterinary Journal*. Vol.24, pp. 161-162.
Carmody, S., Brennan, L., 2010. Effects of pentylenetetrazole-induced seizures on metabolomic profiles of rat brain. *Neurochemistry International*. Vol.56, pp. 340-344.
Caudle, W.M., Bammler, T.K., Lin, Y., Pan, S., Zhang, J., 2010. Using 'omics' to define pathogenesis and biomarkers of Parkinson's disease. *Expert Review of Neurotherapeutics*. Vol.10, pp. 925-942.
Choi, I.Y., Lee, S.P., Guilfoyle, D.N., Helpern, J.A., 2003. In vivo NMR studies of neurodegenerative diseases in transgenic and rodent models. *Neurochemical Research*. Vol.28, pp. 987-1001.
Choi, J.K., Dedeoglu, A., Jenkins, B.G., 2007. Application of MRS to mouse models of neurodegenerative illness. *NMR in Biomedicine*. Vol.20, pp. 216-237.
Cohen, H., Kotler, M., Kaplan, Z., Matar, M.A., Kofman, O., Belmaker, R.H., 1997. Inositol has behavioral effects with adaptation after chronic administration. *Journal of Neural Transmission*. Vol.104, pp. 299-305.
Collignon, G., 2007. Contribution à l'étude épidémiologique de l'enzootie de harper australien en France depuis 2003 chez le cheval. Veterinary Thesis of University of Toulouse.
Colucci-D'Amato, L., Farina, A., Vissers, J.P., Chambery, A., 2011. Quantitative neuroproteomics: classical and novel tools for studying neural differentiation and function. *Stem Cell Reviews*. Vol.7, pp. 77-93.
Cooper, K.L., Meng, Y., Harnan, S., Ward, S.E., Fitzgerald, P., Papaioannou, D., Wyld, L., Ingram, C., Wilkinson, I.D., Lorenz, E., 2011. Positron emission tomography (PET) and magnetic resonance imaging (MRI) for the assessment of axillary lymph node metastases in early breast cancer: systematic review and economic evaluation. *Health Technology Assessment*. Vol.15, pp. iii-iv, 1-134.
Davis, E.P., Buss, C., Muftuler, L.T., Head, K., Hasso, A., Wing, D.A., Hobel, C., Sandman, C.A., 2011. Children's Brain Development Benefits from Longer Gestation. *Frontiers in Psychology*. Vol.2, p. 1.
do-Rego, J.C., Viana, A.F., Le Maitre, E., Deniel, A., Rates, S.M., Leroux-Nicollet, I., Costentin, J., 2006. Comparisons between anxiety tests for selection of anxious and non anxious mice. *Behavioural Brain Research*. Vol.169, pp. 282-288.
Domange, C., 2008. Etude des disruptions métaboliques provoquées chez le modèle murin par l'ingestion d'Hypochoeris radicata (L.), plante toxique pour l'espèce équine. Validation de l'approche métabonomique par des études comportementales et par imagerie cérébrale. Thesis of University of Toulouse.
Domange, C., Canlet, C., Traore, A., Bielicki, G., Keller, C., Paris, A., Priymenko, N., 2008. Orthologous metabonomic qualification of a rodent model combined with magnetic resonance imaging for an integrated evaluation of the toxicity of Hypochoeris radicata. *Chemical Research in Toxicology*. Vol.21, pp. 2082-2096.

Domange, C., Casteignau, A., Collignon, G., Pumarola, M., Priymenko, N., 2010. Longitudinal study of Australian stringhalt cases in France. *Journal of Animal Physiology and Animal Nutrition (Berl)*. Vol.94, pp. 712-720.

Dorman, D.C., Struve, M.F., Norris, A., Higgins, A.J., 2008. Metabolomic analyses of body fluids after subchronic manganese inhalation in rhesus monkeys. *Toxicological Sciences*. Vol.106, pp. 46-54.

Einat, H., Clenet, F., Shaldubina, A., Belmaker, R.H., Bourin, M., 2001. The antidepressant activity of inositol in the forced swim test involves 5-HT(2) receptors. *Behavioural Brain Research*. Vol.118, pp. 77-83.

Einat, H., Karbovski, H., Korik, J., Tsalah, D., Belmaker, R.H., (1999). Inositol reduces depressive-like behaviors in two different animal models of depression. *Psychopharmacology (Berl)*. Vol.144, pp. 158-162.

Fiehn, O., 2001. Combining genomics, metabolome analysis, and biochemical modelling to understand metabolic networks. *Comparative and Functional Genomics*. Vol.2, pp. 155-168.

Fiehn, O., Garvey, W.T., Newman, J.W., Lok, K.H., Hoppel, C.L., Adams, S.H., 2010. Plasma metabolomic profiles reflective of glucose homeostasis in non-diabetic and type 2 diabetic obese African-American women. *PLoS One*. Vol.5, e15234.

Frisoni, G.B., Filippi, M., 2005. Multiple sclerosis and Alzheimer disease through the looking glass of MR imaging. *AJNR American Journal of Neuroradiology*. Vol.26, pp. 2488-2491.

Gardner, S.Y., Cook, A.G., Jortner, B.S., Troan, B.V., Sharp, N.J.H., Campbell, N.B., Brownie, C.F., 2005. Stringhalt associated with a pasture infested with Hypochoeris radicata. *Equine Veterinary Education*. Vol.17, pp. 118-122.

Gay, C.C., Fransen, S., Richards, J., Holler, S., 1993. Hypochoeris-associated stringhalt in North America. *Equine Veterinary Journal*. Vol.25, pp. 456-457.

Gouy, I., Leblond, A., Egron-Morand, G., Cadore, J.L., 2005. Etude de cas de harper australien après sa recrudescence dans la région lyonnaise. *Pratique Vétérinaire Equine*. Vol.37, pp. 53-60.

Griffin, J.L., Salek, R.M., 2007. Metabolomic applications to neuroscience: more challenges than chances? *Expert Review of Proteomics*. Vol.4, pp. 435-437.

Griffith, H.R., den Hollander, J.A., Stewart, C.C., Evanochko, W.T., Buchthal, S.D., Harrell, L.E., Zamrini, E.Y., Brockington, J.C., Marson, D.C., 2007. Elevated brain scyllo-inositol concentrations in patients with Alzheimer's disease. NMR in Biomedicine. Vol.20, pp. 709-716.

Holmes, E., Tsang, T.M., Tabrizi, S.J., 2006. The application of NMR-based metabonomics in neurological disorders. *NeuroRx*. Vol.3, pp. 358-372.

Hughes, R.N., 2004. The value of spontaneous alternation behavior (SAB) as a test of retention in pharmacological investigations of memory. *Neuroscience and Biobehavioral Reviews*. Vol.28, pp. 497-505.

Huntington, P.J., Jeffcott, L.B., Friend, S.C., Luff, A.R., Finkelstein, D.I., Flynn, R.J., 1989. Australian Stringhalt--epidemiological, clinical and neurological investigations. *Equine Veterinary Journal*. Vol.21, pp 266-273.

Jenkins, B.G., Koroshetz, W.J., Beal, M.F., Rosen, B.R., 1993. Evidence for impairment of energy metabolism in vivo in Huntington's disease using localized 1H NMR spectroscopy. *Neurology*. Vol.43, pp. 2689-2695.

Jiang, H., Peng, J., Zhou, Z.Y., Duan, Y., Chen, W., Cai, B., Yang, H., Zhang, W., 2010. Establishing (1)H nuclear magnetic resonance based metabonomics fingerprinting profile for spinal cord injury: a pilot study. *Chinese Medical Journal (Engl)*. Vol.123, pp. 2315-2319.

Jiang, Z., Sun, J., Liang, Q., Cai, Y., Li, S., Huang, Y., Wang, Y., Luo, G., 2011. A metabonomic approach applied to predict patients with cerebral infarction. *Talanta*. Vol.84, pp. 298-304.

Kaddurah-Daouk, R., Kristal, B.S., Weinshilboum, R.M., 2008. Metabolomics: a global biochemical approach to drug response and disease. Annu Rev Pharmacol Toxicol. 48, 653-83.

Kaddurah-Daouk, R., Krishnan, K.R., 2009. Metabolomics: a global biochemical approach to the study of central nervous system diseases. *Neuropsychopharmacology*. Vol.34, pp. 173-186.

Kastrup, O., Wanke, I., Maschke, M., 2005. Neuroimaging of infections. *NeuroRx*. Vol.2, pp. 324-332.

Kitada, K., Akimitsu, T., Shigematsu, Y., Kondo, A., Maihara, T., Yokoi, N., Kuramoto, T., Sasa, M., Serikawa, T., 2000. Accumulation of N-acetyl-L-aspartate in the brain of the tremor rat, a mutant exhibiting absence-like seizure and spongiform degeneration in the central nervous system. *Journal of Neurochemistry*. Vol.74, pp. 2512-2519.

Kofman, O., Agam, G., Shapiro, J., Spencer, A., 1998. Chronic dietary inositol enhances locomotor activity and brain inositol levels in rats. *Psychopharmacology (Berl)*. Vol.139, pp. 239-242.

Kofman, O., Einat, H., Cohen, H., Tenne, H., Shoshana, C., 2000. The anxiolytic effect of chronic inositol depends on the baseline level of anxiety. *Journal of Neural Transmission*. Vol.107, pp. 241-253.

Kouskoumvekaki, I., Panagiotou, G., 2011. Navigating the human metabolome for biomarker identification and design of pharmaceutical molecules. *Journal of Biomedicine and Biotechnology*. Vol.2011, ID 525497.

Le Cao, K.A., Gonzalez, I., Dejean, S., 2009. integrOmics: an R package to unravel relationships between two omics datasets. *Bioinformatics*. Vol.25, pp. 2855-2856.

Levine, J., 1997. Controlled trials of inositol in psychiatry. *European Neuropsychopharmacology*. Vol.7, pp. 147-155.

Li, J., Cui, Z., Zhao, S., Sidman, R.L., 2007. Unique glycerophospholipid signature in retinal stem cells correlates with enzymatic functions of diverse long-chain acyl-CoA synthetases. *Stem Cells*. Vol.25, pp. 2864-2873.

Li, N.J., Liu, W.T., Li, W., Li, S.Q., Chen, X.H., Bi, K.S., He, P., 2010. Plasma metabolic profiling of Alzheimer's disease by liquid chromatography/mass spectrometry. *Clinical Biochemistry*. Vol.43, pp. 992-997.

Liu, J., Wang, H., Zhang, L., Xu, Y., Deng, W., Zhu, H., Qin, C., 2011. S100B transgenic mice develop features of Parkinson's disease. *Archives of Medical Research*. Vol.42, pp. 1-7.

Lutz, N.W., Viola, A., Malikova, I., Confort-Gouny, S., Audoin, B., Ranjeva, J.P., Pelletier, J., Cozzone, P.J., 2007a. Inflammatory multiple-sclerosis plaques generate characteristic metabolic profiles in cerebrospinal fluid. *PLoS One*. Vol.2, e595.

Lutz, N.W., Viola, A., Malikova, I., Confort-Gouny, S., Ranjeva, J.P., Pelletier, J., Cozzone, P.J., 2007b. A branched-chain organic acid linked to multiple sclerosis: first identification by NMR spectroscopy of CSF. *Biochemical and Biophysical Research Communications*. Vol.354, pp. 160-164.

Martin, W.R., 2007. MR spectroscopy in neurodegenerative disease. *Molecular Imaging and Biology*. Vol.9, pp. 196-203.

Masdeu, J.C., 2011. Neuroimaging in psychiatric disorders. *Neurotherapeutics*. Vol.8, pp. 93-102.

Moore, R.E., Kirwan, J., Doherty, M.K., Whitfield, P.D., 2007. Biomarker discovery in animal health and disease: the application of post-genomic technologies. *Biomarker Insights*. Vol.2, pp. 185-196.

Nicholson, J.K., Lindon, J.C., Holmes, E., 1999. 'Metabonomics': understanding the metabolic responses of living systems to pathophysiological stimuli via multivariate statistical analysis of biological NMR spectroscopic data. *Xenobiotica*. Vol.29, pp. 1181-1189.

Nicholson, J.K., Lindon, J.C., 2008. Systems biology: Metabonomics. *Nature*. Vol.455, pp. 1054-1056.

Nowak, K., Mix, E., Gimsa, J., Strauss, U., Sriperumbudur, K.K., Benecke, R., Gimsa, U., 2011. Optimizing a rodent model of Parkinson's disease for exploring the effects and mechanisms of deep brain stimulation. *Parkinson's Disease*. Vol.2011, 414682.

Pears, M.R., Cooper, J.D., Mitchison, H.M., Mortishire-Smith, R.J., Pearce, D.A., Griffin, J.L., 2005. High resolution 1H NMR-based metabolomics indicates a neurotransmitter cycling deficit in cerebral tissue from a mouse model of Batten disease. *The Journal of Biological Chemistry*. Vol.280, pp. 42508-42514.

Pogge, A., Slikker, W., Jr., 2004. Neuroimaging: new approaches for neurotoxicology. *Neurotoxicology*. Vol.25, pp. 525-531.

Porsolt, R.D., Bertin, A., Jalfre, M., 1977. Behavioral despair in mice: a primary screening test for antidepressants. *Archives internationales de pharmacodynamie et de thérapie*. Vol.229, pp. 327-336.

Porsolt, R.D., Bertin, A., Blavet, N., Deniel, M., Jalfre, M., 1979. Immobility induced by forced swimming in rats: effects of agents which modify central catecholamine and serotonin activity. *European Journal of Pharmacology*. Vol.57, pp. 201-210.

Quinones, M.P., Kaddurah-Daouk, R., 2009. Metabolomics tools for identifying biomarkers for neuropsychiatric diseases. *Neurobiology of Disease*. Vol.35, pp. 165-176.

Roberts, M.J., Schirra, H.J., Lavin, M.F., Gardiner, R.A., 2011. Metabolomics: a novel approach to early and noninvasive prostate cancer detection. *Korean Journal of Urology*. Vol.52, pp. 79-89.

Robertson, D.G., 2005. Metabonomics in toxicology: a review. *Toxicological Sciences*. Vol.85, pp. 809-822.

Robertson-Smith, R.G., Jeffcott, L.B., Friend, S.C., Badcoe, L.M., 1985. An unusual incidence of neurological disease affecting horses during a drought. *Australian Veterinary Journal*. Vol.62, pp. 6-12.

Rodgers, R.J., Johnson, N.J., 1995. Factor analysis of spatiotemporal and ethological measures in the murine elevated plus-maze test of anxiety. *Pharmacology Biochemistry and Behavior*. Vol.52, pp. 297-303.

Ross, A.J., Sachdev, P.S., 2004. Magnetic resonance spectroscopy in cognitive research. *Brain Research Brain Research Reviews*. Vol.44, pp. 83-102.

Ross, B., Bluml, S., 2001. Magnetic resonance spectroscopy of the human brain. The Anatomical Record. Vol.265, pp. 54-84.

Rudkin, T.M., Arnold, D.L., 1999. Proton magnetic resonance spectroscopy for the diagnosis and management of cerebral disorders. *Archives of Neurology*. Vol.56, pp. 919-926.

Salek, R.M., Xia, J., Innes, A., Sweatman, B.C., Adalbert, R., Randle, S., McGowan, E., Emson, P.C., Griffin, J.L., 2010. A metabolomic study of the CRND8 transgenic mouse model of Alzheimer's disease. *Neurochemistry International*. Vol.56, pp. 937-947.

Sayre, L.M., Perry, G., Smith, M.A., 2008. Oxidative stress and neurotoxicity. *Chemical Research in Toxicology*. Vol.21, pp. 172-188.

Sinclair, A.J., Viant, M.R., Ball, A.K., Burdon, M.A., Walker, E.A., Stewart, P.M., Rauz, S., Young, S.P., 2009. NMR-based metabolomic analysis of cerebrospinal fluid and serum in neurological diseases--a diagnostic tool? *NMR in Biomedicine*. Vol.23, pp. 123-132.

Slocombe, R.F., Huntington, P.J., Friend, S.C., Jeffcott, L.B., Luff, A.R., Finkelstein, D.K., 1992. Pathological aspects of Australian Stringhalt. *Equine Veterinary Journal*. Vol.24, pp. 174-183.

Song, I.H., Hermann, K., Haibel, H., Althoff, C.E., Listing, J., Burmester, G., Krause, A., Bohl-Buhler, M., Freundlich, B., Rudwaleit, M., Sieper, J., 2011. Effects of etanercept versus sulfasalazine in early axial spondyloarthritis on active inflammatory lesions as detected by whole-body MRI (ESTHER): a 48-week randomised controlled trial. *Annals of the Rheumatic Diseases*. Vol.70, pp. 590-596.

Stoessl, A.J., 2011. Neuroimaging in Parkinson's disease. *Neurotherapeutics*. Vol.8, pp. 72-81.

Tabatabaie, L., Klomp, L.W., Berger, R., de Koning, T.J., 2010. L-serine synthesis in the central nervous system: a review on serine deficiency disorders. *Molecular Genetics and Metabolism*. Vol.99, pp. 256-262.

Takahashi, T., Kitamura, M., Endo, Y., Eto, D., Aoki, O., Kusunose, R., Yoshihara, T., Kai, M., 2002. An outbreak of stringhalt resembling australian stringhalt in Japan. *Journal of Equine Science*. Vol.13, pp. 93-100.

Takeda, H., Tsuji, M., Matsumiya, T., 1998. Changes in head-dipping behavior in the hole-board test reflect the anxiogenic and/or anxiolytic state in mice. *European Journal of Pharmacology*. Vol.350, pp. 21-29.

Tartaglia, M.C., Arnold, D.L., 2006. The role of MRS and fMRI in multiple sclerosis. *Advances in Neurology*. Vol.98, pp. 185-202.

Tate, A.R., Crabb, S., Griffiths, J.R., Howells, S.L., Mazucco, R.A., Rodrigues, L.M., Watson, D., 1996. Lipid metabolite peaks in pattern recognition analysis of tumour in vivo MR spectra. *Anticancer Research*. Vol.16, pp. 1575-1579.

Tate, A.R., Griffiths, J.R., Martinez-Perez, I., Moreno, A., Barba, I., Cabanas, M.E., Watson, D., Alonso, J., Bartumeus, F., Isamat, F., Ferrer, I., Vila, F., Ferrer, E., Capdevila, A., Arus, C., 1998. Towards a method for automated classification of 1H MRS spectra from brain tumours. *NMR Biomedicine*. Vol.11, pp. 177-191.

Toga, A.W., Thompson, P.M., Sowell, E.R., 2006. Mapping brain maturation. *Trends in Neurosciences*. Vol.29, pp. 148-159.

Torre, F., 2005. Clinical diagnosis and results of surgical treatment of 13 cases of acquired bilateral stringhalt (1991--2003). *Equine Veterinarian Journal*. Vol.37, pp 181-183.

Viola, A., Nicoli, F., Denis, B., Confort-Gouny, S., Le Fur, Y., Ranjeva, J.P., Viout, P., Cozzone, P.J., 2004. High cerebral scyllo-inositol: a new marker of brain metabolism disturbances induced by chronic alcoholism. *Magnetic resonance materials in physics, biology, and medicine MAGMA*. Vol.17, pp. 47-61.

Wang, T.J., Larson, M.G., Vasan, R.S., Cheng, S., Rhee, E.P., McCabe, E., Lewis, G.D., Fox, C.S., Jacques, P.F., Fernandez, C., O'Donnell, C.J., Carr, S.A., Mootha, V.K., Florez, J.C., Souza, A., Melander, O., Clish, C.B., Gerszten, R.E., 2011. Metabolite profiles and the risk of developing diabetes. *Nature Medicine*. Vol.17, pp. 448-453.

Wattamwar, P.R., Mathuranath, P.S., 2010. An overview of biomarkers in Alzheimer's disease. *Annals of Indian Academy of Neurology*. Vol.13, S116-123.

Part 6

Prevention, Protection and Monitoring of Neurodegeneration

18

Extract of *Achillea fragrantissima* Downregulates ROS Production and Protects Astrocytes from Oxidative-Stress-Induced Cell Death

Anat Elmann[1], Alona Telerman[1], Sharon Mordechay[1], Hilla Erlank[1], Miriam Rindner[1], Rivka Ofir[2] and Elie Beit-Yannai[3]

[1]*Department of Food Science, Volcani Center, Agricultural Research Organization, Bet Dagan,*

[2]*Dead Sea & Arava Science Center and Department of Microbiology & Immunology Ben-Gurion University of the Negev, Beer-Sheva,*

[3]*Department of Clinical Pharmacology, Faculty of Health Sciences, Ben-Gurion University of the Negev, Beer-Sheva,*

Israel

1. Introduction

Oxidative damage plays a pivotal role in the initiation and progress of many human diseases and also in the development of acute and chronic pathological conditions in brain tissue (Halliwell, 2006; Hyslop et al., 1995; Ischiropoulos & Beckman, 2003; Minghetti, 2005). Compared with other tissues, the brain is particularly vulnerable to oxidative damage due to its high rate of oxygen utilization and high contents of oxidizable polyunsaturated fatty acids (Floyd, 1999; Sastry, 1985). In addition, certain regions of the brain are highly enriched in iron, a metal that is catalytically involved in the production of damaging reactive oxygen species (ROS) (Hallgren & Sourander, 1958). Although ROS are critical intracellular signaling messengers (Schrecka & Baeuerlea, 1991), excess of free radicals may lead to peroxidative impairment of membrane lipids and, consequently, to disruption of neuronal functions, and apoptosis. Among the ROS that are responsible for oxidative stress, H_2O_2 is thought to be the major precursor of highly reactive free radicals, and is regarded as a key factor in both neuronal (Vaudry et al., 2002) and astroglial cell death (Ferrero-Gutierrez et al., 2008). H_2O_2 is normally produced in reactions predominantly catalyzed by superoxide dismutase (SOD) and monoaminoxidases (MAO) A and B in the brain (Almeida et al., 2006; Duarte et al., 2007). As with both Ca^{2+} and NO, H_2O_2 appears to play contradictory roles, in that it is potentially toxic at high concentrations, even though it is a central signaling compound at low concentrations (Miura et al., 2002). Brain cells have the capacity to produce peroxides, particularly H_2O_2, in large amounts (Dringen et al., 2005). Excess of H_2O_2 accumulates during brain injuries and neurodegenerative diseases, and can cross cell membranes to elicit its biological effects intracellularly (Bienert et al., 2006). Although H_2O_2 is generally poorly reactive, it forms highly toxic hydroxyl radicals, which may damage all the major classes of biological macromolecules in the cell, through iron- or copper ion-mediated oxidation of lipids, proteins, and nucleic acids. This capability can partly account for H_2O_2-mediated neuronal and glial cell death. H_2O_2 also induces differential protein activation, which indicates varied biological effects of this molecule. In the mammalian central nervous system (CNS), the transition metal zinc is an endogenous molecule that is localized exclusively to the synaptic vesicles of glutamatergic neurons and that has a special role in modulating synaptic transmission. Chelatable zinc is released into the synaptic cleft with the neurotransmitter during neuronal execution (Assaf & Chung, 1984), and under normal circumstances the robust release of zinc is transient and is efficiently cleared from the synaptic cleft to ensure the performance of successive stimuli. However, in pathological conditions, zinc dyshomeostasis, with consequently elevated levels of extracellular zinc has been recognized as an important factor in the resulting neuropathology (Choi & Koh, 1998; Cote et al., 2005; Li et al., 2009). In neurotransmission, the amount of zinc in the synaptic cleft is in the 10- to 30-μM range, but in pathological conditions that involve sustained neuronal depolarization, e.g., ischemia, stroke, or traumatic brain injury, the levels of extracellular zinc can increase to 100- to 400-μM, at which it can contribute to the resulting neuropathology (Frederickson et al., 2005; Li et al., 2001). *In vivo* and *in vitro* studies showed that, at concentrations that can be reached in the mammalian CNS during excitotoxic episodes, injuries or diseases, zinc is toxic to both neurons and astrocytes (Bishop et al., 2007; Hwang et al., 2008; Kim et al., 1999a; Kim et al., 1999b; Koh et al., 1996; Ryu et al., 2002; Sheline et al., 2000; Stork & Li, 2009). Zinc induces oxidative stress and ROS production, which contribute to both glial cell death (Ryu et al., 2002) and neuronal cell death (Kim et al. 1999a; Kim et al. 1999b). Zinc decreased the GSH content of primary cultures of astrocytes (Kim et al., 2003; Ryu et al., 2002), increased their GSSG content (Kim et al., 2003) and inhibited glutathione reductase activity in these cells (Bishop et al., 2007); furthermore, it slowed the clearance of exogenous H_2O_2 by astrocytes, and promoted intracellular production of ROS (Bishop et al., 2007). Thus, ROS generation, glutathione depletion and mitochondrial dysfunction may be key factors in $ZnCl_2$–induced glial toxicity (Ryu et al., 2002). Astrocytes are the most abundant glial cell type in the brain. They play important roles in maintenance of homeostasis, in provision of metabolic substrates for neurons, and also in coupling cerebral blood flow to neuronal activity. They are prominent in protecting neurons against oxidative stress and cell death, and in providing trophic supports such as the glial cell-line-derived neurotrophic factor (GDNF) (Sandhu et al., 2009). There is evidence that dysfunctional astrocytes can enhance neuronal degeneration by diminishing secretion of trophic factors (Takuma et al., 2004). The study of astrocytes is particularly important, in light of the co- existence of apoptotic death of neurons and astrocytes in damaged brains affected by ischemia and neurodegenerative diseases. Despite their high antioxidative activities, astrocytes exhibit a high degree of vulnerability, and are not resistant to the effects of ROS. They respond to substantial or sustained oxidative stress with increased intracellular Ca^{2+}, loss of mitochondrial potential, and decreased oxidative phosphorylation (Robb et al., 1999). Since astrocytes determine the brain's vulnerability to oxidative injury, and form a tight functional unit with neurons, once astrocyte energy metabolism and antioxidant capacity are impaired, astrocytic death may critically impair neuronal survival (Feeney et al., 2008; Lu et al., 2008). Thus, protection of astrocytes from oxidative insult appears essential to brain function maintenance. Many herb and plant extracts are used as folk medicines for various kinds of diseases and organ dysfunctions. *Achillea fragrantissima* (*Af;* Asteraceae) is a desert plant that for many years has been used as a hypoglycemic medicinal plant in traditional medicine in the Arabian region (Yaniv et al.,

1987), and for the treatment of gastrointestinal disturbances (Segal et al., 1987). The ingredient responsible for the anti-spasmolytic activity was found to be a flavone aglycone named cirsiliol (5,3',4'-trihydroxy-6,7-dimethoxyflavone) that was shown to antagonize the spasmodic effects, inhibit Ca^{2+} influx and stimulate Ca^{2+} release from intracellular stores (Mustafa et al., 1992). In addition, the hydro-alcoholic extract of *Af* was shown to have a remarkable antiviral activity against poliomyelitis-1 virus (Soltan & Zaki, 2009). However, the effects of *Af* in the context of brain injuries and neurodegenerative diseases, have not been studied to date. In a recent study we have found that the ethanolic extract of *Achillea fragrantissima* inhibited lipopolysaccharide (LPS) –induced nitric oxide (NO) production by activated primary microglial cells. This extract also inhibited LPS - elicited expression of the pro-inflammatory cytokines interleukin1β (IL-1β) and tumor necrosis factor-α (TNFα), as well as expression of the proinflammatory enzymes, cyclooxygenase-2 (COX-2) and nitric oxide synthase (iNOS) by these cells (in preparation). Since oxidative stress has become accepted as a suitable target for early therapeutic intervention in brain injuries and neurodegenerative diseases, the present study addressed the astroprotective and antioxidant activities of this plant extract.

2. Materials and methods

2.1 Reagents

Dulbecco's modified Eagle's medium (DMEM), Leibovitz-15 medium, glutamine, antibiotics (10,000 IU/ml penicillin and 10,000 µg/ml streptomycin), soybean trypsin inhibitor, fetal bovine serum (FBS) and Dulbecco's phosphate buffered saline (PBS) (without calcium and magnesium) were purchased from Biological Industries (Beit Haemek, Israel); dimethyl sulfoxide (DMSO) was obtained from Applichem (Darmstadt, Germany); Hydrogen peroxide was obtained from MP Biomedicals (Ohio, USA); 2,2'-Azobis(amidinopropane) (ABAP) was obtained from Wako chemicals (Richmond, VA), and other chemicals including $ZnCl_2$ and 2'7'-dichlorofluorescein diacetate (DCF) were purchased from Sigma Chemical Co. (St Louis, MO, USA).

2.2 Preparation of *Af* Extracts

The plant was collected in the Arava Valley and authenticated. The voucher specimens have been kept in as part of the Arava Rift Valley Plant Collection; VPC (Dead Sea & Arava Science Center, Central Arava Branch, Israel, http://www.deadseaarava-rd.co.il/) under the accession code AVPC0040. Freshly collected plants were dried at 40 °C for three days and extracted in ethanol (96%). The liquid phase was then evaporated off, and the dry material was dissolved in DMSO to a concentration of 100 mg/ml to produce the *Af* extract.

2.3 High performance liquid chromatography (HPLC) conditions

The ethanolic extract of *Af* was subjected to HPLC chromatography. Separation was made using reverse phase column (Betasil C-18, 5 µm, 250 × 0.46 mm; Thermo-Hypersil, UK) by gradient elution with water-acetic acid (97 : 3 V/V) and methanol as described previously (Chen et al., 2010), and detection at 360 nm (Blue line) and 280 nm (Red line) (Fig. 1).

2.4 Liquid chromatography–mass spectrometry (LC–MS) conditions

The ethanolic extract of *Af* was subjected to MS/MS (Fig. 2). The mass spectra were performed on a liquid chromatography-mass spectrometry (LC–MS) Agilent 1100LC series

(Wald- bronn, Germany) and Bruker Esquire 3000plus MS (Bremen, Germany) instrument, operated in the electrospray ionization (ESI) in a positive ion mode. A reverse phase column (BetasilC-18,5 mm, 250 mm x 0.46 mm, Thermo-Hypersil,UK) was used. The MS conditions

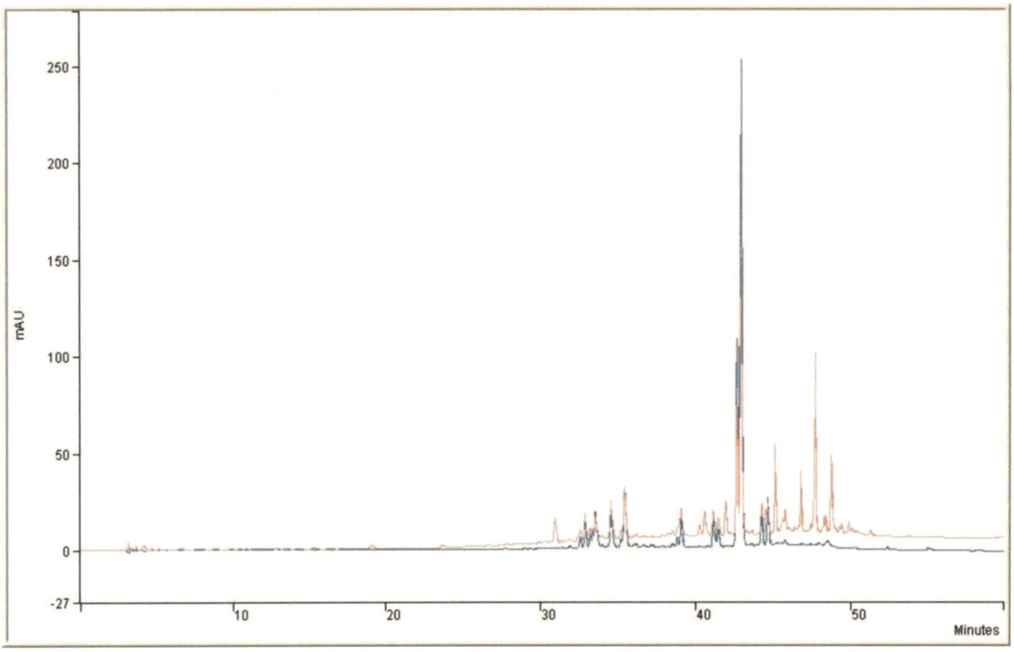

Fig. 1. HPLC analysis of the ethanolic extract of *Af*

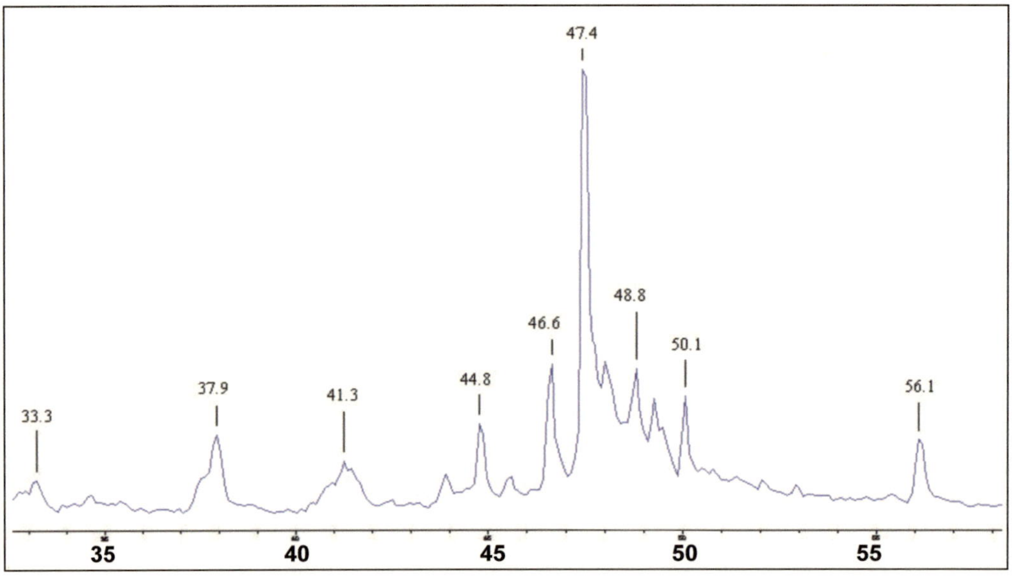

Fig. 2. Liquid chromatography–mass spectrometry (LC–MS) analysis of the ethanolic extract of *Af*

were optimized as follows: API electron spray interface, positive mode polarity, a drying gas flow of 10L/min, an nebulizer gas pressure of 60psi,a drying gas temperature of 300°C, a fragmentor voltage of 0.4V and capillary voltage of 4.5kV.
Four main peaks were identified by ESI-MS: Compound 1, ($C_{27}H_{34}O_{14}Na$), r.t. 50.1, m/z 605 [M+Na+146+146], m/z 582 [M+H+146+146]+, ; suggested as epicatechin-rhamnoside. Compound 2, ($C_{28}H_{33}O_{13}$), r.t. 48.8- m/z 577 [M+H+146+146]+; suggested as Acacetin rhamnoside. Compound 3, ($C_{22}H_{22}O_{10}Na$), r.t. 47.4- m/z 469 [M+Na+162]+, , m/z 447 [M+H+162]+,; suggested as Acacetin-glucoside, m/z 285 [M+H]+ aglycon. Compound 4, ($C_{24}H_{25}O_{12}$), r.t. 46.6- m/z 465 [M+H+162]+, suggested as Quercetin-glucoside, m/z 303 [M+H]+ aglycon.

2.5 Preparation of primary glial cell cultures

Cultures of primary rat glial cells were prepared from cerebral cortices of 1- to 2-day-old neonatal Wistar rats. Briefly, meninges and blood vessels were carefully removed from cerebral cortices kept in Leibovitz-15 medium; brain tissues were dissociated by trypsinization with 0.5% trypsin (10 min, 37 °C, 5% CO_2); and cells were washed first with DMEM containing soybean trypsin inhibitor (100 µg/ml) and 10% FBS and then with DMEM containing 10% FBS. Cells were seeded in tissue culture flasks pre-coated with poly-D-lysine (20 µg/ml in 0.1 M borate buffer pH 8.4) and incubated at 37 °C in humidified air with 5% CO_2. The medium was changed on the second day and every second day thereafter. At the time of primary cell confluence (day 10), microglial and progenitor cells were discarded by shaking (180 RPM, 37 °C) the flasks on a horizontal shaking platform. Astrocytes were then replated on 24-well poly-D-lysine-coated plastic plates, at a density of 1×10^5/well, in DMEM (without phenol red) containing 2% FBS, 2 mM glutamine, 100 U/ml penicillin, and 100 µg/ml streptomycin.
The research was conducted in accordance with the internationally accepted principles for laboratory animal use and care, as found in the US guidelines, and was approved by the Institutional Animal Care and Use Committee of The Volcani Center, Agricultural Research Organization.

2.6 Treatment of astrocytes

Twenty four hours after plating, the original medium in which the cells were grown was aspirated off, and fresh medium was added to the cells. Dilutions of plant extracts first in DMSO and then in the growth medium were made freshly from stock solution just prior to each experiment and were used immediately. The final concentration of DMSO in the medium was 0.2%. Dilutions of H_2O_2 in the growth medium were made freshly from a 30% stock solution immediately prior to each experiment and were used immediately.

2.7 Determination of cell viability

Cell viability was determined using a commercial colorimetric assay (Roche Applied Science, Germany) according to the manufacturer's instructions. This assay is based on the measurement of lactate dehydrogenase (LDH) activity released from the cytosol of damaged cells into the incubation medium.

2.8 Evaluation of intracellular ROS production

Intracellular ROS production was detected using the non-fluorescent cell permeating compound, 2'7'-dichlorofluorescein diacetate (DCF-DA). DCF-DA is hydrolyzed by intracellular esterases and then oxidized by ROS to a fluorescent compound 2'-7'-DCF. Astrocytes were plated onto 24 wells plates (300,000 cells/well) and treated with DCF-DA (20 µM) for 30 min at 37^{0}C. Following incubation with DCF, cultures were rinsed twice with PBS and then re-suspended (1) For measurement of H_2O_2-induced ROS: in DMEM containing 10% FBS, 8 mM HEPES, 2 mM glutamine, 100 U/ml penicillin, and 100 µg/ml streptomycin (2) For measurement of $ZnCl_2$ - induced ROS: in a defined buffer containing 116 mM NaCl, 1.8 mM $CaCl_2$, 0.8 mM $MgSO_4$, 5.4 mM KCl, 1 mM NaH_2PO_4, 14.7 mM $NaHCO_3$, and 10 mM HEPES, pH, 7.4. The fluorescence was measured in a plate reader with excitation at 485 nm and emission at 520 nm.

2.9 Cellular antioxidant activity of *Af* extract

Peroxyl radicals are generated by thermolysis of 2,2'-Azobis(amidinopropane) (ABAP) at physiological temperature. ABAP decomposes at approximately $1.36x10^{-6}s^{-1}$ at 37°C, producing at most $1x10^{12}$ radicals/ml/s (Bowry & Stocker, 1993; Niki et al., 1986; Thomas et al., 1997). Astrocytes were plated onto 24 wells plates (300,000 cells/well) and were incubated for 1 hr with *Af* extract. Then astrocytes were preloaded with DCF-DA for 30 min, washed, and ABAP (0.6 mM final concentration) was then added. The fluorescence, which indicates ROS levels, was measured in a plate reader with excitation at 485 nm and emission at 520 nm.

2.10 Differential pulse voltammetry analysis

Ethanolic extracts were obtained by dissolving 1 g of dry plant powder in 10 ml of ethanol overnight at room temperature. Before performing the differential pulse voltammetry (DPV) analysis, tetrabutylammonium perchlorate was added to the ethanolic extract to final concentration of 1% and the total reducing capacity of the *Af* extracts was analyzed, as described before (Butera et al., 2002). Briefly, the plant extract was placed in a cyclic voltammeter cell equipped with a working electrode (3.2 mm in diameters, glassy carbon), a reference electrode (Ag/AgCl), and an auxiliary electrode (platinum wire). The DPV potential was conducted at a scan rate of 40 mV/s, pulse amplitude 50 mV, sample width 17 ms, pulse width 50 ms, pulse period 200 ms. An electrochemical working station (CH Instruments Inc., 610B, Austin, TX, USA) was used. The output of the DPV experiments was a potential-current curve (Kohen et al., 1999).

2.11 Data analysis

Statistical analyses were performed with one-way ANOVA followed by Tukey-Kramer multiple comparison tests using Graph Pad InStat 3 for windows (GraphPad Software, San Diego, CA, USA).

3. Results

3.1 Protection by the *Af* extract of astrocytes from H_2O_2 -induced cell death

H_2O_2 exposure is used as a model of ischemia reperfusion. The concentration of H_2O_2 used in our experiments (175-200 microM) resembles the concentration reported by Hyslop *et al* to be the concentration of H_2O_2 that appears in the rat striatum under ischemic conditions (Hyslop et al., 1995). In order to characterize the astroprotective potential of the *Af* extract against H_2O_2 -induced oxidative stress, we have assessed changes in intracellular ROS production and in cell viability, using a model in which oxidative stress was induced by the addition of this compound to cultured primary astrocytes. Exposure of normal primary astrocytes with H_2O_2 resulted in a time and concentration dependent astrocytic cell death 20 h later (data not shown). To find out whether the *Af* extract has a protective effect and to determine the optimal concentration of the extract needed for such an effect, astrocytes were pre-incubated with different concentrations of *Af* extract. H_2O_2 was then added, and cytotoxicity was determined after 20 h. Our results showed that the *Af* extract exerted a protective action against H_2O_2 -induced cell death in a dose-dependent manner (Fig. 3). No significant changes were observed in the viability of cells treated with similar concentrations of the *Af* extract in the absence of H_2O_2 (Fig. 3).

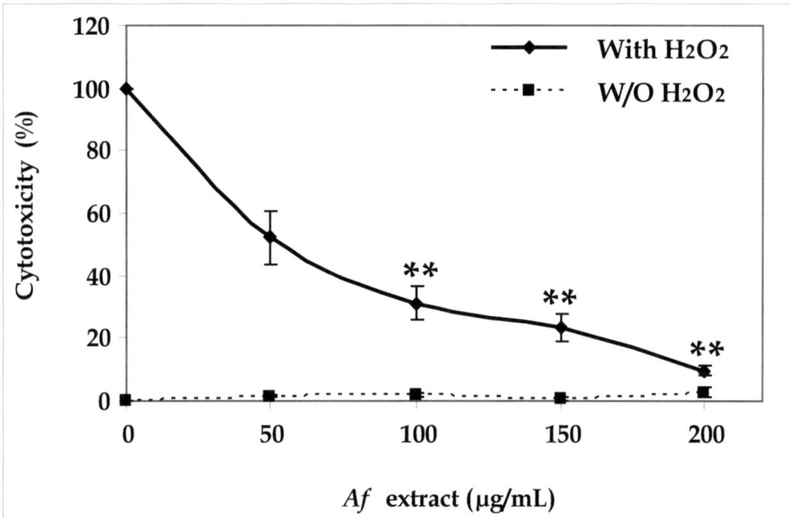

Fig. 3. Protection from H_2O_2-induced astrocytic cell death by different concentrations of the extract of *Af*

Astrocytes were treated with different concentrations of *Af* extract. H_2O_2 (200 µM) was added 2 h after the addition of *Af* extract. Cell death was determined 20 h later. Each point represents the means ± SEM of five experiments (*n* = *20*). $^{**}p<0.001$ compared to cells treated with H_2O_2 alone.

3.2 *Af* extract inhibits H_2O_2- and $ZnCl_2$-induced ROS generation

In order to gain more insight into the mechanisms by which the *Af* extract might exert its protective effects, and to determine whether this extract could inhibit ROS production induced by H_2O_2 and $ZnCl_2$, we assessed the intracellular generation of ROS by these toxic molecules, and tested whether treatment of astrocytes with the *Af* extract affected intracellular ROS levels. For the study of preventive effects against intracellular ROS formation the cells were preloaded with the ROS indicator DCF-DA, and were pretreated with various concentrations of *Af* extract before the application of H_2O_2 or $ZnCl_2$ stress, and ROS formation was determined by reading fluorescence every hour for 4 h. As can be seen in Fig. 4A, H_2O_2 induced ROS production in astrocytes, with the maximum levels produced after 1 h. Pretreatment of astrocytes with the *Af* extract inhibited the H_2O_2-induced elevation of the levels of intracellular ROS in a dose-dependent manner (Fig. 4B). We also found that treatment with $ZnCl_2$ increased ROS generation in astrocytes, and that, similarly to the effect of the *Af* extract on H_2O_2-induced ROS, this extract greatly attenuated $ZnCl_2$-induced ROS generation (Fig. 5).

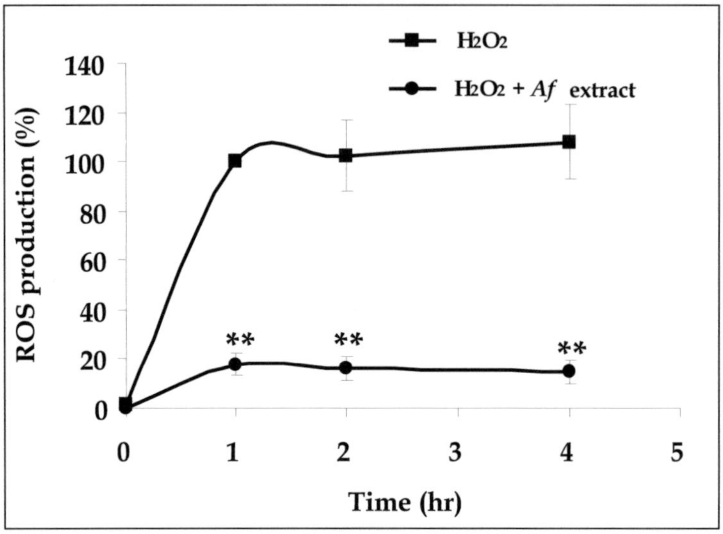

(A)

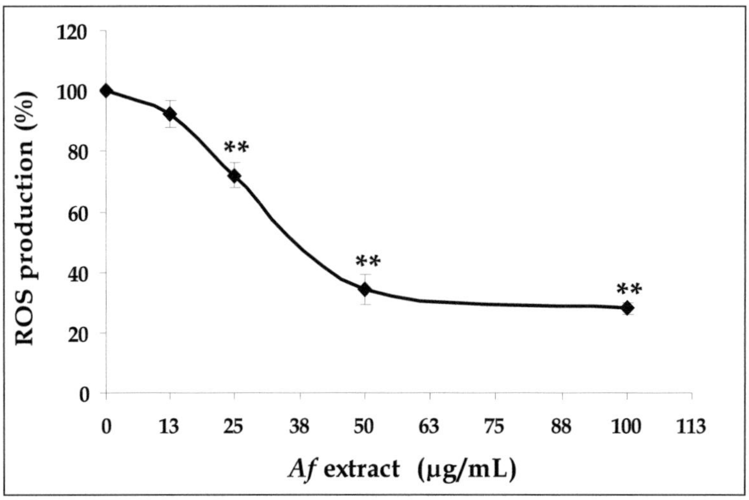

(B)

Fig. 4. The *Af* extract attenuates H_2O_2-induced ROS production in astrocytes

Astrocytes were preloaded with the redox - sensitive DCF-DA for 30 min and washed with PBS. Preloaded astrocytes were then pre-incubated for 2 h with various concentrations of *Af* extract. H_2O_2 (175 µM) was added to the culture and the fluorescence intensity representing ROS production was measured. (A) Pre-incubation with 100 µg/ml *Af* extract and measurements at the indicated time points (B) Pre-incubation with various concentrations of *Af* extract and measurements after 1 h. Each point represents the mean ± SEM of two experiments (n=7). **p<0.001 when ROS production following treatment with H_2O_2+*Af* extract was compared to cells treated with H_2O_2 alone at each of the equivalent time points.

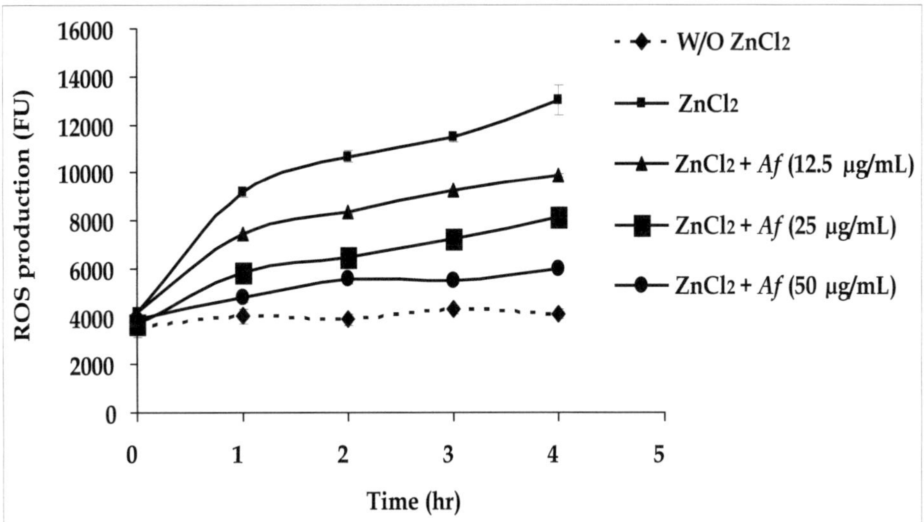

Fig. 5. Zinc induces ROS generation, and the *Af* extract attenuates ROS production following treatment of astrocytes with zinc

Astrocytes were preloaded with DCF-DA for 30 min and washed with PBS. They were then pre-incubated for 2 h with various concentrations of *Af* extract, after which, $ZnCl_2$ (50 µM) was added and the resulting fluorescence signal was measured at the indicated time points. Each point represents the mean ± SEM (n = 7). $p<0.01$ when ROS production following treatment with $ZnCl_2$+*Af* extract was compared to cells treated with $ZnCl_2$ alone at each of the equivalent time points

3.3 *Af* extract reduces 2,2'-azobis(amidinopropane) (ABAP)-mediated peroxyl radicals levels in astrocytes

In addition to H_2O_2, various other species, such as peroxynitrite (ONOO-), nitric oxide (NO·) and peroxyl radicals have been found to oxidize DCFH to DCF in cell culture (Wang & Joseph, 1999), therefore we have used the cellular antioxidant activity assay to measure the ability of compounds present in the *Af* extract to prevent formation of DCF by ABAP-generated peroxyl radicals (Wolfe & Liu, 2007). The kinetics of DCFH oxidation in astrocytes by peroxyl radicals generated from ABAP is shown in Fig. 6A, where it can be seen that ABAP generated radicals in a time-dependent manner, and that treatment of cells with *Af* extract moderated this induction. Fig. 6B shows that the increase in ROS–induced fluorescence was inhibited by *Af* extract in a dose-dependent manner. This indicates that compounds present in the *Af* extract entered the cells and acted as efficient intracellular hydroperoxyl radical scavengers.

3.4 Differential pulse voltammetry (DPV) analysis of *the* antioxidant capacity of *Af* extract

Extract antioxidant capacity was evaluated by differential pulse voltammetry approach (DPV). Voltammetric techniques of analysis are increasingly being used for the determination of many substances of pharmaceutical importance (Zapata-Urzua et al., 2010) as well as of fruit extracts (Butera et al., 2002). These techniques are based on the measurement of current that results from oxidation or reduction at an electrode surface following an applied potential

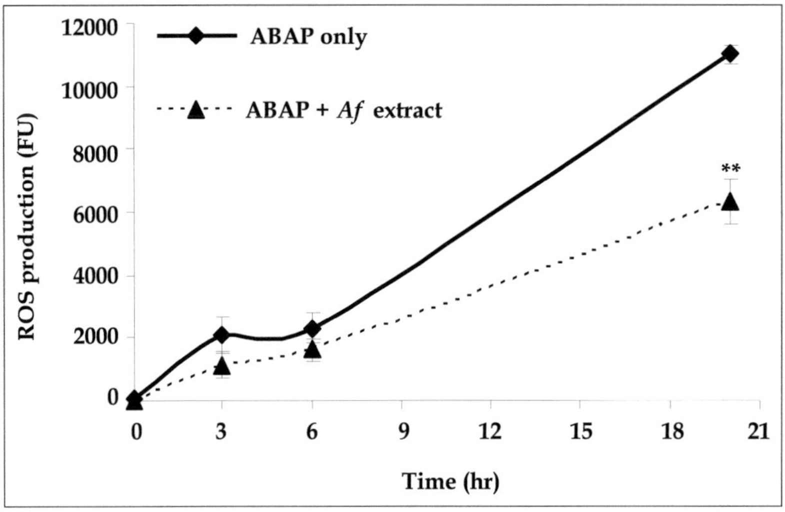

(A)

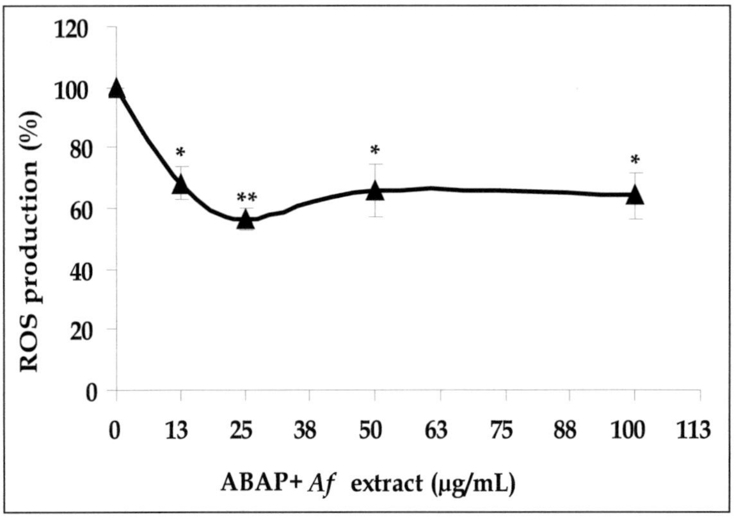

(B)

Fig. 6. Peroxyl radical - induced oxidation of DCFH to DCF in primary astrocytes, and the inhibition of oxidation by *Af* extract

Astrocytes were incubated for 1 h with *Af* extract. They were then preloaded with DCF-DA for 30 min and washed with PBS, after which, 0.6 mM ABAP was added and ROS levels were measured at the indicated time points. Each point represents mean ± SEM of two experiments ($n = 7$). **A.** *Af* extract at 25 μg/ml. **B.** ROS production was measured 20 h after the addition of ABAP *$p<0.01$, **$p<0.001$ compared to cells treated with ABAP only at the equivalent time points.

difference. The DPV technique has excellent resolving power, and is able to differentiate between peaks due to different electroactive species in the same solution which are no more that 50 mV apart (Smyth & Woolfson, 1987). In the present study we have used the DPV approach to analyze the total reducing capacity of the ethanolic *Af* extract. On the potential-current curve generated by DPV, the values of the potential are a characteristic of the antioxidant material and the values of the current are proportional to the amounts of the corresponding antioxidant. Analysis of the *Af* extract by DPV revealed two anodic waves that are caused by two major reducing groups of low-molecular-weight antioxidants, representing the total antioxidants in the extract (Fig. 7). The anodic wave potentials and their corresponding anodic currents, representing the amount of each antioxidant, are presented at Table 1.

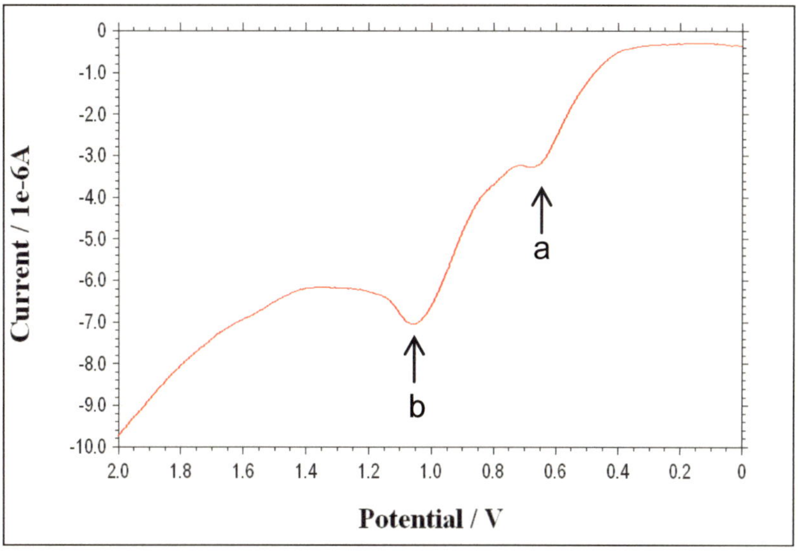

Fig. 7. Representative differential pulse voltammogram of the *Af* extract

Differential pulse voltammetry (DPV) was conducted from E = 0.0 V to final E = 2.0 V at a scan rate of 40 mV/s, pulse amplitude 50 mV, sample width 17 ms, pulse width 50 ms, pulse period 200 ms. Extracts were prepared in duplicate, and each sample was traced three times. **a** - first anodic wave; **b** - second anodic wave.

	Anodic wave a	Anodic wave b
Potential (V ± SD)	0.625±0.003	1.039±0.024
Current (μA ± SD)	3.233±0.251	7.027±0.063

Table 1. Anodic potentials and currents of the ethanolic extracts of *Af*

4. Discussion

The main findings of the present study were that an ethanolic extract of the desert plant *Af* could protect primary cultures of rat brain astrocytes from H_2O_2 -induced cell death, and reduced the levels of intracellular ROS produced after treatment with H_2O_2, $ZnCl_2$ or ABAP. This protective effect of *Af* and the reduction in ROS levels might be mediated by its antioxidant activities (as was demonstrated by the DPV experiments) or by modulation of signals and processes induced by H_2O_2 and $ZnCl_2$. For example, it has been found, that H_2O_2 induced the phosphorylation of ERK1/2, AKT/protein kinase B and ATF-2 in C6 glioma cells (Altiok et al., 2006). It also has been demonstrated that cell death caused by zinc was accompanied by membrane translocation of protein kinase C-alpha (PKC-α), phosphorylation of extracellular signal-regulated kinase (ERK), and activation of group IV calcium-dependent cytosolic phospholipase A_2 ($cPLA_2$) (Chang et al., 2010; Liao et al., 2011). It was also reported that Zn^{2+} bound to and inhibited glutathione reductase and peroxidase, the major enzymes responsible for glutathione (GSH) metabolism and cellular antioxidative defense mechanisms (Mize & Langdon, 1962; Splittgerber & Tappel, 1979).

Hydrogen peroxide also decreased astrocyte membrane fluidity, induced cytoskeletal reorganization, decreased the activities of the antioxidant enzymes catalase and superoxide dismutase (SOD) (Naval et al., 2007), and increased formation of cytonemes and cell-to-cell tunneling nanotube (TNT)-like connections (Zhu et al., 2005). Thus, the *Af* extract might interfere with any or all of the described processes, and enhance the resistance of astrocytes to $ZnCl_2$ and H_2O_2 toxicity, and to oxidative stress. Moreover, defense of glial cells against oxidative damage would be essential for maintaining brain functions.

There are two opportunities for compounds present in *Af* extract to elicit their antioxidant effects in our model: they can act at the cell membrane and break peroxyl radical chain reactions at the cell surface; or they can be taken up by the cell and react intracellularly with ROS. Therefore, the efficiency of cellular uptake and/or membrane binding, combined with the radical-scavenging activity dictates the efficacy of the tested compounds. In order to discriminate between these possibilities, astrocytes were pre-incubated with ABAP, which generates ROS intracellularly. According to our results, which show that *Af* extract inhibited intracellular ROS levels, in addition to other possible activities, compounds present in *Af* extract could enter the cells and react with ROS intracellularly.

Because many low-molecular-weight antioxidants might contribute to the cellular antioxidant defense properties, we analyzed the total antioxidant content of the *Af* extract by the DPV method, which enabled us to demonstrate the presence of two reducing equivalents in the *Af* extract. The advantages of DPV over other voltammetric techniques include excellent sensitivity with a very wide useful linear concentration range for organic species (10^{-6} to 10^{-3} M), short analysis times, simultaneous determination of several analytes, and ease of generating a variety of potential waveforms and measuring small currents.

Our LC-MS analysis identified quercetin-glucoside as one of the major peaks in the *Af* extract. Quercetin glycosides are widely consumed flavonoids that are found in many fruits and vegetables, e.g., onion, and, like other flavonoids, offer a wide range of potential health benefits, including prevention of atherosclerosis and cardiovascular diseases (Peluso, 2006; Terao et al., 2008). In recent years, intestinal absorption and metabolism of quercetin glucosides have been extensively investigated with regard to their bioavailability (Spencer et al., 2004; Walle, 2004). Quercetin glucosides are well absorbed by the small intestine because the presence of a glucose moiety significantly enhances absorption (Arts et al. 2004; Boyer et al., 2005; Hollman & Arts, 2000). In the process of intestinal absorption quercetin-glucosides are subjected to hydrolysis and subsequent conversion into conjugated glucuronides and/or sulfates (Murota & Terao, 2003). A variety of metabolites circulating in the blood-stream were identified (Day et al., 2001; Mullen et al., 2002), and some of them were found to possess a substantial antioxidant activity (da Silva et al., 1998; Manach et al., 1998). It was suggested that metabolites of quercetin glucosides accumulate in the aorta - a target site for its anti-atherosclerotic effect, and attenuate lipid peroxidation that occur in the aorta, along with the attenuation of hyperlipidemia (Kamada et al., 2005; Terao, 1999; Terao et al., 2008).

Two other compounds in the *Af* extract were also identified by LC-MS: acacetin 7-o-rhamnoside, which was also identified in the aerial parts of several plants (El-Wakil, 2007; Sharaf et al., 1997), and acacetin 7-o-glucoside, which was also found in the anti-inflammatory extract of Mcfadyena unguis-cati L. (Aboutabl et al., 2008). All four compounds identified by LC-MS analysis as major peaks in *Af* extract, namely epicatechin-rhamnoside, Acacetin rhamnoside, Acacetin-glucoside, and Quercetin-glucoside, are stable compounds, that under our experimental conditions (ethanol extraction, resolubilization in DMSO, and tissue culture experiments at 37°C and neutral pH) would not react chemically with each other. Chemical interactions between these compounds might occur under high temperatures and extreme pH values.

Several studies have revealed that some herbal medications and antioxidants show promise in prevention of neurodegenerative diseases (Iriti et al., 2010). Substances that can restrict and/or protect brain cells from oxidative stress show promise as potential tools in the therapy of various brain injuries and neurodegenerative diseases. Desert plants survive various stress conditions, including oxidative stress., therefore it is reasonable to suppose that various endogenous molecules present in these plants might also assist animal cells to cope with stresses that develop during pathological conditions.

5. Conclusions

In light of their antioxidant and astroprotective properties, we suggest that *Af* extracts might serve as a new source of beneficial phytochemicals, and should be further evaluated for nutraceutical development as polyvalent cocktails for prevention or treatment of various brain injuries and neurodegenerative diseases, in which oxidative stress and astrocytic cell death form part of the pathophysiology.

6. Acknowledgments

This work was supported by the Chief Scientist of the Ministry of Science, Israel, and by The Israel Science Foundation (grant No. 600/08).

7. References

Aboutabl, E.A., Hashem F.A., Sleem A.A., & Maamoon A.A. (2008). Flavonoids, anti-inflammatory activity and cytotoxicity of *Macfadyena Unguis-Cati* L. *The African Journal of Traditional, Complementary and Alternative medicines (AJTCAM),* Vol.5, No. 1, pp.18-26, ISSN 0189-6016

Almeida, A.M., Bertoncini C.R., Borecky J., Souza-Pinto N.C., & Vercesi A.E. (2006). Mitochondrial DNA damage associated with lipid peroxidation of the mitochondrial membrane induced by Fe2+-citrate. *Anais da Academia Brasileira de Ciências,* Vol.78, No. 3, pp.505-514, ISSN 0001-3765

Altiok, N., Ersoz M., Karpuz V., & Koyuturk M. (2006). *Ginkgo biloba* extract regulates differentially the cell death induced by hydrogen peroxide and simvastatin. *NeuroToxicology,* Vol.27, No. 2, pp.158-163, ISSN 0161-813X

Arts, I.C., Sesink A.L., Faassen-Peters M., & Hollman P.C. (2004). The type of sugar moiety is a major determinant of the small intestinal uptake and subsequent biliary excretion of dietary quercetin glycosides. *British Journal of Nutrition,* Vol.91, No.6, pp.841-847, ISSN 0007-1145

Assaf, S.Y., & Chung S.H. (1984). Release of endogenous Zn2+ from brain tissue during activity. *Nature (London),* Vol.308, No. 5961, pp.734-736, ISSN 0028-0836

Bienert, G.P., Schjoerring J.K., & Jahn T.P. (2006). Membrane transport of hydrogen peroxide. *Biochimica et biophysica acta,* Vol.1758, No. 8, pp.994-1003, ISSN 0005-2736

Bishop, G.M., Dringen R., & Robinson S.R. (2007). Zinc stimulates the production of toxic reactive oxygen species (ROS) and inhibits glutathione reductase in astrocytes. *Free radical biology & medicine,* Vol.42, No. 8, pp.1222-1230, ISSN 0891-5849

Bowry, V.W., & Stocker R. (1993). Tochoferol-mediated oxidation. The prooxidant effect of vitamin E on the radical-initiated oxidation of human low density lipoproteins. *Journal of the American Chemical Society,* Vol.115, No. 14, pp.6029-6044, ISSN 0002-7863

Boyer, J., Brown D., & Liu R.H. (2005). In vitro digestion and lactase treatment influence uptake of quercetin and quercetin glucoside by the Caco-2 cell monolayer. *Nutrition Journal,* Vol.4, No. 1, pp.1, ISSN 1475-2891

Butera, D., Tesoriere L., Di Gaudio F., Bongiorno A., Allegra M., Pintaudi A.M., Kohen R., & Livrea M.A. (2002). Antioxidant activities of sicilian prickly pear (Opuntia ficus indica) fruit extracts and reducing properties of its betalains: betanin and indicaxanthin. *Journal of agricultural and food chemistry,* Vol.50, No. 23, pp.6895-6901, ISSN 0021-8561

Chang, C.Y., Ou Y.C., Kao T.K., Pan H.C., Lin S.Y., Liao S.L., Wang W.Y., Lu H.C., & Chen C.J. (2010). Glucose exacerbates zinc-induced astrocyte death. *Toxicology letters,* Vol.199, No. 1, pp.102-109, ISSN 0378-4274

Chen, H., Zuo Y., & Deng Y. (2010). Separation and determination of flavonoids and other phenolic compounds in cranberry juice by high-performance liquid chromatography. *Journal of Chromatography A,* Vol.913, No. 1-2, pp.387-395, ISSN 0021-9673

Choi, D.W., & Koh J.Y. (1998). Zinc and brain injury. *Annual review of neuroscience,* Vol.21, pp.347-375, ISSN 0147-006X

Cote, A., Chiasson M., Peralta M.R., 3rd, Lafortune K., Pellegrini L., & Toth K. (2005). Cell type-specific action of seizure-induced intracellular zinc accumulation in the rat hippocampus. *The Journal of physiology,* Vol.566, No. 3, pp.821-837, ISSN 0022-3751

da Silva, E.L., Piskula M.K., Yamamoto N., Moon J.H., & Terao J. (1998). Quercetin metabolites inhibit copper ion-induced lipid peroxidation in rat plasma. *FEBS letters,* Vol.430, No. 3, pp.405-408, ISSN 0014-5793

Day, A.J., Mellon F., Barron D., Sarrazin G., Morgan M.R., & Williamson G. (2001). Human metabolism of dietary flavonoids: identification of plasma metabolites of quercetin. *Free radical research,* Vol.35, No. 6, pp.941-952, ISSN 1071-5762

Dringen, R., Pawlowski P.G., & Hirrlinger J. (2005). Peroxide detoxification by brain cells. *Journal of neuroscience research,* Vol.79, No. 1-2, pp.157-165, ISSN 0360-4012

Duarte, T.L., Almeida G.M., & Jones G.D. (2007). Investigation of the role of extracellular H2O2 and transition metal ions in the genotoxic action of ascorbic acid in cell culture models. *Toxicology letters,* Vol.170, No. 1, pp.57-65, ISSN 0378-4274

El-Wakil, E.A. (2007). Phytochemical and molluscicidal investigations of Fagonia arabica. *Zeitschrift für Naturforschung C. A journal of biosciences,* Vol.62, No. 9-10, pp.661-667, ISSN 0939-5075

Feeney, C.J., Frantseva M.V., Carlen P.L., Pennefather P.S., Shulyakova N., Shniffer C., & Mills L.R. (2008). Vulnerability of glial cells to hydrogen peroxide in cultured hippocampal slices. *Brain research,* Vol.1198, pp.1-15, ISSN 0006-8993

Ferrero-Gutierrez, A., Perez-Gomez A., Novelli A., & Fernandez-Sanchez M.T. (2008). Inhibition of protein phosphatases impairs the ability of astrocytes to detoxify hydrogen peroxide. *Free radical biology & medicine,* Vol.44, No. 10, pp.1806-1816, ISSN 0891-5849

Floyd, R. (1999). Antioxidants, oxidative stress, and degenerative neurological disorders. *Experimental Biology and Medicine,* Vol.222, No. 3, pp.236-245, Print ISSN 1535-3702 Online ISSN 1535-3699

Frederickson, C.J., Koh J.Y., & Bush A.I. (2005). The neurobiology of zinc in health and disease. *Nature reviews. Neuroscience,* Vol.6, pp.449-462, ISSN 1471-003X (Print)1471-0048 (Electronic)

Hallgren, B., & Sourander P. (1958). The effect of age on the non-hem iron in the human brain. *Journal of neurochemistry,* Vol.3, pp.41-51, ISSN 1471-4159

Halliwell, B. (2006). Oxidative stress and neurodegeneration: where are we now? *Journal of neurochemistry,* Vol.97, No. 6, pp.1634-1658, ISSN 0022-3042

Hollman, P.C., & Arts L.C. (2000). Review: Flavonols, flavones and flavanols - nature, occurrence and dietary burden. *Journal of the Science of Food and Agriculture,* Vol.80, No. 7, pp.1081-1093, ISSN 0022-5142

Hwang, J.J., Lee S.J., Kim T.Y., Cho J.H., & Koh J.Y. (2008). Zinc and 4-hydroxy-2-nonenal mediate lysosomal membrane permeabilization induced by H2O2 in cultured hippocampal neurons. *Journal of Neuroscience,* Vol.28, No. 12, pp.3114-3122, ISSN 0270-6474

Hyslop, P.A., Zhang Z., Pearson D.V., & Phebus L.A. (1995). Measurement of striatal H_2O_2 by microdialysis following global forebrain ischemia and reperfusion in the rat: correlation with the cytotoxic potential of H_2O_2 in vitro. *Brain Resarch,* Vol.671, No. 2, pp.181-186, ISSN 0006-8993

Iriti, M., Vitalini S., Fico G., & Faoro F. (2010). Neuroprotective herbs and foods from different traditional medicines and diets. *Molecules (Basel, Switzerland),* Vol.15, No. 5, pp.3517-3555, ISSN 1420-3049

Ischiropoulos, H., & Beckman J.S. (2003). Oxidative stress and nitration in neurodegeneration: Cause, effect, or association? *Journal Of Clinical Investigation,* Vol.111, No. 2, pp.163-169, ISSN 0021-9738

Kamada, C., da Silva E.L., Ohnishi-Kameyama M., Moon J.H., & Terao J. (2005). Attenuation of lipid peroxidation and hyperlipidemia by quercetin glucoside in the aorta of high cholesterol-fed rabbit. *Free radical research,* Vol.39, No. 2, pp.185-194, ISSN 1071-5762

Kim, E.Y., Koh J.Y., Kim Y.H., Sohn S., Joe E., & Gwag B.J. (1999a). Zn2+ entry produces oxidative neuronal necrosis in cortical cell cultures. *The European journal of neuroscience,* Vol.11, No. 1, pp.327-334, ISSN 0953-816X

Kim, G.W., Gasche Y., Grzeschik S., Copin J.C., Maier C.M., & Chan P.H. (2003). Neurodegeneration in striatum induced by the mitochondrial toxin 3-nitropropionic acid: Role of matrix metalloproteinase-9 in early blood-brain barrier disruption? *Journal of Neuroscience,* Vol.23, No. 25, pp.8733-8742, ISSN 0270-6474

Kim, Y.H., Kim E.Y., Gwag B.J., Sohn S., & Koh J.Y. (1999b). Zinc-induced cortical neuronal death with features of apoptosis and necrosis: mediation by free radicals. *Neuroscience,* Vol.89, No. 1, pp.175-182, ISSN 0306-4522

Koh, J.Y., Suh S.W., Gwag B.J., He Y.Y., Hsu C.Y., & Choi D.W. (1996). The role of zinc in selective neuronal death after transient global cerebral ischemia. *Science (New York, N.Y.),* Vol.272, No. 5264, pp.1013-1016, ISSN 0036-8075

Kohen, R., Beit-Yannai E., Berry E.M., & Tirosh O. (1999). Overall low molecular weight antioxidant activity of biological fluids and tissues by cyclic voltammetry. *Methods in enzymology,* Vol.300, Oxidants and Antioxidants Part B, pp.285–296, ISSN 0076-6879

Li, H., Swiercz R., & Englander E.W. (2009). Elevated metals compromise repair of oxidative DNA damage via the base excision repair pathway: implications of pathologic iron overload in the brain on integrity of neuronal DNA. *Journal of neurochemistry,* Vol.110, No. 6, pp.1774-1783, ISSN 0022-3042

Li, Y., Hough C.J., Suh S.W., Sarvey J.M., & Frederickson C.J. (2001). Rapid translocation of Zn(2+) from presynaptic terminals into postsynaptic hippocampal neurons after physiological stimulation. *Journal of neurophysiology,* Vol.86, No. 5, pp.2597-2604, ISSN 0022-3077

Liao, S.L., Ou Y.C., Lin S.Y., Kao T.K., Pan H.C., Chang C.Y., Lai C.Y., Lu H.C., Wang W.Y., & Chen C.J. (2011). Signaling cascades mediate astrocyte death induced by zinc. *Toxicology letters,* Vol.204, No. 2-3, pp.108-117, ISSN 0387-4274

Lu, M., Hu L.F., Hu G., & Bian J.S. (2008). Hydrogen sulfide protects astrocytes against H_2O_2-induced neural injury via enhancing glutamate uptake. *Free radical biology & medicine,* Vol.45, No. 12, pp.1705-1713, ISSN 0891-5849

Manach, C., Morand C., Crespy V., Demigne C., Texier O., Regerat F., & Remesy C. (1998). Quercetin is recovered in human plasma as conjugated derivatives which retain antioxidant properties. *FEBS letters,* Vol.426, No. 3, pp.331-336, ISSN 0014-5793

Minghetti, L. (2005). Role of inflammation in neurodegenerative diseases. *Current Opinion In Neurology,* Vol.18, No. 3, pp.315-321, ISSN 1350-7540

Miura, I., Miyamoto K., Nakamura K., & Watanabe Y. (2002). Hydrogen peroxide induced chemokine production in the glia-rich cultured cerebellar granule cells under acidosis. *Life sciences,* Vol.70, No. 7, pp.821-831, ISSN 0024-3205

Mize, C.E., & Langdon R.G. (1962). Hepatic glutathione reductase. I. Purification and general kinetic properties. *The Journal of biological chemistry,* Vol.237, No. 5, pp.1589-1595, ISSN (printed): 0021-9258 (electronic): 1083-351X.

Mullen, W., Graf B.A., Caldwell S.T., Hartley R.C., Duthie G.G., Edwards C.A., Lean M.E., & Crozier A. (2002). Determination of flavonol metabolites in plasma and tissues of rats by HPLC-radiocounting and tandem mass spectrometry following oral ingestion of [2-(14)C]quercetin-4'-glucoside. *Journal of Agriculture and Food Chemistry,* Vol.50, No. 23, pp.6902-6909, ISSN 0021-8561

Murota, K., & Terao J. (2003). Antioxidative flavonoid quercetin: implication of its intestinal absorption and metabolism. *Archives of biochemistry and biophysics,* Vol.417, No. 1, pp.12-17, ISSN 0003-9861

Mustafa, E.H., Abu Zarga M., & Abdalla S. (1992). Effects of cirsiliol, a flavone isolated from Achillea fragrantissima, on rat isolated ileum. *General pharmacology,* Vol.23, No. 3, pp.555-560, ISSN 0306-3623

Naval, M.V., Gómez-Serranillos M.P., Carreteroa M.E., & Villara A.M. (2007). Neuroprotective effect of a ginseng (Panax ginseng) root extract on astrocytes primary culture. *Journal of ethnopharmacology,* Vol.112, No. 2, pp.262-270, ISSN 0378-8741

Niki, E., Saito M., Yoshikawa Y., Yamamoto Y., & Kamiya Y. (1986). Oxidation of lipids XII. Inhibition of oxidation of soybean phosphatidylcholine and methyl linoleate in aqueous dispersions by uric acid. *Bulletin of the Chemical Society of Japan,* Vol.59, pp.471-477, online ISSN: 1348-0634 print ISSN: 0009-2673

Peluso, M.R. (2006). Flavonoids attenuate cardiovascular disease, inhibit phosphodiesterase, and modulate lipid homeostasis in adipose tissue and liver. *Experimental biology and medicine (Maywood, N.J.),* Vol.231, No. 8, pp.1287-1299, ISSN 1535-3702

Robb, S.J., Robb-Gaspers L.D., Scaduto R.C., Thomas A.P., & Connor J.R. (1999). Influence of calcium and iron on cell death and mitochondrial function in oxidatively stressed astrocytes. *Journal of neuroscience research,* Vol.55, No. 6, pp.674-686, ISSN 0360-4012

Ryu, R., Shin Y., Choi J.W., Min W., Ryu H., Choi C.R., & Ko H. (2002). Depletion of intracellular glutathione mediates zinc-induced cell death in rat primary astrocytes. *Experimental brain research,* Vol.143, No. 2, pp.257-263, ISSN 0014-4819

Sandhu, J.K., Gardaneh M., Iwasiow R., Lanthier P., Gangaraju S., Ribecco-Lutkiewicz M., Tremblay R., Kiuchi K., & Sikorska M. (2009). Astrocyte-secreted GDNF and glutathione antioxidant system protect neurons against 6OHDA cytotoxicity. *Neurobiology of disease,* Vol.33, No. 3, pp.405-414, ISSN 0969-9961

Sastry, P. (1985). Lipids of nervous tissue: composition and metabolism. *Progress in lipid resarch,* Vol.24, No. 2, pp.69-176, ISSN 0163-7827

Schrecka, R., & Baeuerlea P.A. (1991). A role for oxygen radicals as second messengers. *Trends in Cell Biology,* Vol.1, No. 2-3, pp.39-42, ISSN 0962-8924

Segal, R.A., Duddeck D.H., & Kajtar M. (1987). The sesquiterpene lactones from *A. fragrantissima. Tetrahedron,* Vol.43, No. 18, pp.4125-4132, ISSN 0040-4020

Sharaf, M., el-Ansari M.A., Matlin S.A., & Saleh N.A. (1997). Four flavonoid glycosides from Peganum harmala. *Phytochemistry (Oxford),* Vol.44, No. 3, pp.533-536, ISSN 0031-9422

Sheline, C.T., Behrens M.M., & Choi D.W. (2000). Zinc-induced cortical neuronal death: contribution of energy failure attributable to loss of NAD(+) and inhibition of glycolysis. *Journal of Neuroscience,* Vol.20, No. 9, pp.3139-3146, ISSN 0270-6474

Smyth, W.F., & Woolfson A.D. (1987). Drug assays--the role of modern voltammetric techniques. *Journal of clinical pharmacy and therapeutics,* Vol.12, No. 2, pp.117-134, ISSN 0269-4727

Soltan, M.M., & Zaki A.K. (2009). Antiviral screening of forty-two Egyptian medicinal plants. *Journal of ethnopharmacology,* Vol.126, No. 1, pp.102-107, ISSN 0378-8741

Spencer, J.P., Abd-el-Mohsen M.M., & Rice-Evans C. (2004). Cellular uptake and metabolism of flavonoids and their metabolites: implications for their bioactivity. *Archives of biochemistry and biophysics,* Vol.423, No. 1, pp.148-161, ISSN 0003-9861

Splittgerber, A.G., & Tappel A.L. (1979). Inhibition of glutathione peroxidase by cadmium and other metal ions. *Archives of Biochemistry and Biophysics,* Vol.197, No. 2, pp.534-542, ISSN: 0003-9861

Stork, C.J., & Li Y.V. (2009). Rising zinc: a significant cause of ischemic neuronal death in the CA1 region of rat hippocampus. *Journal of cerebral blood flow and metabolism,* Vol.29, No. 8, pp.1399-1408, ISSN 0271-678X

Takuma, K., Baba A., & Matsuda T. (2004). Astrocyte apoptosis: implications for neuroprotection. *Progress in Neurobiology,* Vol.72, No.2, pp.111-127, ISSN 0301-0082

Terao, J. (1999). Dietary flavonoids as antioxidants in vivo: conjugated metabolites of (-)-epicatechin and quercetin participate in antioxidative defense in blood plasma. *The Journal of Medical Investigation,* Vol.46, No. 3-4, pp.159-168, ISSN 1343-1420

Terao, J., Kawai Y., & Murota K. (2008). Vegetable flavonoids and cardiovascular disease. *Asia Pacific journal of clinical nutrition,* Vol.17 Suppl 1, pp.291-293, ISSN 0964-7058

Thomas, M.J., Chen Q., Franklin C., & Rudel L.L. (1997). A comparison of the kinetics of low-density lipoprotein oxidation initiated by copper or by azobis (2-amidinopropane). *Free radical biology & medicine,* Vol.23, No. 6, pp.927-935, ISSN 0891-5849

Vaudry, D., Pamantung T.F., Basille M., Rousselle C., Fournier A., Vaudry H., Beauvillain J.C., & Gonzalez B.J. (2002). PACAP protects cerebellar granule neurons against oxidative stress-induced apoptosis. *European Journal of Neuroscience,* Vol.15, No. 9, pp.1451-1460, ISSN 0953-816X

Walle, T. (2004). Absorption and metabolism of flavonoids. *Free Radical Biology and Medicine,* Vol.36, No. 7, pp.829-937, ISSN 0891-5849

Wang, H., & Joseph J.A. (1999). Quantifying cellular oxidative stress by dichlorofluorescein assay using microplate reader. *Free Radical Biology and Medicine,* Vol.27, No. 5-6, pp.612-616, ISSN 0891-5849

Wolfe, K.L., & Liu R.H. (2007). Cellular antioxidant activity (CAA) assay for assessing antioxidants, foods, and dietary supplements. *Journal of Agriculture and Food Chemistry,* Vol.55, No. 22, pp.8896-8907, ISSN 0021-8561

Yaniv, Z., Dafni A., Friedman J., & Palevitch D. (1987). Plants used for the treatment of diabetes in Israel. *Joural of Ethnopharmacology,* Vol.19, No. 2, pp.145-151, ISSN 0378-8741

Zapata-Urzua, C., Perez-Ortiz M., Bravo M., Olivieri A.C., & Alvarez-Lueje A. (2010). Simultaneous voltammetric determination of levodopa, carbidopa and benserazide in pharmaceuticals using multivariate calibration. *Talanta (Oxford),* Vol.82, No. 3, pp.962-968, ISSN 0039-9140

Zhu, D., Tan K.S., Zhang X., Sun A.Y., Sun G.Y., & Lee J.C. (2005). Hydrogen peroxide alters membrane and cytoskeleton properties and increases intercellular connections in astrocytes. *Journal of cell science,* Vol.118, Pt 16, pp.3695-3703, ISSN 0021-9533

19

Quantification of Volumetric Changes of Brain in Neurodegenerative Diseases Using Magnetic Resonance Imaging and Stereology

Niyazi Acer[1], Ahmet Tuncay Turgut[2],
Yelda Özsunar[3] and Mehmet Turgut[4]
[1]*Dept. of Anatomy, Erciyes University School of Medicine, Kayseri,*
[2]*Dept. of Radiology, Ankara Training and Research Hospital, Ankara,*
[3]*Dept. of Radiology, Adnan Menderes University School of Medicine, Aydın,*
[4]*Dept. of Neurosurgery, Adnan Menderes University School of Medicine, Aydın,*
Turkey

1. Introduction

In this chapter, we review the different magnetic resonance imaging (MRI)-based methods used to quantify whole and subcortical brain structures volume, and discuss the relevance of the brain atrophy in different neurodegenerative disseases. Although there are a lot of studies for multiple sclerosis (MS) and dementia of Alzheimer's type (AD) for the brain atrophy using different methods, the optimal method for quantifying atrophy has not been established to date.

In recent years, computed tomography (CT) scanning has been replaced with MRI scanning due to its enhanced soft-tissue resolution, especially for cerebrospinal fluid (CSF)-filled spaces, such as ventricular enlargement in patients with AD. Thus, a transition has occurred from CT to MRI in longitudinal studies investigating the human brain. As a result of development of new neuroimaging methods in clinical practice, volumetric methods started to be more sophisticated depending on various imaging methods (Lim et al., 2000). There are numerous reasons for the aforementioned transition; first of all, unlike CT, MRI has no inherent radiation effect, and secondly, CT underestimates cortical sulcal volume relative to MRI due to poorer resolution and spectral shift artifact on CT (Lim et al., 2000). Due to higher contrast resolution, MRI can better characterize the brain morphology including the size, tissue composition such as gray (or grey) matter and white matter, and shape of different cortical or subcortical neuroanatomic structures (Lim et al., 2000). Nowadays, it is possible to use MRI to visualize and quantify the directional coherence of white matter fibers, called diffusion tensor imaging (DTI), for investigation of connectivity and disconnectivity between different brain regions (Basser et al., 1994). Additionally, MRI equipments are also used to provide functional brain responses with functional MRI (fMRI) and perfusion MRI as in some nuclear medicine neuroimaging methods such as positron emission tomography (PET) and single photon emission computed tomography (SPECT). These methods can provide pathognomonic data of certain structural lesions in AD, as they can demonstrate neuronal activity or receptor characteristics (Small, 2002). High field MRI has started to further depict the regional atrophy patterns AD and other neurodegenerative disorders.

In this chapter, we aim to overview the challenging and exciting radiological methods used for the diagnosis of various neurodegenerative diseases. Specifically, we focus on the neuroimaging techniques in the first part of the chapter, their clinical applications in the second part, and methods for volume estimation including stereological techniques on the last part of the text.

2. Neuroimaging techniques

Primary neuroimaging techniques that are widely used clinically are CT, PET, SPECT, conventional MRI, fMRI, magnetic resonance spectroscopy (MRS), and tractography or DTI. These techniques enlighten different aspects of brain structures or functions (Frey et al., 1999; Small, 2002). An overview of the neuroimaging techniques is following:

2.1 Computed tomography (CT)

CT is the first imaging modality to provide *in vivo* evidence of the brain atrophy in different neurodegenerative diseases. CT images are generated by passing an x-ray beam through the skull or other object (e.g. spine and vertebral column) and it measures the attenuation of an x-ray beam through different body tissues e.g. brain, bone and CSF. Therefore, tissue's appearance will vary according to degree of its attenuation (Frey et al., 1999). The degree of attenuation can be measured numerically as a tissue density number for each voxel (volume element) and then these numbers can be converted to gray scale values and presented visually as pixels (Frey et al., 1999). Among different body tissues, the bone has the highest attenuation and appears white on CT images (Small, 2002). On the other hand, CT study has some limitations such as radiation hazards, inability to differentiate gray and white matter due to low contrast resolution and visualization of the posterior fossa structures, particularly brain stem and cerebellum. Despite to these limitations, quantitative CT still can demonstrate the presence of greater brain atrophy and ventricular dilatation in patients with AD compared with controls (Creasey et al., 1986).

2.2 Single photon emission computed tomography (SPECT)

In SPECT, the scanner determines the site of the photon source following adminstration of an unstable isotope or inhaled/injected tracer and thus an image reflecting cerebral blood flow or receptor distribution is produced (Schuckit et al., 1992). Unfortunately, its spatial resolution is not high enough for imaging deep structures and determination of the source of single photon emitters is difficult (Small, 2002).

2.3 Positron emission tomography (PET)

A PET scanner determines the line along which the photons travel, by recording the simultaneous arrival of two different photons at different detectors, and an image is then constructed from information received by the scanner. Importantly, PET study demonstrates receptor characteristics like density and affinity following injection of receptor ligands labeled with nuclides, in addition to cerebral blood flow. In patients with AD, PET studies using fluorodeoxyglucose have revealed characteristic alterations in cerebral blood flow and metabolism in the parietal, temporal and prefrontal cortices (Mazziotta et al., 1992).

2.4 Conventional magnetic resonance imaging (MRI)

The MRI scanner detects the radiofrequency energy emitted and energy level changes represent different brain structures. Typically, T1-weighted images differentiate gray and white matter, while T2-weighted images delineate white matter hyperintensities. It is reported that spatial resolution for MRI is 1 to 2 mm, less than that of CT (Small, 2002). Fortunately, patients can have multiple MRI scans because it does not involve ionizing radiation. In MRI study, the object is placed in a high field strength magnetic field varying from 0.5 to 3 Tesla (T). Technically, different relaxation times, in addition to proton density, are measured and further manipulations by using various pulse sequences are possible. Today, various MRI techniques such as fast spin echo, high performance gradients, echo planar and diffusion weighted imaging are available for clinical use, in addition to MRI contrast agents, CSF velocity analysis, and interventional MRI (Bradley & Bydder, 1997). Recently, some technical improvements regarding the acquisition and processing of structural data have provided vivid visual representations of the external surface and internal structures of the human brain (Lim et al., 2000). Clinically, the progressive neuronal loss leading to atrophy in neurodegenerative disease increases the value of MRI (Loewe et al., 2002).

2.5 Functional magnetic resonance imaging (fMRI)

With recent developments in MRI techniques, it is also possible to measure brain activity and tissue signal changes, reflecting local changes in oxygenation of haemoglobin, which depend on regional blood perfusion. Technical point of view, the signal intensity of deoxygenated hemoglobin differs from that of oxygenated hemoglobin (Belliveau et al., 1992). This MRI method also called BOLD technique. As a rule, the brain tissue during brain activity does not use this excess oxygen, causing high concentration of oxygenated blood, greater levels of magnetic field homogeneity and higher MRI signal intensity (Wagner et al., 1998). Thus, brain regions receiving greater blood flow during brain activity produce a stronger MRI signal than do other regions and areas of relative brain activity can be easily detected (Small, 2002).

2.6 Diffusion tensor imaging (DTI)

DTI provides detailed information concerning the anatomy of white matter structure in the central nervous system. With use of DTI, visualizations of projections of axonal fibers, i.e. neuronal connectivity, is possible by quantitative evaluation on the anisotropy of water diffusion, local fiber orientation and integrity of white matter tracks (Jones et al., 1999). Technically, DTI visualizes diffusional anisotropy within each voxel as three-dimensional projections of axonal fibers. In patients with AD and other neuropsychiatric disorders, the degree of neuronal connectivity loss is a useful marker in the progression of the disease (Buchsbaum et al., 1998; Ewers et al., 2011). Moreover, recent studies revealed the presence of loss of myelin and axons in patients with AD, particularly periventricular areas (Hanyu et al., 1997; Ewers et al., 2011).

2.7 Magnetic resonance spectroscopy (MRS)

From the technical view, the magnetic resonance spectrum display according to frequency shows different chemical forms of the element such as characteristic peaks, thus reflecting tissue metabolite concentrations (Weiner, 1987; Bothwell & Griffin 2011). As a noninvasive study, MRS provides quantitative regional biochemical and physiologic features of the tissue. To determine *N*-acetylaspartate (NAA) content of hippocampus in patients with AD, some authors used proton MRS (1H MRS) and volumetric MRI (Weiner, 1987; Schuff et al. 1997).

2.8 Improvements in magnetic resonance imaging

2.8.1 Mechanisms of tissue contrast: Pulse sequences

By varying elements of the image acquisition sequence of MRI, it is possible to manipulate the amount of contrast between various tissues. It is well-known that hydrogen atoms are the most important element of the tissue and MRI device demonstrate signals related with free water. Based on proton density and relaxation time of any tissue, different structures will appear in an acquired image. T1 means the time taken for excited nuclei to return to equilibrium, while T2 is an xponential time constant related with the time for the excited nuclei to lose signal (Lim et al., 2000). Technical view of point, the time between radiofrequency pulses (TR) and the amount of time after the pulse called echo time (TE) are important parameters; a long TR and a long TE give T2-weighted image, while a short TR and a short TE gives T1-weighted image. Although T1-weighted spin-echo and inversion recovery sequences have poor definition of CSF/skull margins for reliably measuring intracranial volume, they are used for morphometric studies because they provide good white-gray contrast (Lim et al., 2000).

Sources of contrast other than that based on manipulation of T1, T2, fluid-attenuated inversion recovery (FLAIR) and proton density are used to obtain further information. T1-weighted images are superior to T2-weighted images for the evaluation of atrophy, because T2-weighted ones overestimate the dimensions of ventricles and sulci (Kucharczyk & Henkelman, 1994). On the other hand, T1-weighted imaging gives a clear distinction between grey matter, white matter and CSF; therefore, they are used for quantitative MRI studies of brain morphology, particularly of individual brain structures (Keller & Roberts, 2009) (Fig. 1).

Fast spin echo T2 sequences has been usually used in brain imaging due to their short acquisition time and increased robustness to motion artifacts. In imaging of neurodegenerative disorders like Parkinson-like syndromes, however, gradient echo T2-weighted spin-echo sequences are preferred because they increase the sensitivity for paramagnetic materials (ferritin, melanin etc.). Also, proton-density or FLAIR sequences identify gliosis owing to result of progressive neuronal loss (Loewe et al., 2002). Therefore, T2-weighted imaging may be used for determination of intracranial volume as the increased signal intensity of CSF provides better determination of CSF and the parenchyma of the brain (Keller & Roberts, 2009). Therefore, the type of MRI sequence used is important for volume estimation.

2.8.2 Two-dimensional multi-slice and three-dimensional imaging

Two-dimensional (2D) images are obtained in axial, sagittal and coronal planes (Fig. 1). Image orientation, giving a different view of the brain with optimal visualization of different structures, is described according to radiofrequency pulse excitations and the magnetic gradients in three orthogonal axes. Basically, a mid-sagittal section provides an image of the corpus callosum and the prefrontal cortex, coronal section gives an image of the limbic structures including hippocampus, and axial section gives an image of basal ganglia structures and the lateral ventricular system.

It is important to know that 2D image has a limitation so that only selected slices imaged and therefore a comparison across subjects is difficult, although it may be possible by orienting each slice acquisition relative to a specific anatomic plane. On the other hand, three-dimensional (3D) volume acquisition protocols include the entire brain and they are widely used in psychiatric neuroimaging. Using T1-weighted MRI sections with a good gray/white matter differentiation, the entire brain with 1.5 mm or thinner slices are obtained in 10 minutes or less. As a rule, an in-plane resolution of 1 mm means that each pixel in the image matrix represents 1 mm^2 (Lim et al., 2000).

Quantitative investigations of the brain using MRI may reveal important information about the function and organisation of the brain being studied, recently. MRI has become the method of choice for the examination of macroscopic neuroanatomy in vivo due to excellent levels of image resolution and between tissue contrasts. Estimation of brain compartment volume needs high resolution MRIs for the delineation of anatomical boundaries. With the use of higher magnetic field strength, a better image quality with can be obtained using thinner slices and shorter imaging time. For this reason, many researchers frequently use MRI scanners which are either with 1.5 T or 3 T systems (Fig. 2). Although 3 T systems offer increased resolution of between-tissue contrast (i.e. increased visualisation of the borders between gray matter, white matter and CSF), MRI scans on 1.5 T systems are sufficient for the quantification of relatively small brain structures, such as the hippocampus, amygdala, and deep gray matter nuclei (Keller & Roberts, 2009).

3. Clinical applications

3.1 Dementia syndromes

A number of studies reported that patients with MS have smaller volumes of the parenchyma than in age-matched control subjects (Bermel et al., 2003; Sanfilipo et al., 2005, 2006). The first method used for the estimation of brain atrophy is linear measurement of ventricles or other brain structural dimensions (Smith et al., 2002). In general, MRI studies reveal some differences in the volume of the brain structures in certain neurodegenerative diseases, an inhomogeneous group of neurological diseases with unknown etiology, such as demantia. In such diseases, multiple systems or one system or one group of nuclei may partly or totally be involved (Loewe et al., 2002). Basically, there are two principal pathological processes which determine imaging findings: neuronal or white matter loss and deposition of different compounds. The loss of neurons leads to progressive atrophy associated with white matter loss and gliosis (Kern & Behl, 2009).

Nowadays, dementia is a well-known illness with a high incidence in the aged population. Clinically, there are a number of neurodegenerative diseases causing dementia, including AD, dementia with Lewy bodies, and frontotemporal dementia. Furthermore, dementia picture is also present in some neurodegenerative illnesses including Creutzfeldt-Jakob disease, Huntington's disease, progressive supranuclear palsy, multiple system atrophy, amyotrophic lateral sclerosis, and Parkinson's disease (Loewe et al., 2002; Vitali et al., 2008).

3.1.1 Alzheimer disease (AD)

AD is well-known progressive neurodegenerative pathology, accounting for around 60% of all cases dementia. Clinically, patients with AD have serious cognitive findings related with memory, language, such as confusion, poor judgment, language disturbance, agitation, withdrawal, and hallucinations (Mohs & Haroutunian, 2002).

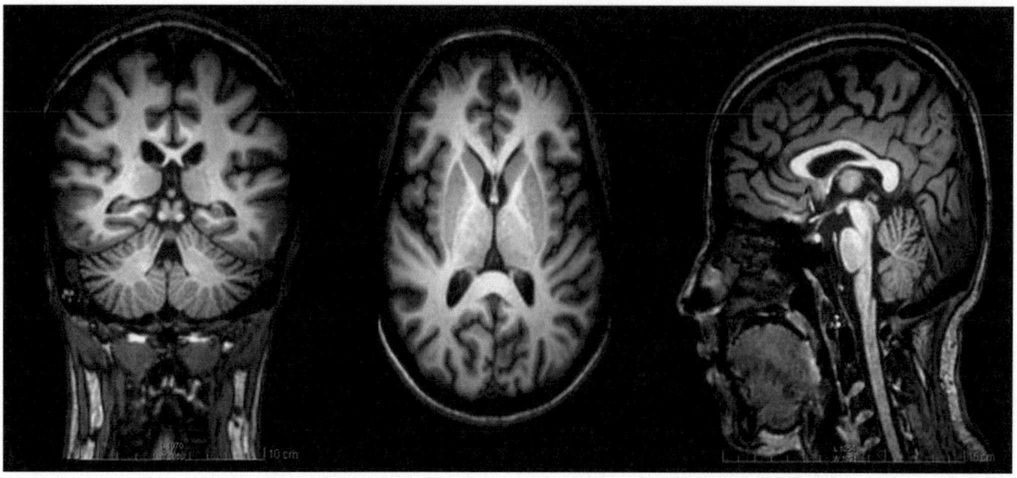

Fig. 1. T1-weighted MRI scans acquired in coronal (left), axial (center) and sagittal (right) planes with 3 T. All images were acquired with a field of view of 25 cm and 256 x 256 matrix, 1-mm slice thickness. Image was acquired using a turbo field echo sequence, gated to achieve an effective TR of >8 ms and TE of 4 ms. Left: Coronal image passing through lateral ventricles and temporal lobes. Center: Axial image passing through the lateral ventricles and basal ganglia. Right: Mid-sagittal image highlighting the corpus callosum, brain stem and cerebellum

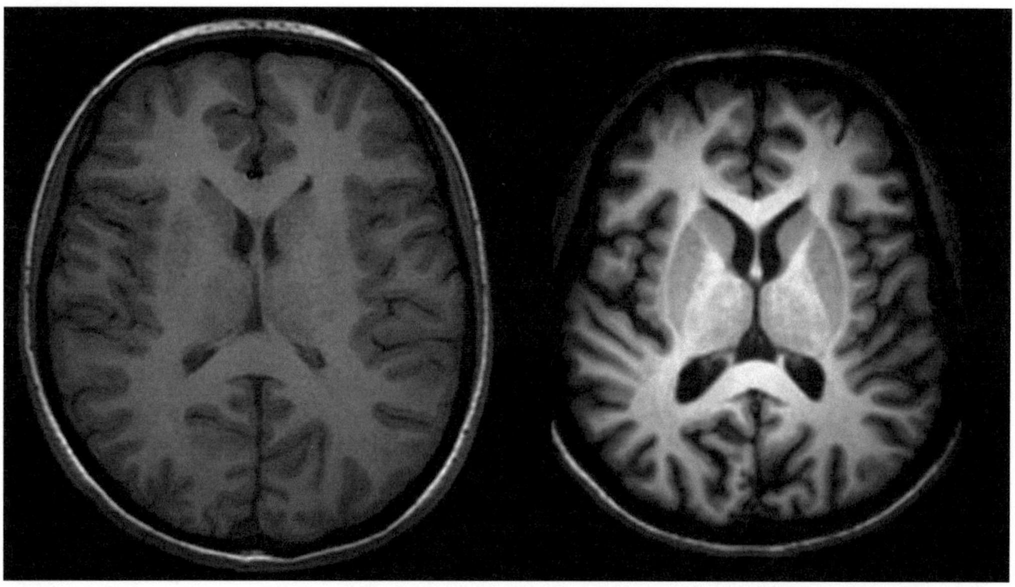

Fig. 2. T1-weighted axial MRIs acquired with 1.5 T (left) and 3T (right) MRI scanners. 3T MRI was acquired with a field of view of 25 cm and 256 x 256 matrix, 1-mm slice thickness. Image was acquired using a turbo field echo sequence, gated to achieve an effective TR of >8 ms and TE of 4 ms. 1.5T MRI was acquired with field of view of 24 cm, 1.5 mm slice thickness. Image was acquired using a spoiled gradient recalled acquisition sequence, gated to achieve an effective TR of >35 ms and TE of 15 ms

Gross examination of the brain in patients with AD demonstrated an obvious atrophy, widening of the sulci, and erosion of the gyri. Histologically, the atrophy of the cortex is associated with significant reductions in the numbers of neurons. Macroscopically, the weight of the brain is decreased compared to normal controls (Masliah et al., 1991). In a previous study using unbiased stereologic sampling techniques, about 50% loss in neurons of the superior temporal gyrus has been reported (Gomez-Isla et al., 1996, 1997). In another study, 40-46% loss of large neurons in the frontal and temporal cortices of specimens has been reported in patients with AD (Terry et al., 1981). In fact, neuronal loss and degeneration are not restricted to the cortex; it may be observed in subcortical nuclei such as the locus ceruleus, raphe aminergic nuclei (Zweig et al., 1988; Chan-Palay & Asan, 1989), and the nucleus basalis of Meynert (Whitehouse et al., 1982). In such cases, synaptic markers such as synaptophysin are significantly reduced in the cerebral cortex, especially the frontal and parietal cortices and in the hippocampus, with increasing age (Nagy et al., 1995).

Radiologically, MRI provides understanding of disease progression in AD and other dementias. Recently, it has been reported that patients with AD have atrophy in parietal lobes, medial temporal lobe and hippocampus on MRI (Loewe et al., 2002, Vitali et al., 2008). The parietal lobe atrophy is observed on axial or coronal T1-weighted or FLAIR sequences with thinning of the posterior part of the body of the corpus callosum on T1-weighted sagittal sequences (Yamauchi et al., 2000). In some studies, decreased hippocampal and entorhinal cortex (ERC) volumes in patients with AD were noted (Appel et al., 2009). Hippocampal atrophy is observed with thin coronal T1-weighted or FLAIR tomographic slices through the medial temporal lobes (Teipel et al., 2003). A lot of quantitative MRI studies indicate that white matter hyperintensities correlate with neuropsychological functioning in both healthy elderly persons and demented patients (Boone et al., 1992; Lopez et al., 1992). Other studies indicate loss of cerebral gray matter (Rusinek et al., 1991), hippocampal and parahippocampal atrophy (Kesslak et al., 1991), and lower left amygdala and ERC volumes in patients with AD (Pearlson et al., 1992; Obrien, 2007).

Recently, a longitudinal study demonstrated that most common neuropathologic findings in elderly patients are neuritic plaques and neurofibrillary tangles (Mohs &Haroutunian, 2002). The presence of these findings before clinical AD diagnosis suggests that *in vivo* methods that directly image these pathognomonic lesions would be useful presymptomatic detection technologies (Mohs & Haroutunian, 2002).

3.1.2 Frontotemporal demantia (FTD)

Frontotemporal demantia (FTD) is as common a cause of dementia. In particular, volumes of some regions of the frontal lobe (the ventromedial and posterior orbital regions of the frontal lobe), the cingulate cortex, and the insula are reduced in patients with the FTD, compared with those of both AD patients and age-matched controls. This feature differentiates this illness from AD as these areas are relatively spared in the latter disease (Rosen et al., 2002). In patients with the semantic variant of FTD, there is a relative preservation of frontal lobe volumes but marked loss of volumes in the temporal lobes (Rosen et al,. 2005, 2006). In clinical practice, FTD includes a group of neurodegenerative diseases characterized by focal atrophy of frontal and anterior temporal lobes and non-AD pathology (Neary et al., 1998; McKhann, 2001; Ratnavalli, 2002).

3.1.3 Dementia with Lewy bodies (DLB)

Dementia with Lewy bodies results a diffuse, irreversible and destructive atrophy (Seppi & Schocke, 2005). Measurement of brain volume to predict atrophy using MRI may be used as a predicter for outcome in different neurodegenerative diseases such as AD. There are a lot of biologic factors influencing cerebral volume measurement such as inflammation and edema, cerebrovascular disease, chronic alcoholism and normal aging (Ron et al., 1982; Molyneux et al., 2000).

3.2 Multiple Sclerosis (MS)

In cases with MS, various measurement techniques revealed atrophy of brain and spinal cord, axonal loss, and Wallerian degeneration (Sharma et al., 2004). Recent studies show that the MS is a destructive disease process and whole-brain atrophy is a valuable marker for the progression of the disease (Sharma et al., 2004).

3.3 Medial temporal lobe epilepsy (MTLE)

In patients with medial temporal lobe epilepsy (MTLE), the atrophy of the hippocampus is often observed on routine MRI. Recently, it has been reported that automatic morphometry can be used as a clinical tool to provide a quantifiable estimation of of hippocampal atrophy in patients with MTLE (Bonilha et al., 2009). Most recently, Henry et al. (2011) suggested that ultrahigh-field-strength MRI revealed prominent atrophy of Ammon horn in patients with MTLE and hippocampal sclerosis.

3.4 Ageing

With increasing age, there are some volumetric changes in the gray matter structures of the temporal lobe, amygdale, and hippocampus, a critical structure for memory in AD, but they are heterogenous, with some regions showing more atrophic changes than others (O'Sullivan, 2009). Recently, it has been reported that it is possible to differentiate ageing from AD with 87% accuracy (Likeman et al., 2005; O'Sullivan, 2009). Some volumetric studies demonstrated that changes in white matter regions provide an early and accurate diagnosis (Davatzikos et al., 2008).

4. Methods for volume estimation

4.1 Manual, automated and semiautomated methods for volume estimation

Use of imaging methods for quantitive volume estimation such as manual, semi-automated and automated methods can provide the capability to reliably detect and identify general and specific structural abnormalities of the brain. Use of these methods can aid to diagnose some specific neurological diseases and facilitate monitoring of the progression of the disease. Quantative measures of the brain atrophy can be clinically relevant and much work has been carried out to establish diagnosis of AD (Furlong, 2008).

At present, a number of manual, semi-automated and automated methods based on conventional MRI are available for measuring whole or regional brain volume. Ideally, the technique for measuring tissue volume should be reproducible, sensitive to subtle modifications, practical, fast and correct. Theoretically, many factors may affect the quantification of brain atrophy using segmentation methods, such as the pulse sequence and the resolution parameters chosen for the acquisition (Horsfield et al., 2003; Sharma et al., 2004).

One of these most important factors is slice thickness. The use of thin slice helps to reduce the partial volume effect and consequently permits a better estimation of tissue volumes. Moreover, high contrast makes segmentation between the different cerebral compartments easier. Depending on the compartment of interest, tissue contrast can be chosen such as CSF/parenchyma or gray/white matter (Grassiot et al., 2009). There are many different segmentation methods for estimating brain volume using manual or automated techniques. Flippi et al. (1998) used manual technique for whole brain volume with MS. Although the manual tracing of brain structure allows brain volume to be estimated, this technique is a time consuming method (Flippi et al., 1998).

Semi-automated techniques, quicker and more reproducible, use various algorithms of brain segmentation from 3D volume (Horsfield et al., 2003). For both semi-automated and automated methods, however, manual defining of brain structures is necessary. In semi-automated methods, manual marking of some anatomical landmarks and an automatic segmentation of the region of interest (ROI) are required, while automated methods are completely user-independent in the determination of various parameters such as brain size and shape. Importantly, experienced raters with detailed knowledge of neuroanatomy are necessary for manual techniques and correct estimations related to the neuroanatomical ROI are possible (Keller & Roberts, 2009).

Automated and semi-automated methods for segmentation and quantification of the brain are used in most studies. More recently, various image analysis tools have been developed, including both automated and semi-automated algorithms, relying on either raw or normalized brain volume assessments (Pelletier et al., 2004). Several previous studies have described automatic segmentation methods using MRIs. Calmon & Roberts (2000) reported a segmentation method for the lateral ventricles on coronal MR images. Stokking et al. (2000) described the development of a morphology-based brain segmentation method for fully automatic segmentation of the brain using T1-weighted MRI data. Webb et al. (1999) reported a method of automatic detection of the hippocampus with atrophy. These methods each segmented one target object on each MRI obtained by different sequences. Therefore, these methods could not segment two or more objects simultaneously on MRIs obtained by a single sequence.

There are two primary methods for manual quantification of brain compartment volume from MRIs, namely stereology in conjunction with point counting and planimetric methods or manual tracing (Acer et al., 2007; Keller & Roberts, 2009). Authors used manual tracing of brain boundaries from MRI scans using various softwares such as Analyze (Biomedical Imaging Resource, Mayo Foundation), BRAINS (Iowa Mental Health Clinical Research Center 2008), and FreeSurfer (Dale et al., 1999; Fischl et al., 1999; Fischl et al., 2002). Manual techniques such as planimetry or tracing methods require the investigator to delineate a brain region based on reliable anatomical landmarks, whilst the software package provides information on volume. Tracing methods require the investigator to trace the brain ROI using a mouse driven cursor throughout a defined number of MRI sections (Keller & Roberts, 2009). The cut surface areas, determined by pixel counting within the traced region, are summed and multiplied by the distance between the consecutive sections traced to estimate the total volume. Although tracing methods represent the most commonly used tool to estimate brain structure volume on MRIs, there are some drawbacks associated this technique (Geuze et al., 2005). Firstly, the time taken to perform manual tracing or manual segmentation methods is significantly longer than stereological point counting methods (Acer et al., 2007, 2008; Keller & Roberts, 2009). Secondly, tracing and manual segmentation methods suffer from the risk of "hand wobble" during the delineation of ROI boundaries on MRI sections (Keller & Roberts, 2009).

The measurement of rates of change requires volume quantification. In general, manual or semi-automated methods have been employed for volume quantification on structural brain

MRIs, but they are generally severely limited in practicality and reliability. For example, a high-resolution 3D brain MRI data set can contain more than 100 slices to cover an entire brain (Keller & Roberts, 2009). Manually delineating tissue boundaries for volumetric measurement can be a tedious and demanding process because of the presence of the extremely complex convoluted structures of the brain. Manual tracing is also well-known to be associated with large subjective variability and low reproducibility. As a result, methods with better reproducibility and higher precision are required for measuring subtle neuro-anatomic changes and these methods are likely to be based on computerized approaches. FreeSurfer is freely available on the World Wide Web (www or commonly known as the Web), it has been widely used in the neuroimaging field. At present, fully automated methods are most often used. Fully automated or semi-automated methods can be applied to a specific ROI (such as the thalamus or the hippocampus) to obtain a regional brain volume (Houtchens et al., 2007).

4.2 Brain segmentation

Brain tissue segmentation of MRIs means to specify the tissue type for each pixel or voxel in a 2D or 3D data set, respectively, on the basis of information available from both MRIs and the prior knowledge of the brain. It is an important preprocessing step in many medical research and clinical applications, such as quantification of tissue volume, visualization and analysis of anatomical structures, multimodality fusion and registration, functional brain mapping, detection of pathology, surgical planning, surgical navigation, and brain substructure segmentation (Suri et al., 2002). So far, various segmentation techniques such as Gaussian mixture models (Ashburner & Friston, 2005), discriminant analysis (Amato et al., 2003), k-nearest neighbor classification (Mohamed et al., 1999), and fuzzy c-means clustering (Pham & Prince, 1999; Suckling et al., 1999; Ahmed et al., 2002; Zhou & Bai, 2007) were used to determine gray and white matter volume. Most recently, it has been reported that "fuzzy" cluster or classifier approaches were found to have a high reliability, accuracy, and validity (Herndon, 1998).

4.3 Image processing and segmentation

Today, medical image processing and segmentation are used to improve the quality of diagnosis. We can calculate the cortical volume and surface area using the Fuzzy C-Means algorithm as a semi-automated segmentation method as described in Figure 3.
Firstly, T1-weighted MRIs are normalized using registration algorithms. Following normalization process, we obtain brain contour to calculate volume and surface area of the brain using image working algorithms. Images of brain are cleared brain contour using morphological image processing. This method involves two major steps and final segmented images result from separation of parenchyma for brain volume and surrounding line for cortical surface area of the brain (Tosun et al., 2004; Ueda et al., 2009; Brouwer et al., 2010; Lui et al., 2010) (Fig. 4).

4.4 Stereological approaches

In general, stereological methods provide quantitative data on 3D structures using 2D images. Stereological methods have been widely applied on MRIs to estimate geometric variables, such as volume and surface area, and various internal brain compartments. The volume of internal brain structure can be obtained using the Cavalieri principle of stereologic approaches.

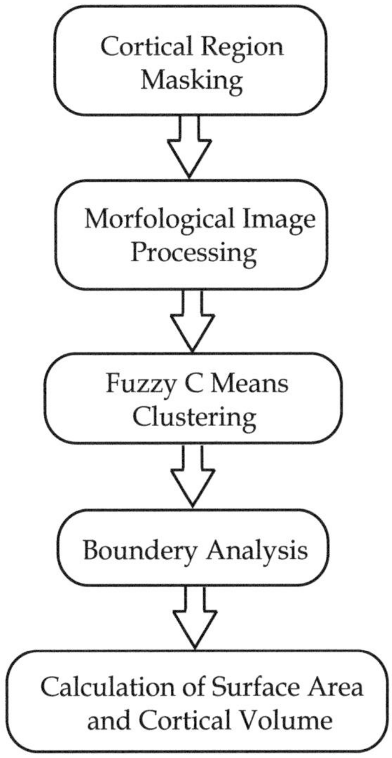

Fig. 3. Brain image segmentation blocks (Nakamura & Fisher, 2009)

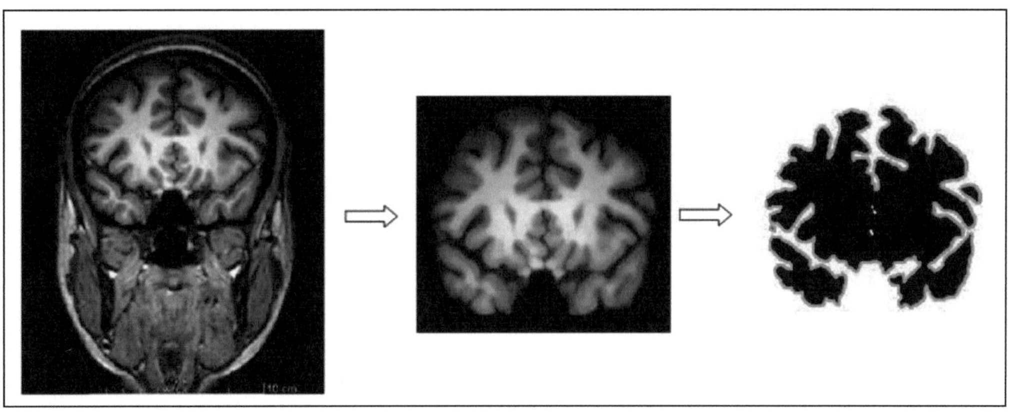

Fig. 4. Segmentation called the Fuzzy C. Left: Original T1-weighted image. Center: Masking and removal of artifacts the outer contour of the brain. Right: Contour of segmented image is outlined

4.4.1 Point-counting method

The Cavalieri method in combination with point counting requires beginning from a uniform random starting within the sectioning interval, a structure of interest is exhaustively sectioned with a series of parallel plane probes a constant distant apart. An unbiased estimate of volume is obtained by multiplying the total area of all sections through the structure by sectioning interval *t* as following:

$$estV = t \times (a_1 + a_2 + .. + a_n) \quad (1)$$

where $a_1, a_2 \ldots a_n$ show the section areas and t is the sectioning interval (Roberts et al., 2000; García-Fiñana et al., 2003).

The point counting method involves overlying each MRI with a regular grid of test points. After each superimposition, the number of test points hitting the structure of interest is counted on each section and we can estimate volume following formula:

$$estV = t \times \left(\frac{a}{p}\right) \times (p_1 + p_2 + .. + p_n) \quad (2)$$

where $p_1, p_2, \ldots p_n$ show point counts and a/p represent the area associated with each test point. To avoid bias, the position of the test system should be uniform randomly (Roberts et al., 2000; García-Fiñana et al., 2003).

In any case, the following formula (Eq.3) can be used for volume estimation from MRIs of the brain (Şahin & Ergür, 2006; Acer et al., 2008):

$$V(pc) = t \times \left[\frac{su \times d}{sl}\right]^2 \times \sum p \quad (3)$$

where 't' is the section thickness, 'su' the scale unit of the printed film, 'd' the distance between the test points of the grid, 'sl' the measured length of the scale printed on the film and 'Σp' is the total number of points hitting the sectioned cut surface areas of the related structures such as the cerebrum.

From stereological point of view, planimetry and point-counting are two different methods for estimating volume based on the Cavalieri principle. The Cavalieri principle may be used for estimating the volume of brain and substructures such as hypocampus, amygdale and thalamus. Therefore, a random beginning is necessary and the object is cut into slices of a known and fixed thickness. The volume is estimated by multiplying the distance between the slices by the total cut area of the structures are under investigation. The cut area of the structures may be estimated by point-counting or planimetry. Nevertheless, the Cavalieri principle in combination with point-counting is ideal for estimating total volumes of various brain and any compartments. Keller et al. (2002, 2007, 2008) and Acer et al. (2008, 2010) have previously applied this technique to obtain volume estimations of various brain structures such as Broca's area, hippocampus, ventricles, cerebral hemisphere, and cerebellum. In these studies, a set of parallel and equidistant MRIs of the brain is randomly selected, and the ROI is directly estimated on each image by randomly superimposing a grid of points, and subsequently, counting the number of points that fall within the ROI (Keller et al., 2002, 2007, 2008; Acer et al., 2008, 2010).

Stereology in combination with point counting has an advantage related with the time taken to estimate volume of brain structures on MRIs. Compared with manual tracing or segmentation methods, this technique is much more time efficient. Another advantage of stereology in combination with point counting is the prediction of the coefficient of error (CE) so that it may be used to identify the optimal parameters of sampling needed to achieve a given precision such as we need the number of MRI sections and the density of the point grid.

Importantly, the stereological approach provides an opportunity for the investigator making appropriate changes on their sampling or estimating procedures. Therefore, the Cavalieri method gives a CE of estimation for each volume assessment. Thus, an investigator may easily observe the potential variability in any given volume measurement. It may cause some problems in accuracy and hence interpretation in the presence of high CE for these measurements. If too few slices or too few points are taken for volume estimation, it is possible to encounter with such problems. The investigator is eligible to change the spacing of points in the grid or the number of slices available in any CT or MR study to provide a reasonable CE value. More importantly, an appropriate grid size and the number of slices required for volume estimation of an object is crucial at the beginning, obviating the need to calculate the CE value for repeated sessions (Sahin et al., 2003; Acer et al., 2008).

In the stereological method, continuous investigator computer interaction is necessary because all points intersecting the cerebral hemispheres should be removed or marked on consecutive MRI sections. For the reliable measurement of each brain structure using stereology in conjunction with point counting, the stereological parameters like grid size and slice gap should be optimized by counting at least 200 points per structure. In a previous study investigating the cerebral hemispheres, a grid size of 15 and slice gap of every 15 sections results in approximately 200 points being counted per hemisphere on frequently acquired 3D T1-weighted images (Mackay et al., 1998; Cowell et al., 2007), and it achieves a CE lower than the optimal 5% (Roberts et al., 2000). It has been reported that stereological volume estimation of a cerebral hemisphere using the Windows based software packages (EASYMEASURE and MEASURE) takes approximately 10 minutes (Keller & Roberts, 2009).

Stereological point counting method involves the random placement of a grid with sufficient resolution in 2D or 3D over the structure of interest and counting the points overlying the ROI. For this method, the requirements are a grid encompassing the region or structure completely, the structure placed with a grid randomly, and an adequate number of points counted on an adequate number of slices. Thus, the stereological point counting approach is very efficient and statistically sound, in addition to providing a CE of the measurement of the volume of the structure of interest.

4.4.2 Worked example for point-counting technique

According to point-counting technique, a square grid of test points is positioned on each MRI section, and all points hitting the cerebrum are counted (Fig. 5).

T = 1.6cm, d = 0.8cm, SU=8 cm, SL=7.8 cm, $\sum P = 796$

$$V(pc) = t \times \left[\frac{su \times d}{sl}\right]^2 \times \sum p$$
$$V = 1.6 \times \left[\frac{8 \times 0.8}{7.8}\right]^2 \times 796 = 856.90 cm^3 \quad (3)$$

In the Cavalieri method in combination with point-counting technique using MRI sections, relationship between numbers of section and counts is given in Table 1.

Section number	1	2	3	4	5	6	7	8	Total Point Counts
Point number	42	72	122	132	129	116	115	68	796

Table 1. Relationship between numbers of section and counts of point in point-counting technique

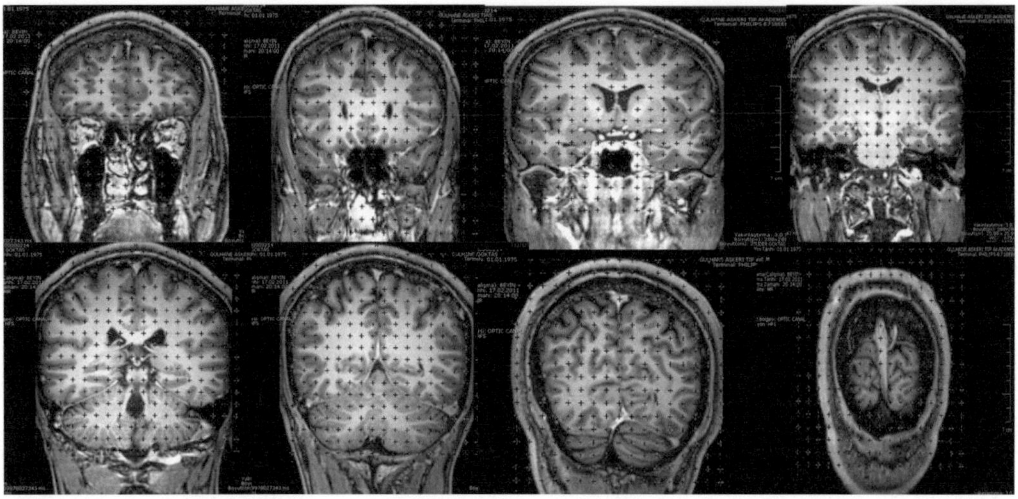

Fig. 5. Acoronal MRI series with a point-counting on it for the estimation of the cerebral volume from first to last section (T=1.6 cm)

4.4.3 Error prediction for point counting technique

The error predictors given below originate from the recent literature (García-Fiñana & Cruz-Orive, 2000; Garcia Finana, 2006; Garcia Finana et al., 2009). In particular, the estimation of volume and variance of the volume estimate for the cerebral volume are calculated as follows.

An unbiased estimator of *Q* can be constructed from a sample of equidistant observations of *f*, with a distance *T* apart, as follows:

$$\hat{Q}_T = T\sum_{k\in Z} f\left(x_0 + kT\right) = T\left(f_1 + f_2 + ... f_n\right) \tag{4}$$

where x_0 is a uniform random variable in the interval [0,*T*) and $\{f_1, f_2, \ldots, f_n\}$ is the set of equidistant observations of *f* at the sampling points which lie in [*a*, *b*]. In many applications, *Q* represents the volume of a structure and *f*(*x*) is the area of the intersection between the structure and a plane that is perpendicular to a given sampling axis at the point of abscissa *x* (García-Fiñana & Cruz-Orive, 2000; Garcia Finana, 2006; Garcia Finana et al., 2009).

This data sample represents the area of cerebrum in cm² on a total of 8 MRI sections a distance *T* = 1.6 cm apart (Table 1).

To estimate Var ($\hat{Q}_T$) via Eq. (5) we have to calculate first $\alpha(q)$, C_0, C_1, C_2 and C_4 (Table 2).

$$\mathrm{var}\left(\hat{Q}_T\right) = \alpha\left(q\right)\left(3C_0 - 4C_1 + C_2\right)T^2 \quad q \in \left[0,1\right] \tag{5}$$

From Eq. (6), we have:

$$C_k \sum_{i=1}^{n-k} f_i f_{i+k}, \quad k = 1,\ 2,\ ...\ n - 1 \tag{6}$$

Equation (5) is an extended version of the variance estimator given in (García-Fiñana & Cruz-Orive, 2004).

Section (i)	P_i	P_i^2	$P_i.P_{i+1}$	$P_i.P_{i+2}$	$P_i.P_{i+4}$
1	42	1764	3024	5124	5418
2	72	5184	8784	9504	8352
3	122	14884	16104	15738	14030
4	132	17424	17028	15312	8976
5	129	16641	14964	14835	0
6	116	13456	13340	7888	0
7	115	13225	7820	0	0
8	68	4624	0	0	0
		87202	81064	68401	36776
Total	796	C_0	C_1	C_2	C_4

Table 2. Calculation of the constants C0, C1, C2, C4

The smoothness constant can be estimated from Eq. (7) as follows:

$$q = \max\left\{0, \frac{1}{2\log 2}\log\left[\frac{(3C_0 - 4C_2 + C_4)}{(3C_0 - 4C_1 + C_2)}\right] - \frac{1}{2}\right\} \tag{7}$$

$$q = \left\{0, \frac{1}{2\log 2}\log\left[\frac{3\times 87202 - 4\times 68401 + 36776}{3\times 87202 - 4\times 81064 + 68401}\right] - \frac{1}{2}\right\} = 0.53$$

We apply Eq. (7) with α = 0.53.
The coefficient α(q) has the following expression (Eq.8):

$$\alpha(q) = \frac{\Gamma(2q+2)\zeta(2q+2)\cos(\pi q)}{(2\pi)^{2q+2}\left(1-2^{2q-1}\right)} \qquad q \in [0,1] \tag{8}$$

where Γ and ζ denote the gamma function and the Riemann Zeta function, respectively.

$$a(0.53) = \frac{\Gamma(2.06)\zeta(2.06)\cos(1.66)}{(2\tau)^{2.06}(1-2^{0.06})} = 0.018$$

Therefore, the estimate of Var ($\hat{Q}_T$) obtained via Eq. (5) is:

$$\begin{aligned} \text{var}(Q_T) &= a(q)(3C_0 - 4C_1 + C_2)T^2 \\ \text{var}(Q_T) &= 0.018 \times (3\times 87202 - 4\times 81064 + 68401) \times (1.6)^2 \\ \text{var}(Q_T) &= 9.2 \end{aligned} \tag{9}$$

We predict the value of CE;

$$CE(Q_T) = \sqrt{9.2 / 856.9} = 0.0103 = 1.03\%$$

In our studies, we calculate the CE values as predictive using the R program. First, by using the statistical package R, codes are developed to calculate the contribution to the predictive

CE (García-Fiñana & Cruze-Orive, 2004). A value of CE lower than 5% is in the acceptable range (Gundersen & Jensen, 1987, and 1999; Sahin et al., 2003). In addition, it is very important to note that an appropriate grid size and the number of slices required for volume estimation of an object is crucial at the beginning.

5. Conclusion

In conlusion, MRI may help to specify the cause of the disease such as the brain atrophy, if a kind of neurodegenerative dissease is present. Unfortunately, however, conventional MRI study not give subsutructural detailed information about cellular and molecular organisation of the brain tissue. On the other hand, it is also possible to define the etiologies of the pathologies using new functional MRI methods, such as diffusion weighted imaging and MRS. Future advances in functional and anatomic neuroimaging techniques provide further insights into certain neurodegenerative disseases of the brain. A combination of different neuroimaging techniques and atrophy correction through MRI, PET and SPECT superimposition may demonstrate functional and morphological features of the brain tissue. In similar to MRI, PET and SPECT are useful in the diagnosis of some neurodegenerative diseases.

By using MRI, the estimation of the brain volume is a well-known entity for the determination of the brain atrophy. Several different methods such as segmentation techniques are available for the estimation of the brain volume, but there are only a few stereological studies using point-counting and planimetric methods. Recently, the Cavalieri principle in combination with point-counting has become popular in the understanding of the pathologies of brain morphology. There is no doubt that determination of the brain atrophy using MRI will be useful in understanding of neurodegenerative diseases, monitoring of disease progression, and treatment of such patients. In conclusion, the Cavalieri principle in combination with point-counting is an ideal method for the estimation of total volume of the brain or any of its compartment for the diagnosis of atrophic neurodegenerative diseases.

Nevertheless, further combinations of new imaging techniques with different methods for volume estimation using a combination of different neuroimaging techniques are needed for early diagnosis and monitorization of course of the disease. It is important to know that these techniques for volume estimation must be reproducible and reliable. The greater accuracy of imaging methods in detection of early neurodegenerative disseases will result in early optimal treatment to delay further cognitive decline.

6. References

Acer, N.; Sahin, B.; Baş, O.; Ertekin, T. & Usanmaz, M. (2007). Comparison of three methods for the estimation of total intracranial volume: stereologic, planimetric, and anthropometric approaches. *Ann Plast Surg* Vol. 58, No. 1, (Jan 2007), pp. 48-53. ISSN 0148-7043

Acer, N.; Sahin, B.; Usanmaz, M., Tatoğlu, H. & Irmak, Z. (2008). Comparison of point counting and planimetry methods for the assessment of cerebellar volume in human using magnetic resonance imaging: a stereological study. *Surg Radiol Anat* Vol. 30, No. 4, (Jun 2008), pp. 335-9. ISSN 0930-1038

Acer, N.; Uğurlu, N.; Uysal, DD.; Unur, E.; Turgut, M. & Camurdanoğlu, M. (2010). Comparison of two volumetric techniques for estimating volume of intracerebral ventricles using magnetic resonance imaging: a stereological study. *Anat Sci Int* Vol. 85, No. 3, (Sep 2010), pp. 131-9. ISSN 1447-6959

Ahmed, MN.; Yamany, SM.; Mohamed, N.; Farag, AA. & Moriarty, T. (2002). A modified fuzzy c-means algorithm for bias field estimation and segmentation of MRI data. *EEE Trans Med Imag* Vol. 21, No. 3, (Mar 2002), pp. 193–199. ISSN 0278-0062

Amato, U.; Larobina, M.; Antoniadis, A. & Alfano, B. (2003). Segmentation of magnetic resonance brain images through discriminant analysis. *J Neurosci Methods* Vol. 131, No. 1-2, (Dec 2003), pp 65–74. ISSN 0165-0270

Appel, J.; Potter, E.; Shen, Q.; Pantol G.; Greig, MT.; Loewenstein, D. & Duara, R. (2009). A comparative analysis of structural brain MRI in the diagnosis of Alzheimer's disease. *Behav Neurol* Vol. 21, No. 1, (Oct 2009), pp. 13–19, ISSN 0953-4180

Ashburner, J. & Friston, KJ. (2005). Unified segmentation. *NeuroImage* Vol. 26, No. 3, (Jul 2005), pp. 839–851. ISSN 1053-8119

Belliveau JW, Kennedy DN, McKinstry RC, Buchinder, BR; Weiskoff, RM; Cohen, MS; Vevea, JM, Brady, TJ. & Rosen BR. (1992). Functional mapping of the human visual cortex by magnetic resonance imaging. *Science* Vol. 254, No. 5032, (Nov 1991), pp. 716–719. ISSN 0036-8075

Basser, PJ.; Mattiello, J. & LeBihan, D. (1994). MR diffusion tensor spectroscopy and imaging. *Biophysics Journal* Vol. 66, No. 1 (Jan 1994), pp. 259-267, ISSN 0006-3495/94/01/259/09

Bermel, RA.; Sharma, J.; Tjoa, CW.; Puli, SR. & Bakshi, R. (2003). A semiautomated measure of whole-brain atrophy in multiple sclerosis. *J Neurol Sci* Vol. 208, No. 1-2, (Apr 2003), pp. 57–65, ISSN 0022-510X

Bothwell, JH. & Griffin JL. (2011). An introduction to biological nuclear magnetic resonance spectroscopy. *Biol Rev Camb Philos Soc* Vol. 86, No. 2, (May 2011), pp. 493-510, ISSN 0006-3231

Brouwer, RM.; Hulshoff, PHE. & Schnack, HG. (2010). Segmentation of MRI brain scans using non-uniform partial volume densities. *NeuroImage* Vol. 49, No. 1, (Jan 2010), pp. 467-477, ISSN 1053-8119

Bradley, WG. Jr. & Bydder, GM. (1997). *Advanced MR Imaging techniques.* Martin Dunitz Ltd, Informa Healthcare; 1 ed., , London. ISBN 978-1853170249

Boone, KB.; Miller, BL.; Lesser, IM.; Mehringer, CM.; Hill-Gutierrez, E.; Goldberg, MA. & Berman, NG. (1992). Neuropsychological correlates of white-matter lesions in healthy elderly subjects. A threshold effect. *Arch Neurol* Vol. 49, No. 5, (May 1992), pp. 549–554, ISSN 0003-9942

Bonilha, L.; Halford, JJ.; Rorden, C.; Roberts, DR.; Rumboldt, Z. & Eckert, MA. (2009). Automated MRI analysis for identification of hippocampal atrophy in temporal lobe epilepsy. *Epilepsia* Vol. 50, No. 2 (Feb 2009) pp. 228-233. ISSN 0013-9580

Buchsbaum, MS.; Tang, CY.; Peled, S.; Gudbjartsson, H.; Lu, D.; Hazlett, EA.; Downhill, J.; Haznedar, M.; Fallon, JH. & Atlas SW. (1998). MRI white matter dianffusion anisotropy and PET metabolic rate in schizophrenia. *Neuroreport* Vol. 9, No. 3 (Feb 1998), pp. 425–430, ISSN 0959-4965

Creasey, H.; Schwartz, M.; Frederickson, H.; Haxby, JV. & Rapoport, SI. (1986). Quantitative computed tomography in dementia of the Alzheimer type. *Neurology* Vol. 36, No. 12 (Dec 1986), pp. 1563-1568. ISSN 0811-8663

Chan-Palay, V. & Asan, E. (1989). Alterations in catecholamine neurons of the locus coeruleus in senile dementia of the Alzheimer type and in Parkinson's disease with and without dementia and depression. *J Comp Neurol* Vol. 287, No. 3, (Sep1989), pp. 373–392, ISSN 0021-9967

Calmon, G. & Roberts, N. (2000). Automatic measurement of changes in brain volume on consecutive 3DMR images by segmentation propagation. *Magn Reson Imaging* Vol. 18, No.4 (May 2000), pp. 439–453, ISSN 0730-725X

Cowell, PE.; Sluming, VA.; Wilkinson, ID.; Cezayirli, E.; Romanowski, CA.; Webb, JA.; Keller, SS.; Mayes, A. & Roberts, N. (2007). Effects of sex and age on regional prefrontal brain volume in two human cohorts. *Eur J Neurosci* Vol. 25, No. 1 (Jan 2007), pp. 307-318, ISSN 0953-816X

Dale, AM.; Fischl, B. & Sereno, MI. (1999). Cortical surface-based analysis I. Segmentation and surface reconstruction. *Neuroimage* Vol. 9, No. 2 (Feb 1999), pp. 179–194, ISSN 1053-8119

Davatzikos, C.; Fan, Y.; Wu, X.; Shen, D. & Resnick, SM. (2008). Detection of prodromal Alzheimer's disease via pattern classification of magnetic resonance imaging. *Neurobiol Aging* Vol. 29, No. 4 (Apr 2008), pp. 514-523, ISSN 0197-4580

Ewers M, Frisoni GB, Teipel SJ, Grinberg LT, Amaro E Jr, Heinsen H, Thompson PM. & Hampel H. (2011). Staging Alzheimer's disease progression with multimodality neuroimaging. *Prog Neurobiol* (in press). ISSN 0301-0082

Fischl, B.; Sereno, MI. & Dale, AM. (1999). Cortical surface-based analysis. II: Inflation, flattening, and a surface-based coordinate system. *Neuroimage* Vol. 9, No. 2 (Feb 1999), pp. 195–207, ISSN 1053-8119

Fischl, B., Salat, DH.; Busa, E.; Albert, M.; Dieterich, M.; Haselgrove, C.; van der Kouwe, A.; Killiany, R.; Kennedy, D.; Klaveness, S.; Montillo, A.; Makris, N.; Rosen, B. & Dale, AM. (2002). Whole brain segmentation: automated labeling of neuroanatomical structures in the human brain. *Neuron* Vol. 33, No. 3 (Jan 2002), pp. 341–355, ISSN 0896-6273

Flippi, M.; Masrtonardo, G.; Rocca, MA.; Pereira, C. & Comi, G. (1998). Quntative volumetric analysis of brain magnetic resonance imaging from patients with multiple sclerosis. *J Neurol Sci* Vol. 158, No. 2 (Jun 1998), pp. 148-153. ISSN 0022-510X

Frey, H.; Lahtinen, A.; Heinonen, T. & Dastidar, P. (1999). Clinical Application of MRI Image Processing in Neurology *IJBEM* Vol. 1, No. 1 (May 1999), pp. 47-53, ISSN 1456-7865

Furlong, C. (2008) Investigation of the precision and accuracy of surface area and volume estimators of the human brain using stereology and magnetic resonance. *Liverpool University.* Doctorate Thesis, (March 2008), England

García-Fiñana, M.; Cruz-Orive, LM.; Mackay, CE.; Pakkenberg, B. & Roberts, N. (2003). Comparison of MR imaging against physical sectioning to estimate the volume of human cerebral compartments. *Neuroimage* Vol. 18, No. 2 (Feb 2003), pp. 505-516, ISSN 1053-8119

García-Fiñana, M. (2006). Confidence intervals in Cavalieri sampling. *J Microsc* Vol. 222, No. 3, (Jun 2006), pp. 146-157, ISSN 0022-2720

García-Fiñana, M.; Keller, SS. & Roberts, N. (2009). Confidence intervals for the volume of brain structures in Cavalieri sampling with local errors. *J Neurosci Methods* Vol. 179, No. 1 (Apr 2009), pp. 71-77, ISSN 0165-0270

García-Fiñana M. & Cruze-Orive LM. (2004). Improved variance prediction for systematic on R. *Statistics* Vol. 38, No. 3, pp. 243-272, ISSN 0233-1888

García-Fiñana, M. & Cruz-Orive, LM. (2000). New approximations for the variance in cavalieri sampling. *J Microsc* Vol. 199, No. 2 (Sep 2000), pp. 224–238, ISSN 0022-2720

Geuze, E.; Vermetten, E. & Bremner, JD. (2005). MR-based in vivo hippocampal volumetrics: 1. Review of methodologies currently employed. *Mol Psychiatry* Vol. 10, No. 2 (Feb 2005), pp. 147-159, ISSN 1359-4184

Gundersen, HJ. & Jensen, EB. (1987). The efficiency of systematic sampling in stereology and its prediction. *J Microsc* Vol. 147, No. 3 (Sep 1987), pp. 229-263, ISSN 0022-2720

Gomez-Isla, T.; Hollister, R.; West, H.; Mui, S.; Growdon, JH.; Petersen, RC.; Parisi, JE. & Hyman, BT. (1997). Neuronal loss correlates with but exceeds neurofibrillary tangles in Alzheimer's disease. *Ann Neurol* Vol. 41, No. 1 (Jan 1997), pp. 17–24, ISSN 0364-5134

Gomez-Isla, T.; Price, JL.; McKeel, DW Jr.; Morris, JC.; Growdon, JH. & Hyman, BT. (1996). Profound loss of layer II entorhinal cortex neurons occurs in very mild Alzheimer's disease. *J Neurosci* Vol. 16, No. 14 (Jul 1996), pp. 4491–4500, ISSN 0270-6474

Grassiot, B.; Desgranges, B.; Eustache, F. & Defer, G. (2009). Quantification and clinical relevance of brain atrophy in multiple sclerosis: a review. *J Neurol* Vol. 256, No. 9 (Sep 2009), pp. 1397-1412, ISSN 0340-5354

Gundersen, HJ.; Jensen, EB.; Kiêu, K. & Nielsen, J. (1999). The efficiency of systematic sampling in stereology reconsidered. *J Microsc* Vol. 193, No. 4 (Mar 1999), pp. 199–211, ISSN 0022-2720

Hanyu, H.; Shindo, H.; Kakizaki D.; Abe, K.; Iwamoto, T. & Takasaki M. (1997). Increased water diffusion in cerebral white matter in Alzheimer's disease. *Gerontology* Vol. 43, No. 6 (Oct 24, 1996), pp. 343–351, ISSN 0304-324X

Henry, TR.; Chupin, M.; Lehéricy, S.; Strupp, JP.; Sikora, MA.; Sha, ZY.; Ugurbil, K. & Van de Moortele, PF. (2011). Hippocampal sclerosis in temporal lobe epilepsy: findings at 7 T. *Radiology* (in press). [Epub ahead of print]. ISSN 0033-8419

Horsfield, MA.; Rovaris, M.; Rocca, MA.; Rossi, P.; Benedict, RH.; Filippi, M. & Bakshi, R. (2003). Whole-brain atrophy in multiple sclerosis measured by two segmentation processes from various MRI sequences. *Neurol Sci* Vol. 216, No. 1 (Dec 2003), pp. 169-177, ISSN 0020-510X

Houtchens, MK.; Benedict, RH.; Killiany, R.; Sharma, J.; Jaisani, Z., Singh, B.; Weinstock-Guttman, B.; Guttmann, CR. & Bakshi, R. (2007). Thalamic atrophy and cognition in multiple sclerosis. *Neurology* Vol. 69, No. 17 (Sep 2007), pp. 1213–1223, ISSN 0028-3878

Herndon, RC., Lancaster, JL., Giedd, JN. & Fox, PT. (1998). Quantification of white matter and gray matter volumes from three-dimensional magnetic resonance golume studies using fuzzy classifiers. *J Magn Reson Imaging* Vol. 8, No. 5 (Sep 1998), pp. 1097-1005, ISSN 1053-1807

Jones, EK.; Simmons, A.; Williams, SCR. & Horsfield, MA. (1999). Non-invasive assessment of axonal fiber connectivity in the human brain via diffusion tensor MRI. *Magn Reson Med* Vol. 42, No. 1 (July 1999), pp. 37–41, ISSN 1522-2594

Keller, SS. & Roberts, N. (2009). Measurement of brain volume using MRI: software, techniques, choices and prerequisites. *Journal of Anthropological Sciences* Vol. 87, pp. 127-151, ISSN 1827-4765

Keller, SS.; Mackay, CE.,; Barrick, TR.; Wieshmann, UC.; Howard, MA. & Roberts N. (2002). Voxel-based morphometric comparison of hippocampal and extrahippocampal abnormalities in patients with left and right hippocampal atrophy. *Neuroimage* Vol. 16, No. 1 (May 2002), pp. 23-31, ISSN 1053-8119

Keller SS.; Highley JR.; Garcia-Finana M.; Sluming V.; Rezaie R. & Roberts N. (2007). Sulcal variability, stereological measurement and asymmetry of Broca's area on MR images. *J Anat* Vol. 211, No. 4 (Oct 2007), pp. 534-555, ISSN 0021-8782

Keller, SS & Roberts, N. (2008). Voxel-based morphometry of temporal lobe epilepsy: An introduction and review of the literature. *Epilepsia* (May 2008), Vol. 49, No. 5, pp. 741-757, ISSN 0013-9580

Kern, A. & Behl, C. (2009). The unsolved relationship of brain aging and late-onset Alzheimer disease *Biochimica et Biophysica Acta (BBA)* Vol. 1790, No. 10, (Oct 2009), pp. 1124-1132, ISSN 0304-4165

Kesslak, JP.; Nalcioglu, O. & Cotman, CW. (1991). Quantification of magnetic resonance scans for hippocampal and parahippocampal atrophy in Alzheimer's disease. *Neurology* Vol. 41, No. 1 (Jan 1991), pp. 51–54, ISSN 0811-8663

Kucharczyk, W. & Henkelman, M. (1994). Visibility of Calcium on MR and CT: can MR show calcium that CT can not?. *AJNR Am J Neuroradiol.* Vol. 15, No. 6 (Jun 1994), pp. 1145–1148, ISSN 0195-6108

Likeman, M.; Anderson, VM.; Stevens, JM.; Waldman, AD.; Godbolt, AK.; Frost, C.; Rossor, MN. & Fox, NC. (2005). Visual assessment of atrophy on magnetic resonance imaging in the diagnosis of pathologically confirmed young-onset demantias. *Arch Neurol* Vol. 62, No. 9 (Sept 2005), pp. 1410-1415, ISSN 0003-9942

Lim, OK.; Rosenbloom, M. & Pfefferbaum, A. (2000). In Vivo Structural Brain Assessment: In: *Psychopharmacology-4th Generation of Progress,* Bloom FE, Kupfer DJ. (Ed.), Part II Clinic section, ISBN 978-0781701662.
http://www.acnp.org/g4/GN401000089/Default.htm

Liu, YS.; Yi, J.; Zhang, H.; Zheng, G. & Paul, JC. (2010). Surface area estimation of digitized 3D objects using quasi-Monte Carlo methods. *Pattern Recogn.* Vol. 43, No. 11 (November 2010), pp. 3900-3909, ISSN 0031-3203

Loewe, C.; Oschatz, E. & Prayer, D. (2002). Imaging of Neurodegenerative Disorders of the Brain in Adults. *Imaging Decisions* Vol. 6, Suplement 1 (Dec 2002), pp. 4-18, ISSN 1617-0830

Lopez, OL.; Becker, JT.; Rezek, D.; Wess, J.; Boller F.; Reynolds CF, 3rd. & Panisset, M. (1992). Neuropsychiatric correlates of cerebral white-matter radiolucencies in probable Alzheimer's disease. *Arch Neurol* Vol. 49, No. 8 (Aug 1992), pp. 828–834, ISSN 0003-9942

Mackay, CE.; Roberts, N.; Mayes, AR.; Downes, JJ.; Foster, JK. & Mann, D. (1998). An exploratory study of the relationship between face recognition memory and the volume of medial temporal lobe structures in healthy young males. *Behav Neurol* Vol. 11, No. 1 (Jan 1998), pp. 3-20, ISSN 0953-4180

Masliah, E.; Terry, R.; Alford, M.; DeTeresa, R. & Hansen, LA. (1991). Cortical and subcortical patterns of synaptophysin-like immunoreactivity in Alzheimer's disease. *Am J Pathol* Vol. 138, No. 1 (Jan 1991), pp. 235–246, ISSN 0002-9440

Mazziotta, JC.; Frackowiak, RSJ. & Phelps, ME. (1992). The use of positron emission tomography in the clinical assessment of dementia. *Semin Nucl Med* Vol. 22, No. 4 (Oct 1992), pp. 233–246, ISSN 0001-2998

McKhann, GM.; Albert, MS.; Grossman, M.; Miller, B.; Dickson, D. & Trojanowski, JQ. (2001). Clinical and pathological diagnosis of frontotemporal dementia: Report of the Work Group on Frontotemporal Dementia and Pick's Disease. *Arch Neurol* Vol. 58, No. 11 (Nov 2001), pp. 1803-1809, ISSN 0003-9942

Mohamed, FB.; Vinitski, S.; Faro, SH.; Gonzalez, CF.; Mack, J. & Iwanaga, T. (1999). Optimization of tissue segmentation of brain MR images based on multispectral 3D feature maps. *Magn. Reson. Imaging* Vol.17, No. 3 (Apr 1999), pp. 403–409, ISSN 0730-725X

Mohs, RC. & Haroutunian, V. (2002) Chapter 82: Alzheimer Disease: From Earliest Symptoms to End Stage, *Neuropsychopharmacology*: pp. 1189-1197. Edited by Kenneth L. Davis, Dennis Charney, Joseph T. Coyle, and Charles Nemeroff. American College of Neuropsychopharmacology The Fifth Generation of Progress

Molyneux, PD.; Kappos, L.; Polman, C.; Pozzilli, C.; Barkhof, F.; Filippi, M.; Yousry, T; Hahn, D.; Wagner, K.; Ghazi, M.; Beckmann, K.; Dahlke, F.; Losseff, N.; Barker, GJ.; Thompson, AJ. & Miller, DH. (2000). The effect of interferon beta-1b treatment on MRI measures of cerebral atrophy in secondary progressive multiple sclerosis. European Study Group on Interferon Beta-1b in Secondary Progressive Multiple Sclerosis. *Brain* Vol. 123, No. 11 (Nov 2000), pp. 2256-2263, ISSN 0006-8950

Nagy, Z.; Esiri, MM.; Jobst, KA.; Morris, JH.; King, EM.; McDonald, B.; Litchfield, S.; Smith, A.; Barnetson, L. & Smith, AD. (1995). Relative roles of plaques and tangles in the dementia of Alzheimer's disease: correlations using three sets of neuropathological criteria. *Dementia* Vol. 6, No. 1 (Jan 1995), pp. 21–31, ISSN 1013-7424

Nakamura, K. & Fisher, E. (2009). Segmentation of brain magnetic resonance iamges for measuremnt of gray matter atrophy in multple sclerosis patients. *Neuroimage* Vol. 44, No. 3 (Feb 2009), pp. 796-776, ISSN 1053-8119

Neary, D,; Snowden, JS.; Gustafson, L.; Passant, U.; Stuss, D.; Black, S.; Freedman, M.; Kertesz, A.; Robert, PH.; Albert, M.; Boone, K.; Miller, BL.; Cummings, J. & Benson, DF. (1998). Frontotemporal lobar degeneration: A consensus on clinical diagnostic criteria. *Neurology* Vol. 51, No. 6 (Dec 1998), pp. 1546-1554, ISSN 0811-8663

Obrien, JT. (2007). Role of imaging techniques in the diagnosis of dementia. *Br J Radiol* Vol. 80, No. 2 (Dec 20074), pp. 71-77, ISSN 0007-1285

O'Sullivan, M. (2009). Patterns of brain atrophy on magnetic resonance imaging and the boundary between ageing and Alzheimer's disease. *Rev Clin Gerontol* Vol. 19, No. 4 (Nov 2009), pp. 295-307, ISSN 0959-2598

Pearlson, GD.; Harris, GJ.; Powers, RE.; Barta, PE.; Camargo, EE.; Chase, GA.; Noga, JT. & Tune, LE. (1992). Quantitative changes in mesial temporal volume, regional cerebral blood flow, and cognition in Alzheimer's disease. *Arch Gen Psychiatry* Vol. 49, No. 5 (May 1992), pp. 402–408. ISSN 0003-990X

Pelletier, D.; Garrison, K. & Henry, R. (2004). Measurement of whole brain atrophy in multiple sclerosis. *J Neuroimaging* Vol. 14, No. 3 (Jul 2004), pp.11S–19S, ISSN 1051-2284

Pham, DL. & Prince, JL. (1999). Adaptive fuzzy segmentation of magnetic resonance images. *IEEE Trans Med Imag* Vol. 18, No. 9 (Sep 1999), pp. 737–752, ISSN 0278-0062

Ratnavalli, E.; Brayne, C.; Dawson, K. & Hodges, JR. (2002). The prevalence of frontotemporal dementia. *Neurology* Vol. 58, No. 11 (Jun 2002), pp. 1615-1621. ISSN 0811-8663

Rusinek, H.; de Leon, MJ.; George, AE.; Stylopoulos, LA.; Chandra, R.; Smith, G.; Rand, T.; Mourino, M. & Kowalski, H. (1991). Alzheimer disease: measuring loss of cerebral gray matter with MR imaging. *Radiology* Vol. 178, No. 1 (Jan 1991), pp. 109–114. ISSN 0033-8419

Rosen, HJ.; Gorno-Tempini, ML.; Goldman, WP.; Perry, RJ.; Schuff, N.; Weiner, M.; Feiwell, R.; Kramer, JH. & Miller, BL. (2002). Patterns of brain atrophy in frontotemporal dementia and semantic dementia. *Neurology* Vol. 58, No. 2 (Jan 2002), pp. 198–208. ISSN 0811-8663

Rosen, HJ.; Allison, SC.; Schauer, GF.; Gorno-Tempini, ML.; Weiner, MW. & Miller, BL. (2005). Neuroanatomical correlates of behavioural disorders in dementia. *Brain* Vol. 128, No. 11 (Nov 2005), pp. 2612–2625. ISSN 0006-8950

Rosen, HJ.; Wilson, MR.; Schauer, GF.; Allison S.; Gorno-Tempini ML.; Pace-Savitsky C.; Kramer JH.; Levenson RW.; Weiner M. & Miller BL. (2006). Neuroanatomical correlates of impaired recognition of emotion in dementia. *Neuropsychologia* Vol. 44, No. 3 (Sep 2005), pp. 365–373, ISSN 0028-3932

Ron, MA.; Acker, W.; Shaw, GK. & Lishman, WA. (1982). Computerized tomography of the brain in chronic alcoholism: a survey and follow-up study. *Brain* Vol. 105, No. 3 (Sep 1982), pp. 497-514. ISSN 0006-8950

Roberts, N.; Puddephat, MJ. & McNulty, V. (2000). The benefit of stereology for quantitative radiology. *Br J Radiol* Vol. 73, No. 871 (Jul 200), pp. 679-697, ISSN 0007-1285.

Sahin, B. & Ergur, H. (2006). Assessment of the optimum section thickness for the estimation of liver volume using magnetic resonance images: a stereological gold standard study. *Eur J Radiol* Vol. 57, No. 1 (Jan 2006), pp. 96-101. ISSN 0720-04X

Sahin, B.; Emirzeoglu, M.; Uzun, A.; Incesu, L.; Bek, Y.; Bilgic, S. & Kaplan, S. (2003). Unbiased estimation of the liver volume by the Cavalieri principle using magnetic resonance images. *Eur J Radiol* Vol. 47, No. 2 (Aug 2003), pp. 164– 170, ISSN 0720-04X

Sanfilipo, MP.; Benedict, RH.; Sharma, J.; Weinstock-Guttman, B. & Bakshi, R. (2005). The relationship between whole brain volume and disability in multiple sclerosis: a comparison of normalized gray vs white matter with misclassification correction. *Neuroimage* Vol. 26, No. 4 (July 2005), pp. 1068–1077. ISSN 1053-8119

Sanfilipo, MP.; Benedict, RH.; Weinstock-Guttman, B. & Bakshi, R. (2006). Gray and white matter brain atrophy and neuropsychological impairment in multiple sclerosis. *Neurology* Vol. 66, No. 5 (Mar 2006), pp. 685–692, ISSN 0811-8663

Schuckit, MA. (1992). An introduction and overview of clinical applications of NeuroSPECT in psychiatry. *J Clin Psychiatry* Vol. 53, Suppl (November 1992), pp. 3–6, ISSN 0160-6689

Schuff, N.; Amend, D.; Ezekiel, F.; Steinman, SK.; Tanabe, J.; Norman, D.; Jagust, W.; Kramer, JH.; Mastrianni, JA.; Fein, G. & Weiner, MW. (1997). Changes of hippocampal N-acetyl aspartate and volume in Alzheimer's disease: a proton MR spectroscopic imaging and MRI study. *Neurology* Vol. 49, No. 6, pp. 1513–1521. ISSN 0811-8663

Seppi, K. & Schocke, MF. (2005). An update on conventional and advanced magnetic resonance imaging techniques in the differential diagnosis of neurodegenerative parkinsonism. *Curr Opin Neurol* Vol. 18, No. 4 (Aug 2005), pp. 370–375. ISSN 1350-7540

Sharma, J.; Sanfilipo , MP.; Benedict, RH.;Weinstock-Guttman, B.; Munschauer, FEIII.. & Bakshi, R. (2004). Whole-brain atrophy in multiple sclerosis measured by automated versus semiautomated MR imaging segmentation. *AJNR Am J Neuroradiol* Vol. 25, No. 6 (Jun 2004), pp. 985–996, ISSN 0195-6108

Small, GW. (2002). Structural And Functional Brain Imaging of Alzheimer Disease. *Neuropsychopharmacology: The Fifth Generation of Progress,* Davis, KL.; Charney, D.; Joyle, J. (Ed). pp. 1232-1242. ISBN 978-0781728379.

Smith, SM.; Zhang, Y.; Jenkinson, M.; Chen, J.; Matthews, PM.; Federico, A. & De Stefano, N. (2002). Accurate, robust, and automated longitudinal and cross-sectional brain change analysis, *Neuroimage* Vol. 17, No. 1 (Sep 2002), pp. 479–489, ISSN 1053-8119

Stokking, R.; Vincken, KL. & Viergever, MA. (2000). Automatic morphology-based brain segmentation (MBRASE) from MRI-T1 data. *Neuroimage* Vol. 12, No. 6 (Dec 2000), pp. 726–738, ISSN 1053-8119

Suckling, J.; Sigmundsson, T.; Greenwood, K. & Bullmore, ET. (1999). A modified fuzzy clustering algorithm for operator independent brain tissue classification of dual echo MR images. *Magn Reson Imaging* Vol. 17, No. 7 (Sep 1999), pp. 1065–1076, ISSN 0730-725X

Suri, JS.; Setarehdan, SK. & Singh, S. (2002). Advanced Algorithmic Approaches to Medical Image Segmentation: *State-of-the-Art Applications in Cardiology, Neurology, Mammography and Pathology*. Spring- Verlag, London/Berlin/Heidelberg, ISBN 978-1-85233-389-8

Terry, RD.; Peck, A.; DeTeresa, R.; Schechter, R. & Horoupian, DS. (1981). Some morphometric aspects of the brain in senile dementia of the Alzheimer type. *Ann Neurol* Vol. 10, No. 2 (Aug 1981), pp. 184–192, ISSN 0364-5134

Teipel, SJ.; Bayer, W.; Alexander, GE.; Bokde, AL.; Zebuhr, Y.; Teichberg, D.; Müller-Spahn, F.; Schapiro, MB.; Möller, HJ.; Rapoport, SI. & Hampel, H. (2003). Regional pattern of hippocampus and corpus callosum atrophy in Alzheimer's disease in relation to dementia severity: evidence for early neocortical degeneration. *Neurobiol Aging* Vol. 24, No. 1 (Jan 2003), pp. 85–94, ISSN 0197-4580

Tosun, D.; Rettmann, ME.; Han, X.; Tao, X., Xu, C.; Resnick, SM., Dzung, LP. & Prince, JL. (2004). Cortical surface segmentation and mapping, *NeuroImage* Vol. 23, Suppl. 1, pp. 108-118, ISSN 1053-8119

Ueda, K.; Fujiwara, H.; Miyata, J.; Hirao, K.; Saze, T.; Kawata, R.; Fujimoto, S., Tanaka, Y., Sawamoto, N.; Fukuyama, H. & Murai T. (2009). Investigating association of brain volumes with intracranial capacity in schizophrenia. *Neuroimage* Vol. 19, No. 3, (Sep 2009), pp. 2503-2508, ISSN 1053-8119

Vitali, P.; Migliaccio, R.; Agosta, F.; Rosen, HJ. & Geschwind, MD. (2008). Neuroimaging in dementia. *Semin Neurol* Vol. 28, No. 4, pp. 467-483. ISSN 0271-8235

Wagner, AD.; Schacter, DL.; Rotte, M.; Koutstaal, W.; Maril, A.; Dale, AM.; Rosen, BR. & Buckner, RL. (1998). Building memories: remembering and forgetting of verbal experiences as predicted by brain activity. *Science* Vol. 281, No. 5380 (Aug 1998), pp.1188-1191, ISSN 0036-8075

Webb, J.; Guimond, A., Eldridge, P.; Chadwick, D.; Meunier, J. & Thirion, JP. (1999). Automatic detection of hippocampal atrophy on magnetic resonance images. *Magn Reson Imaging* Vol. 17, No. 8 (Oct 1999), pp. 1149–1161, ISSN 0730-725X

Weiner, MW. (1987). NMR spectroscopy for clinical medicine, animal models, and clinical examples. *Ann NY Acad Sci* Vol. 508, (November 1987), pp. 287–289, ISSN 1749-6632

Whitehouse, PJ.; Price, DL.; Struble, RG.; Clark, AW.; Coyle, JT. & Delon, MR. (1982). Alzheimer's disease and senile dementia: loss of neurons in the basal forebrain. *Science* Vol. 215, No. 4537 (Mar 1982), pp. 1237–1239, ISSN 0036-8075

Yamauchi, H.; Fukuyama, H.; Nagahama, Y.; Katsumi, Y.; Hayashi, T.; Oyanagi, C.; Konishi, J. & Shio, H. (2000). Comparison of the pattern of atrophy of the corpus callosum in frontotemporal dementia, progressive supranuclear palsy, and Alzheimer's disease. *J Neurol Neurosurg Psychiatry* Vol. 69, No. 5, (Nov 2000), pp. 623–629, ISSN 0022-3050

Zweig, RM.; Ross, CA.; Hedreen, JC.; Steele, C.; Cardillo, JE.; Whitehouse, PJ.; Folstein, MF. & Price, DL. (1988). The neuropathology of aminergic nuclei in Alzheimer's disease. *Ann Neurol* Vol. 24, No. 2, (Aug 1988), pp. 233–242, ISSN 0364-5134

Zhou, Y. & Bai, J. (2007). Atlas-based fuzzy connectedness segmentation and intensity nonuniformity correction applied to brain MRI. *IEEE Trans. Biomed Eng* Vol. 54, No. 1, pp. 122–129, ISSN 0278-0062

20

Acid-Sensing Ion Channels in Neurodegenerative Diseases: Potential Therapeutic Target

Chu Xiang-Ping[1], Wang John Q.[1] and Xiong Zhi-Gang[2]
[1]*Department of Basic Medical Science, University of Missouri-Kansas City, Kansas City, Missouri;*
[2]*Department of Neurobiology, Morehouse School of Medicine, Atlanta, Georgia; USA*

1. Introduction

Under pathological conditions such as tissue inflammation, ischemic stroke, traumatic brain injury, and epileptic seizure, accumulations of lactic acid due to enhanced anaerobic glucose metabolism and the release of proton from ATP hydrolysis result in significant reduction of tissue pH, a condition termed acidosis. Acidosis can activate a distinct family of ion channels: acid-sensing ion channels (ASICs) (Waldmann et al., 1997b), which are heavily expressed in the peripheral sensory and central neurons (Waldmann & Lazdunski, 1998; Krishtal, 2003; Wemmie et al., 2006; Lingueglia, 2007; Xiong et al., 2006, 2007, 2008; Sluka et al., 2009). ASICs belong to the amiloride-sensitive degenerin/epithelial Na^+ channel (DEG/ENaC) superfamily (Kellenberger & Schild, 2002). Four genes (*ACCN1 - 4*) encoding at least six ASIC subunits have been cloned. Each subunit has two transmembrane domains with a large extracellular loop and short intracellular N- and C-termini (Waldmann et al., 1997b). Functional ASICs are trimeric complexes of these subunits (Jasti et al., 2007; Gonzales et al., 2009) and most of these subunits can form homomeric and/or heteromeric channels (Benson et al., 2002; Baron et al., 2002, 2008; Wemmie et al., 2002, 2003; Askwith et al., 2004; Chu et al., 2004, 2006; Xiong et al., 2004; Zha et al., 2006; Sherwood et al., 2011). ASICs are enriched in brain neurons (Alvarez de la Rosa et al., 2003; Wemmie et al., 2003; Xiong et al., 2004; Sherwood et al., 2011), where at least three (ASIC1a, ASIC2a and ASIC2b) of the seven subunits can be found. ASIC1a is the dominant subunit in brain and homomeric ASIC1a and heteromeric ASIC1a/2b channels are permeable to both Na^+ and Ca^{2+} ions (Waldmann et al., 1997b; Yermolaieva et al., 2004; Zha et al., 2006; Sherwood et al., 2011). ASICs are inhibited by the diuretic amiloride, a non-specific ASIC blocker (Waldmann et al., 1997b). The tarantula toxin psalmotoxin 1 (PcTX1) blocks the homomeric ASIC1a (Escoubas et al., 2000) and heteromeric ASIC1a/2b (Sherwood et al., 2011) channels. The roles of ASICs in a variety of neurologic conditions are still under active investigation. ASIC1a channels localize at synapse and contribute to synaptic plasticity, learning/memory, and fear conditioning (Wemmie et al., 2002, 2003, 2004). Activation of Ca^{2+}-permeable homomeric ASIC1a and heteromeric ASIC1a/2b channels is involved in acidosis-mediated ischemic brain injury (Xiong et al., 2004; Pignataro et al., 2007; Sherwood et al., 2011). Moreover, ASIC1a channels play critical roles in neurodegenerative diseases such as multiple sclerosis (Friese et al., 2007; Vergo et al., 2011), Parkinson's (Arias et al., 2008) and Huntington's (Wong et al., 2008) disease and in seizures (Chang et al., 2007; Ziemann et al., 2008) and depression (Coryell et al., 2009). Thus, controlling their activation might ameliorate acidosis-mediated CNS disorders (Xiong et al., 2008). This chapter provides an overview of recent advance in electrophysiological properties as well as pharmacological profiles of ASICs, and their roles in neurodegenerative disorders.

2. Electrophysiological and pharmacological properties of ASICs

2.1 Electrophysiological properties of ASICs

The electrophysiological properties and pharmacological profiles of ASICs have been extensively explored in heterologous expression systems (Chu et al., 2004; Hesselager et al., 2004) and in neurons from different brain regions, such as cortex (Varming, 1998; Xiong et al., 2004; Chu et al., 2004, 2006), hippocampus (Baron et al., 2002; Askwith et al., 2004), striatum (Jiang et al., 2009), cerebellum (Allen & Attwell, 2002), retinal ganglion (Lilley et al., 2004), and spinal cord (Wu et al., 2004; Baron et al., 2008). Fig. 1 shows typical ASIC current mediated by homomeric ASIC1a, 1b, 2a, or 3 channels expressed in CHO cells.

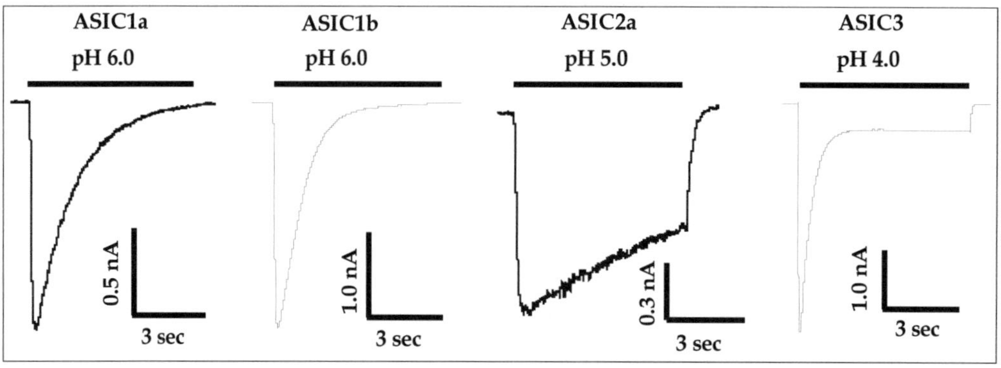

Fig. 1. Acid-triggered inward currents in CHO cells expressing indicated ASIC subunits

Homomeric ASIC1a channels have a pH for half-maximal activation (pH_{50}) between 6.2 and 6.8 (Babini et al., 2002; Benson et al., 2002; Chu et al., 2002; Jiang et al., 2009). Although the precise configuration of ASICs in native neurons is not clear, homomeric ASIC1a and heteromeric ASIC1a/2 channels are the major components in brain neurons (Wemmie et al., 2002; Askwith et al., 2004; Xiong et al., 2004; Jiang et al., 2009; Sherwood et al., 2011). For example, our recent studies have shown that rapid drops in extracellular pH from 7.4 to lower levels (e.g., 6.5, 6.0, 5.0 and 4.0) induced transient inward currents in cultured medium spiny neurons (MSNs) of the mouse striatum (Fig. 2A) (Jiang et al., 2009). The dose-response curve for activation of ASICs revealed a pH_{50} value of 6.25 (Fig. 2B). This pH_{50} value of ASICs in MSNs is comparable to that of homomeric ASIC1a channels (Walmann et al., 1997). The ASIC currents in MSNs had a linear I-V relationship with a reversal potential close to +60 mV (Fig. 2C, D), indicating that ASICs in MSNs are Na^+-selective.

In contrast to homomeric ASIC1a channels, the following properties distinguish rodent ASIC1b from ASIC1a: (1), although the amino acid sequence of approximately 2/3 of the

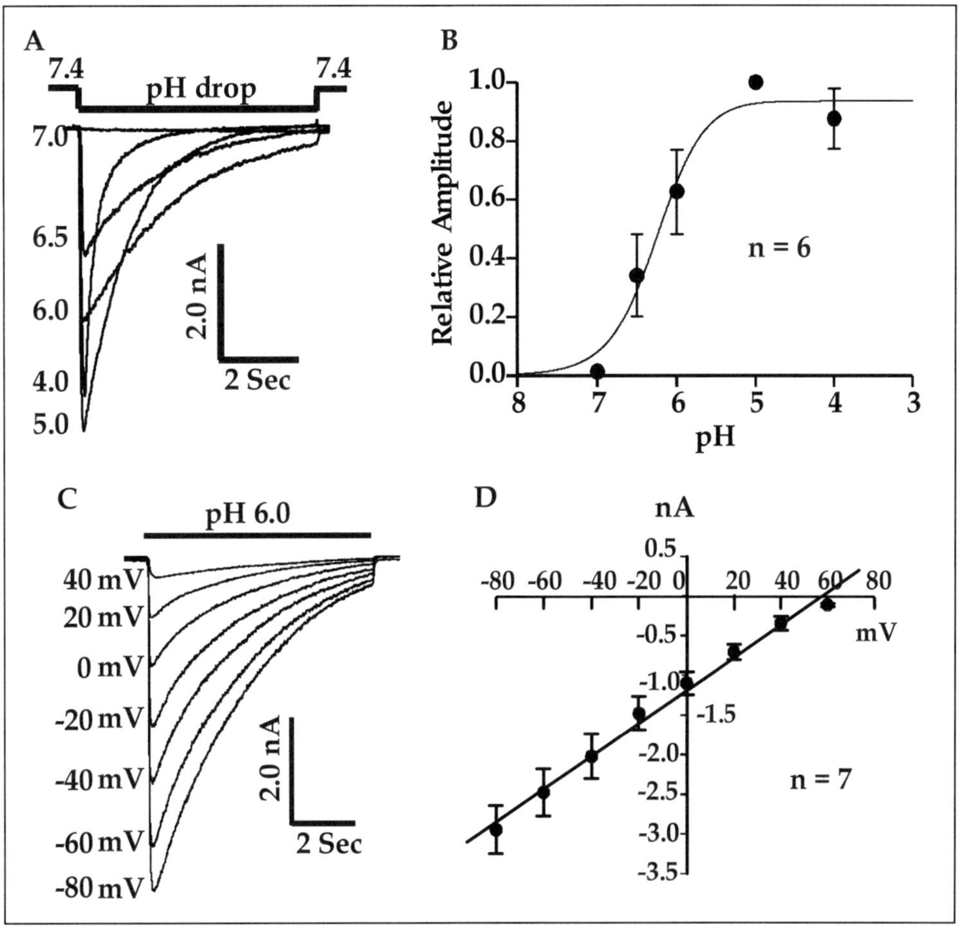

Fig. 2. Electrophysiological properties of ASICs in cultured mouse MSNs. (A) pH-dependent activation of ASIC currentsin in MSNs. (B) Dose-response curve for activation of the currents by pH drops. The pH_{50} value is 6.25 and the Hill coeficient is 0.94. (C) The I-V relationship of acid-activated currents with different holding levels by decreasing the pH from 7.4 to 6.0 in MSNs. (D) The I-V curve. The extrapolated reversal potential is close to 60 mV, which is close to the sodium equilibrium potential

ASIC1a and ASIC1b proteins are identical, there are significant differences in the sequence for the first one third (about 172 amino acids) of the protein beginning at the N terminal; this sequence includes the intracellular N-terminus, the first transmembrane domain, and the proximal part of the ectodomain (Chen et al., 1998; Bassler et al., 2001); (2), the expression of ASIC1b in the nervous system is limited to peripheral sensory neurons, while ASIC1a is also expressed in the CNS; (3), rodent ASIC1b is impermeable to Ca^{2+} while ASIC1a channels have significant Ca^{2+} permeability; Interestingly, a recent study has shown that human ASIC1b channels are permeable to Ca^{2+} (Hoagland et al., 2010); (4), the threshold for activation of ASIC1b current is lower than ASIC1a (~6.5 for ASIC1b and ~7.0 for ASIC1a) and it has lower pH_{50} (5.9); (5), ASIC1b is potentiated by PcTx1(Chen et al., 2006), which is a specific inhibitor of ASIC1a.

Homomeric ASIC2a channels are relatively insensitive to proton, with a pH_{50} of 4.4 (Price et al., 1996; Waldmann et al., 1996; Lingueglia et al., 1997). However, ASIC2a subunits can associate with ASIC1a to form heteromeric channels in brain (Askwith et al., 2004; Chu et al., 2004, 2006; Xiong et al., 2004; Jiang et al., 2009). Different from homomeric ASIC2a subunits, homomeric ASIC2b subunits do not form functional channels by themselves, but can associate with other ASIC subunits to form heteromultimeric channels (Lingueglia et al., 1997; Hesselager et al., 2004; Sherwood et al., 2011). For example, ASIC2b can be associated with ASIC1a to form functional channels and contribute to acidosis-induced neuronal injury (Sherwood et al., 2011).

ASIC3, like ASIC1b (Chen et al., 1998), is expressed primarily in peripheral sensory neurons (Waldmann et al., 1997a; Babinski et al., 1999; Wu et al., 2004; Lingueglia, 2007; Lin et al., 2008). In contrast to other subunits of ASICs, homomeric ASIC3 channels can respond to a large drop of extracellular pH with a transient inactivating current followed by a sustained component (Waldmann et al., 1997a; Sanilas et al., 2009) (Fig. 1). The transient currents are highly sensitive to protons, with a pH_{50} of around 6.5 (Waldmann et al., 1997a; Hesselager et al., 2004). Electrophysiological studies have shown that ASIC3 subunits function as homomeric or heteromeric channels in sensory neurons (Sutherland et al., 2001; Benson et al., 2002; Deval et al., 2004, 2008; Lin et al., 2008; Hattori et al., 2009). They can sense extracellular acidification occurring in physiological and/or pathological processes, such as cutaneous touch, pain perception, inflammation and ischemia (Benson et al., 1999; Immke & McCleskey, 2001; Price et al., 2001; Sutherland et al., 2001; Mamet et al., 2003; Molliver et al., 2005; Sluka et al., 2007; Ikeuchi et al., 2009). For example, ASIC3 channels expressed in cardiac sensory neurons can respond to myocardial ischemia (Benson et al., 1999; Sutherland et al., 2001; Yagi et al., 2006). Further, cutaneous sensory neurons from rats display large ASIC3-like currents when stimulated by moderate acidosis (Deval et al., 2008). Consequently, it is generally accepted that ASIC3 is a sensor of moderate acidosis during ischemia and inflammatory pain in sensory neurons (Lingueglia, 2007).

ASIC4 subunits are expressed in pituitary gland. Similar to ASIC2b, they do not seem to form functional homomeric channels (Aropian et al., 2000; Grunder et al., 2000).

2.2 Pharmacological profiles of ASICs

2.2.1 Amiloride

Amiloride, the potassium-sparing diuretic agent, is a commonly used nonspecific blocker for ASICs. It inhibits the ASIC current and acid-induced increase in intracellular Ca^{2+} ($[Ca^{2+}]_i$) with an IC_{50} of 10–60 μM (Waldmann et al., 1997b; de Weille et al., 1998; Chen et al., 1998; Benson et al., 1999; Chu et al., 2002; Wu et al., 2004; Xiong et al., 2004; Yermolaieva et al., 2004; Jiang et al., 2009). For example, our recent study has shown that amiloride dose-dependently inhibited the ASIC currents in MSNs with an IC_{50} of 13.6 μM (Fig. 3) (Jiang et al., 2009). Unlike the currents mediated by other homomeric ASICs, however, the sustained current mediated by homomeric ASIC3 channels is insensitive to amiloride (Waldmann et al., 1997b; Benson et al., 1999; Yagi et al., 2006). Based on the studies of ENaC, it is believed that amiloride inhibits ASICs by a direct blockade of the channel (Schild et al., 1997; Adams et al., 1999). The pre-TM II region of the channel is critical for the effect of amiloride. Mutation of Gly-430 in this region, for example, dramatically changed the sensitivity of ASIC2a current to amiloride (Champigny et al., 1998). Consistent with its inhibition on the ASIC current, amiloride has been shown to suppress acid-induced pain in peripheral sensory system (Ugawa et al., 2002; Sluka et al., 2003; Jones et al., 2004; Dube et al., 2005), and acidosis-mediated injury of CNS neurons (Xiong et al., 2004; Yermolaieva et al., 2004). However, because of its nonspecificity for other ion channels (e.g., ENaC and T-type Ca^{2+} channels) and ion exchange systems (e.g., Na^+/H^+ and Na^+/Ca^{2+} exchanger), it is less likely that amiloride will be used as a future neuroprotective agent in human subjects. It is worth mentioning that the normal activity of Na^+/Ca^{2+} exchanger, for example, is critical for maintaining the cellular Ca^{2+} homeostasis and the survival of neurons against delayed calcium deregulation caused by glutamate receptor activation (Bano et al., 2005). Inhibition of Na^+/Ca^{2+} exchange by amiloride may therefore compromise normal neuronal Ca^{2+} handling, thus potentiating the glutamate toxicity (Bano et al., 2005).

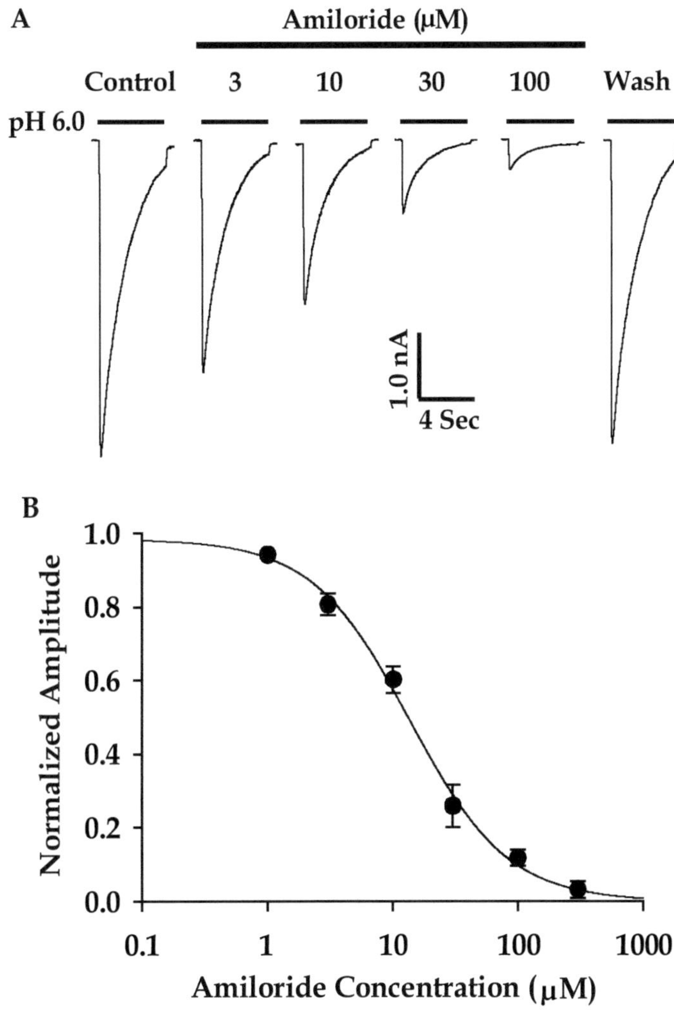

Fig. 3. Dose-dependent blockade of ASIC currents in cultured MSNs by amiloride, a non-specific ASIC blocker. (A) Amiloride dose-dependently inhibits the ASIC currents activated by pH 6.0. (B) Dose-inhibition curve of the acid-induced currents by amiloride. The IC_{50} of amiloride is 13.6 μM

2.2.2 A-317567

A-317567, a small molecule structurally unrelated to amiloride, is another nonselective ASIC blocker (Dube et al., 2005). It inhibits the ASIC1a, ASIC2a, and ASIC3-like currents with an IC_{50} of 2–30 µM. Unlike amiloride, which has no effect on the slow component of the ASIC3 current, A-317567 blocks both the fast and the sustained ASIC3 currents. Also different from amiloride, A-317567 does not show diuresis or natriuresis activity (Dube et al., 2005), suggesting that it is more specific for ASICs than amiloride. Its inhibition of sustained ASIC3 current suggests that it might be potent in reducing acidosis-mediated chronic pain. Indeed, A-317567 has been shown to be effective in suppressing the pain in a rat model of thermal hyperalgesia at a dose tenfold lower than amiloride (Dube et al., 2005).

2.2.3 PcTX1

Being a peptide toxin isolated from venom of the South American tarantula *Psalmopoeus cambridgei*, PcTX1 is a potent and specific inhibitor for homomeric ASIC1a channels (Escoubas et al., 2000). This toxin contains 40 amino acids cross-linked by three disulfide bridges. In heterologous expression systems, PcTX1 specifically inhibits the acid-activated current mediated by homomeric ASIC1a subunits with an IC_{50} of 1 nM (Escoubas et al., 2000). At concentrations that effectively inhibit the ASIC1a current, it has no effect on the currents mediated by other configurations of ASICs (Escoubas et al., 2000), or known voltage-gated Na^+, K^+, Ca^{2+} channels as well as several ligand-gated ion channels (Xiong et al., 2004). Unlike amiloride, which directly blocks the ASICs, PcTX1 acts as a gating modifier. It shifts the channel from its resting state toward the inactivated state by increasing its apparent affinity for protons (Chen et al., 2005). Recently, PcTX1 has also been shown to suppress heteromeric ASIC1a/2b channels (Sherwood et al., 2011).

2.2.4 APETx2

Being a peptide toxin isolated from sea anemone *Anthopleura elegantissima*, APETx2 is a potent and selective inhibitor for homomeric ASIC3 and ASIC3 containing channels (Diochot et al., 2004). The toxin contains 42 amino acids, also cross-linked by three disulfide bridges. It reduces transient peak acid-evoked currents mediated by homomeric ASIC3 channels (Diochot et al., 2004). In contrast to the peak ASIC3 current, the sustained component of the ASIC3 current is insensitive to APETx2. In addition to homomeric ASIC3 channels (IC_{50} = 63 nM for rat and 175 nM for human), APETx2 inhibits heteromeric ASIC3/1a (IC_{50} = 2 µM), ASIC3/1b (IC_{50} = 900 nM), and ASIC3/2b (IC_{50} = 117 nM). Homomeric ASIC1a, ASIC1b, ASIC2a, and heteromeric ASIC3/2a channels, on the other hand, are not sensitive to APETx2 (Diochot et al., 2004).

2.2.5 Nonsteroid anti-inflammatory drugs (NSAIDs)

NSAIDs are the most commonly used anti-inflammatory and analgesic agents. They inhibit the synthesis of prostaglandins (PGs), a main tissue inflammatory substance. A recent study demonstrated that NSAIDs also inhibit the activity of ASICs at their therapeutic doses for analgesic effects (Voilley et al., 2001). Ibuprofen and flurbiprofen, for example, inhibit ASIC1a containing channels with an IC_{50} of 350 µM. Aspirin and salicylate inhibit ASIC3 containing channels with an IC_{50} of 260 µM, whereas diclofenac inhibits the same channels with an IC_{50} of 92 µM. In addition to a direct inhibition of the ASIC activity, NSAIDs also prevent inflammation-induced increase of ASIC expression in sensory neurons (Voilley et al., 2001).

2.2.6 Aminoglycosides (AGs)

AGs (streptomycin, neomycin and gentamicin) are a group of antibiotics that have been shown to block Ca^{2+} channels (Zhou and Zhao, 2002), excitatory amino acid receptors (Pérez et al., 1991), and transient-receptor-potential V1 channels (Raisinghani and Premkumar, 2005). Recently, Garza et al determined the effect of AGs on proton-gated ionic currents in DRG neurons of the rat, and in human embryonic kidney (HEK)-293 cells (Garza et al., 2010). In DRG neurons, streptomycin and neomycin produced a significant, reversible reduction in the amplitude of proton-gated currents in a concentration-dependent manner. In addition, they slowed desensitization rates of ASIC currents. Gentamicin also showed a significant reversible action on the ASIC currents. In HEK-293 cells, streptomycin produced a significant reduction in the amplitude of the proton-gated current, whereas neomycin and gentamicin had no significant effect. These results indicate that ASICs are molecular targets for AGs, which may explain, in part, their effects on excitable cells. Moreover, AGs might potentially represent a novel class of molecules with high affinity, specificity, and selectivity for different ASIC subunits.

2.2.7 Diarylamidines

Diarylamidines have been widely used for the treatment of protozoan diseases such as trypanosomiasis and leishmaniasis since 1930s (Baraldi et al., 2004; Mishra et al., 2007). Recently, Chen and colleges found that four members of the diarylamidines, 4', 6-diamidino-2-phenylindole, diminazene, hydroxystilbamidine and pentamidine strongly inhibit ASIC currents in hippocampal neurons with IC_{50} of 2.8, 0.3, 1.5 and 38 μM, respectively. The inhibitory concentration is much lower than amiloride. Sub-maximal concentrations of diminazene also potently accelerate desensitization of ASIC currents in hippocampal neurons. Diminazene blocks ASIC1a, -1b, -2a, and -3 currents expressed in CHO cells with a rank order of potency 1b > 3 > 2a > or = 1a. This study indicates that diarylamidines represent a novel class of non-amiloride ASIC blockers and suggests that diarylamidines as small molecules may be developed as therapeutic agents in the treatment of ASIC-involved diseases (Chen et al., 2010).

3. Activation of ASICs induces membrane depolarization and increases intracellular Ca^{2+} in brain neurons

Since all ASICs are Na^+-selective channels which have a reversal potential near Na^+ equilibrium potential (+60 mV), activation of ASICs at normal resting potentials produces exclusively inward currents which result in membrane depolarization and the excitation of neurons (Baron et al., 2002; Wu et al., 2004; Jiang et al., 2009). For example, our recent study has shown that a minor drop in extracellular pH from 7.4 to 6.8 induces significant membrane depolarization, which accompanies trains of action potentials (Fig. 4) (Jiang et al., 2009). This acid-induced membrane depolarization is significantly attenuated by either amiloride or PcTX1 (Fig. 4). Tetrodotoxin, a voltage-gated Na^+ channel blocker, has little effect on the membrane depolarization but completely diminished the action potentials triggered by a drop in pH from 7.4 to 6.8. For homomeric ASIC1a channels, acid activation induces Ca^{2+} entry directly through these channels (Walmann et al., 1997b; Chu et al., 2002; Xiong et al., 2004; Yermolaieva et al., 2004). In addition, the ASIC-mediated membrane depolarization may facilitate the activation of voltage-gated Ca^{2+} channels and NMDA receptor-gated channels (Wemmie et al., 2002; Zha et al., 2006), further promoting neuronal excitation and $[Ca^{2+}]_i$ accumulation. The Ca^{2+}-permeability of ASICs in CNS neurons has been characterized using fluorescent Ca^{2+} imaging and ion-substitution protocols (Xiong et al., 2004; Yermolaieva et al., 2004). In mouse cortical, striatal and hippocampal neurons, activation of ASICs by decreasing in extracellular pH induces increases in $[Ca^{2+}]_i$. This acid-induced increase in $[Ca^{2+}]_i$ could be recorded in the presence of a cocktail blocking other voltage-gated and ligand-gated Ca^{2+} channels (Xiong et al., 2004; Jiang et al., 2009), indicating Ca^{2+} entry directly through ASICs. The acid-induced increase in $[Ca^{2+}]_i$ is eliminated by specific and non-specific ASIC1a blockade, or by ASIC1 gene knockout (Xiong et al., 2004; Yermolaieva et al., 2004; Jiang et al., 2009). Consistent with the finding of fluorescent imaging, acid-activated inward current is activated when extracellular solution contains Ca^{2+} as the only conducting cation (Xiong et al., 2004). Thus, homomeric ASIC1a channels constitute an additional and important Ca^{2+} entry pathway for neurons.

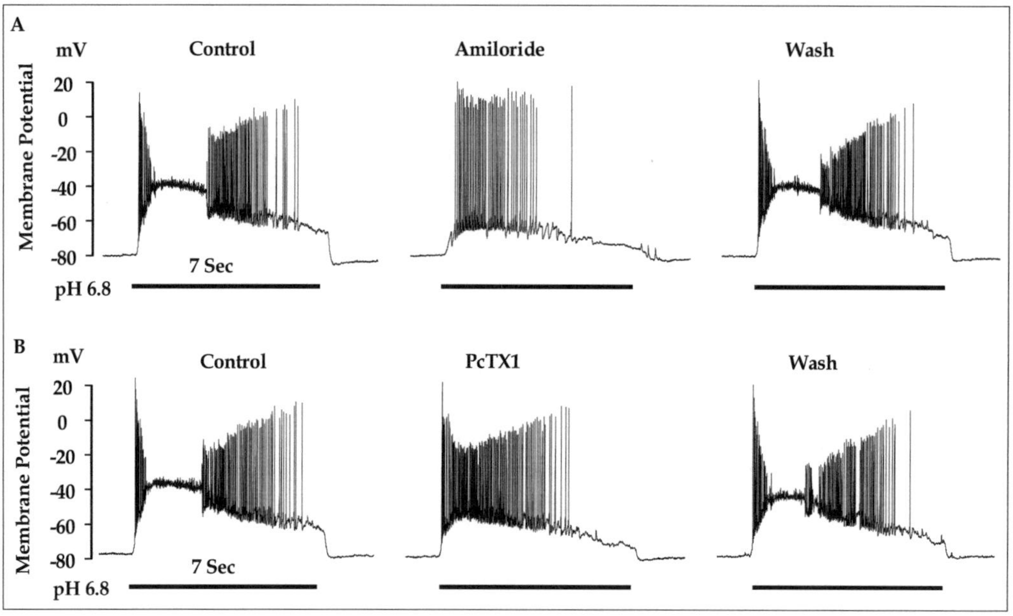

Fig. 4. pH drop triggered membrane depolarization and action potentials by activation of ASICs in cultured MSNs. Membrane depolarization by a drop in pH from 7.4 to 6.8 subsequently triggered trains of action potentials. The membrane depolarization was inhibited by amiloride (A) and PcTX1 (B)

4. Physiological implications of ASICs in the CNS

4.1 ASIC1a channels in synaptic plasticity, learning and memory

A change in pH at the synaptic cleft following synaptic release may render ASICs the opportunity to regulate synaptic transmission. The findings that ASICs are present at synaptic sites and can interact with postsynaptic density protein 95 as well as C kinase 1-interacting proteins (Hruska-Hageman et al., 2002; Wemmie et al., 2002; Zha et al., 2006, 2009) support this notion. Indeed, studies by Wemmie and coworkers have demonstrated that ASIC1a activation is involved in synaptic plasticity, learning and memory (Wemmie et al., 2002). They demonstrated that high frequency stimulation produces long-lasting potentiation of excitatory postsynaptic potentials (EPSP) in hippocampal slices from wild-type mice. However, the potentiation of EPSP decays rapidly to the baseline in slices from ASIC1a null mice. Further studies showed that the NMDA receptor antagonist D-2-Amino-5-phosphonovalerate inhibits EPSP summation in slices from wild-type but not ASIC1a-knockout mice, suggesting that the loss of ASIC1a impaired NMDA-receptor function. ASIC1a disruption does not impair presynaptic vesicle release, as evidenced by normal single evoked EPSPs and paired-pulse facilitation. Interestingly, a later study by Cho and Askwith demonstrated that the presynaptic release probability is increased in cultured hippocampal neurons from the ASIC1 knockout mice (Cho & Askwith, 2008). Although localizations of ASICs at neuronal cell body and postsynaptic sites have been clearly demonstrated (Wemmie et al., 2002; Zha et al., 2006), it remains to be determined whether ASICs are also expressed at presynaptic sites.

4.2 ASIC1a channels in fear-related behavior

ASIC1a is enriched in key structures of fear circuit (e.g. amygdala) (Wemmie et al., 2003). Thus, ASIC1a may influence fear responses. Indeed, Wemmie and colleagues demonstrated that ASIC1-null mice display significant deficits in cue and context fear conditioning (Wemmie et al., 2003). The loss of ASIC1a also reduces unconditioned fear in the open field test, during acoustic startle, and in response to predator odor (Coryell et al., 2007). Overexpressing ASIC1a, on the other hand, increases fear conditioning (Wemmie et al., 2004), but not unconditioned fear responses (Coryell et al., 2008).

Further studies by Wemmie's group suggest that activation of ASIC1a in brain chemosensors contributes to CO_2 induced fear-related behavior (Ziemann et al., 2009). It has long been known that breathing CO_2 triggers panic attacks in patients with panic disorder, and that these patients show an increased sensitivity to CO_2 inhalation (Papp et al., 1993). In addition, patients with increasing hypercarbia due to respiratory failure become extremely anxious. How can CO_2 inhalation contribute to fear behavior and related panic disorders? Wemmie and colleagues have provided evidence that ASIC1a channels are involved (Ziemann et al., 2009). They showed that inhaled CO_2 triggers a drop in brain pH and induces fear behavior in mice. Eliminating or inhibiting ASIC1a significantly limits this activity. Overexpressing ASIC1a in the amygdala rescues the CO_2-induced fear deficit in ASIC1a null mice. Buffering brain pH, on the other hand, attenuates fear behavior, whereas lowering pH in the amygdale reproduces the effect of CO_2. These studies provide a novel molecular mechanism underlying CO_2-induced intense fear and related anxiety/panic disorders and define the amygdala as an important chemosensor that detects hypercarbia/acidosis and initiates behavioral responses (Ziemann et al., 2009).

4.3 ASICs and retinal integrity

pH variations in the retina are involved in the fine-tuning of visual perception. Expression of ASICs in the retina suggests that they might play a role (Lilley et al., 2004). One study by Ettaiche suggested that ASIC2 is important for retinal function and likely protects against light-induced retinal degeneration. They showed that both photoreceptors and neurons of the mouse retina express ASIC2a and ASIC2b. Inactivation of the ASIC2 gene in mice leads to an increased rod electroretinogram of a- and b-waves, indicating an enhanced gain of visual transduction. ASIC2 knockout mice also show more sensitivity to light-induced retinal degeneration. Thus, ASIC2 is likely a negative modulator of rod phototransduction, and that functional ASIC2 channels are beneficial for the maintenance of retinal integrity (Ettaiche et al., 2004). However, since homomeric ASIC2a channels have an extremely low-sensitivity to protons (i.e. pH_{50} of 4.4), it is not clear whether active channel activity is required for this role.

Further studies by Ettaiche and colleagues also suggested an involvement of ASIC1a in retinal physiology (Ettaiche et al., 2006). In situ hybridization and immunohistochemistry detected the expression of ASIC1a in the outer and inner nuclear layers (cone photoreceptors, horizontal cells, some amacrine and bipolar cells) and in the ganglion cell layer. ASIC1a knockdown by antisense oligonucleotides and ASIC1a blockade by relatively specific inhibitor PcTX1 decreased the photopic a- and b-waves and oscillatory potentials. This finding suggests that ASIC1a is involved in normal retinal activity. Interestingly, a recent study by Render and colleagues did not detect any remarkable morphological changes in cone photoreceptors in ASIC1a-/- mice, at least at 5 or 22-27 weeks of age (Render et al., 2010). Thus, the exact role of this subunit in retinal integrity and/or function remains to be determined.

In addition to ASIC1a and ASIC2, a potential role of ASIC3 in retinal function and survival has been reported (Ettaiche et al., 2009). Ettaiche and colleagues demonstrated the presence of ASIC3 in the rod inner segment of photoreceptors, in horizontal and some amacrine cells. ASIC3 is also detected in retinal ganglion cells (RGCs) but contributes little to ASIC currents recorded in cultured RGCs. At 2 - 3 months, knockout mice experienced a moderate enhancement of scotopic electroretinogram a-wave amplitude and a concomitant increase of b-wave amplitude without alteration of retinal structure. Older (8-month-old) mice had large reductions in scotopic a- and b-waves, respectively, and reductions in oscillatory potential amplitudes associated with complete disorganization of the retina and degenerating rod inner segments. At 8 and 12 months of age, GFAP and TUNEL staining revealed an up-regulation of GFAP expression in Müller cells and the presence of apoptotic cells in the inner and outer retina (Ettaiche et al., 2009). Thus, ASIC3 also appears to be required for the maintenance of retina integrity.

5. ASICs in neurodegenerative diseases

5.1 ASIC1 channels and multiple sclerosis

Multiple sclerosis is a neuroinflammatory disease associated with axonal degeneration. Although inflammation and demyelination are the primary features of CNS lesions, axonal degeneration correlates best with clinical deficits in individuals with this disease. It has been suggested that the inflammatory insult leads to axonal degeneration by causing neuronal mitochondrial dysfunction, energy failure and alteration of ion exchange mechanisms (Waxman, 2006). Since excessive accumulation of Na^+ and Ca^{2+} ions is associated with axonal degeneration (Stys & LoPachin, 1998), Friese et al determined whether ASIC1a activation, which is known to cause accumulation of Na^+ and Ca^{2+} ions, contributes to such process in inflammatory lesions of the CNS (Friese et al., 2007). They showed that in an experimental model of autoimmune encephalomyelitis (EAE), ASIC1 null mice exhibit a significantly reduced clinical deficit and axonal degeneration as compared to wild-type mice. Further, pH measurements in the spinal cord of EAE mice display tissue acidosis sufficient to open ASIC1. The ASIC1 gene disruption also shows protective effect in nerve explants in vitro. ASIC blockade by amiloride is equally neuroprotective in nerve explants and in EAE. Thus, ASIC1a may be a potential target for axon degeneration associated with multiple sclerosis.

More recently, Vergo et al., from the same group studied acute and chronic EAE and multiple sclerosis spinal cord and optic nerve tissues to examine the distribution of ASIC1 and its relationship with neuronal and glial damage (Vergo et al., 2011). They found that ASIC1 was upregulated in axons and oligodendrocytes within lesions from mice with acute EAE and from patients with active multiple sclerosis. The expression of ASIC1 was associated with axonal damage as indicated by co-localization with the axonal injury marker beta amyloid precursor protein. Moreover, blocking ASIC1 with amiloride protected both myelin and neurons from damage in the acute model, and when given either at disease onset or, more clinically relevant, at first relapse, ameliorated disability in mice with chronic-relapsing EAE. Together these findings suggest that blockade of ASIC1 has the potential to provide both neuro- and myelo-protective benefits in multiple sclerosis (Vergo et al., 2011).

5.2 ASICs and Parkinson's disease (PD)

PD is characterized by motor impairments and a loss of dopaminergic neurons in the substantia nigra (SNc) (Dauer & Przedborski, 2003). However, the mechanism of neuronal injury is not entirely clear. Previous studies have shown that the vulnerable neurons in this region also express ASIC1a (Wemmie et al., 2003; Pidoplichko & Dani, 2006). Given that PD, like ischemia, is associated with cerebral lactic acidosis, Arias et al tested the effect of ASIC blockade in a mouse model of PD induced by 1-methyl-4-phenyl-1,2,3,6-tetrahydropyridine (MPTP) treatment (Arias et al., 2008). As expected, amiloride was found to protect SNc neurons from MPTP-induced degeneration, and to preserve dopaminergic cell bodies in the SNc. Administration of PcTX venom resulted in a modest effect, attenuating the deficits in striatal DAT binding and dopamine. These findings suggest a potential role for ASICs in the pathogenesis of Parkinson's disease.

5.3 ASICs and Huntington's disease (HD)

HD is a fatal neurodegenerative disorder. Energy metabolism deficit and acidosis have been observed in both *in vitro* and *in vivo* models of HD as well as in the brains of HD patients (Wong et al., 2008). To examine the potential involvement of ASICs in the pathology of HD, Wong et al tested effect of amiloride derivative benzamil both *in vitro* and *in vivo* (Wong et al., 2008). They showed that benzamil markedly reduced the huntingtin-polyglutamine (htt-polyQ) aggregation in an inducible cellular system. In addition, the effect of benzamil was recapitulated in the R6/2 animal model of HD. Further experimentation showed that benzamil alleviated the inhibition of ubiquitin-proteasome system (UPS) activity, resulting in enhanced degradation of soluble htt-polyQ specifically in its pathological range. Blocking the expression of ASIC1a with siRNA also enhanced UPS activity, resulting in decreased htt-polyQ aggregation in the striatum of R6/2 mice. Thus, targeting ASIC1a might be an alternative approach to combat HD and other polyQ-related disorders.

5.4 ASIC1a and Alzheimer's disease (AD)

Based on ASIC1a channels in synaptic plasticity and learning/memory, a recent preliminary study has suggested that a reduced function of ASIC1a channels may contribute to the learning and memory deficit associated with AD (Maysami et al., 2009). In this study, Maysami et al showed that acid-activated currents in mouse cortical neurons and in CHO cells expressing ASIC1a are inhibited by nanomolar concentrations of amyloid beta peptide, a critical player for the pathology of AD. In addition to a reduction of current amplitude, amyloid beta peptide also slows down the activation of the channels. Thus, restoring the activity of ASIC1a channels could be a new intervention for AD.

5.5 ASICs in depression-related behavior

Depression disorders are a highly prevalent condition among adults in general population but the molecular pathways underlying depression are poorly understood. Recent studies by Coryell and colleagues have linked ASIC function to depression-related behavior (Coryell et al., 2009). They demonstrated that genetically disrupting ASIC1a in mice produced antidepressant-like effects in the forced swim test, the tail suspension test, and following unpredictable mild stress. Pharmacologically inhibiting ASIC1a also had antidepressant-like effects. The effects of ASIC1a disruption in the forced swim test were independent and additive to those of several commonly used antidepressants. Restoring ASIC1a to the amygdale of ASIC1a null mice reversed the forced swim test effects. The mechanism underlying the involvement of ASIC1a in depression-related behavior is not clear. It is likely that brain-derived neurotrophic factor (BDNF) is involved since both ASIC1a disruption and inhibition interfere with the ability of stress to reduce BDNF in the hippocampus. Thus, antagonists of ASIC1a channels may have potential for combating human depression.

5.6 ASICs and anxiety disorders

Anxiety disorders are debilitating neuropsychiatric disorders. Current treatments for anxiety disorders include pharmacological agents such as benzodiazepines and selective serotonin reuptake inhibitors. These agents, while effective in many patients, can induce a variety of side effects. Thus, it is necessary to develop a new generation of effective and better-tolerated anxiolytic agents. In this regard, Dwyer et al have shown that ASIC1a inhibitors have an effect in preclinical rodent models of autonomic and behavioral parameters of anxiety (Dwyer et al., 2009). In the stress-induced hyperthermia model, acute administration of ASIC inhibitors PcTX1, A-317567, and amiloride prevented stress-induced elevations in core body temperature. In the four-plate test, acute treatment with PcTX1 and A-317567 produced dose-dependent increases in the number of punished crossings. Further experiment showed that infusion of A-317567 into the amygdala significantly elevated the extracellular levels of GABA, but not glutamate, in this brain region. These findings suggest that ASIC inhibition has anxiolytic-like effects in some behavioral models and that GABAergic mechanisms are involved in the effects.

A recent study also suggests an involvement of ASIC3 in anxiety-like behavior (Wu et al., 2010). Although it is widely accepted that ASIC3 is predominately distributed in the peripheral nervous system, its expression has been found in rat hypothalamus (Meng et al., 2009). Study by Wu and colleagues also reported the expression of ASIC3 in the sensory mesencephalic trigeminal nucleus of mouse brain (Wu et al., 2010). However, whether ASIC3 plays any functional role in the brain was unclear. Wu et al showed that, in anxiety behavior tasks, ASIC3 null mice spent more time in the open arms of an elevated plus maze than did their wild-type littermates. ASIC3 null mice also displayed less aggressiveness toward intruders but more stereotypic repetitive behaviors during resident-intruder testing than did wild-type littermates. Therefore, loss of ASIC3 produces behavioral changes in anxiety and aggression in mice, which suggests that ASIC3-dependent sensory activities might be related to the central process of emotion modulation (Wu et al., 2010).

Although the studies from ASIC1a and ASIC3 knockout mice indicated that ASICs contribute to neuropsychiatric disorders such as depression and anxiety, whether these neurological conditions are associated with significant change in local or global pH in the CNS remains to be determined.

5.7 ASICs in acidosis-mediated ischemic neuronal injury

During neurological conditions such as brain ischemia, increased anaerobic glycolysis due to reduced oxygen supply leads to lactic acid accumulation (Rehncrona, 1985). Accumulation of lactic acid, alone with increased H^+ release from ATP hydrolysis, causes a decrease in pH, resulting in brain acidosis. During brain ischemia, for example, extracellular pH falls to 6.5 or lowers (Rehncrona, 1985; Nedergaard et al., 1991).

Acidosis has long been known to play an important role in ischemic brain injury (Tombaugh & Sapolsky, 1993; Siesjo, et al., 1996), and a direct correlation of brain acidosis with infarct size has been described (Siesjo, 1988). However, the exact mechanism underlying acidosis-mediated neuronal injury remained uncertain. Severe acidosis may cause non-selective denaturation of proteins and nucleic acids (Kalimo et al., 1981); trigger cell swelling through stimulation of Na^+/H^+ and $Cl^-/HCO3^-$ exchangers, which leads to cellular edema and osmolysis (Kimelberg et al., 1990); hinder postischemic metabolic recovery by inhibiting mitochondrial energy metabolism and impairing postischemic blood flow via vascular edema (Hillered et al., 1985). The stimulation of pathologic free radical formation by acidosis has also been described (Rehncrona et al., 1989). At the neurotransmitter level, profound acidosis inhibits astrocytic glutamate uptake, which may contribute to excitatory neuronal injury (Swanson et al., 1995). Marked acidosis, with tissue pH<5.5, may influence neuronal vulnerability indirectly by damaging glial cells (Giffard et al., 1990).

The widespread expression of ASIC1a in the brain, its activation by pH drops to the level commonly seen during ischemia, and its demonstrated role in intracellular Ca^{2+} accumulation suggested a potential involvement of these channels in the pathology of brain injury. Indeed, a number of recent studies have demonstrated an important role for ASIC1a activation in acidosis-mediated neuronal injury (Xiong et al., 2004; Yermolaieva et al., 2004; Gao et al., 2005; Pignataro nt al., 2007; Sherwood et al., 2009, 2011; Gu et al., 2010; Jetti et al., 2010; Li et al., 2010; Mari et al., 2010). In cultured mouse and human cortical neurons, for example, activation of ASICs by acid incubation induced glutamate receptor-independent neuronal injury inhibited by specific ASIC1a blockade, and/or by ASIC1 gene knockout (Xiong et al., 2004; Li et al., 2010). In rodent models of brain ischemia, intracerebroventricular injection of ASIC1a blocker/inhibitor reduced the infarct volume from transient or permanent focal ischemia by up to 60%(Xiong et al., 2004; Pignataro et al., 2007). Similarly, ASIC1 gene knockout produced significant neuroprotection in mice (Xiong et al., 2004). The protection by ASIC1a blockade had a time window of efficacy of up to 5 hours, and the protection persists for at least 7 days (Pignataro nt al., 2007).

More recently, Sherwood et al., found that ASIC2b subunit can form functional channels with ASIC1a in cultured hippocampal neurons, and that the heteromeric ASIC1a/2b channels are calcium-permeable (Sherwood et al., 2011). Further, activation of heteromeric ASIC1a/2b channels contributes to acidosis-induced neuronal death. These data indicate that ASIC2, like ASIC1a, plays a role in acidosis-induced neuronal death and implicate the ASIC1a/2b subtype as a novel pharmacological target to prevent neuronal injury after stroke (Sherwood et al., 2011).

Since activation of NMDA receptors and subsequent Ca^{2+} toxicity have been known to play an important role in ischemic brain injury, the outcome of co-application of both antagonists has also been investigated. Compared to ASIC1a or NMDA blockade alone, co-application of NMDA and ASIC antagonists produced additional neuroprotection, and the presence of ASIC1a blockade prolonged the time window of effectiveness of NMDA blockade (Pignataro nt al., 2007). Thus, ASIC1a represents a novel pharmacological target for ischemic brain injury.

In contrast to ASIC1a, a study by Johnson and colleagues suggests that an increased ASIC2a expression could provide protection against ischemic injury (Johnson et al., 2001). They showed an increased ASIC2a expression in neurons that survived global ischemia. This may be explained by the possibility that increased ASIC2a expression favors the formation of heteromeric ASIC1a/ASIC2a channels with reduced acid-sensitivity and no Ca^{2+} permeability.

5.8 ASIC activation and epileptic seizure activity

A significant drop of brain pH during intense neuronal excitation or seizure activity (Urbanics et al., 1978; Somjen et al., 1984; Simon et al., 1985, 1987; Chesler & Chan, 1988; Chesler & Kaila, 1992) suggests that ASIC activation might occur and activated ASICs then play a role in the generation/maintenance of epileptic seizures. However, the exact role of ASIC activation in seizure generation, propagation, and termination seems controversial.

Babinski and colleagues first reported a change of ASIC1a and ASIC2b expression in the hippocampal area following pilocarpine-induced epilepticus (Biagini et al., 2001), suggesting that the channels containing ASIC1a and ASIC2b subunits might play a role in the pathology of epilepsy.

Later on, a number of studies showed that amiloride, a commonly used non-selective ASIC blocker, has an anticonvulsant property *in vivo* in pilocarpine and pentylenetetrazole models of seizures (Ali et al., 2004, 2006; N'Gouemo, 2008), suggesting that ASIC activation might be proconvulsant. However, since amiloride also inhibits a number of other channels and ion exchange systems, these findings do not define ASICs as a specific target for amiloride to achieve its anti-epileptic action.

Using a number of *in vitro* epilepsy models, a preliminary study by Chang et al provided additional evidence that ASIC1a activation might be proconvulsant (Chang et al., 2007). In a cell culture model of epilepsy, brief withdrawal of the NMDA antagonist kynurenic acid induces a dramatic increase in the firing of action potentials, in addition to a sustained membrane depolarization. ASIC blockade by amiloride and the selective ASIC1a blocker PcTX1 significantly inhibited the increase of neuronal firing and the sustained membrane depolarization. In hippocampal slices, high frequency electrical stimulation or removal of extracellular Mg^{2+} triggers spontaneous seizure-like bursting. Bath perfusion of amiloride and PcTX1 decreased the amplitude and the frequency of these seizure-like bursting activities. Similarly, slices prepared from the brains of ASIC1a knockout mice demonstrated a reduced sensitivity to low extracellular Mg^{2+}-induced or stimulation-evoked seizure activities (Chang et al., 2007).

In contrast, studies by Ziemann and colleagues, performed largely *in vivo*, have suggested that activation of ASIC1a channels is involved in the termination of epileptic seizure activity (Ziemann et al., 2008). An interesting finding by Ziemann and colleagues was that the level of ASIC1a expression is higher in GABAergic interneurons than in excitatory neurons (Ziemann et al., 2008). Therefore, acidosis generated during seizures might produce more

ASIC activation in inhibitory interneurons and facilitate GABAergic transmission, resulting in seizure termination.

The inconsistent data on the role of ASICs in epileptic seizures may result from the use of different epilepsy models. The different ages of animals used may also contribute to the inconsistency since expression and function of ASICs in CNS neurons undergo dramatic developmental changes (Li et al., 2010). In addition, the finding that hippocampal interneurons are highly diverse with dramatically different expression level of ASICs (Weng et al., 2010) adds additional complexity to this subject.

6. Conclusion

ASICs represent new biological components in peripheral sensory and CNS neurons. Increasing evidence indicates the involvement of these channels in both physiological and pathological processes of CNS (Grunder & Chen, 2010). Therefore, targeting these channels may provide novel and effective therapeutic interventions for a number of CNS diseases. In addition to establishing ASIC-specific small molecule antagonists that can easily pass through the blood brain barrier, alternative strategies may consider targeting endogenous modulators that are known to influence the expression and/or activity of these channels.

7. References

Adams, C.M.; Snyder, P.M. & Welsh, M.J. (1999). Paradoxical Stimulation of a DEG/ENaC Channel by Amiloride. *Journal of Biological Chemistry*, Vol. 274, No. 22, pp.15500-15504, ISSN 0021-9258

Akopian, A.N.; Chen, C.C.; Ding, Y. Cesare, P. & Wood, J.N. (2000). A New Member of the Acid-Sensing Ion Channel Family. *Neuroreport*, Vol.11, No.10, pp. 2217 - 2222, ISSN 0959-4956

Ali, A.; Ahmad, F.J.; Pillai, K.K. & Vohora, D. (2004). Evidence of the Antiepileptic Potential of Amiloride With Neuropharmacological Benefits in Rodent Models of Epilepsy and Behavior. *Epilepsy & Behavior*, Vol. 5, No. 3, pp. 322-328, ISSN 1525-5050

Ali, A.; Pillai, K.P.; Ahmad, F.J.; Dua, Y. & Vohora, D. (2006). Anticonvulsant Effect of Amiloride in Pentetrazole-Induced Status Epilepticus in Mice. *Pharmacological Reports*, Vol. 58, No.2, pp. 242-245, ISSN 1734-1140

Allen, N.J. & Attwell, D. (2002). Modulation of ASIC Channels in Rat Crebellar Purkinje Nurons by Ichemia-Rlated Sgnals. *Journal of Phsiology*, Vol. 543, No. 2, pp. 521 - 529, ISSN 0022-3751

Alvarez de la Rosa, D.; Canessa, C.M.; Fyfe, G.K. & Zhang, P. (2000). Structure and Regulation of Amiloride Sensitive Sodium Channels. *Annual Review of Physiology*, Vol. 62, No.1, pp.573-594, ISSN 0066-4278

Arias, R.L.; Sung, M.L.; Vasylyev, D.; Zhang, M.Y.; Albinson, K.; Kubek, K.; Kagan, N.; Beyer, C.; Lin, Q.; Dwyer, J.M.; Zaleska, M.M.; Bowlby, M.R.; Dunlop, J. & Monaghan, M. (2008). Amiloride is Neuroprotective in an MPTP Model of Parkinson's Disease. *Neurobiology of Disease*, Vol. 31, No. 3, pp. 334-341, ISSN 0969-9961

Askwith, C.C.; Wemmie, J.A.; Price, M.P.; Rokhlina, T. & Welsh, M.J. (2004). Acid-Sensing Ion Channel 2 (ASIC2) Modulates ASIC1 H^+-Activated Currents in Hippocampal

Neurons. *Journal of Biological Chemistry*, Vol. 279, No. 18, pp.18296-18305, ISSN 0021-9258

Babini, E.; Paukert, M.; Geisler, H.S. & Grunder, S. (2002). Alternative Splicing and Interaction with Di- and Polyvalent Cations Control the Dynamic Range of Acid-Sensing Ion Channel 1 (ASIC1). *Journal of Biological Chemistry*, Vol. 277, No. 44, pp.41597-41603, ISSN 0021-9258

Bano, D.; Young, K.W.; Guerin, C.J.; Lefeuvre, R.; Rothwell, N.J.; Naldini, L.; Rizzuto, R.; Carafoli, E. & Nicotera, P. (2005). Cleavage of the Plasma Membrane Na^+/Ca^{2+} Exchanger in Excitotoxicity. *Cell*, Vol. 120,No.2, pp. 275-285, ISSN 0092-8674

Baraldi, P.G.; Bovero, A.; Fruttarolo, F.; Preti, D.; Tabrizi, M.A.; Pavani, M.G. & Romagnoli, R. (2004). DNA Minor Groove Binders as Potential Antitumor and Antimicrobial Agents. *Medicinal Research Reviews*, Vol. 24, No. 4, pp. 475-528, ISSN 0198-6325

Baron, A.; Voilley, N.; Lazdunski, M. & Lingueglia, E. (2008). Acid Sensing Ion Channels in Dorsal Spinal Cord Neurons. *Journal of Neuroscience*, Vol.28, No.6, pp.1498-1508, ISSN 0270-6474

Baron, A.; Waldmann, R. & Lazdunski, M. (2002). ASIC-Like, Proton-Activated Currents in Rat Hippocampal Neurons. *Journal of Physiology*, Vol. 539, No.2, pp.485-494, ISSN 0022-3751

Bässler, E.L.; Ngo-Anh, T.J.; Geisler, H.S.; Ruppersberg, J.P. & Gründer, S. (2001). Molecular and Functional Characterization of Acid-Sensing Ion Channel (ASIC) 1b. *Journal of Biological Chemistry*, Vol. 276, No. 36, pp. 33782-33787, ISSN 0021-9258

Benson, C.J.; Eckert, S.P. & McCleskey, E.W. (1999). Acid-Evoked Currents in Cardiac Sensory Neurons: A Possible Mediator of Myocardial Ischemic Sensation. *Circulation Research*, Vol. 84, No. 8, pp. 921-928, ISSN 0009-7330

Benson, C.J.; Xie, J.; Wemmie, J.A.; Price, M.P.; Henss, J.M.; Welsh, M.J. & Snyder, P.M. (2002). Heteromultimers of DEG/ENaC Subunits Form H^+-Gated Channels in Mouse Sensory Neurons. *Proceedings of National Academy of Science U.S.A.*, Vol. 99, No. 4, pp. 2338-2343, ISSN 0027-8424

Benveniste, M. & Dingledine, R. (2005). Limiting Stroke-Induced Damage by Targeting an Acid Channel. *New England Journal of Medicine*, Vol. 352, No. 1, pp. 85-86, ISSN 0028-4793

Biagini, G.; Babinski, K.; Avoli, M.; Marcinkiewicz, M. & Seguela, P. (2001). Regional and Subunit Specific Down-Regulation of Acid-Sensing Ion Channels in the Pilocarpine Model of Epilepsy. *Neurobiology of Disease*, Vol. 8, No. 1, pp.45-58, ISSN 0969-9961

Champigny, G.; Voilley, N.; Waldmann, R. & Lazdunski, M. (1998). Mutations Causing Neurodegeneration in Caenorhabditis Elegans Drastically Alter the PH Sensitivity and Inactivation of the Mammalian H^+-Gated Na^+ Channel MDEG1. *Journal of Biological Chemistry*, Vol. 273, No. 25, pp. 15418-15422, ISSN 0021-9258

Chang, S.Y.; Li, M.H.; Li, T.F.; Chu, X.P.; Lan, J.Q.; Thomson, S.; Jessick, V.; Meller, R.; Simon, R.P. & Xiong, Z.G. (2007). Involvement of Acid-Sensing Ion Channels in the Generation of Epileptic Seizure Activity [abstract]. 37th *Society for Neuroscience Annual Meeting*, 257.5. ISBN 0-916110-04-4, San Diego, California, USA, November 3-7, 2007

Chen, C.C.; England, S.; Akopian, A.N. & Wood, J.N. (1998). A Sensory Neuron Specific, Proton-Gated Ion Channel. *Proceedings of National Academy of Science U.S.A.*, Vol. 95, No. 17, pp.10240 - 10245, ISSN 0027-8424

Chen, X.; Kalbacher, H. & Gründer, S. (2006). Interaction of Acid-Sensing Ion Channel (ASIC) 1 with the Tarantula Toxin Psalmotoxin 1 is State Dependent. *Journal of General Physiology*, Vol.127, No.3, pp.267-76, ISSN 0022-1295

Chen, X.; Kalbacher, H. & Gründer, S. (2005). The Tarantula Toxin Psalmotoxin 1 Inhibits Acid-Sensing Ion Channel (ASIC) 1a by Increasing its Apparent H^+ Affinity. *Journal of General Physiology*, Vol.126, No.1, pp. 71-79, ISSN 0022-1295

Chen, X.; Qiu, L.; Li, M.; Dürrnagel, S.; Orser, B.A.; Xiong, Z.G. & MacDonald, J. F. (2010). Diarylamidines: High Potency Inhibitors of Acid-Sensing Ion Channels. *Neuropharmacology*, Vol. 58, No. 7, pp.1045-1053, ISSN 0028-3908

Chesler, M. & Chan, C.Y. (1988). Stimulus-Induced Extracellular PH Transients in the In Vitro Turtle Cerebellum. *Neuroscience*, Vol. 27, No. 3, pp. 941-948, ISSN 0306-4522

Chesler, M. & Kaila, K. (1992). Modulation of PH by Neuronal Activity. *Trends in Neuroscience*, Vol, 15, No. 10, pp. 396-402, ISSN 0166-2236

Cho, J.H. & Askwith, C.C. (2008). Presynaptic Release Probability Is Increased in Hippocampal Neurons From ASIC1 Knockout Mice. *Journal of Neurophysiology*, Vol. 99, No. 2, pp.426-441, ISSN 0022-3077

Chu, X.P.; Close, N.; Saugstad, J.A. & Xiong, Z.G. (2006). ASIC1a-Specific Modulation of Acid-Sensing Ion Channels in Mouse Cortical Neurons by Redox Reagents. *Journal of Neuroscience*, Vol. 26, No. 20, pp. 5329 - 5339, ISSN 0270-6474

Chu, X.P.; Miesch, J.; Johnson, M.; Root, L.; Zhu, X.M.; Chen, D.; Simon, R.P. & Xiong, Z.G. (2002). Proton-Gated Channels in PC12 Cells. *Journal of Neurophysiology*, Vol. 87, No. 5, pp.2555-2561, ISSN 0022-3077

Chu, X.P.; Wemmie, J.A.; Wang, W.Z.; Zhu, X.M.; Saugstad, J.A.; Price, M.P.; Simon, R.P. & Xiong, Z.G. (2004). Subunit-Dependent High-Affinity Zinc Inhibition of Acid-Sensing Ion Channels. *Journal of Neuroscience*, Vol.24, No. 40, pp. 8678 - 8689, ISSN 0270-6474

Coryell, M.W.; Wunsch, A.M.; Haenfler, J.M.; Allen, J.E.; McBride, J.L.; Davidson, B.L. & Wemmie, J.A. (2008). Restoring Acid-Sensing Ion Channel-1a in the Amygdala of Knock-out Mice Rescues Fear Memory but not Unconditioned Fear Responses. *Journal of Neuroscience*, Vol. 28, No. 51, pp. 13738-13741, ISSN 0270-6474

Coryell, M.W.; Wunsch, A.M.; Haenfler, J.M.; Allen, J.E.; Schnizler, M.; Ziemann, A.E.; Cook, M.N.; Dunning, J.P.; Price, M.P.; Rainier, J.D.; Liu, Z.; Light, A.R.; Langbehn, D.R. & Wemmie, J.A. (2009). Acid-Sensing Ion Channel-1a in the Amygdala, a Novel Therapeutic Target in Depression-Related Behavior. *Journal of Neuroscience*, Vol. 29, No. 17, pp. 5381-5388, ISSN 0270-6474

Coryell, M.W.; Ziemann, A.E.; Westmoreland, P.J.; Haenfler, J.M.; Kurjakovic, Z.; Zha, X.M.; Price, M.; Schnizler, M.K. & Wemmie, J.A. (2007). Targeting ASIC1a Reduces Innate Fear and Alters Neuronal Activity in the Fear Circuit. *Biological Psychiatry*. Vol.62, No. 10, pp.1140-1148, ISSN 0006-3223

Dauer, W. & Przedborski, S. (2003). Parkinson's Disease: Mechanisms and Models. *Neuron*, Vol. 39, No. 6, pp. 889-909, ISSN 0896-6273

Deval, E.; Noël, J.; Lay, N.; Alloui, A.; Diochot, S.; Friend, V.; Jodar, M.; Lazdunski, M. & Lingueglia, E. (2008). ASIC3, A Sensor of Acidic and Primary Inflammatory Pain. *EMBO Journal*, Vol. 27, No. 22, pp. 3047– 3055, ISSN 0261-4189

Diochot, S.; Baron, A.; Rash, L.D.; Deval, E.; Escoubas, P.; Scarzello, S.; Salinas, M. & Lazdunski, M. (2004). A New Sea Anemone Peptide, APETx2, Inhibits ASIC3, A Major Acid-Sensitive Channel in Sensory Neurons. *EMBO Journal,* Vol. 23, No.7, pp.1516-1525, ISSN 0261-4189

Deval, E.; Salinas, M.; Baron, A.; Lingueglia, E. & Lazdunski, M. (2004). ASIC2b-Dependent Regulation of ASIC3, An Essential Acid-Sensing Ion Channel Subunit in Sensory Neurons via the Partner Protein PICK-1. *Journal of Biological Chemistry,* Vol. 279, No. 19, pp. 19531-19539, ISSN 0021-9258

de Weille, J.R.; Bassilana, F.; Lazdunski, M. & Waldmann, R. (1998). Identification, Functional Expression and Chromosomal Localisation of a Sustained Human Proton-Gated Cation Channel. *FEBS Letters,* Vol.433, No.3, pp.257-60, ISSN 0014-5793

Dubé, G.R.; Lehto, S.G.; Breese, N.M.; Baker, S.J.; Wang, X.; Matulenko, M.A.; Honoré, P.; Stewart, A.O.; Moreland, R.B. & Brioni, J.D. (2005). Electrophysiological and In Vivo Characterization of A-317567, a Novel Blocker of Acid Sensing Ion Channels. *Pain,* Vol. 117, No. 1-2, pp. 88-96. ISSN 0885-3294

Dwyer, J.M.; Rizzo, S.J.; Neal, S.J.; Lin, Q.; Jow, F.; Arias, R.L.; Rosenzweig-Lipson, S.; Dunlop, J. & Beyer, C.E. (2009). Acid Sensing Ion Channel (ASIC) Inhibitors Exhibit Anxiolytic-Like Activity in Preclinical Pharmacological Models. *Psychopharmacology (Berl),* Vol.203, No. 1, pp. 41-52, ISSN 1432-2072

Escoubas, P.; de Weille, J.R.; Lecoq, A.; Diochot, S.; Waldmann, R.; Champigny, G.; Moinier, D.; Ménez, A. & Lazdunski, M. (2000). Isolation of a Tarantula Toxin Specific for a Class of Proton-Gated Na^+ Channels. *Journal of Biological Chemistry,* Vol. 275, No. 33, pp. 25116-25121, ISSN 0021-9258

Ettaiche, M.; Deval, E.; Cougnon, M.; Lazdunski, M. & Voilley, N. (2006). Silencing Acid-Sensing Ion Channel 1a Alters Cone-Mediated Retinal Function. *Journal of Neuroscience,* Vol. 26, No. 21, pp.5800-5809, ISSN 0270-6474

Ettaiche, M.; Deval, E.; Pagnotta, S.; Lazdunski, M. & Lingueglia, E. (2009). Acid-Sensing Ion Channel 3 in Retinal Function and Survival. *Investigative Ophthalmology & Visual Science,* Vol. 50, No.5, pp. 2417-2426, ISSN 0146-0404

Ettaiche, M.; Guy, N.; Hofman, P.; Lazdunski, M. & Waldmann, R. (2004). Acid-Sensing Ion Channel 2 is Important For Retinal Function and Protects Against Light-Induced Retinal Degeneration. *Journal of Neuroscience,* Vol. 24, No. 5, pp. 1005-1012, ISSN 0270-6474

Friese, M.A.; Craner, M.J.; Etzensperger, R.; Vergo, S.; Wemmie, J.A.; Welsh, M.J.; Vincent, A. & Fugger, L. (2007). Acid-Sensing Ion Channel-1 Contributes to Axonal Degeneration in Autoimmune Inflammation of the Central Nervous System. *Nature Medicine,* Vol.13, No. 12, pp.1483-1489, ISSN 1078-8956

Gao, J.; Duan, B.; Wang, D.G.; Deng, X.H.; Zhang, G.Y.; Xu, L. & Xu, T.L. (2005). Coupling Between NMDA Receptor and Acid-Sensing Ion Channel Contributes to Ischemic Neuronal Death. *Neuron,* Vol. 48, No.4, pp.635-646, ISSN 0896-6273

Garza, A.; López-Ramírez, O.; Vega, R. & Soto, E. (2010). The Aminoglycosides Modulate the Acid-Sensing Ionic Channel Currents in Dorsal Root Ganglion Neurons from the Rat. *Journal of Pharmacology & Experimental Therapeutics,* Vol. 332, No. 2, pp. 489-499. ISSN 0022-3565

Giffard, R.G.; Monyer, H. & Choi, D.W. (1990). Selective Vulnerability of Cultured Cortical Glia to Injury by Extracellular Acidosis. *Brain Research,* 1990; Vol. 530, No.1, pp. 138-141, ISSN 0006-8993

Gonzales, E.B.; Kawate, T. & Gouaux, E. (2009). Pore Architecture and Ion Sites in Acid-Sensing Ion Channels and P2X Receptors. *Nature,* Vol. 460, No. 7255, pp.599-604, ISSN 0028-0836

Grunder, S. & Chen, X. (2010). Structure, Function, and Pharmacology of Acid-Sensing Ion Channels (ASICs): Focus on ASIC1a. *International Journal of Physiology, Pathophysiology and Pharmacology,* Vol. 2, No.2 , pp. 73-94, ISSN 1944-8171

Grunder, S.; Geissler, H.S.; Bassler, E.L. & Ruppersberg, J.P. (2000). A New Member of Acid-Sensing Ion Channels from Pituitary Gland. *Neuroreport,* Vol.11, No.8, pp. 1607 - 1611, ISSN 0959-4956

Gu, L.; Liu, X.; Yang, Y.; Luo, D. & Zheng, X. (2010). ASICs Aggravate Acidosis-Induced Injuries During Ischemic Reperfusion. *Neuroscience Letters,* Vol. 479, No. 1, pp. 63-68, ISSN 0304-3940

Hattori, T.; Chen, J.; Harding, A.M.; Price, M.P.; Lu, Y.; Abboud, F.M. & Benson, C.J. (2009). ASIC2a and ASIC3 Heteromultimerize to Form PH-Sensitive Channels in Mouse Cardiac Dorsal Root Ganglia Neurons. *Circulation Research,* Vol. 105, No.3, pp. 279-286, ISSN 0009-7330

Hesselager, M.; Timmermann, D.B. & Ahring, P.K. (2004). PH Dependency and Desensitization Kinetics of Heterologously Expressed Combinations of Acid-Sensing Ion Channel Subunits. *Journal of Biological Chemistry,* Vol. 279, No. 12, pp. 11006-11015, ISSN 0021-9258

Hillered, L.; Smith, M.L. & Siesjo, B.K. (1985). Lactic Acidosis and Recovery of Mitochondrial Function Following Forebrain Ischemia in the Rat. *Journal of Cerebral Blood Flow & Metabolism,* Vol. 5, No. 2, pp.259-266, ISSN 0271-678X

Hoagland, E.N.; Sherwood, T.W.; Lee, K.G.; Walker, C.J. & Askwith, C.C. (2010). Identification of a Calcium Permeable Human Acid-Sensing Ion Channel 1 Transcript Variant. *Journal of Biological Chemistry,* Vol. 285, No. 53, pp. 41852-41862, ISSN 0021-9258

Huang, Y. & McNamara, J.O. (2004). Ischemic Stroke: "Acidotoxicity" is a Perpetrator. *Cell,* Vol. 118, No.6, pp.665-666, ISSN 0092-8674

Hruska-Hageman, A.M.; Wemmie, J.A.; Price, M.P. & Welsh, M.J. (2002). Interaction of the Synaptic Protein PICK1 (Protein Interacting with C Kinase 1) with the Non-Voltage Gated Sodium Channels BNC1 (Brain Na^+ Channel 1) and ASIC (Acid-Sensing Ion Channel). *Biochemical Journal,* Vol. 361, No. 3, pp. 443-450, ISSN 0264-6021

Ikeuchi, M.; Kolker, S.J. & Sluka, K.A. (2009). Acid-Sensing Ion Channel 3 Expression in Mouse Knee Joint Afferents and Effects of Carrageenan-Induced Arthritis. *Journal of Pain,* Vol.10, No. 3, pp. 336 - 342, ISSN 1256-5900

Immke, D.C. & McCleskey, E.W. (2001). Lactate Enhances the Acid-Sensing Na+ Channel on Ischemia-Sensing Neurons. *Nature Neuroscience,* Vol.4, No. 9, pp. 869-870, ISSN 1097- 6256

Jasti, J.; Furukawa, H.; Gonzales, E.B. & Gouaux, E. (2007). Structure of Acid-Sensing Ion Channel 1 at 1.9 A Resolution and Low pH. *Nature,* Vol. 449, No. 7160, pp.316-323, ISSN 0028-0836

Jetti, S.K.; Swain, S.M.; Majumder, S.; Chatterjee, S.; Poornima, V. & Bera, A.K. (2010). Evaluation of the Role of Nitric Oxide in Acid Sensing Ion Channel Mediated Cell Death. *Nitric Oxide,* Vol. 22, No. 3, pp. 213-219, ISSN 1089-8603

Jiang, Q.; Li, M.H.; Papasian, C.J.; Branigan, D.; Xiong, Z.G.; Wang, J.Q. & Chu, X.P. (2009). Characterization of Acid-Sensing Ion Channels in Medium Spiny Neurons of Mouse Striatum. *Neuroscience,* Vol.162, No.1, pp. 55 - 66, ISSN 0306-4522

Johnson, M.B.; Jin, K.; Minami, M.; Chen, D. & Simon, R.P. (2001). Global Ischemia Induces Expression of Acid-Sensing Ion Channel 2a in Rat Brain. *Journal of Cerebral Blood Flow & Metabolism,* Vol. 21, No. 6, pp.734-740, ISSN 0271-678X

Jones, N.G.; Slater, R.; Cadiou, H.; McNaughton, P. & McMahon, S.B. (2004). Acid-Induced Pain and its Modulation in Humans. *Journal of Neuroscience,* Vol.24, No. 48, pp. 10974 - 10979, ISSN 0270-6474

Kalimo, H.; Rehncrona, S.; Soderfeldt, B.; Olsson, Y. & Siesjo, B.K. (1981). Brain Lactic Acidosis and Ischemic Cell Damage: 2. Histopathology. *Journal of Cerebral Blood Flow & Metabolism,* Vol. 1, No. 3, pp.313-327, ISSN 0271-678X

Kellenberger, S. & Schild, L. (2002). Epithelial Sodium Channel/Degenerin Family of Ion Channels: a Variety of Functions for a Shared Structure. *Physiological Review,* Vol. 82, No. 3, pp. 735 - 767, ISSN 0031-9333

Kimelberg, H.K.; Barron, K.D.; Bourke, R.S.; Nelson, L.R. & Cragoe, E.J. (1990). Brain Anti-cytoxic Edema Agents. *Progress in Clinical and Biological Research* Vol. 361, No.1, pp. 363-385, ISSN 0361-7742

Krishtal, O. (2003). The ASICs: Signaling Molecules? Modulators? *Trends in Neuroscience,* Vol, 26, No. 9, pp. 477-483, ISSN 0166-2236

Li, M.; Inoue, K.; Branigan, D.; Kratzer, E.; Hansen, J.C.; Chen, J.W.; Simon, R.P. & Xiong, Z.G. (2010). Acid-Sensing Ion Channels in Acidosis-Induced Injury of Human Brain Neurons. *Journal of Cerebral Blood Flow & Metabolism,* Vol. 30, No. 6, pp.1247-1260, ISSN 0271-678X

Li, M.; Kratzer, E.; Inoue, K.; Simon, R.P. & Xiong, Z.G. (2010). Developmental Change in the Electrophysiological and Pharmacological Properties of Acid-Sensing Ion Channels in CNS Neurons. *Journal of Physiology,* Vol. 588, No.20, pp.3883-3900, ISSN 0022-3751

Lilley, S.; LeTissier, P. & Robbins, J. (2004). The Discovery and Characterization of a Proton-Gated Sodium Current in Rat Retinal Ganglion Cells. *Journal of Neuroscience,* Vol. 24, No. 5, pp. 1013 - 1022, ISSN 0270-6474

Lin, Y.W.; Min, M.Y.; Lin, C.C.; Chen, W.N.; Wu, W.L.; Yu, H.M. & Chen, C.C. (2008). Identification and Characterization of a Subset of Mouse Sensory Neurons That Express Acid-Sensing Ion Channel 3. *Neuroscience,* Vol.151, No.2, pp.544-557, ISSN 0306-4522

Lingueglia, E. (2007). Acid-Sensing Ion Channels in Sensory Perception. *Journal of Biological Chemistry,* Vol. 282, No. 24, pp. 17325–17329, ISSN 0021-9258

Lingueglia, E.; de Weille, J.R.; Bassilana, F.; Heurteaux, C.; Sakai, H.; Waldmann, R. & Lazdunski, M. (1997). A Modulatory Subunit of Acid Sensing Ion Channels in Brain and Dorsal Root Ganglion Cells. *Journal of Biological Chemistry,* Vol. 272, No. 47, pp. 29778–29783, ISSN 0021-9258

Lu, Y.; Ma, X.; Sabharwal, R.; Snitsarev, V.; Morgan, D.; Rahmouni, K.; Drummond, H.A.; Whiteis, C.A.; Costa, V.; Price, M.; Benson, C.; Welsh, M.J.; Chapleau, M.W. & Abboud, F.M. (2009). The Ion Channel ASIC2 is Required for Baroreceptor and Autonomic Control of the Circulation. *Neuron,* Vol. 64, No.6, pp. 885-897, ISSN 0896-6273

Mamet, J.; Lazdunski, M. & Voilley, N. (2003). How Nerve Growth Factor Drives Physiological and Inflammatory Expressions of Acid-Sensing Ion Channel 3 in Sensory Neurons. *Journal of Biological Chemistry,* Vol. 278, No. 49, pp. 48907 - 48913, ISSN 0021-9258

Mari, Y.; Katnik, C. & Cuevas, J. (2010). ASIC1a Channels are Activated by Endogenous Protons During Ischemia and Contribute to Synergistic Potentiation of Intracellular Ca(2+) Overload During Ischemia and Acidosis. *Cell Calcium,* Vol. 48, No. 1, pp. 70-82, ISSN 0143-4160

Maysami, S.; Branigan, D.; Simon, R.P. & Xiong, Z,G. (2009). Amyloid Beta Peptide Modulates the Activity of Acid-Sensing Ion Channels in Neurons [abstract]. 39th *Society for Neuroscience Annual Meeting,* 237.8. ISBN 0-916110-04-4, Chicago, Illinois, USA, October 17-21, 2009

Meng, Q.Y.; Wang, W.; Chen, X.N.; Xu, T.L. & Zhou, J.N. (2009). Distribution of Acid-Sensing Ion Channel 3 in the Rat Hypothalamus. *Neuroscience,* Vol. 159, No. 3, pp.1126-1134, ISSN 0306-4522

Mishra, J.; Saxena, A. & Singh, S. (2007). Chemotherapy of Leishmaniasis: Past, Present and Future. *Current Medicinal Chemistry,* Vol. 14, No. 10, pp. 1153-1169, ISSN 0929-8673

Molliver, D.C.; Immke, D.C.; Fierro, L.; Paré, M.; Rice, F.L. & McCleskey, E.W. (2005). ASIC3, An Acid-Sensing Ion Channel, is Expressed in Metaboreceptive Sensory Neurons. *Molecular Pain,* Vol.1, No. 1, pp. 35, ISSN 1744-8069

Nedergaard, M.; Kraig, R.P.; Tanabe, J. & Pulsinelli, W.A. (1991). Dynamics of Interstitial and Intracellular PH in Evolving Brain Infarct. *American Journal of Physiology,* Vol. 260, No. 3, pp. R581-R588, ISSN 0363-6119

N'Gouemo, P. (2008). Amiloride Delays the Onset of Pilocarpine-Induced Seizures in Rats. *Brain Research,* Vol. 1222, No. 1, pp. 230-232, ISSN 0006-8993

Papp, L.A.; Klein, D.F. & Gorman, J.M. (1993). Carbon Dioxide Hypersensitivity, Hyperventilation, and Panic Disorder. *American Journal of Psychiatry,* Vol. 150, No. 8, pp. 1149-1157, ISSN 0002-953X

Pidoplichko, V.I. & Dani, J.A. (2006). Acid-Sensitive Ionic Channels in Midbrain Dopamine Neurons are Sensitive to Ammonium, Which May Contribute to Hyperammonemia Damage. *Proceedings of National Academy of Science U.S.A.,* Vol. 103, No. 30, pp. 11376-11380, ISSN 0027-8424

Pignataro, G.; Simon, R.P. & Xiong, Z.G. (2007). Prolonged Activation of ASIC1a and the Time Window for Neuroprotection in Cerebral Ischaemia. *Brain,* Vol. 130, No.1, pp.151-158, ISSN 0006-8950

Pérez, M.E.; Soto, E. & Vega, R. (1991). Streptomycin Blocks the Postsynaptic Effects of Excitatory Amino Acids on the Vestibular System Primary Afferents. *Brain Research,* Vol. 563, No. 1-2, pp. 221-226, ISSN 0006-8993

Price, M.P.; Lewin, G.R.; McIlwrath, S.L.; Cheng, C.; Xie, J.; Heppenstall, P.A.; Stucky, C.L.; Mannsfeldt, A.G.; Brennan, T.J.; Drummond, H.A.; Qiao, J.; Benson, C.J.; Tarr, D.E.; Hrstka, R.F.; Yang, B.; Williamson, R.A. & Welsh, M.J. (2000). The Mammalian Sodium Channel BNC1 is Required for Normal Touch Sensation. *Nature,* Vol. 407, No. 6807, pp. 1007-1011, ISSN 0028-0836

Price, M.P.; McIlwrath, S.L.; Xie, J.; Cheng, C.; Qiao, J.; Tarr, D.E.; Sluka, K.A.; Brennan, T.J.; Lewin, G.R. & Welsh, M.J. (2001). The DRASIC Cation Channel Contributes to the Detection of Cutaneous Touch and Acid Stimuli in Mice. *Neuron,* Vol. 32, No. 6, pp. 1071-1083, ISSN 0896-6273

Price, M.P.; Snyder, P.M. & Welsh, M.J. (1996). Cloning and Expression of a Novel Human Brain Na^+ Channel. *Journal of Biological Chemistry,* Vol. 271, No.14, pp.7879-7882, ISSN 0021-9258

Raisinghani, M. & Premkumar, L.S. (2005). Block of Native and Cloned Vanilloid Receptor 1 (TRPV1) by Aminoglycoside Antibiotics. *Pain,* Vol. 113, No. 1-2, pp. 123-33, ISSN 0885-3924

Rehncrona, S. (1985). Brain Acidosis. *Annals of Emergency Medicine,* Vol.14, No. 8, pp. 770-776, ISSN 0196-0644

Rehncrona, S.; Hauge, H.N. & Siesjo, B.K. (1989). Enhancement of Iron Catalyzed Free Radical Formation by Acidosis in Brain Homogenates: Differences in Effect by Lactic Acid and CO_2. *Journal of Cerebral Blood Flow & Metabolism,* Vol. 9, No. 1, pp. 65-70, ISSN 0271-678X

Render, J.A.; Howe, K.R.; Wunsch, A.M.; Guionaud, S.; Cox, P.J. & Wemmie, J.A. (2010). Histologic Examination of the Eye of Acid-Sensing Ion Channel 1a Knockout Mice. *International Journal of Physiology,Pathophysiology and Pharmacology,* Vol. 2, No.2 , pp. 69-72, ISSN 1944-8171

Salinas, M.; Lazdunski, M. & Lingueglia, E. (2009). Structural Elements for the Generation of Sustained Currents by the Acid Pain Sensor ASIC3. *Journal of Biological Chemistry,* Vol. 284, No., pp. 31851– 31859, ISSN 0021-9258

Schild, J.H. & Kunze, D.L. (1997). Experimental and Modeling Study of Na+ Current Heterogeneity in Rat Nodose Neurons and Its Impact on Neuronal Discharge. *Journal of Neurophysiology,* Vol. 78, No.6, pp.3198-209, ISSN 0022-3077

Sherwood, T.W. & Askwith, C.C. (2009). Dynorphin Opioid Peptides Enhance Acid-Sensing Ion Channel 1a Activity and Acidosis-Induced Neuronal Death. *Journal of Neuroscience,* Vol.29, No. 45, pp.14371-14380, ISSN 0270-6474

Sherwood, T.W.; Lee, K.G.; Gormley, M.G. & Askwith, C.C. (2011). Heteromeric Acid-Sensing Ion Channels (ASICs) Composed of ASIC2b and ASIC1a Display Novel Channel Properties and Contribute to Acidosis-Induced Neuronal Death. *Journal of Neuroscience,* Vol. 31, No. 26, pp. 9723-9734, ISSN 0270-6474

Siesjo, B.K. (1988). Acidosis and Ischemic Brain Damage. *Neurochemical Pathology* Vol. 9, No. pp.31-88, ISSN 0734-600X

Siesjo, B.K.; Katsura, K. & Kristian, T. (1996). Acidosis-Related Damage. *Advance in Neurology,* Vol. 71, No. 1, pp.209-233, ISSN 0091-3952

Simon, R.P.; Copeland, J.R.; Benowitz, N.L.; Jacob, P. III. & Bronstein, J. (1987). Brain Phenobarbital Uptake During Prolonged Status Epilepticus. *Journal of Cerebral Blood Flow & Metabolism,* Vol. 7, No. 6, pp. 783-788, ISSN 0271-678X

Simon, R.P.; Benowitz, N.; Hedlund, R. & Copeland, J. (1985). Influence of the Blood-Brain PH Gradient on Brain Phenobarbital Uptake During Status Epilepticus. *Journal of Pharmacology & Experimental Therapeutics,* Vol. 234, No. 3, pp. 830-835, ISSN 0022-3565

Sluka, K.A.; Price, M.P.; Breese, N.M.; Stucky, C.L.; Wemmie, J.A. & Welsh, M.J. (2003). Chronic Hyperalgesia Induced by Repeated Acid Injections in Muscle is Abolished by the Loss of ASIC3, but not ASIC1. *Pain,* Vol. 106, No.3, pp. 229-239, ISSN 0885-3924

Sluka, K.A.; Radhakrishnan, R.; Benson, C.J.; Eshcol, J.O.; Price, M.P.; Babinski, K.; Audette, K.M.; Yeomans, D.C. & Wilson, S.P. (2007). ASIC3 in Muscle Mediates Mechanical, but not Heat, Hyperalgesia Associated with Muscle Inflammation. *Pain,* Vol. 129, No. 1-2, pp. 102 - 112, ISSN 0885-3294

Sluka, K.A.; Winter, O.C. & Wemmie, J.A. (2009). Acid-Sensing Ion Channels: A New Target for Pain and CNS Diseases. *Current Opinion in Drug Discovery & Development,* Vol. 12, No.5, pp.693-704, ISSN 1367-6733

Somjen, G.G. (1984). Acidification of Interstitial Fluid in Hippocampal Formation Caused by Seizures and by Spreading Depression. *Brain Research,* Vol. 311, No. 1, pp. 186-188, ISSN 0006-8993

Stys, P.K. & LoPachin, R.M. (1998). Mechanisms of Calcium and Sodium Fluxes in Anoxic Myelinated Central Nervous System Axons. *Neuroscience*, Vol. 82, No. 1, pp. 21-32, ISSN

Sutherland, S.P.; Benson, C.J.; Adelman, J.P. & McCleskey, E.W. (2001). Acid-Sensing Ion Channel 3 Matches the Acid-Gated Current in Cardiac Ischemia-Sensing Neurons. *Proceedings of National Academy of Science U.S.A.,* Vol.98, No. 2, pp.711-766, ISSN 0027-8424

Swanson, R.A.; Farrell, K. & Simon, R.P. (1995). Acidosis Causes Failure of Astrocyte Glutamate Uptake During Hypoxia. *Journal of Cerebral Blood Flow & Metabolism,* Vol. 15, No. 3, pp. 417-424, ISSN 0271-678X

Tombaugh, G.C. & Sapolsky, R.M. (1993). Evolving Concepts About the Role of Acidosis in Ischemic Neuropathology. *Journal of Neurochemistry,* Vol. 61, No. 3, pp. 793-803, ISSN 0022-3042

Ugawa, S.; Ueda, T.; Ishida, Y.; Nishigaki, M.; Shibata, Y. & Shimada, S. (2002). Amiloride-Blockable Acid-Sensing Ion Channels are Leading Acid Sensors Expressed in Human Nociceptors. *Journal of Clinical Investigation,* Vol.110, No. 8, pp.1185-1190, ISSN 0021-9738

Ugawa, S.; Yamamoto, T.; Ueda, T.; Ishida, Y.; Inagaki, A.; Nishigaki, M. & Shimada, S. (2003). Amiloride-Insensitive Currents of the Acid-Sensing Ion Channel-2a

(ASIC2a)/ASIC2b Heteromeric Sour-Taste Receptor Channel. *Journal of Neuroscience,* Vol. 23, No. 9, pp. 3616-3622, ISSN 0270-6474

Urbanics, R.; Leniger-Follert, E. & Lubbers, D.W. (1978). Time Course of Changes of Extracellular H^+ and K^+ Activities During and After Direct Electrical Stimulation of the Brain Cortex. *Pflugers Archiv,* Vol. 378, No.1, pp. 47-53, ISSN 0365-267X

Varming, T. (1999). Proton-Gated Ion Channels in Cultured Mouse Cortical Neurons. *Neuropharmacology,* Vol. 38, No.12 , pp. 1875-1881, ISSN 0028-3908

Vergo, S.; Craner, M.J.; Etzensperger, R.; Attfield, K.; Friese, M.A.; Newcombe, J.; Esiri. M. & Fugger, L. (2011). Acid-Sensing Ion Channel 1 is Involved in Both Axonal Injury and Demyelination in Multiple Sclerosis and Its Animal Model. *Brain,* Vol.134, No. 2, pp. 571-584, ISSN 0006-8950

Voilley, N.; de Weille, J.; Mamet, J. & Lazdunski, M. (2001). Nonsteroid Anti-Inflammatory Drugs Inhibit Both the Activity and the Inflammation-Induced Expression of Acid-Sensing Ion Channels in Nociceptors. *Journal of Neuroscience,* Vol. 21, No. 20, pp. 8026-8033, ISSN 0270-6474

Waldmann, R.; Bassilana, F.; de Weille, J.; Champigny, G.; Heurteaux, C. & Lazdunski, M. (1997a). Molecular Cloning of a Non-Inactivating Proton-Gated Na+ Channel Specific for Sensory Neurons. *Journal of Biological Chemistry,* Vol. 272, No. 34, pp. 20975–20978, ISSN 0021-9258

Waldmann, R. & Lazdunski, M. (1998). H(+)-Gated Cation Channels: Neuronal Acid Sensors in the ENaC/DEG Family of Ion Channels. *Current Opinion in Neurobiology,* Vol. 8, No.3, pp. 418-424, ISSN 0959- 4388

Waldmann, R.; Champigny, G.; Bassilana, F.; Heurteaux, C. & Lazdunski, M. (1997b). A Proton-Gated Cation Channel Involved in Acid-Sensing. *Nature,* Vol. 386, No. 6621, pp.173-177, ISSN 0028-0836

Waldmann, R.; Champigny, G.; Voilley, N.; Lauritzen, I. & Lazdunski, M. (1996). The Mammalian Degenerin MDEG, An Amiloride-Sensitive Cation Channel Activated by Mutations Causing Neurodegeneration in Caenorhabditis Elegans. *Journal of Biological Chemistry,* Vol. 271, No. 18, pp. 10433–10436, ISSN 0021-9258

Waxman, S.G. (2006). Axonal Conduction and Injury in Multiple Sclerosis: the Role of Sodium Channels. *Nature Reviews Neuroscience, Vol.* 7, No.12, pp. 932-941, ISSN 1741-0048

Wemmie, J.A.; Askwith, C.C.; Lamani, E.; Cassell, M.D.; Freeman, J.H., Jr. & Welsh, M.J. (2003). Acid Sensing Ion Channel 1 is Localized in Brain Regions with High Synaptic Density and Contributes to Fear Conditioning. *Journal of Neuroscience,* Vol. 23, No. 13, pp.5496-5502, ISSN 0270-6474

Wemmie, J.A.; Chen. J.; Askwith, C.C.; Hruska-Hageman, A.M.; Price, M.P.; Nolan, B.C.; Yoder, P.G.; Lamani, E.; Hoshi, T.; Freeman, J.H. & Welsh, M.J. (2002). The Acid-Activated Ion Channel ASIC Contributes to Synaptic Plasticity, Learning, and Memory. *Neuron,* Vol. 34, No.3, pp.463-477, ISSN 0896-6273

Wemmie, J.A.; Coryell, M.W.; Askwith, C.C.; Lamani, E.; Leonard, A.S.; Sigmund, C.D. & Welsh, M.J. (2004). Overexpression of Acid-Sensing Ion Channel 1a in Transgenic Mice Increases Acquired Fear-Related Behavior. *Proceedings of National Academy of Science U.S.A.,* Vol. 101, No. 10, pp.3621-3626, ISSN 0027-8424

Wemmie, J.A.; Price, M.P. & Welsh, M.J. (2006). Acid-Sensing Ion Channels: Advances, Questions and Therapeutic Opportunities. *Trends in Neuroscience*, Vol. 29, No. 10, pp. 578-586, ISSN 0166-2236

Weng, J.Y.; Lin, Y.C. & Lien, C.C. (2010). Cell Type-Specific Expression of Acid-Sensing Ion Channels in Hippocampal Interneurons. *Journal of Neuroscience*, Vol. 30, No. 19, pp.6548-6558, ISSN 0270-6474

Wong, H.K.; Bauer, P.O.; Kurosawa, M.; Goswami, A.; Washizu, C.; Machida, Y.; Tosaki, A.; Yamada, M.; Knopfel, T.; Nakamura, T. & Nukina, N. (2008). Blocking Acid-Sensing Ion Channel 1 Alleviates Huntington's Disease Pathology via an Ubiquitin-Proteasome System Dependent Mechanism. *Human Molecular Genetics*, Vol.17, No. 20, pp. 3223-3235, ISSN 0964-6906

Wu, L.J.; Duan, B.; Mei, Y.D.; Gao, J.; Chen, J.G.; Zhuo, M.; Xu, L.; Wu, M. & Xu, T.L. (2004). Characterization of Acid-Sensing Ion Channels in Dorsal Horn Neurons of Rat Spinal Cord. *Journal of Biological Chemistry*, Vol. 279, No. 42, pp. 43716–43724, ISSN 0021-9258

Wu, W.L.; Lin, Y.W.; Min, M.Y. & Chen, C.C. (2010). Mice Lacking Asic3 Show Reduced Anxiety-Like Behavior on the Elevated Plus Maze and Reduced Aggression. *Genes, Brain and Behavior*, Vol. 9, No. 6, pp. 603-614, ISSN 1601-1848

Xiong, Z.G.; Chu, X.P. & Simon, R.P. (2007). Acid Sensing Ion Channels--Novel Therapeutic Targets for Ischemic Brain Injury. *Frontier in Bioscience*, Vol. 12, No. pp. 1376-1386, ISSN 1093-9946

Xiong, Z.G.; Zhu, X.M.; Chu, X.P.; Minami, M.; Hey, J., Wei, W.L.; MacDonald, J.F.; Wemmie, J.A.; Price, M.P.; Welsh, M.J. & Simon, R.P. (2004). Neuroprotection in Ischemia: Blocking Calcium Permeable Acid-Sensing Ion Channels, *Cell*, Vol. 118, No.6, pp. 687-698, ISSN 0092-8674

Xiong, Z.G.; Pignataro, G.; Li, M.; Chang, S.Y. & Simon, R.P. (2008). Acid-Sensing Ion Channels (ASICs) as Pharmacological Targets for Neurodegenerative Diseases. *Current Opinion in Pharmacology*, Vol.8, No. 1, pp.25-32, ISSN 1471- 4892

Xu, T.L. & Xiong, Z.G. (2007). Dynamic Regulation of Acid-Sensing Ion Channels by Extracellular and Intracellular Modulators. *Current Medicinal Chemistry*, Vol. 14, No.16, pp.1753-1763, ISSN 0929-8673

Yagi, J.; Wenk, H.N.; Naves, L.A. & McCleskey, E.W. (2006). Sustained Currents Through ASIC3 Ion Channels at the Modest pH Changes that Occur During Myocardial Ischemia. *Circulation Research*, Vol.99, No. 5, pp. 501 - 509, ISSN 0009-7330

Yermolaieva, O.; Leonard, A.S.; Schnizler, M.K.; Abboud, F.M. & Welsh, M.J. (2004). Extracellular Acidosis Increases Neuronal Cell Calcium by Activating Acid-Sensing Ion Channel 1a. *Proceedings of National Academy of Science U.S.A.*, Vol. 101, No. 17, pp.6752-6757, ISSN 0027-8424

Zha, X.M.; Costa, V.; Harding, A.M.; Reznikov, L.; Benson, C.J. & Welsh, M.J. (2009). ASIC2 Subunits Target Acid-Sensing Ion Channels to the Synapse via an Association with PSD-95. *Journal of Neuroscience*, Vol. 29, No. 26, pp. 8438 - 8446, ISSN 0270-6474

Zha, X.M.; Wemmie, J.A.; Green, S.H. & Welsh, M.J. (2006). Acid-Sensing Ion Channel 1A is a Postsynaptic Proton Receptor That Affects the Density of Dendritic Spines. *Proceedings of National Academy of Science U.S.A.*, Vol. 103, No. 44, pp. 16556-16561, ISSN 0027-8424

Zhou, Y. & Zhao, Z.Q. (2002). Effects of Neomycin on High-Threshold Ca(2+) Currents and Tetrodotoxin-Resistant Na(+) Currents in Rat Dorsal Root Ganglion Neuron. *European Journal of Pharmacology*, Vol. 450, No. 1, pp. 29-35, ISSN 0014-2999

Ziemann, A.E.; Allen, J.E.; Dahdaleh, N.S.; Drebot, I.I.; Coryell, M.W.; Wunsch, A.M.; Lynch, C.M.; Faraci, F.M.; Howard, M.A. III; Welsh, M.J. & Wemmie, J.A. (2009). The Amygdala is a Chemosensor that Detects Carbon Dioxide and Acidosis to Elicit Fear Behavior. *Cell*, Vol.139, No. 5, pp.1012-1021, ISSN 0092-8674

Ziemann, A.E.; Schnizler, M.K.; Albert, G.W.; Severson, M.A.; Howard, M.A. III.; Welsh, M.J. & Wemmie, J.A. (2008). Seizure Termination by Acidosis Depends on ASIC1a. *Nature Neuroscience*, Vol.11, No.7, pp. 816-822, ISSN 1097- 6256

21

Genome Profiling and Potential Biomarkers in Neurodegenerative Disorders

Luca Lovrečić, Aleš Maver and Borut Peterlin
Clinical Institute of Medical Genetics, University Medical Center Ljubljana, Slovenia

1. Introduction

Neurodegenerative disorders (NDG) are incurable, progressive and debilitating conditions resulting from progressive degeneration and death of nerve cells. They are among the most serious health problems faced by modern society. Most of these disorders become more common with advancing age, including Alzheimer's disease and Parkinson's disease. The burden of these neurodegenerative diseases is growing inexorably as the population ages, with incalculable economic and human costs. According to the Global Burden of Disease Study, a collaborative study of the World Health Organization, the World Bank and the Harvard School of Public Health, dementia and other neurodegenerative diseases will be the eighth cause of disease burden for developed regions in 2020 [1, 2]. Also, according to the WHO, neurodegenerative diseases will become the world's second leading cause of death by 2050, overtaking cancer [2]. True, such estimates and predictions need to be taken with caution, but they definitely confirm that neurodegenerative diseases are of an increasing public concern.

Most NDG diseases are characterized by the aggregation of intracellular proteins. Majority of neurodegenerative disorders occur sporadically and are believed to arise through interactions between genetic and environmental factors. Only a small minority belong to familial forms where certain disease occurs due to a mutation of the gene coding for the abnormally aggregating protein.

We differentiate many types of NDG disease, but the lines that separate one from another are often unclear. For instance, symptoms such as motor impairment and dementia may occur in many different types of NDG disease. Motor impairment similar to that seen in Parkinson's disease is not enough to rule out other diagnoses, especially when both motor and cognitive impairment are present. At the time being, there is no such diagnostic test that can clearly indicate the presence, absence, or category of a NDG disease. Individual diagnosis is based on clinical evaluation of the symptoms, with the exception of monogenic NDG diseases, such as Huntington's disease (HD). HD is a single gene disorder and cause is invariably trinucleotide expansion mutation [3].

Definitive diagnosis of certain NDG diseases still relies on neuropathological evaluation. But it has been demonstrated that brain pathology can show marked overlap among the syndromes of age-related cognitive and motor impairment [4]. Also, previous research reports have shown that pathological markers do not always correlate optimally with clinical findings. Some individuals with extensive neuropathology may retain relatively intact neurological function while others with less extensive pathology may be significantly impaired [5, 6]. The neuropathological findings may be the response to other antecedent disease processes and are not necessarily the cause of the underlying disease at the early disease stages. Later, as disease progresses, they probably contribute to disease progression in a positive feedback loop.

Analysis of whole genome transcriptome in brain might give us insights into the disturbed pathways and processes involved in disease onset and progression. Many different mechanisms have been proposed to be dysregulated in NDG diseases. We collected all reported studies to date on brain transcriptome in Parkinson's disease, Alzheimer disease, Huntington disease and Down syndrome and performed an integrated meta-analysis.

2. Background

2.1 Common neurodegenerative disorders – Alzheimer and Parkinson disease

Two most common neurodegenerative diseases, Parkinson's disease (PD) and Alzheimer disease(AD) are believed to be heterogeneous based on the causes - combination of genetic and environmental factors, vast variety in the age at onset, variability in leading symptoms and presenting clinical manifestations, disease progression and responses to different therapies employed. Definitive diagnosis of both, AD and PD still relies on a 'gold standard' post mortem neuropathological evaluation, although a number of clinical and neuropsychological tests are often employed when making a clinical diagnosis. AD is detected with approximately 85–90% accuracy and PD with approximaly 75% accuracy. The pathogenesis of both AD and PD are complex and still remain unexplained in worldwide research community.

It has been recently estimated [7] that 24 million people have dementia worldwide and majority is attributable to AD. The authors emphasized the urgency of better understanding of pathophysiology of the disease in order to improve development of disease-modifying treatment. Due to the age-dependent incidence rate of AD and due to the population ageing, it is foreseen that more than 80 million people will have AD by 2040 [8]. It is a progressive neurologic disease affecting particularly cortical and hippocampal neurons, leading to their irreversible loss [9]. Major clinical signs and symptoms are progressive impairment in memory, judgment, decision making, orientation to physical surroundings, and language. The key pathological characteristics are neuronal loss, β amyloid containing extracellular senile plaques, and neurofibrillary tangles, which are composed of a hyperphosphorylated form of the microtubular protein tau.

PD is the second most prevalent NDG disease after AD. According to available data of European Parkinson's Disease Association (EPDA), there are 6.3 million people with PD worldwide. Prevalence is age-dependent - there are approximately 0.5 to 1 percent of individuals with PD in the age group 65 to 69 years, and 1 to 3 percent of individuals with PD in the group of people older than 80 years [10]. Typical clinical sign is parkinsonism - resting tremor, bradykinesia, rigidity, and postural instability. Neuropathological characteristics are the loss of neurons in the substantia nigra and the presence of neuronal inclusions termed Lewy bodies and Lewy neurites whose main component is aggregated and phosphorylated alpha-synuclein [11].

Important futuristic challenge in the management AD and PD remains the establishment of early diagnosis or even identification of individuals prior to the onset of dementia in AD or resting tremor in PD. This implicates advancement in understanding disease pathogenesis and development of diagnostic approaches, including disease/process specific biomarkers.

2.2 Huntington disease – A model of genetic neurodegenerative disorder

Huntington disease is a late onset, single gene disorder and its cause is invariably trinucleotide expansion mutation, known for almost 2 decades [3]. Clinical characteristics of the disease include progressive motor impairment, cognitive decline and various psychiatric symptoms with the typical age of onset in the third to fifth decade. The disease is fatal after 15-20 years of progressive neurodegeneration [12]. So far, no effective treatment has been available to cure the disease or to slow its progression. Hyperkinesias and psychiatric symptoms may respond well to pharmacotherapy, but neuropsychological deficits and dementia remain untreatable [13]. We are unable to predict the age at onset and to follow the disease progression over short time periods due to the unsensitivity of rating scales. Even more, no useful measures to follow response to symptomatic treatment over short time periods are known. In addition, in the presymptomatic period when preventive treatment and slowing of neurodegeneration might be most effective, we have no measures/markers to monitor those responses and benefits.

Although the responsible gene and mutation were already identified and characterized in 1993, the function of normal huntingtin and the mutation mechanism that leads to neurodegeneration are still not clear. Basic research has demonstrated that the pathogenesis of HD involves recruitment of multiple biochemical pathways like protein degradation, apoptosis, accumulation of misfolded mutated proteins, intracelular signaling, oxidative stress, mitochondrial involvement and in the last years also transcription [14, 15].

2.3 Dementia and Down syndrome

Dementia, common symptom of all three already mentioned neurodegenerative diseases is also a common symptom in individuals with Down syndrome (DS). Most of individuals with DS after about age of 30 have the characteristic plaques and neurofibrillary tangles, associated with AD. As in general population, the prevalence of AD in people with DS increases significantly with age. On the other hand, age-related cognitive decline and dementia in people with DS occurs 30–40 years earlier than in the general population, reaching almost 40% in the 50s [16]. Life expectancy of people with DS continues to increase and therefore, dementia is becoming an important issue.

2.4 Biomarkers

Research in the field of biomarkers is a rapidly growing and developing area in medicine. Everyday advances in genomic, proteomic, metabolomic and epigenomic knowledge and technologies have made their way also in the neuroscientific research area. Biomarkers are very important indicators of normal and abnormal biological processes. By definition, biological marker or biomarker is a characteristic that is objectively measured and evaluated as an indicator of normal biological processes, pathogenic processes, or pharmacologic responses to a therapeutic intervention [17]. Despite the fact that enormous effort and extensive research have been concentrated on this area, there is still a major lack of biomarkers for diagnosis, progression monitoring, response to treatment evaluation, etc. in neurodegenerative disorders such as Alzheimer's disease (AD), Parkinson's disease (PD) and Huntington's disease (HD).

Biomarkers have many valuable applications, such as identification of major neuropathological processes in specific disease, disease detection and monitoring of health status, early efficacy and safety evaluations in *in vitro* studies in tissue samples, *in vivo* studies in animal models, and early-phase clinical trials. They are invaluable as a diagnostic tool for identification of patients with a disease or abnormal condition, as a tool in staging the disease or classification of the extent of disease, as an indicator of disease prognosis and in predicting and monitoring of a clinical response to treatment.

Biomarkers are of extreme relevance in chronic NDG diseases - there are no cures for these diseases, as neurons of the central nervous system cannot regenerate on their own after cell death or damage. Tremendous efforts have been made in recent years to identify the neuropathological, biochemical, and genetic biomarkers of these diseases aiming to establish the diagnosis in earlier stages, to survey the rate of progression, or response to treatment. Currently, the neuropathologic diagnosis is a gold standard, but it can only be made in the form of an autopsy after the patient's death. On the other hand, biomarkers may improve the early diagnosis at a stage when disease-modifying therapies are likely to be most effective, the monitoring of disease progression and the efficacy of any therapeutic intervention [18].

2.5 Brain transcriptome in neurodegenerative disorders

Many different research groups have tried to solve the neuropathophysiological puzzle in PD, AD, HD and DS. Human brain has been extensivelly studied using many approaches, in the last decade also variety of »omic« technologies. Whole-genome gene expression studies in brain of each of four diseases individually have shown changes in transcription of number of genes when compared to normal human brain.

We investigated, reviewed and collected data from all reported studies to date on brain transcriptome in Parkinson's disease, Alzheimer disease, Huntington disease and Down syndrome and performed integrated meta-analysis.

3. Methods

In an attempt to present the alterations consistently reported by studies of brain transcriptome in neurodegenerative diseases, we initially searched for such reports in literature databases, then obtained raw and processed experimental data from microarray data repositories, after which we performed probe level meta-analyses of datasets originating from various studies. In addition, to reveal possible commonalities and shared pathways across various neurodegenerative diseases, we inspected the similarities and differences in gene expression dysregularities occurring in these conditions.

3.1 Study inclusion

Initially, we have searched Medline database (http://www.ncbi.nlm.nih.gov/pubmed) for reports from studies of interest using the search string (transcriptom* OR microarray OR profiling OR Affymetrix OR Agilent OR Illumina OR array) AND (Parkinson's disease OR Parkinsons disease OR Parkinson disease AND Alzheimer's disease OR Alzheimers disease OR Alzheimer disease OR dementia OR Down's syndrome OR Downs syndrome OR Down syndrome OR trisomy 21 OR Huntington's disease OR Huntingtons disease OR Huntington disease) to obtain the complete list of studies reporting results relating to transcriptional alterations in brain tissues affected by neurodegenerative processes.

As we were primarily interested in the studies with microarray experimental results accessible from biological repositories, we then searched Gene Expression Omnibus (GEO) repository (*http://www.ncbi.nlm.nih.gov/geo/*), ArrayExpress database (*http://www.ebi.ac.uk/arrayexpress/*) and Stanford Microarray database (*http://smd.stanford.edu*) for studies with data available in the raw or processed form. As most of the gene expression profiling experiments were performed on Affymetrix platform and to avoid difficulties due to different probe annotations utilized by different microarray manufacturers, only results from experiments performed on the Affymetrix U133 platform were included to facilitate further steps in probe level meta-analysis of microarray data. The detailed information on datasets included in the analyses may be observed in Table 1.

3.2 Microarray data pre-processing and preparation for meta-analysis

All the integration and statistical steps described were performed in R statistical environment version 2.13.1 (http://cran.r-project.org), using Bioconductor version 2.8 packages (available at http://bioconductor.org) [19]. Raw data from all microarray experiments listed in Table 1 was obtained directly from Gene Expression Omnibus (GEO) repository (http://www.ncbi.nlm.nih.gov/geo/) utilizing the GEOquery package for R [20, 21].

Before the meta-analysis of data from selected studies was performed, all the datasets obtained in such manner were inspected for significant inter-array differences in distribution of probe intensities. For this reason, raw datasets were initially examined using arrayQualityMetrics package and where necessary the straightforward quantile normalization functions in the affyPLM package was utilized [30, 31]. Non-specific intensity and interquartile variation filters were applied using methods in genefilter package [19]. Log_2 transformations were applied where discrepancies in data reporting format were observed.

Data collections for each individual neurodegenerative disease were then merged using probeset annotations as the common denominator. Using this approach we avoided potential statistical issues originating from averaging probe intensity values to obtain a single mean intensity value for each gene, possibly disregarding distinct expression of different transcripts from the same gene.

These steps resulted in generation of 4 separate data matrices, each carrying data for a single disease, originating from multiple studies - Alzheimer disease (AD), Down syndrome (DS), Huntington disease (HD) and Parkinson disease (PD) datasets.

3.3 Meta-analysis

Summarized differential expression of genes in each merged dataset was calculated using meta-analysis algorithms incorporated in the RankProd package for R [32]. RankProd uses a non-parametric statistical algorithm that facilitates detection of genes that are consistently highly ranked across microarray datasets originating from various microarray experiments in various studies perfomed on the same condition (ie. disease). As this approach is based on rank statistics in contrast to approaches requiring analyzing absolute intensity values, it allows for inclusion of data originating from different laboratories, differing platforms and potentially studies performed under differing conditions [32].

For analyses of such multi-study data, RPadvance function was utilized in our analyses, with origin parameter set to account for data originating from number of different sources corresponding to the number of different originating study [32]. Here it is important to

GEO Accession	Disease name	Platform	Number of probesets*	Number of array experiments		Tissue	Ref
				Affected tissue	Unaffected tissue		
GSE5281	Alzheimer's disease	Affymetrix HG-U133Plus2	54,675	87	74	Entorhinal cortex Hippocampus Medial temporal gyrus Posterior cingulate cortex Primary visual cortex Superior frontal gyrus	[22]
GSE1297	Alzheimer's disease	Affymetrix HG-U133A	22,283	22	9	Hippocampus	[23]
†GSE16759	Alzheimer's disease	Affymetrix HG-U133Plus2	54,675	4	4	Parietal lobe tissue	[24]
†GSE7307	Parkinson's disease	Affymetrix HG-U133Plus2	54,675	22	45	Caudate Gloubus pallidum Putamen Substantia nigra Subthalamic nucleus Thalamus lateral nuclei Thalamus subthalamic nucleus	NA‡
GSE8397	Parkinson's disease	Affymetrix HG-U133A and Affymetrix HG-U133B	22,283 and 22,645	29 and 29	18 and 18	Substantia nigra Frontal cortex	[25]
GSE7621	Parkinson's disease	Affymetrix HG-U133Plus2	54,675	16	9	Substantia nigra	[26]
GSE3790	Huntington's disease	Affymetrix HG-U133A and Affymetrix HG-U133B	22,283 and 22,645	114	87	Cerebellum Frontal cortex Caudate nucleus	[27]
†GSE1397	Down syndrome	Affymetrix HG-U133A	22,283	9	9	Cerebrum Cerebellum Astrocyte samples	[28]
GSE5390	Down Syndrome	Affymetrix HG-U133A	22,283	7	8	Dorsolateral prefrontal cortex	[29]

* According to data obtained from the GEO site

† The dataset included some microarray experiments not related to the scope of this study and those were omitted from the analyses

‡ The study related to listed GEO entry was not yet published

Table 1. Detailed information on studies included in meta-analysis

stress that we have faced the issue of multiple studies simultaneously reporting differential expression in several different anatomical brain parts. As we wanted to facilitate the discovery of differentially expressed genes in diseased tissue in comparison to control samples, we set the origin parameter to take into account these considerations and regard such data as originating from different sources, thereby avoiding comparisons of gene expression between different brain regions rather than between affected and unaffected samples. Afterwards, P-values and q-values were obtained by performing 100 permutation cycles of complete originating datasets. An arbitrary P-value cut-off for significance of differential gene expression was then set at $P<0.05$.

3.4 Investigating intersections between datasets and gene set enrichment analyses

Resulting ordered lists of differentially expressed probesets were subsequently investigated for overlap between AD, DS, HD and PD datasets. Top 1000 genes from each dataset were used and intersections between combinations of two, three and four datasets were obtained. Venn diagrams in the results section were produced using Venny utility available at *http://bioinfogp.cnb.csic.es/tools/venny/index.html*. Furthermore, to gain insight in functional properties of genes in the intersections, gene set enrichment analyses (GSEA) were performed, utilizing GOstats package for R and investigating significant (uncorrected $p<0.05$) over- or underrepresentation of GeneOntology (GO) and KEGG terms annotating genes occurring in the intersections [33-36]. Additionally, DAVID tool (http://david.abcc.ncifcrf.gov/) was used to reveal the functional annotation clusters related to intersecting genes [37]. Required annotation conversions were performed using the hgu133plus.db package from Bioconductor annotation package collection and using biomaRt package for R in combination with Ensembl Biomart service (http://www.biomart.org/) [38, 39].

4. Results

Alltogether, our data collection comprised of data from 9 whole-genome expression studies, performed on samples from 4 neurodegenerative conditions (AD, DS, HD and PD). Collectively, 200, 33, 201, and 186 microarray analysed samples were included in the investigations of AD, DS, HD and PD, respectively, which accounted for 620 separate experiments included overall. A slight predominance of experiments performed on case tissues was noted in most of the experiements with summary case:control ratio amounting to 1,2:1 (339 affected tissues and 281 unaffected tissues included).

Separate analyses of datasets for each NDG disorder have revealed significant perturbances in expression profiles of several genes. When arbitrary permutation p-value cut-off was set at 0.05 for upregulated genes, 5701 probesets attained significance in the AD dataset, 3291 in DS dataset, 4174 in the HD dataset and 3043 in the PD dataset. In the downregulated gene group the $p<0.05$ significance was reached for 5496 probesets in the AD dataset, 2983 probesets in the DS dataset, 4079 in the HD dataset and 3410 in the PD dataset. A detailed view of the distribution of significance values of the top 10,000 ordered differentially expressed genes may be observed in Figure 1 for each of the NDG disorders.

The resulting numbers of significant results are inflated by the effect of multiple testing and therefore the q- values were also estimated as described in the article by Breitling et al [40]. The numbers of upregulated probesets with estimated q-values below 0.05 were 3775 for AD, 1496 for DS, 3182 for HD and 1894 for PD datasets. The numbers of downregulated probesets meeting this criterion were 3624 in AD, 652 in DS, 3065 in HD and 2541 probesets in the PD dataset.

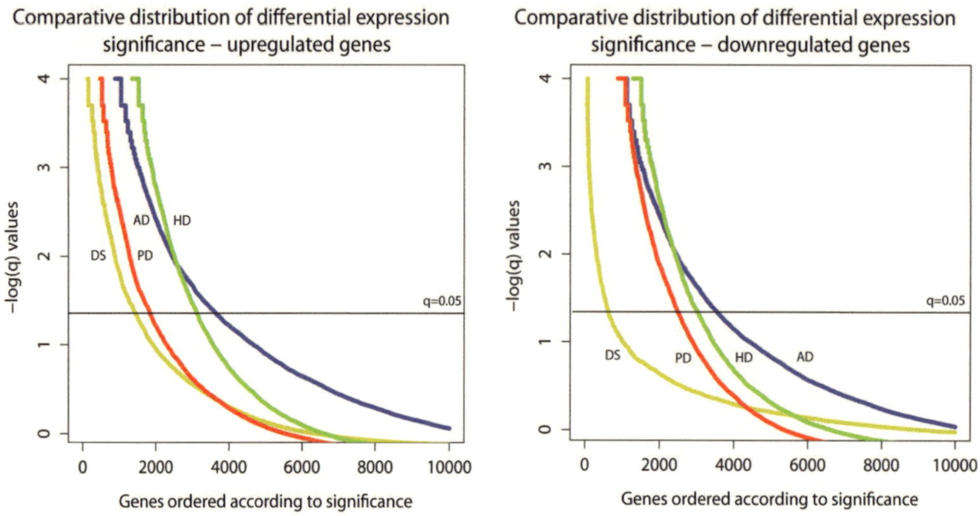

Fig. 1. Distribution of significance estimations for differential expression in 4 neurodegenerative disorders

An extent of global perturbation of the transciptome may be compared, with AD displaying the greatest extent of differentially expressed genes (blue line) and DS displaying the lowest extent, especially in the case of genes displaying downregulation.

4.1 Common patterns of differential expression in neurodegenerative disorders

Comparisons of comformity between profiles of transcriptome perturbations in four neurodegenerative diseases was initially performed by inspecting lists of top 1000 DE (differentially expressed) probesets for each condition and subsequently obtaining probesets (and genes) found to be differentially expressed simultaneously in several conditions.

The numbers of overlapping probesets may be observed in Figure 2. The largest overlap was observed between between the PD and HD lists, with altogether 338 (33.8%) upregulated and 267 (26.7%) downregulated genes differentially expressed in both conditions. Detailed overview of the extent of overlap between pairs of top DE gene list may be observed in Figure 3. A notable number of probesets was DE in all four conditions: 44 upregulated and 16 downregulated as presented in Figure 2a and 2b.

4.2 Comparative functional analyses of differential expression profile in neurodegenerative diseases

Calculations of gene set enrichment profile of upregulated and downregulated sets of genes presented here, were performed using hypergeometric test in the GOstats package. The profiles of DE genes were first calculated for each disorder separately, and afterwards every intersection between combinations of four sets of DE genes was evaluated.

Results of interests from separate GSEA analyses are presented in Table2(a-d) for top 1000 downregulated DE gene sets (the data for upregulated GSEA are not shown). Several GO biological process annotations appeared in all of the four analyses, most notably terms related to synaptic transmission and to cognitive processes.

We have also investigated the extent of similarity of GSEA profiles across four diseases. Top 200 enriched GO terms were inspected in each neurodegenerative disorder and compared for matching terms in pair with other three disorders. Greatest similarity was observed between GSEA terms annotating downregulated genes in all four disorders, which may be observed in more detail in Figure 4. As previously observed for overlapping genes, greatest overlap was observed between PD and HD GO profiles in the upregulated (40.0% overlap) and downregulated sets (59.5% overlap).

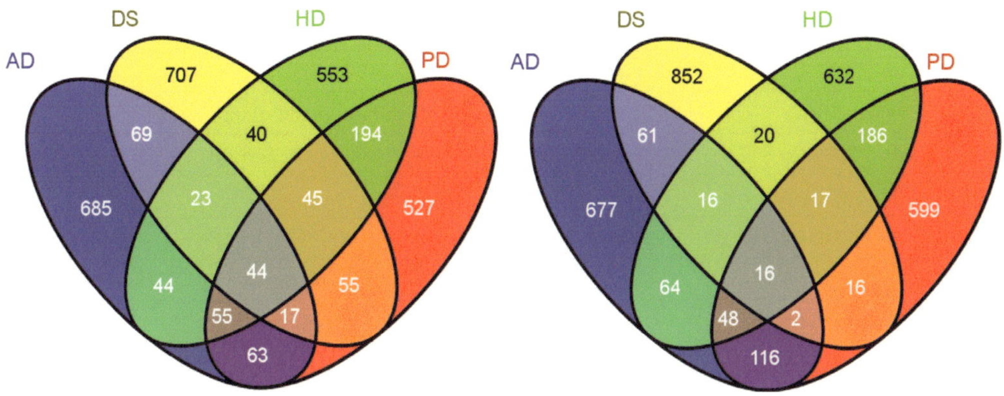

Fig. 2. Number of probesets overlapping between four sets of top 1000 DE upregulated (2a) and of top 1000 DE downregulated (2b) genes

Please note the abbreviations: Alzheimer disease (AD), Down syndrome (DS), Huntington disease (HD) and Parkinson disease (PD).

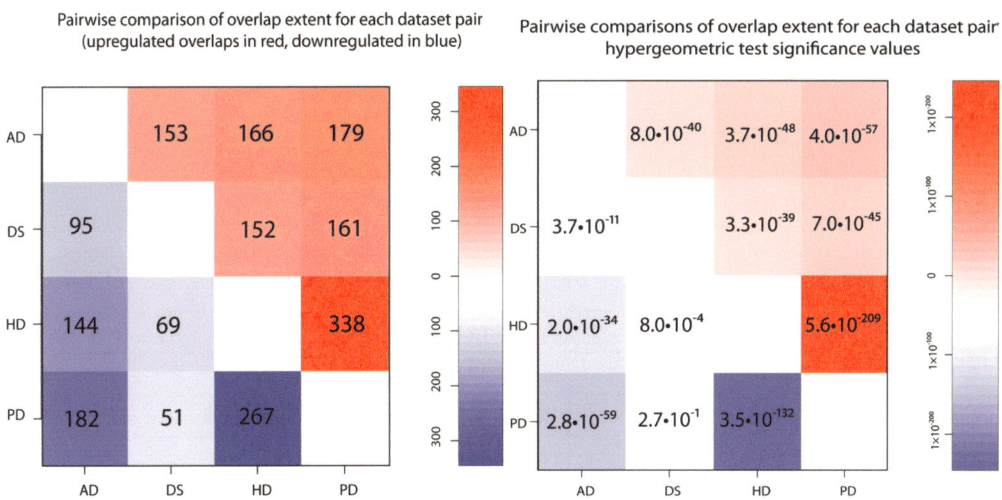

Fig. 3. a) Pairwise overlaps between lists of top DE upregulated (in red) and downregulated genes (in blue). Color intensiy of each square is proportional to size of overlap between a pair of DE gene lists. b) Pairwise overlaps between lists of top DE upregulated (in red) and downregulated genes (in blue). Color intensiy of each square is proportional to the value of -logp value obtained by performing hypergeometric test

GOBPID Accession	P-value	Count of genes annotated	Term
GO:0007268	1,01E-10	61	synaptic transmission
GO:0019226	1,49E-09	63	transmission of nerve impulse
GO:0035637	1,49E-09	63	multicellular organismal signaling
GO:0044282	2,61E-07	68	small molecule catabolic process
GO:0051443	5,09E-07	17	positive regulation of ubiquitin-protein ligase activity
GO:0019752	9,12E-07	70	carboxylic acid metabolic process
GO:0009144	1,82E-06	46	purine nucleoside triphosphate metabolic process
GO:0051438	5,03E-06	17	regulation of ubiquitin-protein ligase activity
GO:0007017	9,55E-06	35	microtubule-based process
GO:0007611	1,65E-05	18	learning or memory
GO:0030330	4,23E-05	16	DNA damage response, signal transduction by p53 class mediator
GO:0031398	4,70E-05	17	positive regulation of protein ubiquitination

Table 2a Alzheimer disease (downregulated genes). GOBPID stands for GeneOntology biological process ID

GOBPID Accession	P-value	Count of genes annotated	Term
GO:0007268	3,47E-37	90	synaptic transmission
GO:0019226	2,02E-35	93	transmission of nerve impulse
GO:0007267	5,12E-29	110	cell-cell signaling
GO:0007399	8,47E-15	113	nervous system development
GO:0007611	6,38E-13	25	learning or memory
GO:0007610	1,09E-12	46	behavior
GO:0050890	5,29E-12	25	cognition
GO:0048666	2,05E-10	59	neuron development
GO:0006836	2,24E-10	23	neurotransmitter transport
GO:0006811	9,51E-10	73	ion transport
GO:0001505	1,00E-09	21	regulation of neurotransmitter levels
GO:0031175	3,23E-09	52	neuron projection development
GO:0032940	9,52E-09	50	secretion by cell
GO:0048667	1,66E-08	46	cell morphogenesis involved in neuron differentiation
GO:0022008	3,13E-08	67	neurogenesis

Table 2b Huntington's disease (downregulated genes). GOBPID stands for GeneOntology biological process ID

GOBPID Accession	P-value	Count of genes annotated	Term
GO:0007268	4,16E-17	68	synaptic transmission
GO:0051234	1,99E-16	229	establishment of localization
GO:0019226	1,34E-15	70	transmission of nerve impulse
GO:0035637	1,34E-15	70	multicellular organismal signaling
GO:0006836	9,40E-14	29	neurotransmitter transport
GO:0009259	8,03E-13	58	ribonucleotide metabolic process
GO:0009144	1,47E-12	55	purine nucleoside triphosphate metabolic process
GO:0007399	8,20E-11	115	nervous system development
GO:0001505	8,41E-11	24	regulation of neurotransmitter levels
GO:0072521	9,91E-11	69	purine-containing compound metabolic process
GO:0007269	1,05E-10	20	neurotransmitter secretion
GO:0006753	2,95E-10	73	nucleoside phosphate metabolic process
GO:0009117	2,95E-10	73	nucleotide metabolic process
GO:0007267	3,23E-10	82	cell-cell signaling
GO:0015980	9,19E-10	39	energy derivation by oxidation of organic compounds

Table 2c Parkinson's disease (downregulated genes). GOBPID stands for GeneOntology biological process ID

GOBPID Accession	P-value	Count of genes annotated	Term
GO:0048856	6,65E-11	173	anatomical structure development
GO:0007267	2,83E-08	65	cell-cell signaling
GO:0050877	6,86E-07	69	neurological system process
GO:0050789	1,60E-06	318	regulation of biological process
GO:0022008	3,01E-06	58	neurogenesis
GO:0030182	3,71E-06	53	neuron differentiation
GO:0007399	4,91E-06	82	nervous system development
GO:0048839	8,26E-06	14	inner ear development
GO:0009887	1,69E-05	42	organ morphogenesis
GO:0007186	1,76E-05	41	G-protein coupled receptor protein signaling pathway
GO:0051716	2,70E-05	194	cellular response to stimulus
GO:0003001	4,34E-05	24	generation of a signal involved in cell-cell signaling
GO:0010903	5,15E-05	3	negative regulation of very-low-density lipoprotein particle remodeling
GO:0007268	7,44E-05	35	synaptic transmission
GO:0048667	7,44E-05	35	cell morphogenesis involved in neuron differentiation
GO:0007165	9,36E-05	165	signal transduction
GO:0048666	1,73E-04	41	neuron development

Table 2d Down's syndrome (downregulated genes). GOBPID stands for GeneOntology biological process ID

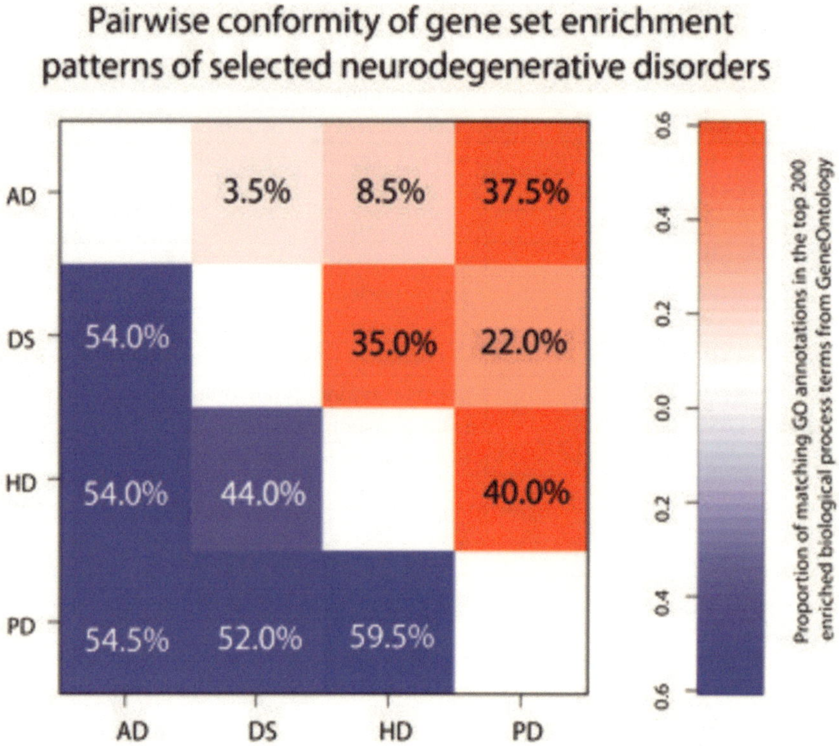

Fig. 4. Pairwise comparison of GO terms between pairs of datasets representing four neurodegenerative diseases. Percentages were calculated by dividing the number of GO terms overlapping by the number of all GO terms included in the overlapping analysis (N=200). GO terms annotating upregulated genes are presented in shades of red color and those annotating downregulated genes in blue

5. Conclusion

We have shown that whole-genome transcription analysis might be useful for identification and clarification of pathophysiological mechanisms in neurodegenerative diseases. We have used innovative approach of comparing and integrating experiment results from different NDG diseases and provided new important insights into the common NDG processes. Elucidation of these mechanisms holds important potential for future prediction and development of new useful treatments as well as for identification of biomarkers of neurodegeneration.

When comparisons of intersections between groups of top DE genes were performed, the greatest overlap was found between DE genes in brain samples of patients with HD and PD, which is possibly in accordance with their primary manifestation in movement disturbances related to function of basal ganglia. On the other hand, this similarity is surprising, as the known etiological agents in HD and PD differ significantly, one disorder being a consequence of monogenic disruption and other being a complex disorder with heterogeneous combination of genetic and environmental factors [41]. Surprisingly high is also the profile overlap between AD and PD, which present as clinically somewhat distinct entities. Recently however, it has been becoming progressively more obvious that the two disorders share not only a significant proportion of clinical elements (movement disorder, cognitive decline, mood and psychiatric disorders) but also share common pathophysiological pathways [42]. These results potentially suggest that clinical distinction between disease entities may not be perfect projection of actual processes at cellular and molecular level. Additionally, in contrast to expectation, however, the lowest overlap was observed between samples from patients with DS and AD, especially as these conditions have been known to share NDG pathways related to amyloid beta deposition in neurons. Reasons for lower extent of overlap may be found in significant differences in the age of patients from whom the brain samples were obtained for studies of DS in comparison with AD. Additionally, it is important that in most instances, a complete triplication of genes located on chromosome 21 may dominate genes commonly dysregulated in DS and AD [29]. Also, the number of brain tissue samples samples profiled in microarray experiments was by far the lowest among other types of NDG diseases investigated in our survey. Therefore, before final answer regarding this finding is obtained, more studies investigating transcriptional alterations in DS brain samples must be performed.

Several GO categories appeared to be consistently singled out in GSEA analyses of separate and overlapping genes DE in NDG disorders. Interestingly several terms were related to processes previously associated with neuron degeneration [42], most prominently GO terms: synaptic transmission (GO:0007268), neurogenesis (GO:0022008) and terms related to higher cognitive processes (GO:0007611). Dysfunctional synaptic transmission (as in glutamate exitotoxicity) and defects in neurogenesis have been previously repeatedly shown to be related to various NDG diseases [42-44]. It is interesting that although disturbances in neuroinflammatory mechanisms have been proposed as a possible causative factor in a number of NDG diseases, our analysis of intersecting genes dysregulated in brain samples of these conditions did not single out a particular common inflammatory pathogenetic pathway. This notion may be interpreted in the light of previously recognized differences in complement-activating immunogenic activity of plaques in different NDG diseases, resulting in absence of commonly overlapping inflammatory genes and GO terms [42].

When we investigated the compatibility of functional profiles between four NDG diseases, we have found greatest overlaps between sets of GO terms annotating genes characterized by downregulation in NDG diseases, where an overlap greater than 40% was observed in all of the pairwise comparisons of the sets of top 200 enriched GO terms. Again, the greatest functional conformance was noted between top downregulated genes in HD and PD as well as AD and PD dataset pairs. Notable overlap was also observed in the functional profiles of upregulated genes, where we noted good functional conformity between DS and HD datasets in addition to HD-PD and AD-PD functional overlaps.

It is important to stress that genome-wide expression studies included in this survey are inherently burdened by important statistical issues that predominantly originate from the issue of testing a large number of variables on a relatively small population of biological replicates (ie. study subjects) [45]. For this reason we attempted to gain a more complete account of biological alterations in neurodegenerative diseases by merging data from several different studies investigating transcriptional changes in brain samples of distinct neurological conditions (AD, DS, HD and PD) [46]. This increased the number of biological replicates considerably, allowing for potentially more reliable calling of DE genes in these conditions. There are, however, important downsides to this approach: the studies included were performed under differing conditions in different institutions and by different research staff. Even more important is the great heterogeneity between brain tissue samples investigated. We have attempted to circumvent these issues by using appropriate RankProd meta-analysis methods, nevertheless these results must be interpreted in light of these considerations.

Nevertheless it is still difficult to differentiate between the causal changes in transcriptome in contrast to changes resulting from previous damage to neural tissue. It is possible, however, that the similarities in transcriptome profile between clinically and pathologically distinct entities suggest a common response to an unknown initial damaging stimulus. We propose that in future, integration of various data such as genomic in combination with transcriptomic data should provide a way to delineate possible mechanisms, where genetic predisposition results in manifestation of transcriptional imbalances, consequently resulting in observed phenotype. Genome-wide expression profiling may however direct further research attempts into a particular direction. Also, there are other "omics" approaches besides transcriptomics and integrating all of them is future challenge.

6. References

[1] C.J.L. Murray ADL, *The Global Burden of Disease*. 1996, World Health Organisation: Geneva.

[2] Menken M, Munsat TL, Toole JF. The global burden of disease study: implications for neurology. *Arch Neurol* 2000; 57(3): p: 418-20.

[3] A novel gene containing a trinucleotide repeat that is expanded and unstable on Huntington's disease chromosomes. The Huntington's Disease Collaborative Research Group. *Cell* 1993; 72(6): p: 971-83.

[4] Schneider JA, Arvanitakis Z, Bang W, Bennett DA. Mixed brain pathologies account for most dementia cases in community-dwelling older persons. *Neurology* 2007; 69(24): p: 2197-204.

[5] Pathological correlates of late-onset dementia in a multicentre, community-based population in England and Wales. Neuropathology Group of the Medical Research Council Cognitive Function and Ageing Study (MRC CFAS). *Lancet* 2001; 357(9251): p: 169-75.

[6] Prohovnik I, Perl DP, Davis KL, et al. Dissociation of neuropathology from severity of dementia in late-onset Alzheimer disease. *Neurology* 2006; 66(1): p: 49-55.

[7] Ballard C, Gauthier S, Corbett A, et al. Alzheimer's disease. *Lancet*; 377(9770): p: 1019-31.

[8] Forlenza OV, Diniz BS, Gattaz WF. Diagnosis and biomarkers of predementia in Alzheimer's disease. *BMC Med*; 8: p: 89.

[9] McKhann G, Drachman D, Folstein M, et al. Clinical diagnosis of Alzheimer's disease: report of the NINCDS-ADRDA Work Group under the auspices of Department of Health and Human Services Task Force on Alzheimer's Disease. *Neurology* 1984; 34(7): p: 939-44.

[10] Nussbaum RL, Ellis CE. Alzheimer's disease and Parkinson's disease. *N Engl J Med* 2003; 348(14): p: 1356-64.

[11] Spillantini MG, Schmidt ML, Lee VM, et al. Alpha-synuclein in Lewy bodies. *Nature* 1997; 388(6645): p: 839-40.

[12] Harper PS. Huntington's disease. Major Problems in Neurology. 1996, London: W.B. Saunders Company Ltd.

[13] Bonelli RM, Hofmann P. A systematic review of the treatment studies in Huntington's disease since 1990. *Expert Opin Pharmacother* 2007; 8(2): p: 141-53.
[14] Harjes P, Wanker EE. The hunt for huntingtin function: interaction partners tell many different stories. *Trends Biochem Sci* 2003; 28(8): p: 425-33.
[15] Sugars KL, Rubinsztein DC. Transcriptional abnormalities in Huntington disease. *Trends Genet* 2003; 19(5): p: 233-8.
[16] Holland AJ, Hon J, Huppert FA, Stevens F, Watson P. Population-based study of the prevalence and presentation of dementia in adults with Down's syndrome. *Br J Psychiatry* 1998; 172: p: 493-8.
[17] Biomarkers and surrogate endpoints: preferred definitions and conceptual framework. *Clin Pharmacol Ther* 2001; 69(3): p: 89-95.
[18] Henley SM, Bates GP,Tabrizi SJ. Biomarkers for neurodegenerative diseases. *Curr Opin Neurol* 2005; 18(6): p: 698-705.
[19] Gentleman RC, Carey VJ, Bates DM, et al. Bioconductor: open software development for computational biology and bioinformatics. *Genome Biol* 2004; 5(10): p: R80.
[20] Barrett T, Edgar R. Gene expression omnibus: microarray data storage, submission, retrieval, and analysis. *Methods Enzymol* 2006; 411: p: 352-69.
[21] Sean D, Meltzer PS. GEOquery: A bridge between the Gene Expression Omnibus (GEO) and BioConductor. *Bioinformatics* 2007; 23(14): p: 1846-7.
[22] Liang WS, Dunckley T, Beach TG, et al. Gene expression profiles in anatomically and functionally distinct regions of the normal aged human brain. *Physiol Genomics* 2007; 28(3): p: 311-22.
[23] Blalock EM, Geddes JW, Chen KC, et al. Incipient Alzheimer's disease: microarray correlation analyses reveal major transcriptional and tumor suppressor responses. *Proc Natl Acad Sci U S A* 2004; 101(7): p: 2173-8.
[24] Nunez-Iglesias J, Liu CC, Morgan TE, Finch CE, Zhou XJ. Joint genome-wide profiling of miRNA and mRNA expression in Alzheimer's disease cortex reveals altered miRNA regulation. *PLoS One* 2010; 5(2): p: e8898.
[25] Moran LB, Duke DC, Deprez M, et al. Whole genome expression profiling of the medial and lateral substantia nigra in Parkinson's disease. *Neurogenetics* 2006; 7(1): p: 1-11.
[26] Lesnick TG, Papapetropoulos S, Mash DC, et al. A genomic pathway approach to a complex disease: axon guidance and Parkinson disease. *PLoS Genet* 2007; 3(6): p: e98.
[27] Hodges A, Strand AD, Aragaki AK, et al. Regional and cellular gene expression changes in human Huntington's disease brain. *Hum Mol Genet* 2006; 15(6): p: 965-77.
[28] Mao R, Wang X, Spitznagel EL, Jr., et al. Primary and secondary transcriptional effects in the developing human Down syndrome brain and heart. *Genome Biol* 2005; 6(13): p: R107.
[29] Lockstone HE, Harris LW, Swatton JE, et al. Gene expression profiling in the adult Down syndrome brain. *Genomics* 2007; 90(6): p: 647-60.
[30] Kauffmann A, Gentleman R, Huber W. arrayQualityMetrics--a bioconductor package for quality assessment of microarray data. *Bioinformatics* 2009; 25(3): p: 415-6.
[31] Heber S,Sick B. Quality assessment of Affymetrix GeneChip data. *OMICS* 2006; 10(3): p: 358-68.
[32] Hong F, Breitling R, McEntee CW, et al. RankProd: A bioconductor package for detecting differentially expressed genes in meta-analysis. *Bioinformatics* 2006; 22(22): p: 2825-7.

[33] Falcon S, Gentleman R. Using GOstats to test gene lists for GO term association. *Bioinformatics* 2007; 23(2): p: 257-8.
[34] Ashburner M, Ball CA, Blake JA, et al. Gene ontology: Tool for the unification of biology. The Gene Ontology Consortium. *Nat Genet* 2000; 25(1): p: 25-9.
[35] Ogata H, Goto S, Sato K, et al. KEGG: Kyoto Encyclopedia of Genes and Genomes. *Nucleic Acids Res* 1999; 27(1): p: 29-34.
[36] Mootha VK, Lindgren CM, Eriksson KF, et al. PGC-1alpha-responsive genes involved in oxidative phosphorylation are coordinately downregulated in human diabetes. *Nat Genet* 2003; 34(3): p: 267-73.
[37] Huang da W, Sherman BT, Lempicki RA. Systematic and integrative analysis of large gene lists using DAVID bioinformatics resources. *Nat Protoc* 2009; 4(1): p: 44-57.
[38] Durinck S, Spellman PT, Birney E, Huber W. Mapping identifiers for the integration of genomic datasets with the R/Bioconductor package biomaRt. *Nat Protoc* 2009; 4(8): p: 1184-91.
[39] Durinck S, Moreau Y, Kasprzyk A, et al. BioMart and Bioconductor: A powerful link between biological databases and microarray data analysis. *Bioinformatics* 2005; 21(16): p: 3439-40.
[40] Breitling R, Armengaud P, Amtmann A, Herzyk P. Rank products: A simple, yet powerful, new method to detect differentially regulated genes in replicated microarray experiments. *FEBS Lett* 2004; 573(1-3): p: 83-92.
[41] Feany MB. ASIP Outstanding Investigator Award Lecture. New approaches to the pathology and genetics of neurodegeneration. *Am J Pathol* 2010; 176(5): p: 2058-66.
[42] Grunblatt E. Commonalities in the genetics of Alzheimer's disease and Parkinson's disease. *Expert Rev Neurother* 2008; 8(12): p: 1865-77.
[43] Palomo T, Archer T, Beninger RJ, Kostrzewa RM. Gene-environment interplay in neurogenesis and neurodegeneration. *Neurotox Res* 2004; 6(6): p: 415-34.
[44] Shankar GM, Walsh DM. Alzheimer's disease: synaptic dysfunction and Abeta. *Mol Neurodegener* 2009; 4: p: 48.
[45] Allison DB, Cui X, Page GP, Sabripour M. Microarray data analysis: from disarray to consolidation and consensus. *Nat Rev Genet* 2006; 7(1): p: 55-65.
[46] Cahan P, Rovegno F, Mooney D, et al. Meta-analysis of microarray results: challenges, opportunities, and recommendations for standardization. *Gene* 2007; 401(1-2): p: 12-8.

22

Immunization with Neural-Derived Peptides as a Potential Therapy in Neurodegenerative Diseases

Humberto Mestre and Antonio Ibarra
Universidad Anahuac Mexico Norte
Mexico

1. Introduction

There is a nosological dilemma when it comes to classifying what comprises a neurodegenerative disease (NDD). Degeneration - purely speaking - is to go from a higher to a lower level of functioning; it is deterioration from normalcy. Neurons are the functional elements of the nervous system. Then degeneration of the nervous system consists of a decrease or loss in the function of neurons. Not necessarily an atrophy, which consists of the death of a particular population of neurons. Clinically, NDD are comprised of progressive dementias, progressive ataxias, disorders in posture and movement, muscle weakness, and progressive blindness. The common characteristic in all of these pathologies is their chronicity. Each and every one of the aforementioned diseases consists of a chronic progression towards the loss of a particular function. However, this definition does not include a limit on temporality. Nosologically speaking neurodegeneration could include several other pathologies from an acute time frame. NDD can further be divided into an acute and chronic classification. Chronic diseases such as: amyotrophic lateral sclerosis (ALS), Alzheimer disease (AD) and Parkinson disease (PD) were the common conception of NDD. The latter was sustained until acute traumatic injuries to the central nervous system (CNS) were found to cause generalized inflammation and other phenomena that lead to degeneration. Examples of CNS injury that cause this secondary degeneration are: global or focal cerebral ischemia (stroke), spinal cord injury (SCI), and traumatic brain injury (TBI). The similarities in neurodegenerative processes between these and chronic NDD allows us to classify them within acute NDD. Neurodegeneration previously consisted of progressive atrophic disorders but has now expanded into the study of all pathophysiological processes that deteriorate the CNS. As a whole, NDD are the cause of many deaths around the world. In the US, stroke, traumatic injuries (such as: SCI and TBI), AD, and PD are within the top 15 causes of mortality, averaging 350,000 deaths per year (Xu et al., 2007). Although NDD have an elevated mortality their greatest impact is on morbidity, affecting 50 million Americans each year and generating a large amount of federal spending (Brown et al., 2005). Every year $144 billion USD are spent on AD alone, and that is excluding the spending required for the other 600 neurological disorders that have been described (Alzheimer's Association, 2010; Meek et al., 1998). The elevated prevalence and incidence require a large initiative to research the hallmarks of these diseases. Until now, our understanding of NDD is quite complex but there is still a lot to uncover. Research is normally directed towards the NDD with the most impact on society such as: ALS, AD and PD. Due to the increased availability of information on the previous diseases this chapter will only discuss these diseases within the chronic NDD section. In order to find treatment opportunities for each one of these diseases we must first understand the basic pathophysiology. ALS is a progressive degeneration of upper and lower motor neurons in the brain and spinal cord. This atrophy eliminates the brain's control over muscle movements and causes them to weaken and become paralyzed. Progressive muscular paralysis causes the inability to move, swallow, and eventually, breathe (Angelov et al., 2003). AD is a progressive disorder characterized by memory loss and severe cognitive decline. This degeneration is caused by excessive accumulations of extracellular amyloid beta peptide, which forms plaques in the hippocampus and cerebral cortex, leading to neuronal death (Frenkel et al., 2005; Butovsky et al., 2006). PD is a chronic progressive disease characterized by motor symptoms (tremor, rigidity and bradykinesia) and nonmotor symptoms (e.g. autonomic, mood and cognitive). These clinical hallmarks are attributed to the degeneration of nigrostraital dopaminergic neurons and other structures in the brainstem, cortex, and subcortex (Laurie et al., 2007). Multiple sclerosis (MS) is an inflammatory autoimmune CNS demyelinating disease that is thought to be perpetrated by myelin-reactive lymphocytes. Demyelination of the CNS causes the loss of function of the affected tract (Stuve et al., 2006). MS is considered an autoimmune disease and not a NDD because there is no direct neuronal death only demyelination. The nosology of NDD excludes MS from our study but it still shares very similar immune pathophysiology and most of the therapies mentioned are derived or designed for use in MS. The inflammatory component of acute injury to the CNS provided new insight into the autoimmune response propagated after a CNS insult. These findings gave immune cells a crucial role in the protection and regeneration of the injured CNS, as well as a role in chronic progressive NDD. Further insight into the immunological component of neurodegenerative diseases provides us with new mechanisms where we are able to intervene in order to resolve these disorders. One of these mechanisms is protective autoimmunity (PA). PA is a new concept where autoreactive mechanisms are being modulated in order to promote neuroprotection. Dr. Michal Schwartz from the Weizmann Institute of Science in Israel originally conceived this concept. Infiltration of immune cells after CNS injury was traditionally regarded as pathological. This view was based on the fact that immune cell-infiltration has been exclusively identified with inflammation, and that inflammation is generally harmful to the injured CNS. However, recent studies indicate that a well-controlled innate and adaptive immune response is essential for the repair of the injured tissue. These results brought about research into immunomodulatory therapies in several NDD. In acute NDD and MS, recent findings have suggested that the inflammatory response is strongly modulated by an autoimmune reaction directed against neural constituents, specifically against myelin basic protein (MBP), one of the most abundant and immunogenic proteins in the CNS (Butovsky et al., 2001; Ibarra et al., 2003; Popovich et al., 1996; Sospedra & Martin, 2005). Dr. Schwartz started to modulate the action of myelin-specific autoreactive lymphocytes by immunizing with MBP. This strategy improved tissue preservation, neuronal survival and motor recovery after acute SCI (Hauben et al., 2000a; Hauben et al., 2000b). PA also proved to be a T cell-dependent response that is genetically determined (Kipnis et al., 2001) and triggered as a physiological response to CNS trauma (Yoles et al., 2001). However, immunizing animals with self-antigens (i.e. MBP) induced an autoimmune disease known as experimental autoimmune encephalomyelitis (EAE, animal model of MS). Therefore, a different way of eliciting PA had to be obtained in order to prevent this complication. Studies suggested that immunizing with a weaker version of the self-antigen could solve the problem, these type of antigens became known as altered peptide ligands (APL). Vaccinating with APL would generate PA without degenerative autoimmunity. In the study of NDD, APL were derived from neural constituents and were therefore coined under the term neural-derived peptides (NDP). The success in the development of these immunomodulatory peptides has inspired a lot of research into their possible therapeutic applications in both chronic and acute NDD. These applications will be described in detail throughout this chapter.

2. Role of immune cells and their potential therapeutic effect

The CNS has long been considered to be an immunologically privileged location. The blood-brain barrier (BBB) was thought to maintain blood-borne cells of both the innate and adaptive immune system out of the CNS. This hypothesis assumed that microglia were the only innate immune cells of the CNS. During damage, microglia became activated and functioned as destructive inflammatory cells indistinguishable from infiltrating macrophages. Immune cells were thought to contribute to the increase in tissue damage during CNS disease (Bethea et al., 1998; Blight, 1992; Dusart et al., 1994; Popovich et al., 1997). The idea was supported by the following: i) CNS trauma activates T lymphocytes against neural constituents, and ii) the passive transfer of myelin autoreactive T cells caused EAE in previously healthy rats (Popovich et al., 1996). The notion was sustained in such a way that the complete inhibition of these responses was proposed as a potential therapeutic intervention, and remains to this day as the predominant clinical approach (Lopez-Vales et al., 2005; Popovich et al., 1999). However, it is now clear that these cells have a pivotal role in CNS repair (Hammarberg et al., 2000; Hashimoto et al., 2007; Hendrix & Nitsch, 2007; Moalem et al., 1999; Rapalino et al., 1998; Turrin & Rivest, 2006; Yin et al., 2003). In the healthy CNS the microglia is in a resting state where its morphology consists of a small cell soma and numerous branching processes, known as resting/ramified state. The ramifications are dynamic structures that enable the cell to sample and monitor its microenvironment (Nimmerjahn et al., 2005; Raivich, 2005). Resting microglia express CD45 (leukocyte common antigen), CD14, and CD11b/CD18 (Kreutzberg, 1996). Under duress, microglial expression patterns are modified from a monitoring role to one of protection and repair. Microglia begin to express key surface receptors such as: CD1, lymphocyte function-associated antigen 1 (LFA-1), intracellular adhesion molecule 1 (ICAM-1), and vascular cell adhesion molecule 1 (VCAM-1). Besides changing their surface receptor repertoire they begin to secrete: inflammatory cytokines such as TNFα and interleukins IL-1β and IL-6, chemokines like macrophage inflammatory protein (MIP-1α), monocyte chemoattractant protein (MCP-1), and interferon inducible protein 10 (IP-10). This change in microenvironment changes the resting/ramified state of the microglia into an amoeboid/phagocytic state. The activated state of microglia has beneficial functions during NDD such as: scavenging neurotoxins, removing cellular debris, and the secretion of trophic factors that promote neuronal survival (Frank-Cannon et al., 2009). During CNS injury, if microglia come in contact with products of the adaptive immune response such as interferon gamma (IFN-γ) and IL-4 it will acquire a phenotype that has antigen presenting cell (APC)-like qualities. This phenotype expresses major histocompatibility complex II (MHC-II) and B 7.2 receptors, giving it the ability to interact with elements of the adaptive immune response. As an APC, microglia can hold dialogue with T cells and are capable of releasing neurotrophic factors (BDNF, NT-3, NGF) and scavenging toxic neurotransmitters and reactive oxygen species (ROS) that endanger the tissue (Li et al., 2007; Schwartz et al., 2003). However, the chronic and uncontrolled activation of microglia increases the permeability of the BBB and elevates the amount of infiltrating blood-borne immune cells (Schmid et al., 2009). This promotes the activation of microglial cells into a destructive phenotype characterized by the production of high levels of nitric oxide (NO, a potent free radical), as well as TNFα, and cyclooxygenase 2 (COX2) (Franciosi et al., 2005; Lee et al., 2007; Shaked et al., 2004). In this phenotype microglia express low amounts of MHC-II and are thus incapable of communicating with the adaptive immune system, an important condition to promote neuroprotection (Schwartz et al., 2003; Shaked et al., 2004). In addition, T lymphocytes are recruited in small amounts and very late. The lack of T cell-mediated activation of microglia results in an uncoordinated release of additional pro-inflammatory cytokines, exacerbating the damage (Bethea et al., 1999; Lopez-Vales et al., 2006; Pan et al., 2003; Resnick et al., 1998; Schwartz et al., 2003; Vanegas & Schaible, 2001). The best way to elicit a T cell-mediated activation of microglial cells is through neural autoreactive T cells. This assures that T cells arrive to the CNS and activate microglia into their protective phenotype propagating the beneficial effects mentioned above (Figure 1). PA has proven to yield clinical improvements in the treatment of several NDD.

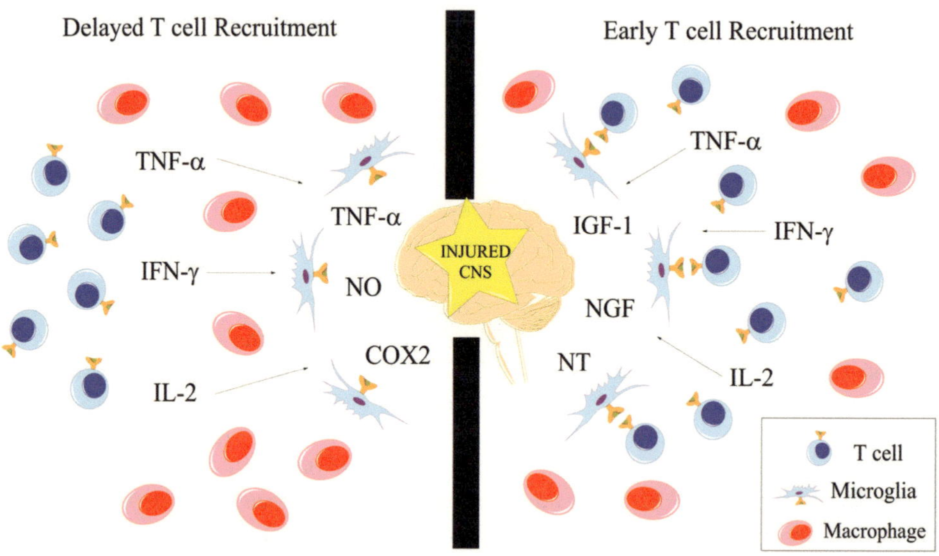

Fig. 1. T cell recruitment into the injured CNS

Left panel: An uncontrolled response where T cells are recruited very late allows the activation of microglia into a destructive phenotype. This is characterized by the release of nitric oxide (NO) and proinflammatory molecules like tumor necrosis factor alfa (TNF-α) and cyclooxygenase-2 (COX2). Under these circumstances, T cells intensify the inflammatory response and exacerbate neurodegeneration. *Right panel:* When the autoreactive response is elicited by immunizing with NDP there is an earlier and larger arrival of T cells. With this approach, microglial cells undergo a T cell-mediated activation into a protective phenotype. This regulated activation releases molecules that promote neuroprotection and neuroregeneration such as: neurotrophins (NT), nerve growth factor (NGF), and insulin-like growth factor 1 (IGF-1). The early arrival of T cells due to immunization with NDP regulates the response so that we can obtain the benefits and not the detriments of the immune response.

3. Modulation of the immune response using neural-derived peptides

Immunomodulation is an idea from the past that looks more promising than ever. It is a change in the body's normal physiological immune response to a specific antigen. This modulation changes the way the immune system would normally respond to an event and replaces it with an alternate desired response. The modification of immune responses is different from agents that suppress the immune response (such as corticosteroids). Immunomodulation has already become a reality. For example, IFN-γ is used in patients with chronic granulomatous disease (Farhoudi et al., 2003), IFN-β is used in patients with multiple sclerosis (Kumpfel et al., 2007), and IL-2 in patients with AIDS and metastatic melanoma (Davey et al., 1997; Terando et al., 2003). Aside from this, numerous vaccines use adjuvants to achieve the desired immune response (Partidos et al., 2004; Petrovsky & Aguilar, 2004). Modulation of the immune response as a therapeutic strategy is a promising alternative for several diseases. PA allows us to speculate that it is better to modulate the immune response rather than eliminating it. In chronic NDD, patients require a competent immune response to fend off pathogens and evade complications due to infections. The ablation of the immune response is usually done with steroids or immunosuppressants, which severely affect the patient's ability to initiate an adequate immune response. In the acute form of NDD the immune system is vital in the return to homeostasis. Immune cells extract cellular debris, reestablish blood flow, secrete neurotrophic factors and eliminate pathogens. All these beneficial effects are lost when the immune response is inhibited using immunosuppressant therapy. Accordingly, it seems only logical that the immune response is essential in NDD. In line with this, it is realistic to envision that the harmful effects exerted by immune cells could be reverted or changed to promote beneficial actions. In order to achieve this goal, it is crucial to avoid or at least diminish the activation of microglial cells by means of the classic pathway (destructive phenotype). For this purpose, an earlier and larger arrival of T cells to the site of injury should be promoted. The opportune and adequate arrival of these cells will favor the activation of microglia under the bases of a protective phenotype (Shaked et al., 2004). A simple way of making this possible is by immunizing with the same antigen that induces the autoreactive response: neural antigens. With this approach, an important number of microglial cells will acquire the protective phenotype and will then release molecules that instead of increasing damage will promote neuroprotection. Thus, we will obtain the benefits and not the detriments of this immune response. The present strategy proposes the modulation of the immunological response by boosting an autoreactive reaction. This could be a bit conflicting for general understanding since it is common to associate autoimmunity with disease. However, at present, it is very clear that autoimmunity is a physiological phenomenon perfectly compatible with homeostasis (Schwartz & Cohen, 2000). Furthermore, autoimmunity has been proposed as a useful and beneficial event (Hauben et al., 2005). Therefore, PA is a protective strategy where autoimmunity is the main player in providing beneficial effects during CNS injury.

4. Modulation of protective autoimmunity with no risk of autoimmune disease

As it was mentioned before, the possibility of inducing an autoimmune disease after vaccination with neural constituents is perhaps the main complication of this therapy. In order to solve this issue, immunizations are done with NDP. NDP are analogs of immunogenic epitopes with one (or a few) substitution(s) at specific amino acid positions of neural peptides (NP). The variation between the amino acid sequence is essential for contact with the T cell receptor (TCR) during antigen processing. This variation allows them to compete for TCR binding and to interfere with the necessary sequence of events required for T cell activation. The interference caused by NDP in TCR antigen recognition could affect T cell differentiation or induce a state of anergy (Nel & Slaughter, 2002). The specificity and avidity of the TCR with its ligand is determined by the primary sequence of the antigenic peptide. That particular sequence affects its binding to the complementary-determining regions of the TCR and the peptide-binding groove of the HLA molecule (Garboczi et al., 1996). A small variation in amino acid sequence can alter its ability to interact with either the MHC-II or TCR receptor molecule. This competition thereby converts an agonist peptide into a partial agonist or even an antagonist (Jameson & Bevan, 1995). Agonist peptides engage in high-affinity interactions with the TCR and induce a robust T cell response; whereas partial agonists or antagonists engage in lower affinity interactions that lead to altered or inhibitory responses (Jameson & Bevan, 1995; Kersh & Allen, 1996). Stimulation of naïve CD4+ T cells with an agonist peptide induces sufficient assembly of signaling complexes to allow activation of the IL-2 promoter and support a Th1 differentiation pathway. In contrast, the signals generated by APL activation are generally insufficient to induce IL-2 synthesis and therefore will not cause activation. That lack of IL-2 production might induce an anergic state or a skewing of the Th1/Th2 differentiation (Nel & Slaughter, 2002). Some APL are already being explored for neurological diseases (Figure 2). These peptides are derived from MBP-encephalitogenic epitopes. A group of them (G91, A96 and A91) have already been tested in animal models (Hauben et al., 2001). Importantly, immunized animals did not present clinical signs of EAE. A91 is a peptide derived from MBP (sequence 87-99), where the lysine residue at position 91 is replaced for alanine. This NDP cross-reacts with the original encephalitogenic epitope of MBP but it activates weak self-reactive T cells thus inducing autoimmunity without developing EAE. Immunizing with A91 inhibits EAE but neither causes anergy nor clonal deletion (Gaur et al., 1997). During antigenic presentation, A91 works as a partial agonist that instead of inducing a Th1 response promotes a Th2 differentiation pathway. This preference for the Th2 phenotype may be responsible for the elimination of the Th1-dependent response observed in EAE. Studies also indicate that post-injury injection of bone marrow-derived dendritic cells pulsed with A91, induce the same significant beneficial effects (Hauben et al., 2003). This indicates that the APC properties of the dendritic cell are enough to activate anti-A91 CD4+ T cells that are responsible for the elevated neuroprotection. To further support the use of immunomodulatory NDP, our laboratory examined the effects of combining immunizations with A91 and methylprednisolone (MP). The use of corticosteroids, such as MP, is the only therapeutic agent currently available for the treatment of a variety of NDD, primarily CNS trauma. In our study, a high dose of MP was administered together with an A91 immunization after SCI. As expected, MP eliminated the beneficial effects of A91. Nevertheless, when vaccination with A91 was delayed for 48 h after injury, there was no interference with its effect by the anti-inflammatory action of MP injected immediately after

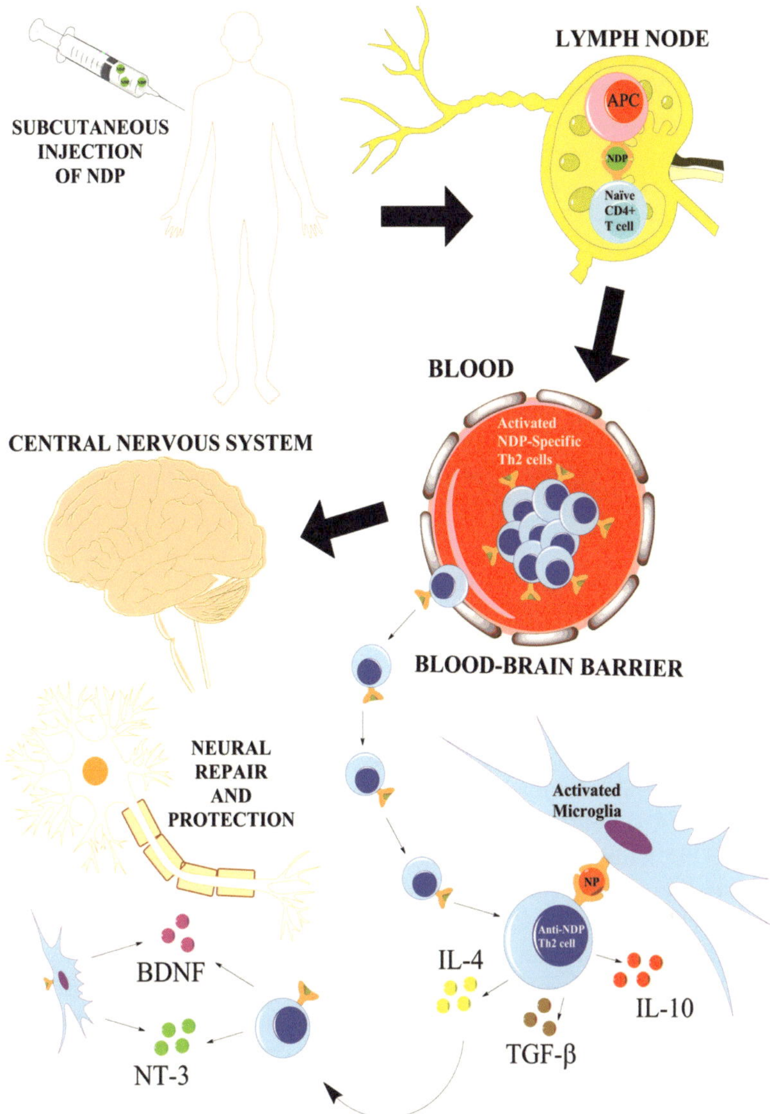

Fig. 2. Immunization with NDP causes repair and protection of the injured CNS Immunizing with NDP causes a peculiar adaptive immune response. The similarity of NDP with neural peptides (NP) causes T cell activation to deviate towards a Th2 phenotype. These NDP-reactive T cells are released into systemic blood flow where they can hone towards the site of injury. Once these autoreactive T cells infiltrate into the CNS, they come in contact with glial cells and activate microglia into a neuroprotective phenotype. Activated microglia function as antigen presenting cells (APC) and present NP to anti-NDP Th2 cells producing anti-inflammatory cytokines like interleukin- 4 and -10 (IL-4, IL-10) and transforming growth factor beta (TGF-β). This T cell-mediated anti-inflammatory effect further ameliorates the degenerative phenomena developed after CNS insult. These cells have also been shown to produce neurotrophic factors implicated in neuroregeneration like neurotrophin-3 (NT-3) and brain-derived neurotrophic factor (BDNF)

SCI (Ibarra et al., 2004). This finding suggests that vaccination with A91 is neuroprotective even if administered 48 h after injury, and that the effect of MP over the immune system is transient and does not interfere with later therapy even if that treatment is immune related. These results offer another interesting benefit of NDP-induced PA, and that is the clinical plausibility of these therapies. In the clinical setting, CNS trauma and pathology is diagnosed long after the moment of incidence. NDP-induced PA is functional even when administered 48 h after the development of NDD and works as an adjuvant in traditional clinical treatment protocols (MP administration post-CNS trauma). It appears that the beneficial effect of the vaccination with A91 will not necessarily be neutralized by concomitant treatment with MP. It is worth mentioning that one of the most prevailing adverse effects observed after NDP immunization is immediate-type hypersensitivity reactions. This undesirable effect is generally associated with the immune deviation toward Th2 phenotype. These observations should stimulate further research into which patients are most likely to benefit from this therapy. Taking into consideration all of the data, therapeutic vaccination with NDP appears to be a promising strategy that could be adapted for treatment in several NDD.

5. Effect of immunizing with neural-derived peptides

In the study of neuroprotection, the term autoreactivity is immediately associated with increased cell death, inhibition of neuroprotective mechanisms and a worse clinical outcome after CNS injury. However, our understanding of the immune system's role in the pathological CNS has changed drastically in the last couple of years. The old school of thought indicated that the immune response was responsible for the exacerbation of neurodestructive phenomenon, so the first line of defense was immunosuppression. The recent findings of PA suggested that the immune response was not only needed after an insult to the CNS but it also had a beneficial neuroprotective role in most NDD. This radical change in information forces us to reevaluate the existing treatment protocols for all NDD. If PA is present in a number of CNS diseases then the use of NDP immunizations is a reasonable treatment option. The use of NDP-induced PA results in the generation of a prevalent Th2 phenotype. These cell types have shown to have the most overwhelming neuroprotective effect in the CNS. The influential roles that these cells have on the outcome of disease have made them the goal of therapy development. The increase in Th2-inducing interventions has been studied in ALS, AD, PD, SCI, TBI, and stroke; it has even been proposed as a treatment for neurodevelopmental disorders such as Rett syndrome (Ben-Zeev et al., 2011). There are many different approaches to the induction of autoreactive Th2 lymphocytes some of these are: glatiramer acetate (GA, Coplymer-1, Cop-1, Copaxone), A91, poly-YE, p472 (Nogo-A-derived peptide). However, the only FDA-approved use of NDP-induced PA is GA under the brand name Copaxone for the treatment of MS. GA, also known as Cop-1, is the most studied of all APL-based therapies. Cop-1 is a synthetic polypeptide consisting of the amino acids tyrosine, glutamate, alanine and lysine that shows cross-reactivity with MBP (Schori et al., 2001; Kipnis & Schwartz, 2002). While the exact mechanism of Cop-1 is still not clearly elucidated, there is reason to believe that it induces Th2 differentiation, which later goes on to mediate neuroprotection (Aharoni et al., 2003; Aharoni et al., 2000). Although Th2 induction is the primary effect, immunization with Cop-1 also results in a Th1 cell deviation. This effect may seem paradoxical in nature but these pro-inflammatory Th1 cells are responsible for a sustained release of BDNF, NT-3, and NT-4

(Ziemssen, 2002, 2005). This Th1-mediated effect also induces astrocyte and neuronal production of these neurotrophic factors through a bystander effect (Aharoni et al., 2005). However, the effect of Cop-1 is not only mediated by its direct effect on CD4+ lymphocytes but also of its effect on APC, especially dendritic cells (DC). A recent study demonstrated that Cop-1 induced a Th2 response by modulating the APC function of DC. They demonstrated that DC exposed to Cop-1 during maturation had an impaired capacity of secreting IL-17p70 (the main Th1-polarizing cytokine). This effect resulted in the induction of a population with an increased frequency of effector Th2 cells that secreted IL-4 (Sanna et al., 2006; Vieira et al., 2003). Although the main components of NDP-induced PA are superficially understood, more research initiatives should be taken to better understand the therapeutic potential of these peptides. Most of the studies published use Cop-1 as the NDP, but the use of alternate peptide sequences such as A91 must be better understood. Nonetheless, there should be a constant effort to develop shorter, cheaper and more efficacious peptide sequences so that the true potential of NDP can be unlocked. Few studies have been conducted on the use of NDP in NDD.

5.1 Chronic neurodegenerative diseases

5.1.1 Amyotrophic lateral sclerosis

There have been many attempts to halt the progression of ALS by blocking different mediators of cytotoxicity (Ludolph et al., 2000). Because not all ALS patients have the defective SOD1 gene, motor neuron death is taken as the hallmark of disease because it is common to all cases of ALS. The animal model of ALS is acute peripheral nerve axotomy (Liu & Martin, 2001; Martin et al., 2000). The only drug currently used to slow down the progression of ALS is riluzole. Riluzole blocks the release of the excitatory neurotransmitter glutamate that can be toxic in elevated concentrations and is fundamental to ALS pathophysiology (Doble & Kennel, 2000; Meininger et al., 2000). In this study conducted by Angelov *et al.*, mice treated with Cop-1 (using a different regimen than MS) show more motor neuron survival in the acute and chronic phases of ALS (Angelov et al., 2003). In the study, mice were subjected to a unilateral facial nerve axotomy. They were then immunized with Cop-1 and assessed. The results showed that vaccination with Cop-1 protected against motor neuron death induced after facial nerve axotomy. Transection of the facial nerve in the adult mouse is known to cause an easily visible late degeneration of axotomized motor neurons (Sendtner et al., 1996). Eight weeks after axotomy, mice immunized with Cop-1 had significantly larger numbers of motor neurons compared to PBS-immunized controls. Studies also indicated that immunization with Cop-1 preserved the activity of axotomized motor neurons. The study concluded that there was an elevated preservation of facial nerve motor neurons but the next step was to confirm that these were still functional. Using biometrical analysis of the mice's whisking patterns they found that Cop-1-treated animals exhibited significantly better facial nerve functionality than controls. The previous results demonstrated that Cop-1-immunized ALS mice benefited from improved motor neuron survival and the preservation of their function after facial nerve axotomy. A mice strain that expresses human mutant SOD1 gene develops a motor disease that closely resembles human ALS. The loss of motor function eventually causes death because of the lack of muscular respiratory control. Angelov *et al.* concluded that treatment with Cop-1 immunizations resulted in an increased survival of the ALS mice. Immunizations with Cop-1 proved to be an adequate and efficacious therapy in an animal model of ALS. A small phase II study was held in human patients with ALS that finished with inconclusive results.

Most patients demonstrated adverse reactions at the site of immunization and elevated lymphocyte proliferation. Although the results showed promise, efforts must be taken to increase the sample size and scrutinize the possible mechanisms through which Cop-1 exerts its protective effects (Gordon et al., 2006). These small but conclusive examples of NDP-induced PA in ALS provide us with enough proof to understand the possible therapeutic advantages. The study of Cop-1 in ALS is still in its beginning and should therefore be a priority in the coming years for NDD researchers. The maximal benefits of PA in ALS have not yet been achieved.

5.1.2 Alzheimer disease

Previous studies proved that immunotherapy in AD via amyloid beta (Aβ) antibodies reduced the levels of Aβ plaques in transgenic mice. However, a human trial with Aβ antibodies caused severe adverse reactions in the form of meningoencephalitis (Nicoll et al., 2003; Orgogozo et al., 2003). A study done by Frenkel et al. postulated that meningoencephalitis was very similar to EAE. They decided to test if amyloid precursor protein-transgenic (APP-Tg) mice were more susceptible to develop EAE. They concluded that EAE lowered the levels of Aβ in APP-Tg mice using antibody-independent mechanisms. As a follow-up they decided to see if they could achieve the low Aβ levels without causing EAE. GA or Cop-1 was an FDA-approved treatment for relapsing-remitting MS and was known to cause an autoreactive response without developing EAE. They were able to reproduce the amyloid load achieved in EAE using immunization with GA (Frenkel et al., 2005). Butovsky et al performed a more directed study, towards the analysis of PA in AD. This work found that Aβ activated microglia supports neurogenesis when stimulated by IL-4. This means that a Th2 phenotype will result in the overexpression of IL-4 and increased neurogenesis after microglial activation with Aβ. Vaccination with autoreactive T cells besides aiding in neurogenesis helped in the elimination of the Aβ plaque in APP-Tg mice. The increase in neurogenesis and the removal of the Aβ plaques resulted in the counteraction of the cognitive decline normally seen in AD (Butovsky et al., 2006). The vaccination with NDP has proven to be of paramount importance in the treatment of yet another NDD. This data is also an indicator of the urgency with which these therapies should be developed, standardized, and translated into clinical trials where they can bear fruits to human disease.

5.1.3 Parkinson disease

Immunological studies in PD are controversial. The animal model is 1-methyl-4-phenyl-1,2,3,6-tetrahydropyridine (MPTP) intoxication (Benner et al., 2004; Laurie et al., 2006). This intoxication depletes dopaminergic neurons in the substantia nigra pars compacta (SNpc), simulating PD. The complication arises because MPTP toxicity also destroys the animal's immune system, causing significant changes in spleen size and diminished numbers of CD3+ T cells 7 days after intoxication (Benner et al., 2004). The alterations in normal immune response impede the researcher's ability to analyze the role of the immune system in PD. However, researchers bypass this complication by cell subset replacements. The use of NDP in PD has been briefly evaluated by several studies from the same laboratory. All studies use the MPTP toxicity model of PD and use adoptive transfer of T cells from Cop-1-immunized mice. In the first study of Benner et al. Cop-1-immunity was found to confer dopaminergic neuroprotection after MPTP intoxication. Animals that received the adoptive transfer of

Cop-1-reactive T cells exhibited a much smaller reduction in the number of SNpc dopaminergic neurons. For the functional analysis of dopaminergic circuits they quantified tyrosine hydroxylase (TH) density. The loss of TH density was significantly less in Cop-1-immunized mice than in controls. Unfortunately, even in Cop-1 immunized mice, the loss of TH density was up to 72%. However, the conclusion was that Cop-1-reactive T cell passive immunization protected neuronal dopamine metabolism as well as structural neuronal elements and its projections. Complementary analysis stated that transferred lymphocytes were readily observed both in ventral midbrains and striata of MPTP mice. The study was also interested in evaluating microglial activation due to the fact that these cells are considered to be pathological in this NDD. To assess microglial activation they analyzed the Mac-1 gene using real time RT-PCR. Results showed that Cop-1 splenocytes are capable of attenuating MPTP-induced microglial reactions and in turn limiting their neurodestructive processes. In accordance to previously demonstrated concepts, the beneficial effects of Cop-1 immunizations were T cell-dependent. Treatment with NDP also increased the expression of the neurotrophic factor GDNF. All results demonstrate the beneficial effects of immunizing with Cop-1 in PD (Benner et al., 2004). A similar study by Laurie et al. corroborated the results observed by Benner and co-workers. Although similar results were obtained, the latter was able to recollect new data. The study concluded that anti-Cop-1 CD4+ T cell transfer into MPTP intoxicated mice exerted its reparative effects in a dose dependent manner. Also this study attributed the neuroprotection to a particular subset of T lymphocytes, CD4+ T cells. This further implicated T helper cells as the main player in PA. In order to support that PA is T cell-dependent, authors' transplanted Cop-1 specific antibodies to MPTP intoxicated mice to see if this conferred neuroprotection, as expected the effects of Cop-1 are CD4+ T cell-dependent (Laurie et al., 2006). This study reiterates the outstanding potential that NDP-induced PA holds in the outcome of PD. Nonetheless, this topic deserves more investigation as to identify the effect of a normal functional immune system and not just the evaluation through substitution studies.

5.2 Acute neurodegenerative diseases

5.2.1 Cerebral ischemia

Immunization with NDP has also proved to be beneficial in cases of focal and global cerebral ischemia. There have been several studies of oral and nasal tolerization with neural constituents (Becker et al., 1997; Frenkel et al., 2003); however, only a few have resorted to NDP. There are primarily two studies that analyze the effects of this Th2-induced response after middle cerebral artery occlusion. The first by Ziv et al. used poly-YE, a high molecular weight (22 to 45 kDa) copolymer that was shown to exert modulatory effects on the immune system (Cady et al., 2000; Vidovic & Matzinger, 1988). This peptide demonstrated abilities to downregulate regulatory T cell functions and allows effector T cell activation. The study showed that a single immunization with poly-YE produced long-lasting clinical and behavioral benefits, along with neuroprotection and increased neurogenesis, starting from the subacute phase. They also found that poly-YE was beneficial even when administered 24 hours after occlusion. The effects of poly-YE immunization were long lasting as animals showed less residual impairment against controls even after 6 weeks. Histological analysis indicated that poly-YE attenuated cell loss in the hippocampus where PBS-treated rats showed large numbers of necrotic cells. The reduction in cell necrosis induced by poly-YE was so dramatic that the ipsilateral and contralateral sides were indistinguishable.

Immunization with poly-YE had a significant neuroprotective effect after stroke, but authors' also wanted to evaluate its neuroregenerative properties. They found that poly-YE promotes neurogenesis after stroke as they saw an overall increase in the number of newly formed neurons in the dentate gyri of treated animals. The results presented in this study showed that the administrations of poly-YE as late as 24 hours after the induction of ischemic stroke greatly improved subsequent recovery. It had a positive effect on the neurological outcome of stroke, delayed degeneration, and enhanced the repair of damaged structures. Also, the therapeutic window (24 hours) seemed to be significantly wider than most of the current candidate therapies for stroke, giving it much more clinically translational value (Ziv et al., 2007). A separate study in our laboratory examined the effect of Cop-1 immunizations on the outcome of ischemic stroke, using the middle cerebral artery occlusion model. Results suggested that Cop-1 significantly improved the neurological outcome of animals after stroke. Histolopathological assessment also demonstrated a decrease in infarct size and infarct volume in Cop-1-treated animals (Ibarra et al., 2007). The results of both studies do not necessarily elucidate the mechanisms through which NDP-induced PA exerts its protective effects in focal cerebral ischemia but they provide evidence of its neuroprotective, and even neuroregenerative, properties. These studies provide NDP-induced PA with another consequential benefit, and that is the wide therapeutic window. Immunizations with NDP in the treatment of stroke require exhaustive research before they reach clinical trial potential but these preliminary results are an enormous step closer.

5.2.2 Traumatic CNS injury

Traumatic CNS injury can be broken down into two compartments: TBI and SCI. A study by Kipnis et al. found that immunizing with Cop-1 after traumatic brain injury had a better outcome on neurological and histological evaluations after injury (Kipnis et al., 2003). TBI triggers self-destructive processes, like other injuries to the CNS. Kipnis et al. studied mice with closed head injury and determined that the immune system plays a key role in the spontaneous recovery. The trauma-induced deficit was reduced, both functionally and anatomically, by post-traumatic vaccination with Cop-1. Several studies have been published on the use of NDP in SCI. Hauben et al. used immunization with a variety of myelin-associated peptides, including those derived from Nogo-A, can be used to evoke a T cell-mediated response that promotes recovery. They show that neuronal degeneration after incomplete spinal cord contusion in rats was substantially reduced, and hence recovery was significantly promoted, by posttraumatic immunization with Nogo-A-derived, p472 (Hauben et al., 2001). Our laboratory has also demonstrated the beneficial effect of immunizing with NDP (A91) on motor recovery and neuronal survival after SCI (Martiñon et al., 2007). Furthermore, we have determined some of the mechanisms of action of NDP-induced PA. In a recent study we found that immunization with Cop-1 and A91 exerted its neuroprotective effect through the inhibition of lipid peroxidation (LP). Animals were immunized with A91 seven days before injury. With the aim of inducing the functional elimination of CNS-specific T cells, animals were tolerized against SC-protein extract and thereafter subjected to a SCI. The lipid-soluble fluorescent products were used as an index of LP and were assessed after injury. Immunization with NDP reduced LP after SCI. Functional elimination of CNS-specific T cells avoided the beneficial effect induced by PA (Ibarra et al., 2010). A consequential study hypothesized that LP was caused by an unregulated production of ROS seen after CNS injury. The main ROS produced during the secondary phase of damage after trauma is NO. When NO is produced in an unregulated fashion it can react with other free radicals such as superoxide anion and produce peroxynitrite a powerful neurotoxic substance. We determined that the decrease in lipid peroxidation was caused by an inhibition in the synthesis of NO after immunization with NDP after SCI (unpublished data). Our results supported our hypothesis and allowed us to corroborate the data with expression analysis. We used real time RT-PCR to also demonstrate a reduction in the expression of the enzyme implicated in post-injury synthesis of NO, the inducible form of nitric oxide synthase (iNOS) (unpublished data). By determining that A91 reactive T cells also secrete NT-3 and IL-4 after SCI, making them a Th2 phenotype, we further substantiate the PA hypothesis. Immunizing with NDP deviates the Th response down a Th2 pathway increasing the synthesis of molecules such as IL-4 and IL-10 and secretion of neurotrophic factors like NT-3. Finally, we have found that the severity of injury would determine the strength and the effect of the PA response (unpublished data). This new data adds more factors into the induction of an autoreactive response. Our study noticed that animals that sustained a non-complete injury to the spinal cord had an increased recovery when immunized with A91. These autoreactive T cells also secreted BDNF and had greater recognition for A91 in vitro. On the other hand, animals that sustained complete or severe SCI did not recover even after A91-immunization. Unexpectedly, these animals did not even possess a clonal response to A91, meaning they were not even able to recognize the antigen in vivo, even with an adjuvant. This indicates that animals that sustained a severe or complete injury to the spinal cord are severely immunosuppressed and may therefore not engage a true PA response (unpublished data). This data that has just surfaced indicates that the neuroimmunological components of CNS disease require much more research in order to elucidate this unknown mechanisms. Even further, we must continue to delve into this immunosuppression caused by severe injury. The study of the body's physiology under duress shows us some of the mechanisms it possesses that could help in regenerating the CNS during disease. Immunization with NDP has proven to be an excellent therapeutical intervention in SCI and several other NDD, providing it with reasonable necessity to continue research on the topic.

6. Improving the beneficial effect of protective autoimmunity

Even though the positive effect of immunizing with NDP has rendered significant results, it is possible to potentiate this effect. The improvement of this strategy would yield a better functional recovery and, thereby, a better quality of life for NDD-affected individuals. It is clear that several damaging mechanisms take place during the acute phase of injury. Unfortunately, NDP-induced PA develops after a few days of immunization. Before PA sets in, the neural tissue is unprotected; therefore, the best approach is a combination of neuroprotective strategies. A therapeutic intervention tailored to each specific time point of injury pathophysiology. This approach will ameliorate one or more of the destructive events and may improve the functional outcome even more than PA alone. Excessive production of ROS from the beginning of CNS injury causes lipid peroxidation LP (Hall, 1994). Peroxidation of membrane lipids affects the integrity of the cell membrane and is the most damaging mechanism. The unregulated synthesis of free radicals offers a potential intervention route for the treatment of NDD. An example of this is the use of glutathione monoethyl ester (GSHE). This cell-permeant derivative of glutathione (GSH) is an antioxidant that limits the effect of ROS on the bi-lipid membrane. GSH has shown neuroprotective properties after SCI (Guizar-Sahagun et al., 2005; Santoscoy et al., 2002). Aside from this effect, GSH supports the proliferation, growth, and differentiation of immune cells. Moreover, GSH is actually required for many specific T cell functions, including DNA replication and IL-2 synthesis (Kidd., 1997). The amount of GSH determines the magnitude of the immunological response (Droge et al., 1994) as well as its depletion inhibits normal function (Kidd, 1997). According to the data presented above, the addition of GSHE to NDP immunizations could significantly improve neuroprotection. The antioxidant properties of GSH will cover the overproduction of ROS from the beginning of injury while it could also assist in inducing a better PA response. A previous work carried out in our laboratory, examined the effect of this combination and demonstrated that the addition of GSHE to NDP immunizations induced earlier and better motor recovery after SCI compared to immunizations alone (Martinon et al., 2007). This effect was observed in animals subjected to either a contusive or a compressive SCI. The substantial improvement observed in treated animals allowed them to attain weight-supported plantar steps. This recovery is of great relevance when translating this treatment into a clinical setting. Motor improvement significantly correlated with increased axonal myelination as well as a marked survival of rubrospinal neurons. Besides finding adjuvant therapies for NDP-induced PA we wanted to see if multiple immunizations would increase the beneficial effect. We examined the effect of double immunizations and their effect on PA. Contrary to our expectations, double immunizations abolished the neuroprotective effect of single dose NDP-induced PA. The findings support the notion that the second immunization after SCI has a negative effect on PA. Rather than strengthening the protective effect, it eliminated it. This phenomenon was probably secondary to anergy since double immunization did not induce cell death (Martinon et al., 2007). According to the present data, the use of NDP and GSHE in SCI is a promising strategy. Further studies are necessary in order to establish the efficacy of this therapy and its potential applications into other NDD. Another attempt of synergistic therapeutic interventions is the use of GA with IFN-β-1a in MS (Lublin & Reingold, 2001). The development of adjuvant and synergistic therapies will aid in the optimization of NDP-induced PA allowing us to tackle the pathophysiology of several NDD.

7. Conclusion

The concept of PA revolutionized the way we saw the immune system in several different diseases. We figured out that it was more important to modulate the response than to eliminate it. With the logarithmic explosion in knowledge we must now hold these conclusions. The use of NDP and their effect on the immune response have proven to be helpful in several different pathologies, particularly in NDD. Using the information that we have recollected across the years, the mechanisms through which NDP-induced PA exerts its effects is everyday less obscure. Unfortunately, due to hypersensitivity reactions and heterogeneous responses among patients NDP have not been taken to their maximum potential. Unfortunately, PA is developed under the bases that the immune system is healthy and will function normally following an insult to the CNS. However, MS is an autoimmune disease, a case where the immune system is fatally skewed. This paradox forces us to adopt a revolutionary idea such as PA and apply it to NDD. The application of NDP-induced PA to the field of NDD can yield insurmountable results and therefore we urge the scientific community to aid in continuing to shed light on these once obscure mechanisms in order to make this therapeutic intervention efficacious and safe. The ultimate goal is to help the suffering and the complications of human disease.

8. References

Aharoni, R.; Eilam, R.; Domev, H.; Labunskay, G.; Sela, M. & Arnon, R. (2005). The immunomodulator glatiramer acetate augments the expression of neurotrophic factors in brains of experimental autoimmune encephalomyelitis mice. *Proceedings of the National Academy of Sciences of the United States of America,* Vol.102, No.52, (December 2005), pp. 19045-19050, ISSN 0027-8424

Aharoni, R.; Kayhan, B.; Eilam, R.; Sela, M. & Arnon, R. (2003). Glatiramer acetate-specific T cells in the brain express T helper 2/3 cytokines and brain-derived neurotrophic factor in situ. *Proceedings of the National Academy of Sciences of the United States of America,* Vol.100, No.24, (November 2003), pp. 14157-14162, ISSN 0027-8424

Aharoni, R.; Teitelbaum, D.; Leitner, O.; Meshorer, A.; Sela, M. & Arnon, R. (2000). Specific Th2 cells accumulate in the central nervous system of mice protected against experimental autoimmune encephalomyelitis by copolymer 1. *Proceedings of the National Academy of Sciences of the United States of America,* Vol.97, No.21, (October 2000), pp. 11472-11477, ISSN 0027-8424

Alzheimer's Association. (2010). Alzheimer's disease facts and figures. *Alzheimer's & dementia,* Vol.6, No.2, (March 2010), pp. 158-194. ISSN 1552-5279

Angelov, D.N.; Waibel, S.; Guntinas-Lichius, O.; Lenzen, M.; Neiss, W.F.; Tomov, T.L.; Yoles, E.; Kipnis, J.; Schori, H.; Reuter, A.; Ludolph, A. & Schwartz, M. (2003). Therapeutic vaccine for acute and chronic motor neuron diseases: implications for amyotrophic lateral sclerosis. *Proceedings of the National Academy of Sciences of the United States of America,* Vol.100, No.8, (April 2003), pp. 4790-4795, ISSN 0027-8424

Becker, K.J.; McCarron, R.M.; Ruetzler, C.; Laban, O.; Sternberg, E.; Flanders, K.C. & Hallenbeck, J.M. (1997). Immunologic tolerance to myelin basic protein decreases stroke size after transient focal cerebral ischemia. *Proceedings of the National Academy of Sciences of the United States of America,* Vol.94, No.20, (September 1997), pp. 10873-10878, ISSN 0027-8424

Ben-Zeev, B.; Aharoni, R.; Nissenkorn, A. & Arnon, R. (2011). Glatiramer acetate (GA, Copolymer-1) an hypothetical treatment option for Rett syndrome. *Medical Hypotheses,* Vol.76, No.2, (February 2011), pp. 190-193, ISSN 1532-2777

Benner, E.J.; Mosley, R.L.; Destache, C.J.; Lewis, T.B.; Jackson-Lewis, V.; Gorantla, S.; Nemachek, C.; Green, S.R.; Przedborski, S. & Gendelman, H.E. (2004). Therapeutic immunization protects dopaminergic neurons in a mouse model of Parkinson's disease. *Proceedings of the National Academy of Sciences of the United States of America,* Vol.101, No.25, (June 2004), pp. 9435-9440, ISSN 0027-8424

Bethea, J.R.; Castro, M.; Keane, R.W.; Lee, T.T.; Dietrich, W.D. & Yezierski, R.P. (1998). Traumatic spinal cord injury induces nuclear factor-kappaB activation. *The Journal of Neuroscience,* Vol.18, No.9, (May 1998), pp. 3251-3260, ISSN 0270-6474

Bethea, J.R.; Nagashima, H.; Acosta, M.C.; Briceno, C.; Gomez, F.; Marcillo, A.E.; Loor, K.; Green, J. & Dietrich, W.D. (1999). Systemically administered interleukin-10 reduces tumor necrosis factor-alpha production and significantly improves functional recovery following traumatic spinal cord injury in rats. *Journal of Neurotrauma,* Vol.16, No.10, (October 1999), pp. 851-863, ISSN 0897-7151

Blight, A.R. (1992). Macrophages and inflammatory damage in spinal cord injury. *Journal of Neurotrauma,* Vol.9, No.1, (March 1992), pp. 83-91, ISSN 0897-7151

Brown, R.C.; Lockwood, A.H. & Sonawane, B.R. (2005). Neurodegenerative diseases: an overview of environmental risk factors. *Environmental health perspectives,* Vol.113, No.9, (September 2005), pp. 1250-1256, ISSN 0091-6765

Butovsky, O.; Hauben, E. & Schwartz, M. (2001). Morphological aspects of spinal cord autoimmune neuroprotection: colocalization of T cells with B7--2 (CD86) and prevention of cyst formation. *The FASEB journal,* Vol.15, No.6, (April 2001), pp. 1065-1067, ISSN 0892-6638

Butovsky, O.; Koronyo-Hamaoui, M.; Kunis, G.; Ophir, E.; Landa, G.; Cohen, H. & Schwartz, M. (2006). Glatiramer acetate fights against Alzheimer's disease by inducing dendritic-like microglia expressing insulin-like growth factor 1. *Proceedings of the National Academy of Sciences of the United States of America,* Vol.103, No.31, (August 2006), pp. 11784-11789, ISSN 0027-8424

Cady, C.T.; Lahn, M.; Vollmer, M.; Tsuji, M.; Seo, S.J.; Reardon, C.L.; O'Brien, R.L. & Born, W.K. (2000). Response of murine gamma delta T cells to the synthetic polypeptide poly-Glu50Tyr50. *Journal of Immunology,* Vol.165, No.4, (August 2000), pp. 1790-1798, ISSN 0022-1767

Davey, R.T.,Jr.; Chaitt, D.G.; Piscitelli, S.C.; Wells, M.; Kovacs, J.A.; Walker, R.E.; Falloon, J.; Polis, M.A.; Metcalf, J.A.; Masur, H.; Fyfe, G. & Lane, H.C. (1997). Subcutaneous administration of interleukin-2 in human immunodeficiency virus type 1-infected persons. *The Journal of infectious diseases,* Vol.175, No.4, (April 1997), pp. 781-789, ISSN 0022-1899

Doble, A. & Kennel, P. (2000). Animal models of amyotrophic lateral sclerosis. *Amyotrophic lateral sclerosis and other motor neuron disorders,* Vol.1, No.5, (December 2001), pp. 301-312, ISSN 1466-0822

Droge, W.; Schulze-Osthoff, K.; Mihm, S.; Galter, D.; Schenk, H.; Eck, H.P.; Roth, S. & Gmunder, H. (1994). Functions of glutathione and glutathione disulfide in immunology and immunopathology. *The FASEB journal,* Vol.8, No.14, (November 1994), pp. 1131-1138, ISSN 0892-6638

Dusart, I.; Morel, M.P. & Sotelo, C. (1994). Parasagittal compartmentation of adult rat Purkinje cells expressing the low-affinity nerve growth factor receptor: changes of pattern expression after a traumatic lesion. *Neuroscience,* Vol.63, No.2, (November 1994), pp. 351-356, ISSN 0306-4522

Farhoudi, A.; Siadati, A.; Atarod, L.; Tabatabaei, P.; Mamishi, S.; Khotaii, G.; Armin, Sh. & Shirvani, F. (2003). Para Vertebral Abscess and Rib Osteomyelitis due to Aspergillous Fumigatus in a Patient with Chronic Granulomatous Disease. *Iranian journal of allergy, asthma, and immunology,* Vol.2, No.1, (March 2007), pp. 13-15, ISSN 1735-1502

Franciosi, S.; Choi, H.B.; Kim, S.U. & McLarnon, J.G. (2005). IL-8 enhancement of amyloid-beta (Abeta 1-42)-induced expression and production of pro-inflammatory cytokines and COX-2 in cultured human microglia. *Journal of neuroimmunology,* Vol.159, No.1-2, (February 2005), pp. 66-74, ISSN 0165-5728

Frank-Cannon, T.C.; Alto, L.T.; McAlpine, F.E. & Tansey, M.G. (2009). Does neuroinflammation fan the flame in neurodegenerative diseases? *Molecular neurodegeneration,* Vol.4, (n.d.), pp. 47, ISSN 1750-1326

Frenkel, D.; Huang, Z.; Maron, R.; Koldzic, D.N.; Hancock, W.W.; Moskowitz, M.A. & Weiner, H.L. (2003). Nasal vaccination with myelin oligodendrocyte glycoprotein reduces stroke size by inducing IL-10-producing CD4+ T cells. *Journal of immunology*, Vol.171, No.12, (December 2003), pp. 6549-6555, ISSN 0022-1767

Frenkel, D.; Maron, R.; Burt, D.S. & Weiner, H.L. (2005). Nasal vaccination with a proteosome-based adjuvant and glatiramer acetate clears beta-amyloid in a mouse model of Alzheimer disease. *The Journal of clinical investigation*, Vol.115, No.9, (September 2005), pp. 2423-2433, ISSN 0021-9738

Garboczi, D.N.; Ghosh, P.; Utz, U.; Fan, Q.R.; Biddison, W.E. & Wiley, D.C. (1996). Structure of the complex between human T-cell receptor, viral peptide and HLA-A2. *Nature*, Vol.384, No.6605, (November 1996), pp. 134-141, ISSN 0028-0836

Gaur, A.; Boehme, S.A.; Chalmers, D.; Crowe, P.D.; Pahuja, A.; Ling, N.; Brocke, S.; Steinman, L. & Conlon, P.J. (1997). Amelioration of relapsing experimental autoimmune encephalomyelitis with altered myelin basic protein peptides involves different cellular mechanisms. *Journal of neuroimmunology*, Vol.74, No.1-2, (April 1997), pp. 149-158, ISSN 0165-5728

Gordon, P.H.; Doorish, C.; Montes, J.; Mosley, R.L.; Diamond, B.; Macarthur, R.B.; Weimer, L.H.; Kaufmann, P.; Hays, A.P.; Rowland, L.P.; Gendelman, H.E.; Przedborski, S. & Mitsumoto, H. (2006). Randomized controlled phase II trial of glatiramer acetate in ALS. *Neurology*, Vol.66, No.7, (April 2006), pp. 1117-1119, ISSN 0028-3878

Guizar-Sahagun, G.; Ibarra, A.; Espitia, A.; Martinez, A.; Madrazo, I. & Franco-Bourland, R.E. (2005). Glutathione monoethyl ester improves functional recovery, enhances neuron survival, and stabilizes spinal cord blood flow after spinal cord injury in rats. *Neuroscience*, Vol.130, No.3, (n.d.), pp. 639-649, ISSN 0306-4522

Hall, E.D.; McCall, J.M. & Means, E.D. (1994). Therapeutic potential of the lazaroids (21-aminosteroids) in acute central nervous system trauma, ischemia and subarachnoid hemorrhage. *Advances in pharmacology*, Vol.28, (n.d.), pp. 221-268, ISSN 1054-3589

Hammarberg, H.; Lidman, O.; Lundberg, C.; Eltayeb, S.Y.; Gielen, A.W.; Muhallab, S.; Svenningsson, A.; Linda, H.; van Der Meide, P.H.; Cullheim, S.; Olsson, T. & Piehl, F. (2000). Neuroprotection by encephalomyelitis: rescue of mechanically injured neurons and neurotrophin production by CNS-infiltrating T and natural killer cells. *The Journal of Neuroscience*, Vol.20, No.14, (July 2000), pp. 5283-5291, ISSN 0270-6474

Hashimoto, M.; Sun, D.; Rittling, S.R.; Denhardt, D.T. & Young, W. (2007). Osteopontin-deficient mice exhibit less inflammation, greater tissue damage, and impaired locomotor recovery from spinal cord injury compared with wild-type controls. *The Journal of Neuroscience*, Vol.27, No.13, (March 2007), pp. 3603-3611, ISSN 0270-6474

Hauben, E.; Butovsky, O.; Nevo, U.; Yoles, E.; Moalem, G.; Agranov, E.; Mor, F.; Leibowitz-Amit, R.; Pevsner, E.; Akselrod, S.; Neeman, M.; Cohen, I.R. & Schwartz, M. (2000). Passive or active immunization with myelin basic protein promotes recovery from spinal cord contusion. *The Journal of Neuroscience*, Vol.20, No.17, (September 2000), pp. 6421-6430, ISSN 0270-6474

Hauben, E.; Gothilf, A.; Cohen, A.; Butovsky, O.; Nevo, U.; Smirnov, I.; Yoles, E.; Akselrod, S. & Schwartz, M. (2003). Vaccination with dendritic cells pulsed with peptides of myelin basic protein promotes functional recovery from spinal cord injury. *The Journal of Neuroscience*, Vol.23, No.25, (September 2003), pp. 8808-8819, ISSN 0270-6474

Hauben, E.; Ibarra, A.; Mizrahi, T.; Barouch, R.; Agranov, E. & Schwartz, M. (2001). Vaccination with a Nogo-A-derived peptide after incomplete spinal-cord injury promotes recovery via a T-cell-mediated neuroprotective response: comparison with other myelin antigens. *Proceedings of the National Academy of Sciences of the United States of America*, Vol.98, No.26, (December 2001), pp. 15173-15178, ISSN 0027-8424

Hauben, E.; Nevo, U.; Yoles, E.; Moalem, G.; Agranov, E.; Mor, F.; Akselrod, S.; Neeman, M.; Cohen, I.R. & Schwartz, M. (2000). Autoimmune T cells as potential neuroprotective therapy for spinal cord injury. *Lancet*, Vol.355, No.9200, (January 2000), pp. 286-287, ISSN 0140-6736

Hauben, E.; Roncarolo, M.G.; Nevo, U. & Schwartz, M. (2005). Beneficial autoimmunity in Type 1 diabetes mellitus. *Trends in immunology*, Vol.26, No.5, (May 2005), pp. 248-253, ISSN 1471-4906

Hendrix, S. & Nitsch, R. (2007). The role of T helper cells in neuroprotection and regeneration. *Journal of Neuroimmunology*, Vol.184, No.1-2, (March 2007), pp. 100-112, ISSN 0165-5728

Ibarra, A.; Correa, D.; Willms, K.; Merchant, M.T.; Guizar-Sahagun, G.; Grijalva, I. & Madrazo, I. (2003). Effects of cyclosporin-A on immune response, tissue protection and motor function of rats subjected to spinal cord injury. *Brain Research*, Vol.979, No.1-2, (July 2003), pp. 165-178, ISSN 0006-8993

Ibarra, A.; Garcia, E.; Flores, N.; Martinon, S.; Reyes, R.; Campos, M.G.; Maciel, M. & Mestre, H. (2010). Immunization with neural-derived antigens inhibits lipid peroxidation after spinal cord injury. *Neuroscience Letters*, Vol.476, No.2, (May 2010), pp. 62-65, ISSN 0304-3940

Ibarra, A.; Hauben, E.; Butovsky, O. & Schwartz, M. (2004). The therapeutic window after spinal cord injury can accommodate T cell-based vaccination and methylprednisolone in rats. *The European Journal of Neuroscience*, Vol.19, No.11, (June 2004), pp. 2984-2990, ISSN 0953-816X

Jameson, S.C. & Bevan, M.J. (1995). T cell receptor antagonists and partial agonists. *Immunity*, Vol.2, No.1, (January 1995), pp. 1-11, ISSN 1074-7613

Kersh, G.J. & Allen, P.M. (1996). Essential flexibility in the T-cell recognition of antigen. *Nature*, Vol.380, No.6574, (April 1996), pp. 495-498, ISSN 0028-0836

Kidd, P.M. (1997). Glutathione: systemic protectant against oxidative and free radical damage. *Alternative Medicine Review.*, Vol.1, (n.d.), pp. 155-176, ISSN 1089-5159

Kipnis, J.; Nevo, U.; Panikashvili, D.; Alexandrovich, A.; Yoles, E.; Akselrod, S.; Shohami, E. & Schwartz, M. (2003). Therapeutic vaccination for closed head injury. *Journal of Neurotrauma*, Vol.20, No.6, (June 2003), pp. 559-569, ISSN 0897-7151

Kipnis, J. & Schwartz, M. (2002). Dual action of glatiramer acetate (Cop-1) in the treatment of CNS autoimmune and neurodegenerative disorders. *Trends in Molecular Medicine*, Vol.8, No.7, (July 2002), pp. 319-323, ISSN 1471-4914

Kipnis, J.; Yoles, E.; Schori, H.; Hauben, E.; Shaked, I. & Schwartz, M. (2001). Neuronal survival after CNS insult is determined by a genetically encoded autoimmune response. *The Journal of Neuroscience*, Vol.21, No.13, (July 2001), pp. 4564-4571, ISSN 0270-6474

Kreutzberg, G.W. (1996). Microglia: a sensor for pathological events in the CNS. *Trends in Neurosciences*, Vol.19, No.8, (August 1996), pp. 312-318, ISSN 0166-2236

Kumpfel, T.; Schwan, M.; Pollmacher, T.; Yassouridis, A.; Uhr, M.; Trenkwalder, C. & Weber, F. (2007). Time of interferon-beta 1a injection and duration of treatment affect clinical side effects and acute changes of plasma hormone and cytokine levels in multiple sclerosis patients. *Multiple Sclerosis*, Vol.13, No.9, (November 2007), pp. 1138-1145, ISSN 1352-4585

Laurie, C.; Reynolds, A.; Coskun, O.; Bowman, E.; Gendelman, H.E. & Mosley, R.L. (2007). CD4+ T cells from Copolymer-1 immunized mice protect dopaminergic neurons in the 1-methyl-4-phenyl-1,2,3,6-tetrahydropyridine model of Parkinson's disease. *Journal of Neuroimmunology*, Vol.183, No.1-2, (February 2007), pp. 60-68, ISSN 0165-5728

Lee, K.H.; Yun, S.J.; Nam, K.N.; Gho, Y.S. & Lee, E.H. (2007). Activation of microglial cells by ceruloplasmin. *Brain Research*, Vol.1171, (September 2007), pp. 1-8, ISSN 0006-8993

Li, L.; Lu, J.; Tay, S.S.; Moochhala, S.M. & He, B.P. (2007). The function of microglia, either neuroprotection or neurotoxicity, is determined by the equilibrium among factors released from activated microglia in vitro. *Brain Research*, Vol.1159, (July 2007), pp. 8-17, ISSN 0006-8993

Liu, Z. & Martin, L.J. (2001). Isolation of mature spinal motor neurons and single-cell analysis using the comet assay of early low-level DNA damage induced in vitro and in vivo. *The Journal of Histochemistry and Cytochemistry*, Vol.49, No.8, (August 2001), pp. 957-972, ISSN 0022-1554

Lopez-Vales, R.; Garcia-Alias, G.; Fores, J.; Udina, E.; Gold, B.G.; Navarro, X. & Verdu, E. (2005). FK 506 reduces tissue damage and prevents functional deficit after spinal cord injury in the rat. *Journal of Neuroscience Research*, Vol.81, No.6, (September 2005), pp. 827-836, ISSN 0360-4012

Lopez-Vales, R.; Garcia-Alias, G.; Guzman-Lenis, M.S.; Fores, J.; Casas, C.; Navarro, X. & Verdu, E. (2006). Effects of COX-2 and iNOS inhibitors alone or in combination with olfactory ensheathing cell grafts after spinal cord injury. *Spine*, Vol.31, No.10, (May 2006), pp. 1100-1106, ISSN 0362-2436

Lublin, F.D. & Reingold, S.C. (2001). Placebo-controlled clinical trials in multiple sclerosis: ethical considerations. National Multiple Sclerosis Society (USA) Task Force on Placebo-Controlled Clinical Trials in MS. *Annals of Neurology*, Vol.49, No.5, (May 2001), pp. 677-681, ISSN 0364-5134

Ludolph, A.C.; Meyer, T. & Riepe, M.W. (2000). The role of excitotoxicity in ALS--what is the evidence? *Journal of Neurology*, Vol.247 Suppl 1, (March 2000), pp. I7-16, ISSN 0340-5354

Martin, L.J.; Price, A.C.; Kaiser, A.; Shaikh, A.Y. & Liu, Z. (2000). Mechanisms for neuronal degeneration in amyotrophic lateral sclerosis and in models of motor neuron. *International Journal of Molecular Medicine*, Vol.5, No.1, (January 1999), pp. 3-13, ISSN 1107-3756

Martinon, S.; Garcia, E.; Flores, N.; Gonzalez, I.; Ortega, T.; Buenrostro, M.; Reyes, R.; Fernandez-Presas, A.M.; Guizar-Sahagun, G.; Correa, D. & Ibarra, A. (2007). Vaccination with a neural-derived peptide plus administration of glutathione improves the performance of paraplegic rats. *The European Journal of Neuroscience*, Vol.26, No.2, (July 2007), pp. 403-412, ISSN 0953-816X

Meek, P.D.; McKeithan, K. & Schumock, G.T. (1998). Economic considerations in Alzheimer's disease. *Pharmacotherapy*, Vol.18, No.2, (March-April 1998), pp. 68-73, ISSN 0277-0008

Meininger, V.; Lacomblez, L. & Salachas, F. (2000). What has changed with riluzole? *Journal of Neurology*, Vol.247, (December 2001), pp. 19-22, ISSN 0340-5354

Moalem, G.; Leibowitz-Amit, R.; Yoles, E.; Mor, F.; Cohen, I.R. & Schwartz, M. (1999). Autoimmune T cells protect neurons from secondary degeneration after central nervous system axotomy. *Nature Medicine*, Vol.5, No.1, (January 1999), pp. 49-55, ISSN 1078-8956

Nel, A.E. & Slaughter, N. (2002). T-cell activation through the antigen receptor. Part 2: role of signaling cascades in T-cell differentiation, anergy, immune senescence, and development of immunotherapy. *The Journal of Allergy and Clinical Immunology*, Vol.109, No.6, (June 2002), pp. 901-915, ISSN 0091-6749

Nicoll, J.A.; Wilkinson, D.; Holmes, C.; Steart, P.; Markham, H. & Weller, R.O. (2003). Neuropathology of human Alzheimer disease after immunization with amyloid-beta peptide: a case report. *Nature Medicine*, Vol.9, No.4, (April 2003), pp. 448-452, ISSN 1078-8956

Nimmerjahn, A.; Kirchhoff, F. & Helmchen, F. (2005). Resting microglial cells are highly dynamic surveillants of brain parenchyma in vivo. *Science*, Vol.308, No.5726, (May 2005), pp. 1314-1318, ISSN 0036-8075

Orgogozo, J.M.; Gilman, S.; Dartigues, J.F.; Laurent, B.; Puel, M.; Kirby, L.C.; Jouanny, P.; Dubois, B.; Eisner, L.; Flitman, S.; Michel, B.F.; Boada, M.; Frank, A. & Hock, C. (2003). Subacute meningoencephalitis in a subset of patients with AD after Abeta42 immunization. *Neurology*, Vol.61, No.1, (July 2003), pp. 46-54, ISSN 0028-3878

Pan, W.; Zhang, L.; Liao, J.; Csernus, B. & Kastin, A.J. (2003). Selective increase in TNF alpha permeation across the blood-spinal cord barrier after SCI. *Journal of Neuroimmunology*, Vol.134, No.1-2, (January 2003), pp. 111-117, ISSN 0165-5728

Partidos, C.D.; Beignon, A.S.; Briand, J.P. & Muller, S. (2004). Modulation of immune responses with transcutaneously deliverable adjuvants. *Vaccine*, Vol.22, No.19, (June 2004), pp. 2385-2390, ISSN 0264-410X

Petrovsky, N. & Aguilar, J.C. (2004). Vaccine adjuvants: current state and future trends. *Immunology and Cell Biology*, Vol.82, No.5, (October 2004), pp. 488-496, ISSN 0818-9641

Popovich, P.G.; Guan, Z.; Wei, P.; Huitinga, I.; van Rooijen, N. & Stokes, B.T. (1999). Depletion of hematogenous macrophages promotes partial hindlimb recovery and neuroanatomical repair after experimental spinal cord injury. *Experimental Neurology*, Vol.158, No.2, (August 1999), pp. 351-365, ISSN 0014-4886

Popovich, P.G.; Stokes, B.T. & Whitacre, C.C. (1996). Concept of autoimmunity following spinal cord injury: possible roles for T lymphocytes in the traumatized central nervous system. *Journal of Neuroscience Research*, Vol.45, No.4, (August 1996), pp. 349-363, ISSN 0360-4012

Popovich, P.G.; Wei, P. & Stokes, B.T. (1997). Cellular inflammatory response after spinal cord injury in Sprague-Dawley and Lewis rats. *The Journal of Comparative Neurology*, Vol.377, No.3, (January 1997), pp. 443-464, ISSN 0021-9967

Raivich, G. (2005). Like cops on the beat: the active role of resting microglia. *Trends in Neurosciences*, Vol.28, No.11, (November 2005), pp. 571-573, ISSN 0166-2236

Rapalino, O.; Lazarov-Spiegler, O.; Agranov, E.; Velan, G.J.; Yoles, E.; Fraidakis, M.; Solomon, A.; Gepstein, R.; Katz, A.; Belkin, M.; Hadani, M. & Schwartz, M. (1998). Implantation of stimulated homologous macrophages results in partial recovery of paraplegic rats. *Nature Medicine*, Vol.4, No.7, (July 1998), pp. 814-821, ISSN 1078-8956

Resnick, D.K.; Graham, S.H.; Dixon, C.E. & Marion, D.W. (1998). Role of cyclooxygenase 2 in acute spinal cord injury. *Journal of Neurotrauma*, Vol.15, No.12, (December 1999), pp. 1005-1013, ISSN 0897-7151

Sanna, A.; Fois, M.L.; Arru, G.; Huang, Y.M.; Link, H.; Pugliatti, M.; Rosati, G. & Sotgiu, S. (2006). Glatiramer acetate reduces lymphocyte proliferation and enhances IL-5 and IL-13 production through modulation of monocyte-derived dendritic cells in multiple sclerosis. *Clinical and Experimental Immunology*, Vol.143, No.2, (February 2006), pp. 357-362, ISSN 0009-9104

Santoscoy, C.; Rios, C.; Franco-Bourland, R.E.; Hong, E.; Bravo, G.; Rojas, G. & Guizar-Sahagun, G. (2002). Lipid peroxidation by nitric oxide supplements after spinal cord injury: effect of antioxidants in rats. *Neuroscience Letters*, Vol.330, No.1, (September 2002), pp. 94-98, ISSN 0304-3940

Schmid, C.D.; Melchior, B.; Masek, K.; Puntambekar, S.S.; Danielson, P.E.; Lo, D.D.; Sutcliffe, J.G. & Carson, M.J. (2009). Differential gene expression in LPS/IFNgamma activated microglia and macrophages: in vitro versus in vivo. *Journal of Neurochemistry*, Vol.109 Suppl 1, (May 2009), pp. 117-125, ISSN 0022-3042

Schori, H.; Kipnis, J.; Yoles, E.; WoldeMussie, E.; Ruiz, G.; Wheeler, L.A. & Schwartz, M. (2001). Vaccination for protection of retinal ganglion cells against death from glutamate cytotoxicity and ocular hypertension: implications for glaucoma. *Proceedings of the National Academy of Sciences of the United States of America*, Vol.98, No.6, (March 2001), pp. 3398-3403, ISSN 0027-8424

Schwartz, M. & Cohen, I.R. (2000). Autoimmunity can benefit self-maintenance. *Immunology Today*, Vol.21, No.6, (June 2000), pp. 265-268, ISSN 0167-5699

Schwartz, M.; Shaked, I.; Fisher, J.; Mizrahi, T. & Schori, H. (2003). Protective autoimmunity against the enemy within: fighting glutamate toxicity. *Trends in Neurosciences*, Vol.26, No.6, (June 2003), pp. 297-302, ISSN 0166-2236

Sendtner, M.; Gotz, R.; Holtmann, B.; Escary, J.L.; Masu, Y.; Carroll, P.; Wolf, E.; Brem, G.; Brulet, P. & Thoenen, H. (1996). Cryptic physiological trophic support of motoneurons by LIF revealed by double gene targeting of CNTF and LIF. *Current Biology*, Vol.6, No.6, (June 1996), pp. 686-694, ISSN 0960-9822

Shaked, I.; Porat, Z.; Gersner, R.; Kipnis, J. & Schwartz, M. (2004). Early activation of microglia as antigen-presenting cells correlates with T cell-mediated protection and repair of the injured central nervous system. *Journal of Neuroimmunology*, Vol.146, No.1-2, (January 2003), pp. 84-93, ISSN 0165-5728

Sospedra, M. & Martin, R. (2005). Immunology of multiple sclerosis. *Annual Review of Immunology*, Vol.23, (n.d.), pp. 683-747, ISSN 0732-0582

Stuve, O.; Youssef, S.; Weber, M.S.; Nessler, S.; von Budingen, H.C.; Hemmer, B.; Prod'homme, T.; Sobel, R.A.; Steinman, L. & Zamvil, S.S. (2006). Immunomodulatory synergy by combination of atorvastatin and glatiramer acetate in treatment of CNS autoimmunity. *The Journal of Clinical Investigation*, Vol.116, No.4, (April 2006), pp. 1037-1044, ISSN 0021-9738

Terando, A.; Sabel, M.S. & Sondak, V.K. (2003). Melanoma: adjuvant therapy and other treatment options. *Current Treatment Options in Oncology*, Vol.4, No.3, (June 2003), pp. 187-199, ISSN 1534-6277

Turrin, N.P. & Rivest, S. (2006). Molecular and cellular immune mediators of neuroprotection. *Molecular Neurobiology*, Vol.34, No.3, (December 2007), pp. 221-242, ISSN 0893-7648

Vanegas, H. & Schaible, H.G. (2001). Prostaglandins and cyclooxygenases [correction of cycloxygenases] in the spinal cord. *Progress in Neurobiology*, Vol.64, No.4, (July 2001), pp. 327-363, ISSN 0301-0082

Vidovic, D. & Matzinger, P. (1988). Unresponsiveness to a foreign antigen can be caused by self-tolerance. *Nature*, Vol.336, No.6196, (November 1988), pp. 222-225, ISSN 0028-0836

Vieira, P.L.; Heystek, H.C.; Wormmeester, J.; Wierenga, E.A. & Kapsenberg, M.L. (2003). Glatiramer acetate (copolymer-1, copaxone) promotes Th2 cell development and increased IL-10 production through modulation of dendritic cells. *Journal of Immunology*, Vol.170, No.9, (May 2003), pp. 4483-4488, ISSN 0022-1767

Xu, J.Q.; Kochanek, K.D.; Murphy, S.L. & Tejada-Vera, B. (2007). *Deaths: Final data for 2007.* Hyattsville, MD: National Center for Health Statistics. 2010.

Yin, Y.; Cui, Q.; Li, Y.; Irwin, N.; Fischer, D.; Harvey, A.R. & Benowitz, L.I. (2003). Macrophage-derived factors stimulate optic nerve regeneration. *The Journal of Neuroscience*, Vol.23, No.6, (March 2003), pp. 2284-2293, ISSN 0270-6474

Yoles, E.; Hauben, E.; Palgi, O.; Agranov, E.; Gothilf, A.; Cohen, A.; Kuchroo, V.; Cohen, I.R.; Weiner, H. & Schwartz, M. (2001). Protective autoimmunity is a physiological response to CNS trauma. *The Journal of Neuroscience*, Vol.21, No.11, (June 2001), pp. 3740-3748, ISSN 0270-6474

Ziemssen, T.; Kumpfel, T.; Klinkert, W.E.; Neuhaus, O. & Hohlfeld, R. (2002). Glatiramer acetate-specific T-helper 1- and 2-type cell lines produce BDNF: implications for multiple sclerosis therapy. Brain-derived neurotrophic factor. *Brain*, Vol.125, No.Pt 11, (November 2002), pp. 2381-2391, ISSN 0006-8950

Ziemssen, T.; Kumpfel, T.; Schneider, H.; Klinkert, W.E.; Neuhaus, O. & Hohlfeld, R. (2005). Secretion of brain-derived neurotrophic factor by glatiramer acetate-reactive T-helper cell lines: Implications for multiple sclerosis therapy. *Journal of the Neurological Sciences*, Vol.233, No.1-2, (June 2005), pp. 109-112, ISSN 0022-510X

Ziv, Y.; Finkelstein, A.; Geffen, Y.; Kipnis, J.; Smirnov, I.; Shpilman, S.; Vertkin, I.; Kimron, M.; Lange, A.; Hecht, T.; Reyman, K.G.; Marder, J.B.; Schwartz, M. & Yoles, E. (2007). A novel immune-based therapy for stroke induces neuroprotection and supports neurogenesis. *Stroke*, Vol.38, No.2 Suppl, (February 2007), pp. 774-782, ISSN 0039-2499

23

Neurodegenerative Disease Monitoring Using a Portable Wireless Sensor Device

Paul Bustamante[1,2],
Gonzalo Solas[1] and Karol Grandez[1]
[1]*CEIT University of Navarra*
[2]*Tecnun University of Navarra*
Spain

1. Introduction

Neurodegenerative diseases are characterized by progressive loss of neurons in the central nervous system. The disorders are clinically well-defined as a disease-related dementia, Alzheimer's disease the most typical case, or as a movement disorder, Parkinson's disease (PD). The risk of developing these diseases increases significantly with age: Parkinson's disease affects 1% of the population over 65 years of age, rising to 2% for those over 80 years.

Parkinson's disease is a common neurodegenerative disorder that often impairs motor skills and speech of the patient. PD is characterized by muscle rigidity, tremor, slowing of physical movement (bradykinesia) and in extreme cases, loss of physical movement (akinesia). In particular, PD is due to a loss of dopaminergic neurons (related to the neurotransmitter dopamine), and subcortical neurons in the brain. Replacement therapy with dopaminergic drugs (levodopa, pramipexole) effectively reverses all the symptoms and signs of the disease. After a changeable period of time, however, this excellent initial response to dopaminergic treatment is complicated by the appearance of disorders known as motor response complications (MRC). These complications are divided into two main categories: (i) fluctuations in motor response and (ii) the emergence of abnormal involuntary movements known as levodopa-induced dyskinesias (LID) (Konitsiotis, 2005).

Generally, motor fluctuations appear first as a shortening of the initially soft and lasting dopaminergic response. For patients with advanced PD, a few hours after the administration of medication the patient begins to notice the reappearance of signs and symptoms of the disease. This is known as "end of dose deterioration" or "wearing off". This may happen several times a day, so the patient can actually spend several hours per day in an "off" state. During the short visit with the neurologist, the patient may appear to be well and thus the neurologist misses the symptoms related to wearing off. As a result, changes in the recent drug treatment availability do not take place in time. It is now well known that early treatment of wearing-off fluctuations delay the onset of more severe complications in the future, as well as the appearance of LID. Therefore any strategy that can detect early changes associated with wearing off would provide a valuable clinical tool that would allow early treatment interventions.

The quantitative assessment of the human body and motor movement disorders has been a topic of great interest for decades. Advanced equipment has been used to study various pathologies of the motor performance of the human body. However, sophisticated equipment alone is not a guarantee for success in the detection and analysis of motor disorders. In many situations, deficiencies in motor performance are not always frequent and motor disorders can occur only in very specific situations that are difficult to imitate or reproduce in a laboratory. The underlying testing and monitoring processes have not experienced the innovation and advancement required to fulfil the needs that such detection and analysis present.

Amyotrophic lateral sclerosis (ALS), often referred to as "Lou Gehrig's Disease," is a progressive neurodegenerative disease that affects nerve cells in the brain and the spinal cord. Motor neurons reach the spinal cord from the brain, and from the spinal cord to the muscles throughout the body. The progressive degeneration of the motor neurons in ALS causes these motor neurons to die and when this happens the ability of the brain to initiate and control muscle movement is lost. With voluntary muscle action progressively affected, patients in the later stages of the disease may become totally paralyzed.

The cases for Parkinson disease and ALS are expected to double worldwide by the year 2020 (Von Campenhausen et al., 2005). Proper medical care of these patients is becoming increasingly complex and expensive. Lengthy hospital stays for monitoring and adjustment of the patients' treatment and the problems related with it, contribute to cost increase and morbidity due to the hospitalization itself. But there is a clinical deficit of objective data on which neurologists can base the assessment and care of patients with chronic neurologically-based movement disorders.

2. Patient monitoring

The patient monitoring is a technique that has become popular in recent years in the field of research, and soon the number of actual implementations in clinics and hospitals will begin to increase. Monitoring of patients is not new, in fact, today there are many hospitals that supply devices (thermometers, gauges, pulse and blood pressure, pulse oximetry, electrocardiogram, electro-devices, etc). The disadvantage of these devices is their large size and weight, and the little mobility they offer. The key innovation lies in one word: continuous monitoring. It consists of a series of devices and techniques designed to monitor, continuously and for a period of time established by the specialists, the physiological parameters of the patient. The specific values and the time evolution of these parameters allow a more precise analysis of the evolution of the disease, and therefore more effective treatment.

There are two main factors that have contributed to the rise of this technology. On one hand, the development of new physiological sensors that allow the measurement of more and more parameters related to the human body. Advances in biological, chemical, electrical and mechanical sensor technologies have led to their wider use as wearable sensors or implants. Improvements in the manufacture of sensors and techniques for nano-engineering, along with parallel advances in technology of microelectromechanical systems (MEMS) offer the potential for implantable or attachable sensors getting smaller.

On the other hand, the popularization of wireless sensor networks (WSN) and the recent advances in their use as body sensor networks (BSN), has been another key development for recent continuous monitoring of patients (Yick et al., 2008). The human body is a complex interior environment that responds and interacts with its external environment, but is somehow "independent." The monitoring of the human body using a wireless sensor network can be achieved by attaching the sensors to the body (or even implanted in the tissues).

The wireless sensor networks are formed by a group of sensor nodes with certain capacity for sensing environment variables and transmitting them wirelessly. These nodes allow forming ad-hoc networks without an established physical infrastructure or a centralized management. These kinds of networks are known for being easy to deploy and for being auto configurable.

The majority of the researches carried out in the field of wireless sensor networks are focused on the network architecture, as well as on the communication protocols within the network. But few advances have been made in the development of novel sensor node architectures. The efforts are focused on the miniaturization of the nodes and the reduction of the energy consumption (Anastasi et al., 2009).

The objective of the work described in this chapter is to develop a single device which could be used in several application fields, due to its capability of being able to acquire signals coming from different types of sensors. Apart from that, the treatment of the data can be carried out in multiple ways, as the device is equipped with an SD card, a RF transceiver (IEEE 802.15.4 specification compliant) and a USB connector, for communication as well as for charging functions.

In order to test its versatility, an application field has been chosen and several tests have been carried out related to that field. More concretely, the application field that has been selected the validity of the objectives proposed in this work has been e-Health, and thus, a continuous monitoring system has been developed.

3. System architecture

The study of the state of the art shows that the devices and methods developed so far for the testing activities in patients affected by PD and ALS lack the most important characteristics of the device described in this article:

- **Accuracy**: the data provided by the device show exact values for the parameters the doctors are interested in. They are not based on subjective appreciation of the performance of the tests carried out by the patients.
- **Ease of use**: both for the clinicians and for the patients. The patient can carry out the tests without having to move from their own homes. And the data is stored in a PC, which offers the possibility of sending it to the hospital via Internet, for the doctors to analyze the results.
- **Frequency**: the ease of use of the system makes it possible to carry out more frequent tests, so the tracking of the variations of the motor functions of the patients is more accurate.
- **Versatility**: using the devices presented in this article, several different tests can be performed, and in each test, several parameters can be measured. For example, for the finger tapping case, both the speed and the regularity (periodicity) can be obtained, which enriches the results of the test and enhances the analysis and the conclusions obtained with it.

In order to comply with this characteristics or requirements, in this work we describe the system developed, which is based on the architecture shown in Fig. 1.

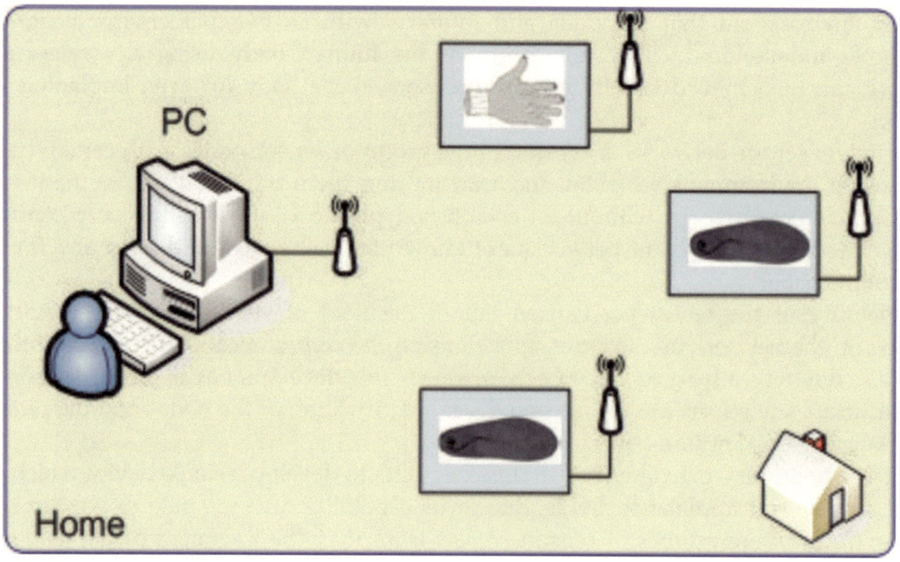

Fig. 1. System architecture

The whole system architecture is composed of four main building blocks:

- **Sensorized glove**: this glove is equipped with five sensors, which are attached to it. Each sensor is a FSR sensor and is connected to the circuit with a simple interface, done with a division resistor. When the user presses the FSR sensor, its resistance varies, and it is converted in voltage, in order to be acquired by the A/D converter.
- **Sensorized insole**: each insole is designed with five FSR sensors, in order to measure the area where the patient puts more pressure and to analyse the way he/she walks.
- **Hardware device**: this is the main development of the present research work. It consists of a tiny electronic circuit, based on a low cost and low energy microprocessor (PIC), protected by a case specifically designed for it. Its main functions are the acquisition and processing of the signals coming from the sensors, and transmitting them to the PC via the USB connection. The selected microprocessor has an 8 channel 10 bit A/D converter and an USB interface, which can be easily programmed and this allows saving space with another chip converter.
- **PC application**: the fourth component of the system architecture is in charge of receiving the data sent by the hardware device via the USB connection, storing and visualizing them, using a graphical user interface. This application was done in Windows with Visual C++ environment.

4. Device architecture

The main aim of the system is to gather data from any kind of sensor in order to store those data in an SD card or transmit them to Base Central Unit (BCU), connected to PC through USB connection. The SD card gives the system the possibility of having longer recording periods which allows the device to be used at a further distance from the BCU.

The data gathered and stored in the SD by the system is downloaded to a PC, by USB connection or by the radio transceiver, which operates in the 2.4GHz ISM band, using the BCU.

4.1 FSR sensors

The sensors used in this work have been Force Sensitive Resistors (FSR). A force-sensitive resistor (alternatively called a force-sensing resistor) has a variable resistance as a function of applied pressure. In this sense, the term "force-sensitive" is misleading - a more appropriate one would be "pressure-sensitive", since the sensor's output is dependent on the area on the sensor's surface to which force is applied.
The sensors used in this work are manufactured by Tekscan, and are constructed of two layers of substrate film. On each layer, a conductive material (silver) is applied, followed by a layer of pressure-sensitive ink (Vecchi et al., 2000). Adhesive is then used to laminate the two layers of substrate together to form the force sensor. The active sensing area is defined by the silver circle on top of the pressure-sensitive ink. Silver extends from the sensing area to the connectors at the other end of the sensor, forming the conductive leads. Fig. 2 shows a picture of the Tekscan FSR sensor.

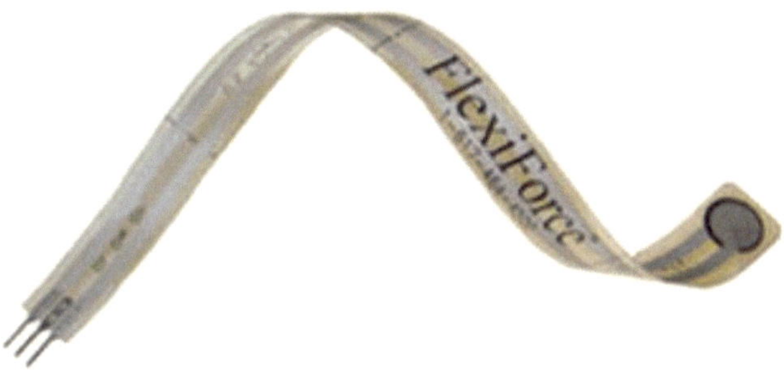

Fig. 2. Tekscan FSR sensor

After choosing Force Sensitive Resistors (FSR) as transducers, both a sensorized glove and an insole have been designed, and then used to carry out several tests related to Parkinson Disease (PD) and Amyotrophic lateral sclerosis (ALS).

4.2 Hardware architecture

The design of the device was related to its main functionality explained above. Measurements obtained from sensors are transmitted through wires to an IDC connector located at one edge of the device. This connector allows these inputs to be connected to A/D channels extended from the CPU. An interface stage is needed for each input due to sensors, done basically with some operational amplifiers and passive filters.
The architecture of the approach presented in this work is shown in Fig. 3. The CPU of the portable wireless device is the 18LF4550, a Microchip PIC18 Microcontroller with nanoWatt technology. It is an 8-bit System On-chip mainly featured by USB and SPI communication interfaces; it has a maximum number of 13 input A/D channels; each with a 10-bit resolution. It is also characterized for its low power consumption in deep-sleep mode, ideal to work as sensor node in monitoring applications. Also, this CPU has an RTC (Real Timer Clock), ideal for use in applications where is necessary to store the data sample time.
Analogical input signals attached to the IDC connector are converted into digital values which are put in an established frame structure according to a particular protocol. The frame arranged is ready to be transmitted via USB or RF.

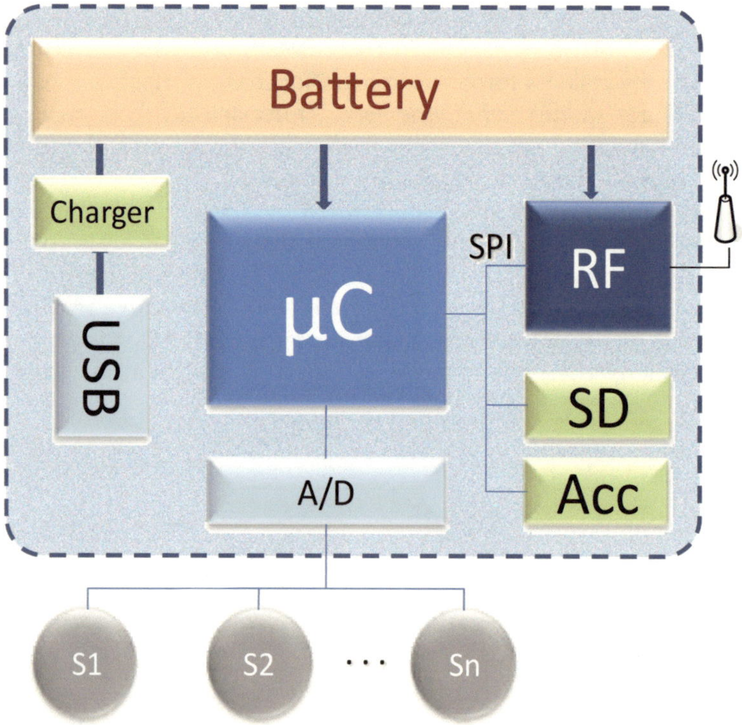

Fig. 3. Wireless device architecture

The USB device module is a mini-USB 2.0 compliant allowing fast transmission of data. It allows also charging the battery using a standard chip with a LED to monitor the charging action.

The device has also 3 more LEDs, whose main functionality is to indicate states in the program or can be programmed for different functions.

The device is designed also to use a 3-axis accelerometer in case it was needed; it also offers the option to record data in a micro-SD card placed in the bottom side. In order to increase the time access to the SD card, which means saving power, a proprietary system files access was implemented, based on the standard FAT32.

The wireless device has a radio frequency chip, the MRF24J40, from Microchip, which works in the 2.4GHz and has a SPI interface to communicate with the CPU. This chip was mainly chosen due to its IEEE 802.15.4 specification compliant (Hardware CSMA-CA mechanism, Automatic ACK response and support RSSI/LQI), additionally it has a hardware security engine and offers a low power consumption: 2uA in sleep mode, 22mA in TX mode (at +0dBm) and 18mA in RX mode.

The distribution of the device's components is illustrated in Fig. 4, where the left side shows the layout of the PCB and the distribution of the chips on the device. On the right side the connection procedure of the device with different kinds of sensors through a sensor interface is shown. This connection is possible by using the IDC connector, which includes pins for a VCC signal, the GND and 10 signals which are directed to the A/D converter. That was done due the fact that the main functionality of this device is to be a multifunctional wireless device.

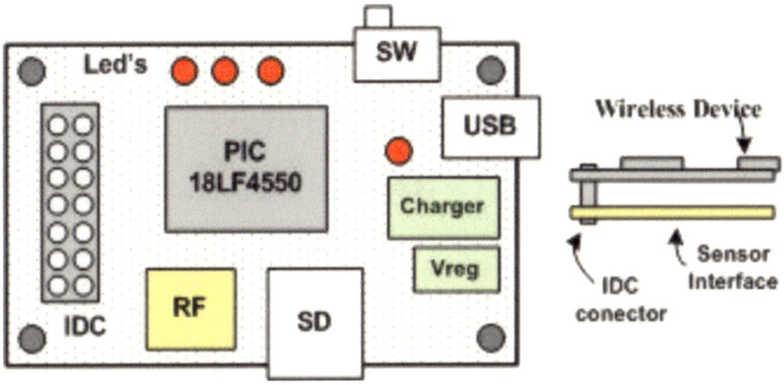

Fig. 4. PCB layout and sensor interface

4.3 Embedded software

The developed software to be embedded into the device has a modular scheme. This design allows the software to be independent from the platform and also gives flexibility.

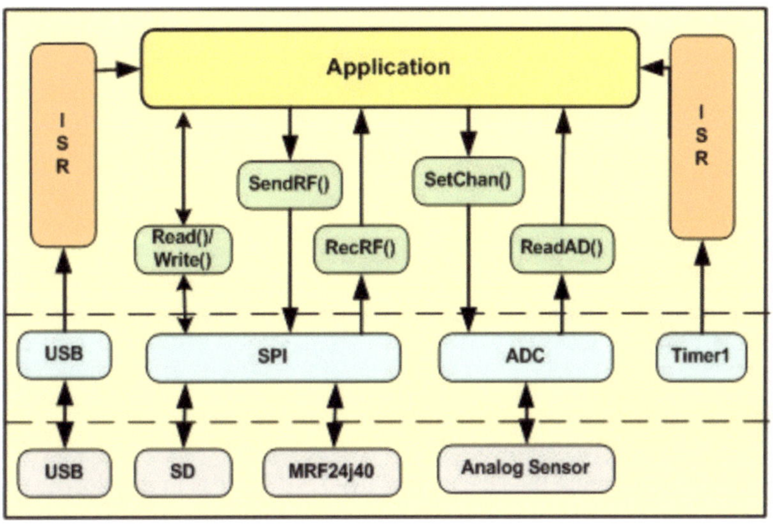

Fig. 5. Embedded software architecture

The whole software structure is divided in 4 layers as depicted in Fig. 5. The layers are separated by dotted lines and a short description for each one is given below:

- **Physical level**: is the lowest level and it depends on the hardware directly. The modules present in this level correspond to the physical modules of the node; these are the force sensors, accelerometer (not mounted), the USB port, the mini-SD slot (optional) and the RF module, which is controlled by the CPU using the SPI bus.
- **Controller level**: the functions developed in this level permit the application level to invoke controller functions. The ADC module converts analogical signals from the force sensors to digital, and the SPI allows communications of the CPU with the accelerometer and the mini-SD card and the RF chip. In this layer the set of USB and RTC (Real Time Clock) functions are also included.

- **Interface level**: this layer is the interface between controller and application; it contains the main functions that the device performs during its duty cycle. These functions range from reading ADC channels or communicating through the SPI interface, to sending and receiving data from the USB, the SD card and the RF chip. Interruption routines are also developed in this layer.
- **Application level**: this is the top level layer and executes related actions according to received interruptions (external switches or internal interruptions).

4.4 Data frame

The structure of the data frame, which is sent by RF or USB, is composed of a header which contains the ID of the device, followed by 4 bytes, indicating the measurement time, and a byte which indicates the length of the data.
Fig. 6 shows the data frame enclosed information of the measurements taken; the first two bytes give information about the frequency of sampling and the next byte gives the number of sensors measured. According to this last parameter, the rest of bytes corresponding to each sensor in groups of two bytes due to the 10-bit conversion configuration of the A/D converter.

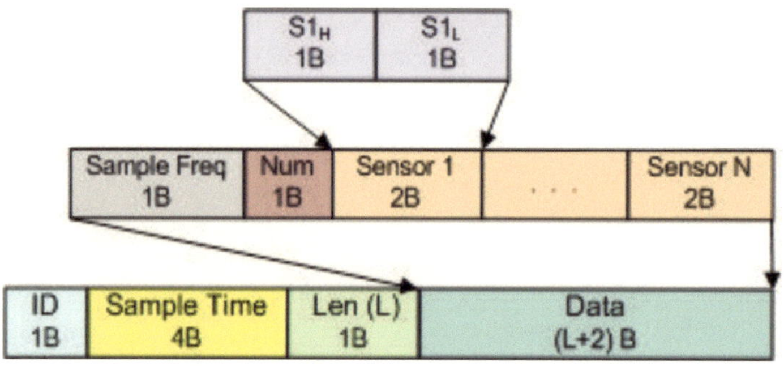

Fig. 6. Data frame

5. Device test in ALS disease

One of the ways of overcoming the lack of data in ALS disease is to develop new easy-to-use testing devices, which can be left in the patient's own home and used to carry out periodic tests without having to go to hospital to do so. The comfortable testing processes and devices make the patients more willing to wear them outside the home, and this leads to a wider amount of data available for the doctors.
Two of the more widely used tests with neurodegenerative disease patients are the Finger Tapping Test (FTT) (Jobbágy et al., 2005) and the Hand-grip Strength Test (Long, 1970). In the case of the FTT, the patient is asked to tap two of the fingers of one hand as quick as possible, and the main parameter measured by the doctors is the tapping frequency. On the other hand, in the hand grip strength test the measured parameter is the force the patient is capable of apply when grabbing an object.
The Finger Tapping Test (FTT), originally developed as part of the Halstead Reitan Battery (HRB) of neuropsychological tests, is a simple measure of motor speed and motor control and is used in neuropsychology as a sensitive test for brain damage (Christianson & Leathem, 2004). Although motor functioning in humans is controlled by many areas of the

brain, the motor strip rostral to the central sulcus is the most important, and the functioning of this area is reflected directly in the FTT. As well as direct motor effects, the speed, co-ordination, and pacing requirements of finger tapping can be affected by levels of alertness, impaired ability to focus attention, or slowing of responses. Tapping frequency can distinguish patients with motor dysfunctions of cerebella, basal ganglia, and cerebral origins from normal subjects.

At the onset of ALS the symptoms may be so slight that they are frequently overlooked. With regard to the appearance of symptoms and the progression of the illness, the course of the disease may include muscle weakness. Muscle weakness is a hallmark initial sign in ALS, occurring in approximately 60% of patients. The hands and feet may be affected first, causing difficulty in lifting, walking or using the hands for the activities of daily living such as dressing, washing and buttoning clothes.

ALS is a very difficult disease to diagnose. To date, there is no one test or procedure to ultimately establish the diagnosis of ALS. Methods for the evaluation of strength in people with ALS include a clinical neurological exam, manual muscle testing (MMT) (Aitkens et al., 1989), and rating scales. These methods are subjective and lack sensitivity to detect small changes. The purpose of the Hand Grip Strength Test is to measure the maximum isometric strength of the hand and forearm muscles.

The devices and methods used so far for the proposed tests have not had any significant improvement or innovation for many years. Traditional ways of performing the tests are still used.

For the finger tapping test, several methods have been proposed and used. The standard method consists of asking the patients to start with the finger tapping process and an examiner using a stopwatch to keep track of the 10-second trial interval. Electronic devices which are based on the same testing methodology have been marketed. The electronic device has an internal timer that starts on the first tap and stops counting taps when the 10 seconds have elapsed. The use of automatic timing is intended to increase the accuracy of testing (McDermid, 2000).

Other devices used, which can be found in the literature, include precision image-based motion analyzer and passive marker-based movement analyzer (Jobbágy et al., 2005); the Halstead-Reitan finger tapping test (HRFTT), developed and manufactured by Reitan Neuropsychological Laboratory, which uses an electronic counter and a tapping key; finger tapping devices containing pressure sensors (Soichiro et al., 2004); systems consisting of accelerometers and touch sensor (Yokoe et a., 2009) (Okuno et al., 2007).

In the case of the hand-grip strength measurement, the innovations carried out in recent years have been even poorer. The most usual way to carry out this specific test is by using hand-grip and pinch-force dynamometers, which offer very poor information about the way the hand grabs objects. Electromyography has been also used in some studies (Long, 1970).

In this work we have used our wireless device to carry out both of the tests. It is integrated in a system consisting of the mentioned device, a sensorized glove (see Fig. 7) which is worn by the patient, and a PC or base station, which is in charge of receiving the data sent by the device, and visualizing them graphically in order to be analyzed by the doctors.

As mentioned before, the sensors used in this test have been Force Sensitive Resistors (FSR). The approach followed in this research work has been the one of attaching several sensors to a glove. This design allows complying with one of the key characteristics identified in the system architecture section: versatility. We consider that this design is more versatile in order to allow carrying out different type of tests and obtaining a wide range of results.

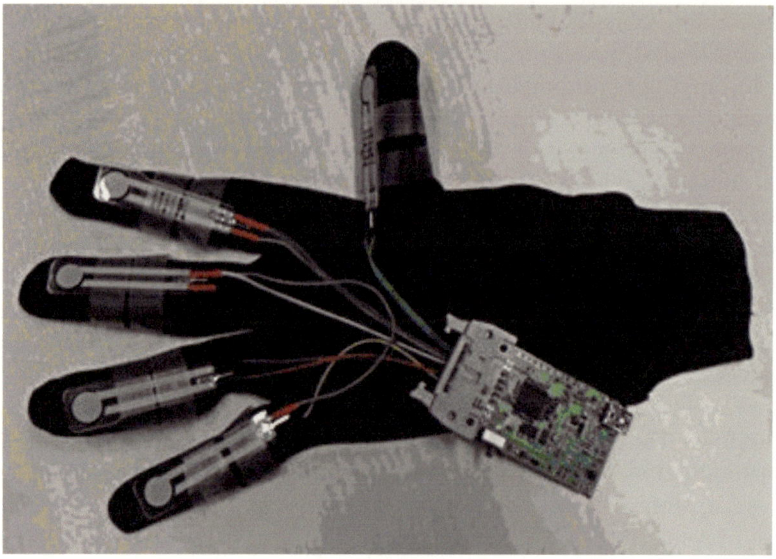

Fig. 7. Sensorized Glove attached to the wireless device

5.1 PC application

In order to gather the data and to be analyzed, a PC application was designed. It has been developed in Visual C++ using the Object Oriented Programming methodology (OOP), which is based in classes. The architecture is shown in Fig. 8. There are five blocks; the most important ones are the USB process and the graphical routines.

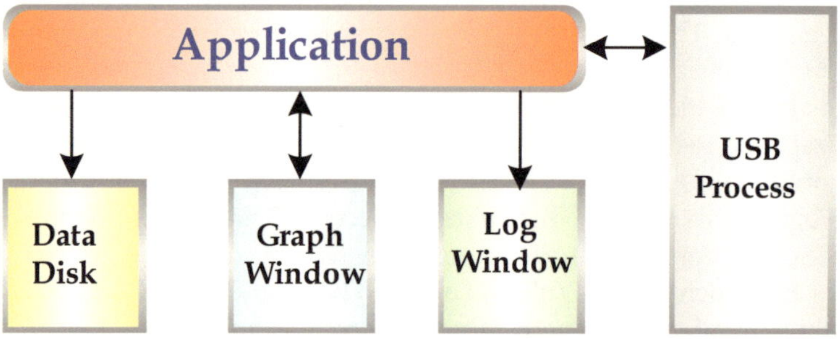

Fig. 8. PC application diagram

The data obtained by the hardware device after gathering and processing the signals coming from the FSR sensor, are sent via the USB connection to a PC, where an application is running. This application receives the data and visualizes and stores them.

Due the fact that the data rate of the device is low (less than 1KBps), the HID protocol has been implemented in the Sensor Device, providing the PC application an easier method of gathering the data, because most operating systems recognize standard USB HID devices, like keyboards and mice, without needing a special driver. In this way, the software can run in any compatible PC with Windows XP Operating System installed.

The application has some functionality that makes it easier for the doctors to analyze the data gathered by the hardware device. These functionalities are:

- **Start/Stop**: this button allows the exact moment in which the test starts and ends to be controlled. When the test starts, a new process is created in the application, which is constantly controlling the USB communications with the device, and passing the gathered data to the GUI window.
- **Zoom**: the zooming tool enables the signals corresponding to the force applied by the patient's each of the fingers to be visualised more accurately. It is also possible to analyze only one finger in the application or to compare with other tests carried out previously.
- **Log**: the application enables a registry or log with the messages corresponding to the events that appear during the testing process (communication states) to be visualised.
- **Files**: the application allows the data in files with ".csv" format to be saved, in order to edit and analyze later in a PC program such as Excel. Also, in the new version of the program, it is possible to save in a Matlab binary format, as some clinicians have experience with that mathematical tool.
- **Options**: in this option, the user can configure the device, by changing the sample frequency, the date of the device in order to maintain well synchronized, etc.

5.2 Hand-grip results

Fig. 9 shows a screen capture of the PC application, where a hand-grip force test is being carried out. As it can be seen in that figure, the force signal corresponding to each of the fingers is plotted using a different colour. That way the analysis of the graph is easier for the clinicians, where they can see for example that the patient has more force with one finger.

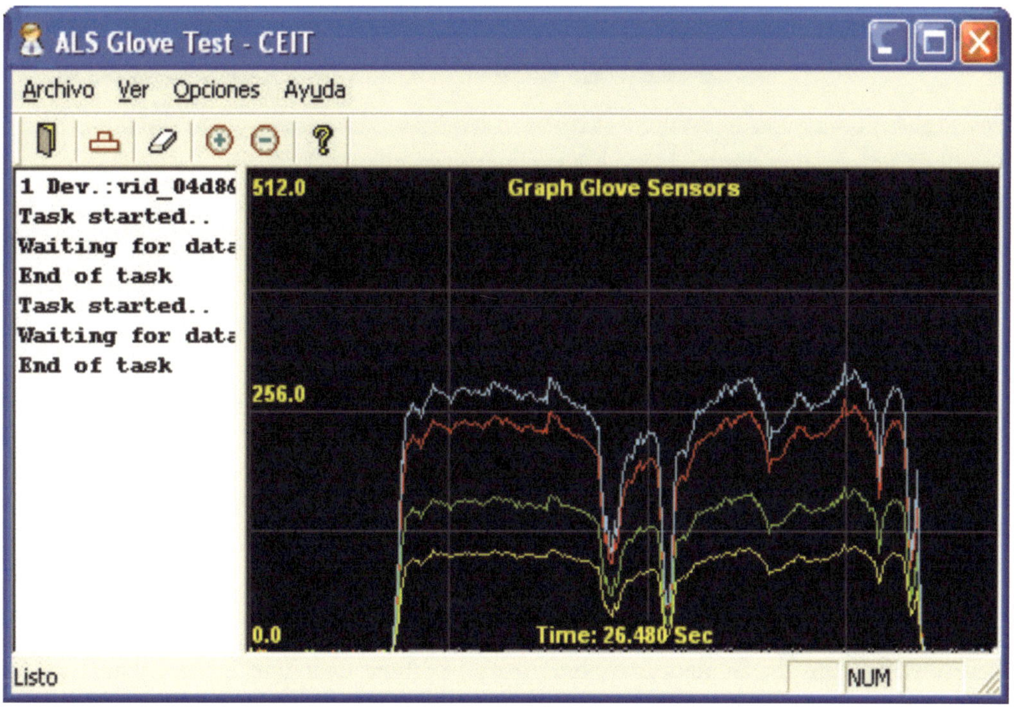

Fig. 9. PC application showing hand-grip force test results

5.3 Finger tapping results

The main innovation of this system is that it can measure both the frequency of the tapping and the force the patient applies when carrying out the test. Fig. 10 shows a screen capture of the PC application used to visualize the results in real-time, in which an ongoing finger tapping test can be seen.

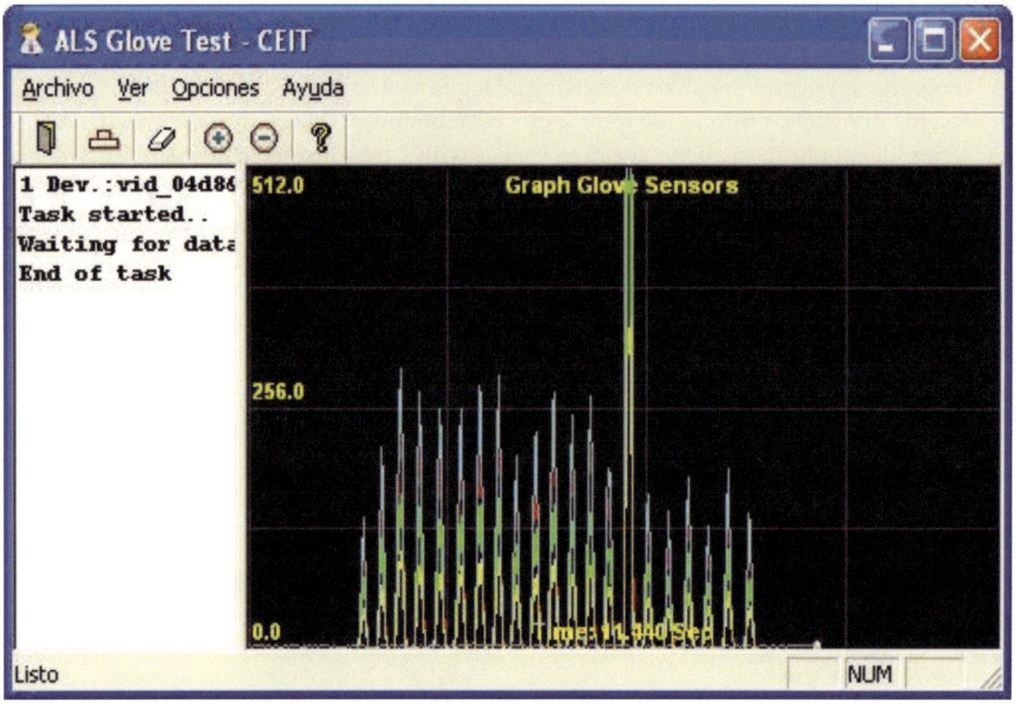

Fig. 10. PC application showing Finger-Tapping test results

Another key point of this finger-tapping test system compared to the existing ones is that the test can be performed using any of the five fingers of the hand. That way, two kinds of finger tapping tests can be carried out: one in which the fingers the patient uses most are involved in the testing process, and another one in which the patient uses the fingers that he or she is less likely to use.

6. Device's test in gait analysis

One of the ways of measuring and quantifying the movement disorders is performing gait analysis. Although several techniques and methods have been developed and used for years, all of them are based on hospitalizing patients and using in-hospital equipment.

Several interviews and meetings held with experts in neurology show that the most common way to carry out the gait analysis is by using sensorized ground platforms, as well as video cameras, in order to capture movement, where the two main disadvantages of these methods are the limited, and short period of time over which the patient can be monitored; and the fact of the monitoring process being carried out in a controlled environment, in which the patient may feel safe.

Recent advances on gait analysis of PD patients include portable digital monitoring systems. These systems allow gathering data by the patient themselves, wearing sensors at home and outside home. The developments performed to date are based on tiny electronic circuits which gather and transmit data coming from sensors, mainly accelerometers (Kauw-A-Tjoe et al., 2007).

Combining the advantages of both approaches used till date (sensorized ground platforms and portable monitoring devices) a gait monitoring system has been developed, using our wireless sensor device. For the approach presented in this test, Force Sensitive Resistors (FSR) sensors have also been selected. Regarding the location of the sensors on the insole, several medical considerations have to be taken into account. As shown in Fig. 11, the most interesting zones to place the sensors are three: the plantar area, the heel and one in the middle. These zones are the ones in which most of the force is applied and, thus, the zones from which more information can be obtained.

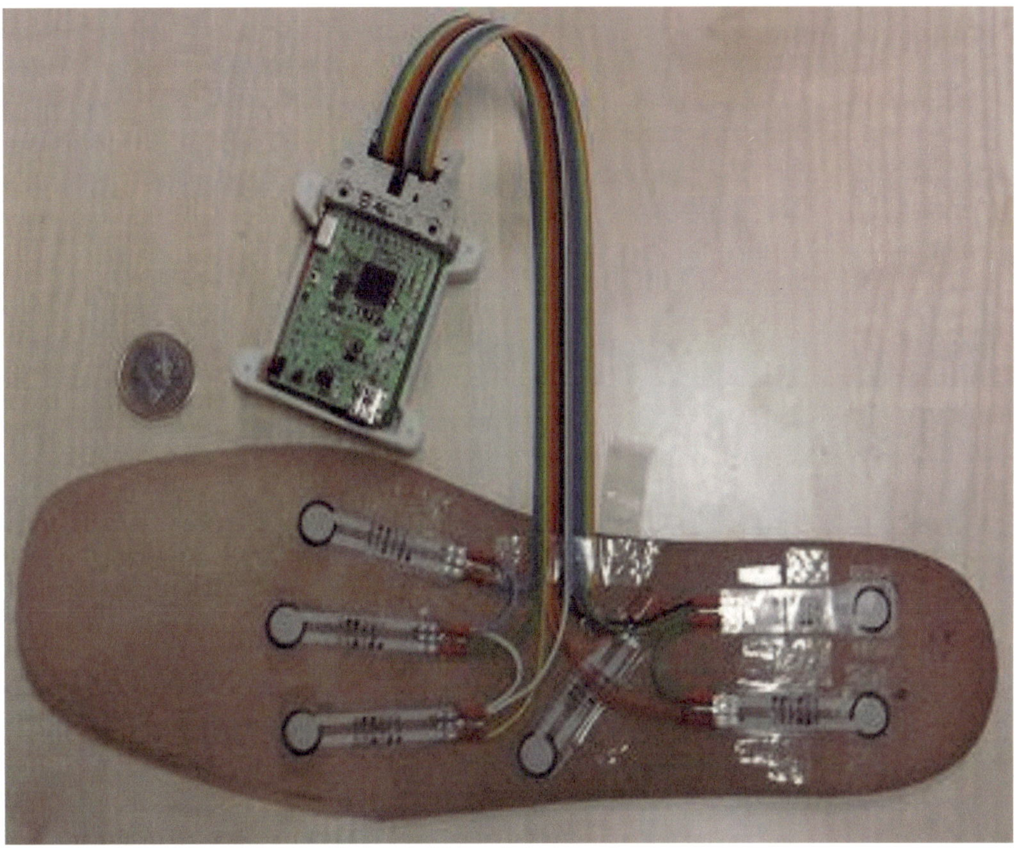

Fig. 11. Insole with the FSR sensors and wireless sensor device

6.1 Gait analysis results

The test methodology carried out consists of several tests performed on patients affected by PD and on healthy individuals. Two people from each group participated in the tests, and each of them carried out three repetitions, in order to avoid random results.

The parameters to be measured are the amplitude of the signal of each sensor (i.e., the force of the step) and the frequency of the signal, which gives an idea of the cadence of the gait. Table 1 shows the results obtained, where it can be seen that parkinsonian people has more frequency in their steps than healthy people. Fig. 11 shows the results for 2 sensors, gathered on the gait of a healthy person. The signal with the greater amplitude corresponds to a sensor located in the heel and the other one to the plantar area.

Samples		Results	
		Amplitude(V)	Central frequency (Hz.)
Non-Parkinsonian	1	2.64	0.88
	2	2.42	0.82
Parkinsonian	1	1.64	1.76
	2	1.76	1.85

Table 1. Results of the test in patients

A delay can be noted between the two signal in Fig. 12. This is due to the nature of the step in a normal gait. Another difference lies in the amplitude of the signals and this is because most of the weight rests on the heel. On the other hand, Fig. 13 shows the analogous results for a Parkinsonian individual.

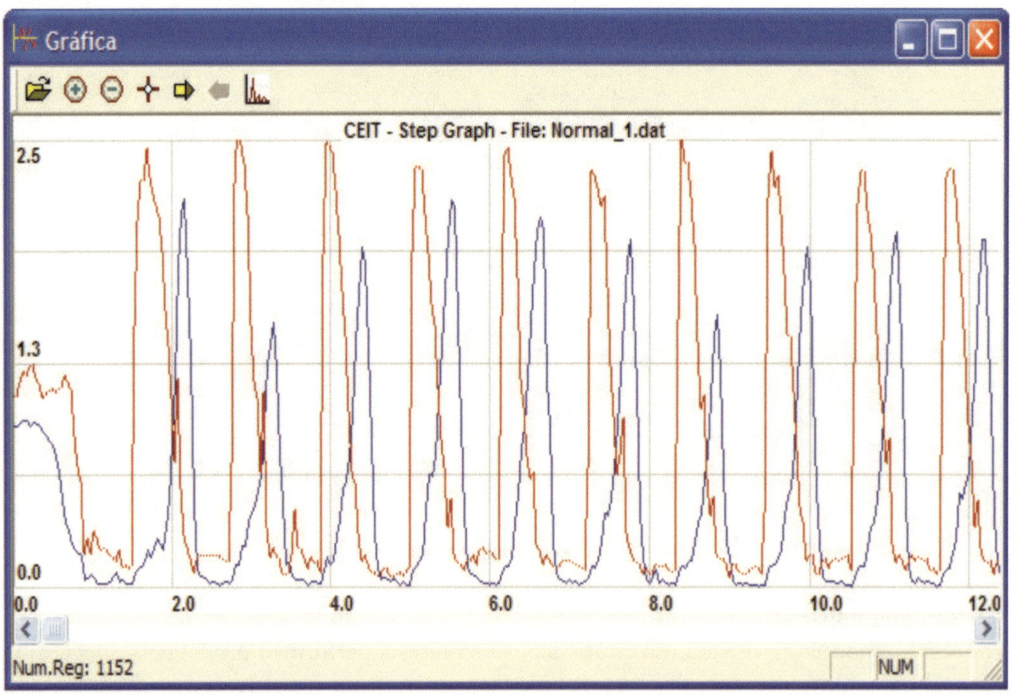

Fig. 12. Signal of a non-Parkinsonian individual over a temporal axis

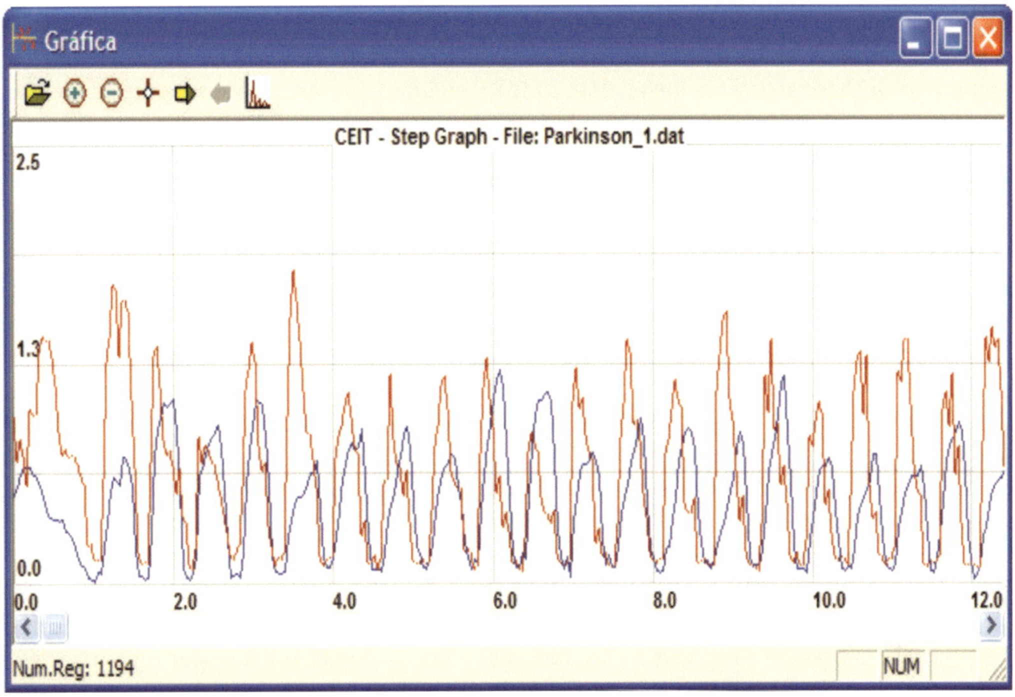

Fig. 13. Signal of a Parkinsonian patient

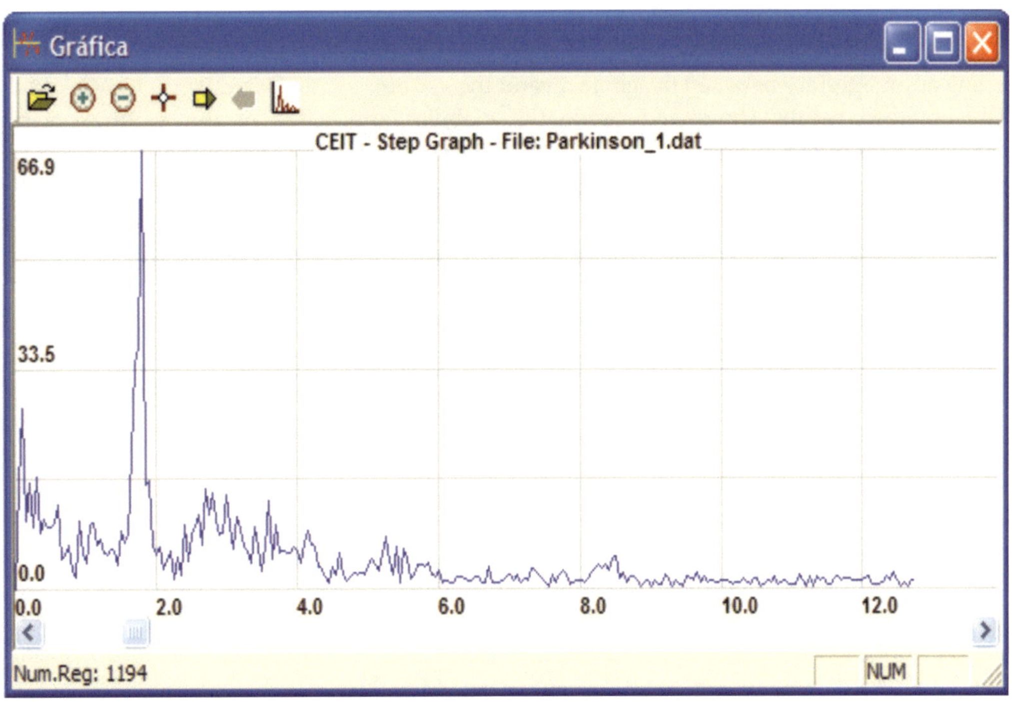

Fig. 14. FFT Signal of a Parkinsonian patient

As Fig. 13 shows, there is no delay between signals which suggests that this is due to the typical short steps of a Pakinsonian patient. Two more interesting conclusions are that the amplitude of these signals is lower than in the previous case, and the frequency is greater, around twice as much. This can be seen in Fig. 14, where the FFT of the Parkinsonian patient's signal is plotted.

7. Conclusion

The design of a tiny wireless sensor node platform has been carried out in this work. This device is mainly featured with its multifunctional functionality which has been proven in this paper on e-Health applications, specifically on tests related to patients affected by neurodegenerative diseases.

The presented work is based on the development of two specific tests for the treatment and analysis of Parkinson Disease (PD) and Amyotrophic Lateral Sclerosis (ALS). For each, the device has a different sensorized platform according to the nature of the performed test. Collected data from sensors can be either transmitted online through RF or downloaded via USB to a PC, or just stored in a card memory for a further download and analysis of data. A sensorized glove allows two tests to be carried out, mostly used on ALS patients; those are the hand-grip and the finger tapping tests. In the same way an insole with sensors located strategically is used to carry out a gait analysis which is one of the ways of measuring the movement disorders in parkinsonian people.

Results from both kinds of tests can be visualized and analyzed with the PC application developed in this work which also proves the versatility of the whole designed system. This application provides useful tools for the analysis of results; it was designed taking into account clinicians feedback as part of the work under the scope of the PERFORM project, acting as an interface between the clinician and the system.

The obtained results show and prove the viability and value of the multifunctional characteristics of the designed device. Additionally, by using the several tools provided by the PC application tools, important parameters can be obtained such as the frequency of a signal through the implemented FFT calculation function, the correlation among sensor signals in terms of phase and magnitude, the customization in the selection of specific signals and the zoom tool for a better appreciation of data.

These functionalities of the PC application allow clinician to obtain valuable conclusions like the stability of the gait (from the harmonics of the signals), the relation between air and ground time of the step (in PD analysis), the finger tapping frequency, the relation between the force applied by the different fingers, or the recording of the periods of time in which the patient is in "on" or "off" state.

Future work, which remains to be done is to focus on the accelerometer not mounted in this work. This component will provide relevant information for the gait analysis mainly helping to determine orientation and acceleration parameters of the patient.

8. Acknowledgement

This work is partly funded by the ICT programme of the European Commission (PERFORM Project: FP7-ICT-2007-1-215952)

9. References

Aitkens, S., Lord, J., Bernauer, E., Fowler, W.M. Jr, Lieberman, J.S., Berck, P. (1989). Relationship of manual muscle testing to objective strength measurements. *Muscle & Nerve*. Vol. 12, No. 3, (March 1989), pp. (173-177), ISSN 1097-4598.

Anastasi, G., Conti, M., Di Francesco, M., & Passarella, A. (2009). Energy conservation in wireless sensor networks: A survey. *Ad Hoc Networks*. Vol. 7, No. 3, (May 2009), pp. (537-568), ISSN 1570-8705.

Christianson, M. K., Leathem, J. M. (2004). Development and Standardisation of the Computerised Finger Tapping Test: Comparison with other finger tapping instruments. *New Zealand Journal of Psychology*, Vol. 33, No. 2, (July 2004), pp. (44-49), ISSN 0112-109X.

Jobbágy Á., Harcos, P., Karoly, R., & Fazekas, G. (2005). Analysis of finger-tapping movement. *Journal of Neuroscience Methods*, Vol. 141, No. 1, (January 2005), pp. (29–39), ISSN 0165-0270.

Kauw-A-Tjoe, R.G., Thalen, J., Marin-Perianu, M., & Havinga, P. (2007). SensorShoe: Mobile Gait Analysis for Parkinson's Disease Patients, *Proceedings of the 9th International Conference on Ubiquitous Computing (UbiComp 2007)*, ISBN: 3-540-74852-0, Innsbruck (Austria), September 2007.

Konitsiotis, S. (2005). Novel pharmacological strategies for motor complications in Parkinson's disease. *Expert Opinion on Investigational Drugs*, Vol. 14, No. 14, (April 2005), pp. (377-399), ISSN 1354-3784.

Long, C. (1970). Intrinsic-extrinsic muscle control of hand in power grip and precision handling - an electromyographic study. *Journal of bone and joint surgery - American volume*. Vol. 52, No. 5, (1970), pp. (853-859), ISSN 0021-9355.

McDermid, R. (2000). A comparison of alternative devices of the finger tapping test. *Archives of Clinical Neuropsychology*, Vol. 15, No. 8, (November 2000).

Okuno, R., Yokoe, M., Fukawa, K., Sakoda, S., & Akazawa, K. (2007). Measurement system of finger-tapping contact force for quantitative diagnosis of Parkinson's disease, *Proceedings of the 29th Annual International Conference of the IEEE Engineering in Medicine and Biology Society EMBS 2007*, ISBN 978-1-4244-0788-3, Lyon (France), August 2007

Soichiro, M., Hisayoshi, O., Akira, K., Hironori, S., & Ko, K. (2004). Quantitative analysis of cerebellar ataxia with a finger tapping device containing a pressure sensor. *Neurological Medicine*, Vo1.61, No. 1, pp. (99-101), ISSN0386-9709.

Vecchi, F., Freschi, C., Micera, S., Sabatini, A. M., & Dario, P. (2000). Experimental evaluation of two commercial force sensors for applications in biomechanics and motor control, *Proceedings of the 5th IFESS Annual Conference*, ISBN 4-9980783-1-3, Aalborg (Denmark), June 2000.

Von Campenhausen, S., Bornschein, B., Wick, R., Bötzel, K., Sampaio, C., Poewe, W., Oertel, W., Siebert, U., Berger, K., & Dodel, R. (2005). Prevalence and incidence of Parkinson's disease in Europe. *European Neuropsychopharmacology*, Vol. 15, No. 4, (August 2005), pp. (473-490), ISSN 0924-977X.

Yick, J., Mukherjee, B., & Ghosal, D. Wireless sensor network survey. *Computer Networks (Elsevier)*. Vol. 52, No. 12, (August 2008), pp. (2292-2330), ISSN 1389-1286.

Yokoe, M., Okuno, R., Hamasakib, T., Kurachic, Y., Akazawaf, K., & Sakoda, S. (2009). Opening velocity, a novel parameter, for finger tapping test in patients with Parkinson's disease. *Parkinsonism Related Disorders*, Vol. 15, No. 6, (July 2009), pp. (440-444), ISSN 1353-8020